FIFTH EDITION

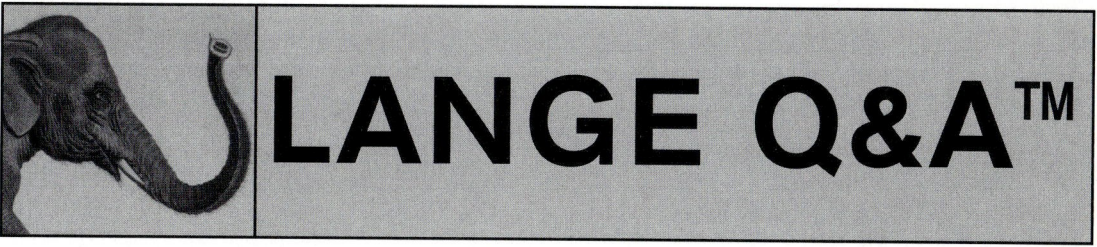

LANGE Q&A™

PHYSICIAN ASSISTANT

Anthony A. Miller, PhD (candidate), PA-C
Associate Professor & Director
Division of Physician Assistant Studies
Shenandoah University
Winchester, Virginia

Albert F. Simon, DHSc, PA-C
Associate Professor and Chair
Department of Physician Assistant Studies
A.T. Still University of Health Sciences
Mesa, Arizona

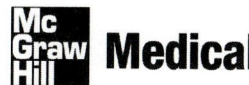
McGraw Hill Medical

New York   Chicago   San Francisco   Lisbon   London
Madrid   Mexico City   New Delhi
San Juan   Seoul   Singapore   Sydney   Toronto

Lange Q&A™: Physician Assistant, 5ed.

1 2 3 4 5 6 7 8 9 0   QPD/QPD   0 9 8 7 6

ISBN 13: 978-0-07-146476-5, ISBN 10: 0-07-146476-X

Notice

Medicine is an ever-changing science. As new research and clinical experience broaden our knowledge, changes in treatment and drug therapy are required. The authors and the publisher of this work have checked with sources believed to be reliable in their efforts to provide information that is complete and generally in accord with the standards accepted at the time of publication. However, in view of the possibility of human error or changes in medical sciences, neither the authors nor the publisher nor any other party who has been involved in the preparation or publication of this work warrants that the information contained herein is in every respect accurate or complete, and they disclaim all responsibility for any errors or omissions or for the results obtained from use of the information contained in this work. Readers are encouraged to confirm the information contained herein with other sources. For example and in particular, readers are advised to check the product information sheet included in the package of each drug they plan to administer to be certain that the information contained in this work is accurate and that changes have not been made in the recommended dose or in the contraindications for administration. This recommendation is of particular importance in connection with new or infrequently used drugs.

This book was set in Palatino by Techbooks.
The editors were Michael Brown and Christie Naglieri.
The production supervisor was Catherine H. Saggese.
Project management was provided by Techbooks.
Quebecor/Dubuque was printer & binder.

This book is printed on acid-free paper.

Library of Congress Cataloging-in-Publication Data

Lange Q & A for the physician assistant / [edited by] Anthony A. Miller, Albert F. Simon.—5th ed.
    p. ; cm.
    Rev. ed. of: Appleton & Lange's review for the physician assistant / [edited by] Anthony A. Miller, Albert F. Simon. 4th ed. c2002.
    Includes bibliographical references and index.
    ISBN 0-07-146476-X (softcover)
    1. Physicians' assistants—Examinations, questions, etc.   I. Miller, Anthony A.   II. Simon, Albert F.   III. Appleton & Lange's review for the physician assistant.   IV. Title: Lange Q and A for the physician assistant.   V. Title: Q & A for the physician assistant.
    [DNLM: 1. Physician Assistants—Examination Questions. W 18.2 L2737 2006]
R697.P45A67 2006
610.73′72069076—dc22

2006048100

To my mother for always being there.
To Ting-Yu for being my inspiration, my friend and greatest supporter.
To Jason, Matt and Sarah for being the best children a father could hope for.
And to Joe, Grace, Simon, Adeline, Josephine & Helen for the joy you bring.

AAM

To Mike and Rob: Still the greatest in my life
To Doreen: thanks for believing in me and being the wonderful friend, inspiration and partner that you are, please remember I will always believe in you too.

AFS

To our colleagues and students: thank you for continuing to inspire us

AAM & AFS

Contents

Contributors

Frank Acevedo, MS, PA-C
Assistant Professor & Associate Director
Department of Physician Assistant Studies
New York Institute of Technology
Old Westbury, NY

Joel W. Bunn, MMS, PA-C
Emergency Medicine and Interventional Radiology
Conemaugh Memorial Medical Center
Johnstown, Pennsylvania
Instructor of Emergency Medicine/Radiology
Department of Physician Assistant Services
Saint Francis University
Loretto, Pennsylvania

Rachel A. Carlson, MSBS, PA-C
Assistant Professor
Physician Assistant Studies
Shenandoah University
Physician Assistant, Valley Health Urgent Care
  Center
Winchester, Virginia

James F. Cawley, MPH, PA-C
Professor and Director
Physician Assistant/Master of Public Health Program
School of Public Health and Health Services
George Washington University
Washington, District of Columbia

Michelle DiBaise, MPAS, PA-C
Adjunct Assistant Professor
Physician Assistant Program
Arizona School of the Health Sciences
A.T. Still University
Mesa, Arizona

Raymond Eifel, MS, PA-C
Assistant Professor
Division of Physician Assistant Studies
Shenandoah University
Winchester, Virginia

Catherine A. Gillespie, DHSc, MPAS, PA-C
Associate Director, Assistant Professor
Physician Assistant Department
Gannon University
Erie, Pennsylvania

Constance M. Goldgar, MS, PA-C
Associate Director
Physician Assistant Program
Department of Family and Preventative
  Medicine
University of Utah
Salt Lake City, Utah

Michelle Heinan, EdD, PA-C
Dean
School of Health Sciences
Argosy University
Eagan, Minnesota

Mary Lapidus Hewett, MS, PA-C
Assistant Professor
Medical University of South Carolina
Physician Assistant, Roper/Saint Francis
  Hospital
Charleston, South Carolina

Nancy Ivansek, MA, PA-C
Newbury Family Practice
Newbury, Ohio

Robert W. Jarski, PhD, PA-C
Professor
School of Health Sciences
Oakland University
Rochester, Michigan

Brenda L. Kaminski, MPH, PA-C
Assistant Professor
Division of Physician Assistant Studies
Shenandoah University
Winchester, Virginia

Matthew A. McQuillan, MS, PA-C
Assistant Professor
Physician Assistant Program
University of Medicine and Dentistry of New Jersey
Physician Assistant, The Doctor Is In
Piscataway, New Jersey

Carla J. Moschella, MS, RD, PA-C
Assistant Professor & Academic Coordinator
Department of Physician Assistant Studies
Massachusetts College of Pharmacy and Health
  Sciences
Boston, Massachusetts

Raymond Pavlick, PhD
Associate Professor
Department of Physician Assistant Studies
Arizona School of Health Sciences
AT Still University
Mesa, Arizona

Paula B. Phelps, MHE, PA-C
Associate Professor
Physician Assistant Program
Idaho State University
Physician Assistant, Southeast Idaho Health
  Department
Pocatello, Idaho

*Maura Polansky, MS, PA-C
Director, Physician Assistant Educational Programs
Physician Assistant, M.D. Anderson
  Cancer Center
University of Texas
Houston, Texas

Jill Reichman, MPH, PA-C
Associate Director & Associate Professor
Physician Assistant Program
University of Medicine and Dentistry of New Jersey
Piscataway, New Jersey

Christina M. Robohm, MS, PA-C
Director of Admissions
Child Health Associate/Physician Assistant
  Program
Assistant Professor
Department of Pediatrics
University of Colorado at Denver and Health
  Sciences Center
Aurora, Colorado

Rebecca Lovell Scott, PhD, PA-C
Lecturer
Northeastern University
Physician Assistant, Cape Cod Community Health
  Center and Free Clinic
Mashpee, Massachusetts

Michel Statler, MLA, PA-C
Associate Director
Physician Assistant Program
Midwestern University
Glendale, Arizona

Susan L. Symington, MPAS, PA-C
Physician Assistant
La Loma Internal Medicine and Pediatrics
Litchfield Park, Arizona

Gary R. Uremovich, MS, MPAS, PA-C
Assistant Professor
Kettering College of Medical Arts
Physician Assistant; Charlotte Eye, Ear, Nose
  and Throat
Charlotte, North Carolina

Bryan D. Walker, MHS, PA-C
Division of Neuroradiology
Georgetown University Hospital
Washington, District of Columbia

Mary L. Warner, MMSc, PA-C
Assistant Dean and Program Director
Physician Associate Program
Yale School of Medicine
New Haven, Connecticut

* The author would like to acknowledge the assistance of Katherine Kennon, MS, PA-C, during the writing of this chapter.

Reviewers

Donna M. Agnew, MSPAS, PA-C
Assistant Professor
Physician Assistant Program
Department of Medical Science &
    Community Health
Arcadia University
Glenside, Pennsylvania

J. Dennis Blessing, PhD, PA-C
Associate Dean for South Texas Programs
School of Allied Health Sciences
Professor & Chair
Department of Physician Assistant Studies
The University of Texas Health Science
    Center at San Antonio
San Antonio, Texas

J. Glenn Forister, MPAS, PA-C
Assistant Clinical Professor
Department of Physician Assistant Studies
The University of Texas Health Science
    Center at San Antonio
San Antonio, Texas

Jennifer A. Holycross, MPAS, PA-C
Academic Coordinator & Assistant Professor
Physician Assistant Program
Butler University—Clarian Health
Indianapolis, Indiana

Richard D. Muma, PhD, MPH, PA-C
Chair & Associate Professor
Department of Physician Assistant
Wichita State University
Wichita, Kansas

David Paulk, EdD, PA-C
Academic Coordinator
Physician Assistant Program
Department of Medical Science &
    Community Health
Arcadia University
Glenside, Pennsylvania

Preface

In this fifth edition of *Lange Q&A: Physician Assistant*, we have responded to the changing aspects of health care by including many of the new treatments and diagnostic tests from modern medical practice in extensively updated questions, while maintaining the basic format and quality our readers have grown to expect. With this edition, overall 60% of the questions are new or substantially revised, a new chapter on preventive medicine has been added, and we have expanded the total number of questions in the book and web based practice test by over 100. An exciting change in this edition are the web based practice tests so you can experience an electronic testing format similar to the one found on the certifying examination. Visit www.PAeasy.com for information on pricing and subscription terms. Further revisions have been made to respond to changes in the format and blueprint of the NCCPA certification examination.

We believe that you will find this review book a helpful and useful resource as you prepare for your initial or recertification examination. In addition, you will find *Appleton & Lange Outline Review for the Physician Assistant* an additional helpful resource for its content outlines and additional questions and answers. The *Outline Review* provides an easy to read summary of the major topics you will find on the national certification examination. Your comments and constructive criticisms are welcome and will be considered in future editions.

We would like to thank our families, friends, and co-workers for their support, encouragement, and patience during the long hours spent working on this project. We also wish to thank Michael Brown, Maya Barahona, and Christie Naglieri from McGraw-Hill for their editorial assistance and our contributors for their hard work and dedication. Finally, we thank you, the readers, for choosing this book as one of your resources. We wish you success on the examination.

Your comments and constructive criticisms are welcome and will be considered in future editions. Please send your comments to *PA@mcgraw-hill.com*. Note the title of the book in the subject line.

Anthony A. Miller, PhD (Candidate), PA-C
Albert F. Simon, DHS, PA-C

Introduction

This book has been designed as a study aid to review for the Physician Assistant National Certification and Recertification Examination. Here, in one package, is a comprehensive review resource with more than 1100 questions presented in the format seen in the national examinations. Each question is answered with a referenced, paragraph-length answer. The entire book has been organized by specialty area to help evaluate your areas of relative strength and weakness and to further direct your study effort with the available references.

ORGANIZATION

This book is divided into seven major sections preceded by an Introduction and a chapter on test-taking tips and techniques. Chapter 1 provides helpful hints on how to prepare for and take certification examinations. Section I, Chapters 2 through 12, reviews the major areas of internal medicine using the question-and-answer format. Sections II through V cover the major subspecialty areas and pharmacology. Section VI, Surgery, is subdivided into five chapters (13 through 17) covering its subspecialties and Chapter 18, which is new in this edition, covers Preventive Medicine.

This introduction provides information on question types, methods for using this book, and specific information on the national certifying and recertifying examinations. The reader is also urged to consult the National Commission on Certification of Physician Assistants' web site for up-to-date information on the examination procedures and content. The web site is *www.nccpa.net*.

QUESTIONS

The National Certifying Examination is made up of "one best answer–single item" questions. In addition, some questions have illustrative materials (graphs, x-rays, tables) that require understanding and interpretation on your part. Finally, some of the items are stated in the negative. In such instances, we have printed the negative word in capital letters (eg, "All of the following are correct EXCEPT"; "Which of the following choices is NOT correct"; and "Which of the following is LEAST correct"). These items are discouraged, and now there are very few. Many examinees will not encounter a negative question when they take the certifying exams.

One Best Answer–Single Item Question

This type of question presents a problem or asks a question and is followed by four to five choices, only one of which is entirely correct. The directions preceding this type of question will generally appear as below:

DIRECTIONS (Questions 1 through 7): Each of the numbered items or incomplete statements in this section is followed by answers or by completions of the statement. Select the ONE lettered answer or completion that is BEST in each case.

An example for this item type follows:

1. An obese 21-year-old woman complains of increased growth of coarse hair on her lip, chin, chest, and abdomen. She also notes menstrual irregularity with periods of amenorrhea. Which of the following is the most likely cause?

(A) polycystic ovary disease
(B) an ovarian tumor
(C) an adrenal tumor
(D) Cushing's disease
(E) familial hirsutism

In this type of question, choices other than the correct answer may be partially correct, but there can be only one best answer. In the question above, the key word is "most." Although ovarian tumors, adrenal tumors, and Cushing's disease are causes of hirsutism (described in the stem of the question), polycystic ovary disease is a much more common cause. Familial hirsutism is not associated with the menstrual irregularities mentioned. Thus, the most likely cause of the manifestations described can only be "(A) polycystic ovary disease."

Answers, Explanations, and References

In each of the sections of this book, the question sections are followed by a section containing the answers, explanations, and references for the questions. This section (1) tells you the answer to each question; (2) gives you an explanation, reviews the reason the answer is correct, and supplies background information on the subject matter (and in most cases, the reason the other answers are incorrect); and (3) tells you where you can find more in-depth information on the subject matter in other books and journals. We encourage you to use this section as a basis for further study and understanding.

If you choose the correct answer to a question, you can read the explanation for reinforcement and to add to your knowledge of the subject matter (remember that the explanations usually tell not only why the answer is correct, but often also why the other choices are incorrect). If you choose the wrong answer to a question, you can read the explanation for an instructional review of the material in the question. Furthermore, you can note the reference cited, look up the complete source in the references at the end of the chapter (eg, Tanagho EA, McAninch JW, eds. *Smith's General Urology*. 16th ed. New York, NY: McGraw-Hill; 2004.), and refer to the pages cited for a more in-depth discussion.

Practice Test

A comprehensive practice test covers and reviews all the topics covered in the book. A web-based version is also available at www.PAeasy.com; visit the site for pricing and subscription terms. The format

for the Practice Test provides you the opportunity for self-assessment in a format similar to that expected for the certifying examination, with the subject areas integrated. Specific instructions for how to take the Practice Test are given later.

HOW TO USE THIS BOOK

There are two logical ways to get the most value from this book. We will call them Plan A and Plan B.

In Plan A, you go straight to the Practice Test and complete it according to the instructions given. This will be a good indictor of your initial knowledge of the subject and will help to identify specific areas for preparation and review. You can then use the earlier chapters of the book to help you improve your relative weak points.

In Plan B, you go through each section checking off your answers and then comparing your choices with the answers and discussions in the book. Once you have completed this process, you can take the Practice Test and see how well prepared you are. If you still have a major weakness, is should be apparent in time for you to take remedial action. Plan B can be accomplished by using the book itself or using the tutorial format for the chapter examinations found on www.PAeasy. com.

In Plan A, by taking the Practice Test first, you get quick feedback regarding your initial areas of strength and weakness. You may find that you have a good command of the material, indicating that perhaps only a cursory review of each section is necessary. This, of course, would be good to know early in your exam preparation. On the other hand, you may find that you have many areas of weakness. In this case, you could then focus on these areas in your review—not just with this book, but also with appropriate textbooks. (It is, however, unlikely that you will not study prior to taking the National Boards, especially since you have this book.) Therefore, it may be more realistic to take the Practice Test after you have reviewed the first seven sections (as in Plan B). This is likely to provide you with a more realistic type of testing situation, as very few of us merely sit down to a test without studying. In this case, you will have done some reviewing (from superficial to in-depth) and your Practice Test will reflect this study time. If, after reviewing the first seven sections and taking the Practice Test, you still have some weaknesses, you can then go back to the first of these sections and supplement your review with the reference texts.

We hope that through careful use of this book, whether through Plan A or Plan B, you find this text a useful and beneficial study guide.

SPECIFIC INFORMATION ON THE EXAMINATIONS

The official source for all information on the certification or recertification process is the National Commission on Certification of Physician Assistants, Inc. (NCCPA), Suite 800, 157 Technology Parkway, Norcross, Georgia 30092. This organization is comprised of representatives from the major organizations of medicine, including the American Academy of Physician Assistants and the Physician Assistant Education Association. Their function is to formulate and administer the annual certification examination and to provide the means for recertification.

Eligibility requires completion of a Physician Assistant program that is accredited by the Accreditation Review Commission on Education for the Physician Assistant (ARC-PA). Details regarding registration are available from the NCCPA.

The entry-level examination (PANCE) consists of 360-questions addressing all aspects of physician assistant education, including anatomy, physiology, history taking, physical examination, laboratory and radiographic interpretation, as well as treatment modalities. Tips for improving your score on the exam are provided in Chapter 1. Currently, the recertification (PANRE) examination consists of 300 questions constructed in a similar format as the entry-level examination. An alternative pathway (Pathway II) for recertification exists and may provide practicing PAs with a choice for recertification. More details on this option are found through the NCCPA web site www.nccpa.net or the American Academy of Physician Assistants via their web site at www.aapa.org.

CHAPTER 1

Test-Taking Skills: Tips and Techniques

Robert W. Jarski, PhD, PA-C

To become certified and maintain their recertification status, physician assistants are required to successfully respond to multiple-choice questions that appear on Board exams. Passing these exams requires not only medical knowledge but also test-taking skills. By providing examples, helpful explanations, and opportunities for experience and practice, this chapter will help the physician assistant student or graduate prepare for the Board exams and use effective test-taking strategies for answering the types of questions found on these standardized tests.

For initial certification, new graduates are required to complete and pass the Physician Assistant National Certifying Exam (PANCE). This 360-item multiple-choice exam covers primary-care medical knowledge. For recertification, graduates are required to complete, in addition to a prescribed number of continuing medical education credits, one of the recertification exams, either the Physician Assistant National Recertifying Exam (PANRE), which contains 300 multiple-choice questions, or Pathway II Recertification Exam, completed at home via a Web-based examination.

These exams are designed by the National Commission on Certification of Physician Assistants (NCCPA). The PANCE and PANRE are timed, multiple-choice tests that are presented and answered on a computer screen in local commercial testing centers. Information about exam development and scoring is available at the NCCPA Web site (http://www.nccpa.net).

Three conditions are generally necessary for successfully passing multiple-choice exams: (1) knowing about or recognizing the medical information contained in the questions; (2) using appropriate test-taking skills and strategies; and (3) avoiding situations that are likely to cause mistakes or impede performance. Test anxiety is an example. Pathway II does not involve time pressure, but any standardized exam can produce anxiety that leads to error. However, remembering that most test questions were created by clinicians like yourself who aim to be fair can help you keep the exam's purpose in perspective. Multiple-choice questions are limited in what they can evaluate; they generally assess only fundamental cognitive knowledge (Ballantyne, 2002; Burton and Miller, 1999) and test-wise individuals use strategies that enable them to respond correctly to these types of questions.

The fact is, written tests—even at their psychometric "best"—are crude evaluation devices (Ballantyne, 2002; Burton and Miller, 1999; Snelbecker, 1985). Multiple-choice questions cannot reflect a clinician's total fund of clinical skills. For example, patient rapport and the mechanics of examining patients are not accurately measured through multiple-choice questions. These questions can, however, successfully measure certain cognitive or knowledge skills. Computer-administered and scored exams have limited assessment capabilities. Test taking is a discrete skill that is different from clinical skills, and expert clinicians are not necessarily expert test takers.

Clinicians who must pass standardized tests should master the skill of test taking the same way they have mastered clinical skills. This may be accomplished by practicing the methods suggested in this chapter, answering the questions in the chapters at www.PAeasy.com. Reading and answering questions directly on a computer screen may be unfamiliar to some physician assistants, and learning to become accustomed and at ease with this format are skills well worth mastering prior to test time.

This chapter primarily presents information based on objective studies and sound psychological principles of test taking, perception, and recall (York University, 2005; U.S. Department of Education, 1986; Snelbecker, 1985). The chapter is organized in four sections: (1) what to do when preparing for the exam; (2) what to do during the exam; (3) illustrative questions; and (4) "do's" and "don'ts" that bring together the strategies explained in the previous three sections.

Objectives

In this chapter, the student or graduate physician assistant will

1. Identify proven techniques from the psychology of learning and educational measurement that will enhance test performance
2. Identify information from testing theory that will help avoid "careless" errors
3. Practice using clues to help identify correct and incorrect responses to exam questions

WHAT TO DO WHEN PREPARING FOR THE EXAM

Getting into Practice

To develop test-taking skills, you must *actively* practice what you will be doing on the test, that is, answering multiple-choice questions. Reading and reviewing without active practice are rarely sufficient. To become proficient in suturing wounds, you need to not only *read* about suturing, but also *practice* suturing. Some physician assistants have not taken a written exam in weeks, months, or years. Do not attempt to sit for Board exams without practicing answering multiple-choice questions any sooner than you would suture a facial laceration without having sutured skin in weeks, months, or years. Responding to questions similar to those encountered on the Boards presented on a computer screen is online content at www.PAeasy.com.

Areas to Emphasize

Although you may enjoy studying the areas relating directly to your own practice specialty, the task at hand is to pass the Boards. This is best accomplished by achieving a fundamental knowledge of all the medical disciplines represented on the exam. Therefore, it is suggested that you direct your studying to the primary care areas with which you are *least* familiar.

The certification and recertification exams are divided into two general dimensions: (1) organ systems, and the disorders and assessments physician assistants encounter; and (2) the knowledge and skills physician assistants should exhibit (NCCPA, 2005). Up-to-date knowledge and skill content areas by percentages, additional testing categories, and a sampling of the diseases and disorders that are included are available on the NCCPA Web site (www.nccpa.net).

As you prepare, you are strongly encouraged to write several of your own test questions. Those who do so frequently comment that their questions were surprisingly similar to those on the Boards. This occurs because only a limited amount of knowledge is amenable to the written exam format. In addition to identifying clinical information that is likely to be tested, you will also gain valuable insight into the logic of test item construction, which in turn helps you to select the intended correct answers from among the foils.

Scheduling Preparation Time

Using a planner, schedule specific periods for test preparation, setting aside specific times for actively reviewing and answering multiple-choice questions. Regular preparation over several months is preferred to cramming; studying just before the exam is usually nonproductive.

For the recertification exam, the amount of preparation needed depends largely on your practice. If your knowledge in primary care family medicine is current, you will need less preparation time than a physician assistant practicing a subspecialty. Primary care knowledge will enhance test performance because in designing the Boards it is assumed that all physician assistants should have fundamental and broad knowledge in primary-care medicine regardless of specialty.

The usual learning aids, such as the use of mnemonics, are highly recommended. The reader is referred to appropriate references for general information about study skills (California Polytechnic State University, 2005; Virginia Tech, 2005; York University, 2005). The remainder of this chapter addresses specific information about the Board exams.

WHAT TO DO DURING THE EXAM

Meeting Your Physical Needs

Your anticipated physical and environmental needs during the testing period should be considered when sitting for the PANCE or PANRE. Arriving early may allow you to select a computer terminal in an optimal location. If permitted, choose one that has few or no distractions, avoiding places near doorways and thoroughfares. Repeated interference can hinder your test performance.

Observe the lighting conditions. Extremely bright fore and overhead lights or glare on computer screens have been reported. Examine the conditions when you arrive and, if possible, request a terminal that meets your needs.

Temperature extremes may be possible. Therefore, dress in layers that will allow you to be comfortable if the temperature is too low or too high. The room situation and your own thermoregulatory mechanisms may change over the course of the day, so be prepared and avoid conditions that may prevent your best performance. In addition, you may wish to consider bringing ear plugs if you are easily distracted by environmental noises.

The exam is divided into several blocks of questions, approximately 60 questions per block for the PANRE and 90 questions per block for the PANCE. Even though the time frame within each block is conveniently provided on the computer screen, you are responsible for the amount of time taken between blocks and completing all blocks within the designated timeframe. (See "Time Allowance" below.) Therefore, you should take a watch in case a clock is not easily visible. (Digital or calculator watches are not permitted.)

You are entitled to a comfortable and quiet environment. However, be alert for potential distractions and make reasonable requests that may be honored by the testing center.

Consider Your Nutritional Needs

Consider nutritional and other personal needs. It is recommended that a heavy meal not be eaten within 2 hours prior to the exam, but a complex carbohydrate snack approximately 30 minutes before test time and between blocks may be beneficial. You may also wish to bring with you packaged drinks and other supplies, such as tissues and cough drops. Although these items are not allowed in the testing room, keep snacks, food for lunch, and drinks handy for breaks taken between blocks of questions.

Get Proper Rest

Your exam performance should reflect your knowledge fund rather than mental and physical endurance. You are encouraged to experience the energy required for answering hundreds of multiple-choice questions by using the online testing at www.PAeasy.com.

Recent electroencephalographic data show that lacking 1 hour of sleep less than the normal 8 hours required by most adults results in brainwave patterns similar to consuming one alcoholic drink; a 2-hour deficit may be similar to legal levels of intoxication (Hammond, 2005). No one could be expected to perform optimally on an exam while intoxicated! Lacking even 1 hour of sleep can be expected to impede your test performance. Try to get adequate sleep and rest before the exam by practicing the same sleep hygiene advice given to patients.

Time Allowance

One advantage of the Pathway II exam is the absence of time pressure. On the other exams, you are allowed a specified number of hours to complete the test on exam day. The amount of time you spend on breaks for rest, bathroom breaks, and meals between blocks of questions is up to you, but you must complete the entire exam within the designated time frame. You may check the number of questions per block and the number of blocks for the entire exam on the NCCPA Web site. www.PAeasy.com.

Before beginning each block of questions, calculate the average amount of time you can spend on each question. Typically you have 1 minute per question. Never go over the calculated time limit on your first attempt at each question. If you do not know an answer, you can mark it by clicking on the appropriate icon and returning to it at the end of the block. Always allow for a few extra minutes at the end for returning to marked items and checking your answers. Your subconscious processes items you have previously encountered while you work on other questions. Also, clues often appear in other items. (See Test Mechanics below.)

Maintain a Positive Attitude

Set yourself up for success by maintaining a positive, confident attitude. Remind yourself that you prepared as best you could, practice other self-coaching suggestions presented here, and use others that have been successful for you in the past.

Do not become discouraged by questions you cannot answer. Many test items are, by design, those that have been answered incorrectly by a large number of test takers. Test questions with a predetermined discrimination level are retained for use in future exams. If too many test takers answer a particular test item correctly, it is not used again. Therefore, many of the items you will be answering are those that other test takers have failed. So keep in mind that there will be a number of questions you are not expected to answer correctly.

Also, be aware that some experimental questions appear on standardized exams. Experimental questions are those being field-tested, and they are not counted in your score. Because you do not know which items these are, assume that any absurd question is experimental. Try not to become irate or unnecessarily concerned about any question.

Self-coaching and imaging or visualization techniques are helpful for all test takers (Davis et al, 2000; Rossman, 2000). Stress management methods may be especially useful for anxious test takers (Davis et al, 2000; Benson and Stuart, 1993). Most professional athletes and stage performers master and routinely use these techniques to manage their stress and avoid situations likely to interfere with optimal performance.

Techniques should be learned and practiced several weeks before the exam and used the day of the exam. These techniques will not bring to mind medical information you have never studied, but they help you retrieve learned information and avoid exam errors due to extreme stress. Effectively managing stress generally results in improved concentration and the ability to reason logically. The suggested techniques may be learned through special courses and by consulting appropriate references (Davis et al, 2000; Benson and Stuart, 1993; Rossman, 2000). Certain brief imaging procedures and breathing techniques described by Davis et al (2000) may be used for relaxing and improving concentration during the exam.

Keeping Your Concentration

During the exam, think of nothing except the questions in front of you. When working in the operating room, you concentrate on the operative field. Similarly, give the exam your full, serious, and undivided attention. Problems at work or home should be left at the exam room doorstep knowing you will later have the opportunity to return to them. Your one and only task during the exam period is to answer questions to the best of your ability.

Test Mechanics

The mechanics of navigating through the computer-administered Board exams may be unfamiliar to most. However, the instructions are explained in detail and practice opportunities are provided on the NCCPA Web site. To conserve your mental focus and energy on exam day, and to maximize the time allotted for rest between blocks, it is helpful to thoroughly master the test instructions well before exam day on a computer without any time constraints. Never find yourself confused because you arrived at the testing center uninformed. In addition, always read the instructions as you begin each section of the exam.

Once you are into the exam, if you do not know the answer to a question, mark it on the computer screen. You will be able to return to it at the end of the block. Unanswered questions are counted incorrect, so it is beneficial to answer the questions you plan to return to, just in case you run out of time at the end. Continue answering the questions you know. Frequently, you will find clues in other questions. In addition, your subconscious will have processed the questions you marked. It has been found that a great deal of information is successfully stored in your memory, but information *retrieval* is often the problem during exam time. Retrieval is enhanced by getting proper rest before the exam, using well-practiced stress management skills, and varying mental tasks during the exam to help keep your mind fresh and alert.

Should You Change Your Answer?

Contrary to some popular misconceptions, if you doubt an answer selection and want to change it, it is suggested that you do so. In numerous studies across disciplines examining thousands of changed responses, answers were changed approximately twice as often from incorrect responses to correct ones (York University, 2005; Welch and Leichner, 1988; Fabrey and Case, 1985). It might not seem this way because we tend to remember mistakes when we have changed answers from right to wrong, but pay no attention to the times we changed answers correctly. On the other hand, if you really have no idea which response is correct and you find yourself purely guessing, perhaps your first instinct will have been accurate. However, if you do have a reason to change your answer, you will probably change from an *incorrect* to a *correct* response.

Answering by Elimination

Answering multiple-choice questions resembles the process of elimination used when arriving at a diagnosis from a differential diagnosis list. Selecting an answer on the exam by the process of elimination increases the probability of choosing the correct response. Using the stem of the question, form a sentence with each choice provided. After reading the stem, it may be helpful to think out the answer before examining the foils. However, be cautioned against selecting the first answer you think is correct; consider *all* possibilities before making a final selection.

Most test questions have in common the following anatomic features: (1) one choice is easily recognized as an outlier and incorrect; (2) two choices appear plausible as either slightly off the topic or the opposite of the correct answer (e.g., artery versus arteriole, left versus right hemithorax); and (3) two choices are correct, but one is better than the other.

The test taker's job is to first (1) eliminate the outlier; next (2) identify the two plausible choices and reject them after weighing them against the two that are more likely to be correct; and finally (3) select the better answer of the remaining two. As with a differential diagnosis, this job is most effectively accomplished through the process of elimination.

By using the process of elimination, almost anyone can eliminate the outlier. By doing so, the probability of selecting the wrong answer by guessing alone is now decreased by 20%. If the two plausible but incorrect choices are identified, you now have two remaining items, and the more correct choice should be selected. At this point, even a pure guess will have a 50-50 chance of being correct. When in doubt, play the odds to your advantage.

Always Triage First

Some exam questions involve dangerous, invasive, expensive, or potentially harmful choices. On the exam, as in real life, you must be alert for such errors. Screen each and every question for potentially harmful or invasive choices. Just as patients are triaged, you should similarly triage each test item encountered. There are three question categories that should be identified.

The first is the "friendly" question—the one that assesses your medical knowledge simply by asking for information. The second category includes those questions designed to trap. Unlike the "friendly" question, the item designed to trap has a preconceived attractor or distracter that may catch the test taker off guard. The third type of question is the one containing a potentially harmful choice. It may refer to a treatment, procedure, finding, or diagnosis.

The third category might not be necessarily tricky, but the test item writer had in mind a possible pitfall that must *not* be selected. Examples of each question type are presented and discussed in the Illustrative Questions presented below.

Some General Hints

Certain "hints" of test taking apply to most multiple-choice questions. These hints are not, however, as likely to work on standardized exams as on other tests, but they may be useful as a last resort instead of guessing randomly.

The choices "all of the above" or "none of the above" have an increased probability of being correct. If a single-answer multiple-choice question contains two alternatives that mean exactly the same thing, they probably are both incorrect.

Finally, if you must make a pure guess, (C) is most likely the correct choice. The next most likely choice is (B). Board exam test writers try to guard against these probabilities, but the odds might prove useful to you if all else fails.

ILLUSTRATIVE QUESTIONS

You may encounter the following types of questions on Board exams. Each example presented illustrates a strategy to help identify correct choices. As always, first triage each question and identify its category as (1) friendly, (2) designed to identify a harmful choice, or (3) designed to trap.

The Oversimplification

Some questions appear tricky because you think, "No question could be this simple!" If you really know the answer to a question, answer it without belaboring or looking for booby traps that are not there. The following is an example.

A 22-year-old woman presents with abdominal pain and fever of 2 days' duration. During the digital pelvic exam, she experiences exquisite pain when the cervix is moved. This suggests a diagnosis of

(A) uterine fibroids

(B) vaginitis

(C) peritonitis

(D) cystitis

(E) cervical carcinoma

The item least likely to cause pain, (E), is eliminated. Any of the remaining four are possibilities, but peritonitis of any etiology is usually a safe diagnostic consideration. Do not get bogged down considering the unlikely diagnostic possibilities when an obvious choice is present. The oversimplification in this case is the correct answer, (C).

The Oversimplification
That Is Dangerous by Omission

As always, triage questions for traps. In the following question, the correct choice is an oversimplification that is dangerous by omission.

A painless testicular mass is found in an otherwise normal 29-year-old. Which of the following diagnoses should be pursued?

(A) varicocele

(B) carcinoma

(C) furuncle

(D) torsion

(E) strangulation

Choices (C), (D), and (E) are ruled out because they usually are painful. (A) and (B), however, usually are painless. Because of its prognosis if left untreated, a testicular mass should be considered cancer until proven otherwise. Not to do so would be considered a life-threatening omission. The correct choice is (B).

Always screen questions for dangerous or critical choices whether harmful by omission or commission. A potentially harmful choice may present itself as an oversimplification.

Clues from Logic

Sometimes a logical (and correct) answer is contained in the stem, as shown in the following example.

The diagnosis of congenital hip dislocation is made

(A) in utero

(B) at birth

(C) at 6 weeks of age

(D) at 6 months of age

(E) fluoroscopically

The term *congenital* means "present at birth." This is when the diagnosis of congenital hip dislocation is made. The correct choice is (B).

Clues from Related Areas

Similar to clues from logic, knowledge about related disciplines can provide additional hints.

An obese 45-year-old woman presents with acute genital pain. Upon examination you find a 2- to 3-cm soft mass in the right labia majora. This is most likely

(A) marked lymphadenopathy

(B) an inguinal hernia

(C) a femoral hernia

(D) a femoral aneurysm

(E) neurofibroma

If the mass were located in the scrotum of an obese man, you would probably not miss the common diagnosis of inguinal hernia. Remembering from developmental anatomy that the labia majora and scrotum are corresponding tissues, (B) would be selected as the correct response, even if the test taker had minimal knowledge about surgical emergencies.

The "Odd" Choice

This test taking clue is demonstrated by way of two examples. The first example comes from psychiatry.

Which of the following is **NOT** a sign of transsexualism?

(A) rejecting one's anatomic sex

(B) sex identity problems during childhood

(C) dressing in clothing of the opposite sex

(D) aversion toward one's own genitalia

(E) sex identity problems during adolescence

Transsexualism is considered pathological because the patient considers a serious and invasive procedure preferable to living as his/her designated gender. Each choice except (C) implies pathology—rejecting one's own anatomy, sex identity problems, and aversion. The odd choice, (C), has, however, no associated pathology and is the correct response.

The second example follows.

A 65-year-old man complains of burning pain in the distal extremities especially upon exposure to heat.

Upon examination, the hands and feet are warm and erythematous. The findings are most consistent with

- (A) diabetes mellitus
- (B) arteriosclerosis
- (C) Raynaud's phenomenon
- (D) thromboembolism
- (E) erythromelalgia

With the limited amount of information provided in the stem, it is unlikely that you can differentiate precisely among the choices provided. Your only clue is the odd choice. Even if you are unfamiliar with the infrequently seen problem of erythromelalgia, notice that choices (A) through (D) are associated with problems causing impaired circulation and cold extremities. "Erythro" or "red" implies *increased* circulation and warmth. (E), the odd choice among the options provided, is the correct answer.

Qualifying Words

Test-item stems containing qualifying words, such as *most*, *more*, *usually*, *often*, *less*, *seldom*, and *few*, will sometimes lead you to the correct answer.

You see in the outpatient clinic a 32-year-old man whom you suspect is suffering from alcohol withdrawal. The most likely finding would be

- (A) visual hallucinations
- (B) auditory hallucinations
- (C) fine motor tremors
- (D) major motor seizures
- (E) autonomic hyperactivity

Any of the above may be seen with alcohol withdrawal. However, fine motor tremors are the most common by far. The stem contains a qualifying word suggesting (C) as the correct choice.

If a qualifying word appears among the choices presented, it deserves special attention. Words such as *best*, *entirely*, *completely*, *always*, and *all* imply that something is always true; words such as *worst*, *never*, *no*, and *none* imply that something is never true. In clinical practice, *always* and *never* are rarely correct.

The Overqualified Choice

To make an answer acceptable, test-item writers sometimes must qualify a choice to the point at which the savvy test taker recognizes the ploy. The following example illustrates an overqualified choice.

In a 66-year-old emphysematous man with a 100-pack-per-year smoking history, clubbing is most appropriately described as

- (A) discoloration
- (B) a flattened angle between the dorsal surface of the distal phalanx and the proximal nail
- (C) an abnormal inwardly curved nail
- (D) a measurably increased eponychium

The overqualified (lengthy) choice, (B), is likely to be correct, as in this example.

However, remember the "odd choice" described above! Sometimes the very short "odd choice" is correct. You will recognize this variation because it will be attractively precise and succinct. Having at least some knowledge about the item, you will identify it as accurate.

Strange Terms

Choices containing completely unfamiliar words are likely to be distracters. Do not assume that you somehow missed an important chapter of Harrison's or that there is a gap in your education. If the choice appears completely bizarre, the test item writer was probably scraping the barrel for a distracter.

On a routine peripheral blood smear from a 13-year-old boy, you see a nucleated cell that is filled with bright red granules and is approximately three times the diameter of a typical red blood cell. This should be recognized as a (an)

- (A) Franz-Kulig cell
- (B) myelocyte
- (C) eosinophil
- (D) Olson cell
- (E) Kupffer cell

Choices (A), (D), and (E) are completely fictitious. The test item writer obviously did not lack imagination. (B) is familiar—remember basic anatomy or hematology? However, identifying a myelocyte on the peripheral smear is not basic primary care which the Board exam covers. Physician assistants should recognize the morphology and significance of an eosinophil; thus, the correct response is (C).

"Apple Pie" Choices

There are some responses to which no one would object. Consider the following test question.

When evaluating a 23-year-old woman with vaginal bleeding, the most important clinical information is gained from the

- (A) prothrombin time
- (B) partial thromboplastin time
- (C) CBC and iron studies
- (D) physical exam
- (E) detailed history

A patient's history provides a clinician's best information and is almost never incorrect. (E) is an "apple pie" choice.

The "apple pie" choice, however, can also be used by test-item writers to set traps.

The most important physical exam component(s) in the emergency evaluation of an unconscious patient is (are)

- (A) body symmetry
- (B) a carefully performed and prompt neurological exam
- (C) the cardiopulmonary exam
- (D) vital signs
- (E) blood gases

The initial triage of this question would identify it as a "trap" question because of the critical nature of the scenario combined with an incorrect "apple pie" choice. Blood gases are promptly dismissed because they are not physical exam components, for which the stem asks. (B) appears attractive because of its "apple pie" component. Nevertheless, remember your ABCs of emergency care! The correct response is (D).

Hints from Inconsistencies in Terminology

Grammar inconsistencies between the stem and a choice (e.g., tense, number, gender) are usually recognized by expert educational evaluators who screen Board exam test questions. You will, therefore, seldom encounter this type of "hint" on Board exams, although it will be found more frequently in classroom situations. Hints due to inconsistencies in terminology are more frequent than other types and you may benefit from being alert for this inconsistency.

A 19-year-old unconscious motorcycle accident victim with suspected multiple trauma is brought to the emergency room. The most significant physical findings usually will result from

- (A) undressing the patient
- (B) a prompt neurological exam

- (C) interviewing the family
- (D) interviewing a witness to the accident
- (E) all the above

Choices (C) and (D) can be excluded because they refer to historical, not physical, findings. This also excludes foil (E). Although indicated, at this point of presentation, the neurological exam is too focused. A more general, overall assessment provides the best clinical information. Therefore, critical, life-saving information across organ systems may be gained from observing the patient. Choice (A) is correct. Similarly, choice (E), blood gases, in the previous example was eliminated because it was inconsistent with the information asked for in the stem.

Rank Orders

When given a list of numbers or other rank orders, the correct response most often occurs somewhere between the extremes, as shown in these examples.

A 17-year-old woman presents with a history of pelvic discomfort during menses. Through questioning, you determine that the amount of blood lost during each cycle is normal. The amount of her blood loss would be approximately

- (A) 25 mL
- (B) 35 mL
- (C) 70 mL
- (D) 100 mL
- (E) 125 mL

Here is the second example.
In reviewing the chart of a 45-year-old man, you notice a past diagnosis of chronic schizophrenia. To be termed *chronic*, this disorder was present for at least

- (A) 3 months
- (B) 1 year
- (C) 2 years
- (D) 3 years
- (E) 4 years

Most test-item writers try to bury the correct answer somewhere in the middle. (C) is the correct answer in each example.

As with hints from inconsistencies in terminology, this clue does not work as often on Board exams as it does on classroom tests. Educational evaluators try to randomize the position of correct responses as much as possible. However, when in doubt, it is better to avoid the extremes when presented with rank-ordered options.

DO'S AND DON'TS

The following do's and don'ts summarize some of the important points made earlier in this chapter.

DO practice what you will be doing during the exam, that is, answering multiple-choice questions on a computer. Answering these questions is a skill different from knowing clinical information. Get into practice for answering Board questions by actually answering similar questions. This is imperative for the clinician who has not taken a written or computer-based exam recently.

DO direct your studying to the primary care areas with which you are *least* familiar. Passing the Boards is best accomplished by achieving a fundamental knowledge level in each medical discipline assessed on the exam.

DO write your own multiple-choice questions. Not only will you gain insights into the mechanics of test-item writing and correctly answering questions, but also it is likely that many of your items will resemble actual Board exam questions.

DO get adequate sleep and rest before the exam. Some individuals elect to stay at a hotel located near the testing center in order to help get a good night's sleep and to avoid being late due to traffic conditions.

DO dress comfortably in layers that prepare you for temperature extremes, hot or cold. Coats or jackets may not be allowed.

DO arrive alert, calm, and well-rested.

DO bring beverages, food for lunch and between-question block snacks. They are not allowed in the exam room but may be checked outside and accessed during breaks.

DO reread instructions provided by the testing agency the night before to ensure you arrive on time, at the right place, and with the right supplies. Recheck directions to the test center.

DO review in detail the information on the PANCE or PANRE content, instructions and format found at www.nccpa.net

DO remember to bring admissions materials (such as your permit and government-issued identification).

DO examine the computer station you are assigned. Be alert for glare or other lighting problems, and potential traffic flow as others arrive and leave throughout the day.

DO consider that the proctor is there to support you. Ask for any reasonable support or change of computer location that will help you do your best.

DO pace yourself, allowing a calculated amount of time per question. In your time allocation, allow for some extra minutes at the end for returning to items you have marked as unsure.

DO avoid situations that might put you in an unfavorable mindset before the exam. For example, if you anticipate heavy highway traffic, arrive at the exam site a day early. If disturbances bother you during an exam, come early and request a computer in a far corner of the testing room. Let nothing interfere with your best possible performance on the day of the exam.

DO relate test questions to your own practice and experience. Test-item writers are people who have derived many of the test questions from their own clinical experience. What would *you* expect a primary care physician assistant to know? Use this mindset to understand the goal of a question and to keep a positive attitude throughout the exam.

DO practice effective stress management techniques daily several weeks before the exam. During the exam, slow breathing always induces a parasympathetic response that will calm the mind, and increase your concentration and focus. If you have any tendency for test anxiety, participate in programs designed to help you do your best.

DO change your answer if you have a good reason to do so. You are twice as likely to change from an incorrect response to a correct one. However, if you are only playing a hunch with no information about the topic at all, your first "gut" reaction might be correct.

DO triage each and every question before selecting your answer. Evaluate it as a question designed: (1) to test knowledge in a "friendly" way; (2) to trap by including common pitfalls; or (3) to evaluate your knowledge about potentially dangerous choices. In the first case, the apparent oversimplification is probably the correct choice. In questions designed to trap, beware of the "apple pie" choice—by omission or commission.

DO use the process of elimination. Your job is to find the single best answer. As with a patient's differential diagnosis, this usually is done by *elimination*. Avoid choosing an answer until after you have considered all of the choices.

DO read the question stem and combine it with each foil to form a sentence. After doing this, use the process of elimination to arrive at the final answer.

DO mark items if you are not sure of the answer. Return to these items when you finish the question block.

DO make *educated* guesses, if you must guess. Use the information provided in this chapter to help in your decision. By also using your medical knowledge and judgment, your chances will be much improved.

DO be alert for qualifying words such as *most, more, usually, often, less, seldom,* and *few,* which will sometimes lead you to the correct answer.

DO eliminate choices containing completely unfamiliar words as distracters. If the choice appears completely unfamiliar, it is probably incorrect.

DO consider "apple pie" choices as probably correct. However, beware that they may also be used to trap.

DO consider choices that are different from the others—the "odd choice." This may involve the choice having the "odd" meaning or the "odd" length—long or short. The overqualified choice often is correct.

DO select item (C) when purely guessing. It is most frequently the correct response on many one-choice-only multiple-choice questions. If you eliminate (C) as a possibility, (B) is the next most likely choice. This is a "last-ditch" strategy that works more often on classroom tests than on Board exams.

DO select "all the above" or "none of the above" as a last-ditch strategy. When appearing as choices, they are more likely to be correct.

DO consider taking the exam as a positive experience. Keep your motivation high through self-coaching and imaging techniques. Use recommended stress management methods, especially if you are anxious when taking tests.

DO plan to reward yourself for a good performance after the exam. This facilitates a positive attitude.

DON'T cram at the last minute. This kind of preparation will not be adequate for an exam that covers mostly primary care breadth rather than depth.

DON'T eat a large meal within 2 hours of the beginning of the exam. Be well nourished, but not full.

DON'T leave any item blank at the end of the exam. Unanswered items will be counted wrong.

DON'T discuss the exam during the administration, during breaks, or after the exam; this adds to anxiety and may result in disqualification or revocation of your certification.

DON'T become irate over seemingly absurd questions. Answer them to the best of your ability, realizing that they probably are experimental questions that will not affect your score. Other test takers probably will also consider them absurd.

DON'T guess randomly. Even if you are completely unsure of the answer to a question, use the hints suggested in this chapter to increase the probability of guessing the correct response. Make educated, not random, guesses.

DON'T think of anything except the exam in front of you. Think of it as your "operative field." Concentrate on giving your best possible performance.

REFERENCES

Ballantyne C. *Multiple Choice Tests.* The Teaching and Learning Centre of Murdoch University, Perth Western Australia, 2002.

Benson H, Stuart EM. *The Wellness Book.* New York: Birch Lane Press; 1993.

Burton RF, Miller DJ. Statistical modelling of multiple-choice and true/false tests. *Bath* December 1999:399–411.

Davis M, Eshelman ER, McKay M. *The Relaxation and Stress Reduction Workbook.* Oakland, CA: New Harbinger Publications; 2000.

Fabrey L, Case SM. Further support for changing multiple-choice answers. *J Med Educ.* June 1985: 60(6);488–490.

Rossman ML. *Guided Imagery for Self-Healing.* Tiburon, CA: H.J. Kramer, Inc; 2000.

Snelbecker GE. *Learning Theory, Instructional Theory and Psychoeducational Design.* Lanham, MD: University Printers of America; 1985.

U.S. Department of Education. *What Works: Research about Teaching and Learning.* Washington, DC: U.S. Department of Education; 1986.

Welch J, Leichner P. Analysis of changing answers on multiple-choice examination for nationwide sample of Canadian psychiatry residents. *J Med Educ.* February 1988:63(6);133–135.

Academic Skills Center: Study Skills Library, California Polytechnic State University. 2005. URL: http://www.sas.calpoly.edu.

Counselling and Development Centre, York University. 2005. URL: http://www.yorku.ca.

Hammond DC, International Society for Neurological Regulation. 2005. URL: http://www.isnr.org.

Study Skills Self-help Information: Online Study Skills Workshops, Virginia Polytechnic Institute and State University. 2005. URL: http://www.ucc.vt.edu.

NCCPA Connect, National Commission on Certification of Physician Assistants. 2005. URL: http://www.nccpa.net.

SECTION I
Internal Medicine Topics

CHAPTER 2

Cardiology
Questions
Mary Warner, MMSc, PA-C

DIRECTIONS (Questions 1 through 44): Select the ONE lettered answer or completion that is BEST in each case.

Questions 1 through 44

1. A patient with a long history of innocent palpitations comes to the clinic complaining now of presyncopal symptoms. She is admitted for evaluation and definitive therapy. Which condition is an indication for implantation of a permanent cardiac pacemaker in this patient?

    (A) first degree AV block
    (B) mobitz Type I heart block with a heart rate of 72
    (C) third degree heart block
    (D) sinus tachycardia with occasional SVT

2. A patient with a history of bradycardia and occasional bursts of ventricular tachycardia is admitted for a pacemaker combined with an implanted cardioverter/defibrillator (ICD). What is the most common complication historically associated with this device?

    (A) development of pacemaker syndrome
    (B) inappropriate discharge of shock
    (C) pericarditis
    (D) bronchospasm

3. One of the potential complications of percutaneous coronary revascularization and atherectomy is perforation of the coronary artery as a result of instrumentation. What is the rate of this complication?

    (A) 1%
    (B) 5%
    (C) 8%
    (D) 11%

4. Your patient's wife calls asking for advice. Her husband was admitted this morning with acute coronary syndrome and the doctors are recommending he have coronary artery bypass grafting (CABG). What are the indications for bypass versus percutaneous coronary intervention?

    (A) patients should have bypass if they have two lesions both with 80% occlusion
    (B) patients should have bypass if they have one lesion with 95% occlusion and diabetes
    (C) patients should have bypass if they have triple vessel disease
    (D) patients have bypass if they have two lesions both with >95% occlusion

5. The use of a bioprosthetic valve replacement versus a mechanical valve is based on several key factors. One of the important factors to consider relates to the patient's age. In which age range would a surgeon most likely consider using a mechanical valve for valvular replacement?

(A) 55 to 65 years of age
(B) 66 to 75 years of age
(C) 76 to 82 years of age
(D) older than 83 years

6. A 62-year-old female comes into the office complaining of substernal chest pain and diaphoresis. Her ECG indicates ST elevation in leads II, III, and AVF. What is the next step of care for this patient?

(A) obtain a stat chest radiograph
(B) start a verapamil drip
(C) have the patient chew an aspirin
(D) repeat the ECG

7. Which of the following is an absolute contraindication for the use of thrombolytic therapy?

(A) systolic pressure at or greater than 170
(B) age greater than 72
(C) active peptic ulcer disease
(D) active internal bleeding

8. Anticoagulation therapy for a mechanical valve should target what international normalized ratio (INR) range?

(A) 1.0 to 2.0
(B) 2.1 to 3.0
(C) 2.5 to 3.5
(D) 3.5 to 4.5

9. Indications for aortic aneurysm repair include

(A) an asymptomatic aneurysm greater than 5.5 cm
(B) 5 cm aneurysm in a patient with coronary artery disease
(C) an asymptomatic aneurysm of 3.4 cm in diameter
(D) 4 cm aneurysm in a patient with a recent CVA

10. Which of the following risk factors is not associated with increased peri-operative mortality in a patient undergoing CABG?

(A) underlying congestive heart failure
(B) presence of diabetes mellitus
(C) advanced age >80
(D) history of sustained ventricular tachycardia

11. Early thrombolytic therapy reduces mortality and limits myocardial infarction size. Four thrombolytic agents have been evaluated extensively in acute infarction. Which antithrombolytic agent should be avoided if the patient previously received it?

(A) streptokinase
(B) retaplase
(C) alteplase (t-PA)
(D) anistreplase (APSAC)

12. Conservative management of arterial peripheral vascular disease (PVD) includes

(A) papaverine
(B) pentoxifylline
(C) calcium channel blockers
(D) alpha-adrenergic blockers

13. The definitive treatment of aortic dissection that involves the ascending aorta (Type A) should include

(A) conservative therapy, admit to the step-down unit
(B) emergent operative intervention
(C) admit to the ICU and follow with IV labetolol
(D) serial CT scans to follow changes

14. A pregnant woman in her second trimester, with no previous history of hypertension is seen in the clinic and found to have hypertension. At what diastolic pressure would you begin pharmacological intervention?

(A) 80 mm Hg
(B) 85 mm Hg
(C) 90 mm Hg
(D) >100 mm Hg

15. A 62-year-old female with pulmonary hypertension called 911 complaining of sweating and difficulty in breathing. Upon arrival to her home the paramedics found her to have pallor, diaphoresis, tachypnea, hypotension, and tachycardia. Her pulse oxymetry was 89%, so they gave her a non-rebreather oxygen mask and transported her to the ED. She was not complaining of angina. The ED physician assistant noted her to be in acute distress with elevated jugular venous pressure, a medial heave, a tender palpable liver, a systolic murmur of tricuspid regurgitation, and an S4 gallop. ECG demonstrated right axis deviation and RV hypertrophy with no STT changes. Her ABG demonstrated a low PaO_2 and a low $PaCO_2$. What is her likely diagnosis?

   (A) acute coronary syndrome
   (B) cor pulmonale
   (C) heart failure
   (D) pulmonary embolus

16. A 33-year-old healthy female during a routine physical examination was found to be hypertensive with a blood pressure of 150/98 mm Hg 3 months ago. She has no family history of hypertension but her provider was concerned, so she was started on ACE inhibitors. Her blood pressure improved slightly but on a routine blood draw her creatinine is noted to be 2.3. She is asymptomatic but is noted to have an abdominal bruit. Based on her history and laboratory evaluation which of the following is her most likely diagnosis?

   (A) essential hypertension
   (B) isolated systolic hypertension
   (C) secondary hypertension
   (D) pheochromocytoma

17. A 55-year-old college professor complains of recent occipital headaches that are noted in the morning and subside later in the day. She has noted that over the past 6 months she tires easily. She has a family history of hypertension but denies all other risk factors. Her blood pressure in the clinic is noted to be 172/108 mm Hg. How would you classify her hypertension?

   (A) essential hypertension
   (B) secondary hypertension related to primary aldosteronism
   (C) secondary hypertension related to Cushing's syndrome
   (D) accelerated hypertension

18. A 73-year-old with a history of rheumatic fever and coronary atherosclerosis presents to the emergency department with dyspnea on exertion and orthopnea. He called 911 because he could not catch his breath. On examination, he has JVD, hepatic congestion and peripheral edema. A blowing holosystolic murmur along the left sternal border that is intensified during a Valsalva maneuver is noted. Atrial fibrillation is noted on his ECG. What is his most likely diagnosis?

   (A) aortic stenosis
   (B) mitral regurgitation
   (C) mitral stenosis
   (D) tricuspid regurgitation

19. A retired operating room nurse comes to the clinic complaining of a dull ache in her legs after prolonged standing. She notes her legs feel heavy and she has mild ankle edema when she spends the day shopping. The aching pain and the edema resolve spontaneously if the patient elevates her legs. She denies calf tenderness or dyspnea. Physical examination reveals +1 ankle edema bilaterally. What is her most likely diagnosis?

   (A) deep venous thrombosis
   (B) lymphedema
   (C) varicose veins
   (D) intermittent claudication

20. What is the most common primary tumor that metastasizes to the heart?

   (A) leukemia
   (B) lymphoma
   (C) prostate
   (D) malignant melanoma

21. A 77-year-old male walks to work every day. One month ago he developed buttock and thigh pain after walking two blocks. The patient is now limited to one block and then he must sit down to alleviate symptoms. He denies pain with weight bearing but notes the pain only after he walks. He denies any recent injury or fall. What is the most likely diagnosis for this patient?

    (A) spinal stenosis
    (B) aortoiliac occlusive disease
    (C) myalgias
    (D) popliteal occlusive disease

22. A 55-year-old male presents to the ED with chest pain that started 30 minutes ago, diaphoresis, and nausea. An ECG shows ST elevation in I, AVL, and V2 though V6. What is the diagnosis?

    (A) inferior infarction
    (B) lateral infarction
    (C) anterior infarction
    (D) posterior infarction

23. A 64-year-old female presents to the office with an ulcer on the anterior aspect of the right leg. She presents to the office because yesterday she shopped all day yesterday and has also developed significant edema. The tissue of her leg appears very thin and has brownish pigmentation noted anteriorly. What is the most likely diagnosis?

    (A) venous insufficiency
    (B) arterial insufficiency
    (C) complications of diabetes mellitus
    (D) peripheral neuropathies

24. A 35-year-old Asian male presents to your office with burning pain and numbness in his right hand. The patient admits the pain intensifies when working with his hands and may continue for several minutes upon resting. This process has been occurring for 1 month and now he has developed a persistent ulcer on the nail margin of his right thumb. He has a twenty-pack year history of smoking. He denies using any medications or any illegal drug or alcohol abuse. What is the most likely diagnosis?

    (A) venous insufficiency
    (B) thromboangiitis obliterans
    (C) Raynaud's phenomenon
    (D) acute arterial thrombosis

25. A 34-year-old female with a history of tobacco use comes to the emergency department complaining of severe substernal anginal symptoms. She has never had these symptoms before. She states that she has been watching TV this afternoon and the pain was not related to physical exertion. ECG demonstrates ST elevation. What is this patient's most likely diagnosis?

    (A) acute coronary syndrome
    (B) stable angina
    (C) unstable angina
    (D) Prinzmetal's angina

26. What is the most common primary tumor of the heart?

    (A) atrial myxoma
    (B) rhabdomyoma
    (C) fibrous histiocytoma
    (D) hemangioma

27. Patients with systemic lupus erythematosus have a predilection to which cardiac abnormality?

    (A) congestive heart failure
    (B) acute myocardial infarction
    (C) abdominal aortic dissection
    (D) pericarditis

28. A 72-year-old male comes to the hospital complaining of fatigue and generalized weakness that has been getting worse over the past month or so. He denies angina, palpitations but complains of a 3-day history of dyspnea. He denies any changes in his weight. He has weak pulses and distant heart sounds. His ECG demonstrates sinus bradycardia and prolongation of his QT interval. His chest x-ray demonstrates a water-bottle appearance of the cardiac silhouette with pleural effusions. What is his most likely underlying diagnosis?

(A) diabetes mellitus
(B) hypothyroidism
(C) hyperthyroidism
(D) pheochromocytoma

29. What ECG change may be noted when a patient has a potassium level of 6.0 meq/L?

(A) prolongation of the ST segment
(B) peaked T waves
(C) loss of P waves
(D) prominent U waves

30. The most common site of arterial aneurysm is

(A) infrarenal aorta
(B) suprarenal aorta
(C) ascending aortic arch
(D) descending thoracic aorta

31. An 82-year-old female with a history of hypertension and coronary artery disease presents to the ED with orthopnea and dyspnea on exertion. She denies angina. Over the past several days, she has noted a worsening of her dyspnea and now sleeps using 4 pillows. She now complains of dyspnea when she climbs the stairs to her bedroom. On physical examination you note her to be comfortably resting in the sitting position, her vitals are within normal, she has 3 cm of JVD and 4+ pitting edema. She is not using accessory muscles and her pulse oximetry is 92% on room air. She has normal heart sounds other than an S4. Rales are heard at the bases of her lung fields bilaterally; there is dullness to percussion over the lung bases as well. What is the laboratory test that you should order to confirm her diagnosis?

(A) arterial blood gas
(B) cardiac echocardiogram
(C) dobutamine stress test
(D) CBC and troponin levels

32. A 74-year-old female is admitted to the hospital for further evaluation of her syncopal episodes after a Holter monitor reveals two runs of sustained ventricular tachycardia. While in the hospital her ECG tracing reveals multi-focal premature ventricular contractions. She has no symptoms or ECG evidence that suggests coronary disease. What study would you recommend to evaluate her ventricular excitability?

(A) repeat the ECG
(B) electrophysiology study
(C) dobutamine stress test
(D) transesophageal echocardiogram

33. The differential diagnosis of a patient with an ECG demonstrating prominent U waves includes

(A) potassium depletion
(B) calcium depletion
(C) digitalis toxicity
(D) hypothermia

34. A 45-year-old patient with a history of hypertension, diabetes mellitus and cocaine abuse presents to the emergency department with acute 10/10, non-radiating, substernal chest pain. She denies recent cocaine use but appears very anxious and irritable. ECG reveals sinus tachycardia with no other significant changes. Which test(s) should be ordered to determine if this patient is suffering from acute coronary syndrome?

(A) arterial blood gases
(B) CPK enzymes
(C) troponin levels
(D) AST and ALT

35. A patient in the ED who is suspected as having cardiac ischemia has an initial troponin level of 0.08 ng/dL. What can be concluded by this finding?

    (A) the patient is having a myocardial infarction
    (B) this is a normal lab result, so the patient may be discharged
    (C) this is a normal finding but a repeat level must be obtained
    (D) this level confirms the patient is suffering from angina

36. A 48-year-old patient with a past history of ionizing radiation to the chest wall presents to the ED with dyspnea and fatigue. Physical examination reveals tachycardia, 4 cm JVD and slight peripheral edema of the extremities. ECG shows low voltage QRS complexes and CXR demonstrates normal lung fields and cardiac silhouette. What test should be ordered next in this patient?

    (A) Holter monitor
    (B) echocardiogram
    (C) cardiac catheterization
    (D) stress test

37. The most likely diagnosis of a patient with right bundle branch block and left hemiblock on ECG is

    (A) acute coronary syndrome
    (B) severe hypotension
    (C) myocarditis
    (D) endocarditis

38. A febrile patient with petechiae and a new onset murmur of aortic regurgitation should have which of the following diagnostic tests to determine if surgical intervention is required?

    (A) Holter monitor
    (B) transthoracic echocardiogram
    (C) cardiac catheterization
    (D) transesophageal echocardiogram

39. Radiographic findings associated with aortic dissection include

    (A) widened mediastinum
    (B) pneumothorax
    (C) consolidation in the right lower lobe
    (D) pleural effusion on the right side

40. Which of the following ECG findings is associated with tetralogy of Fallot?

    (A) right ventricular hypertrophy
    (B) right axis deviation with an rSr' pattern
    (C) left ventricular hypertrophy
    (D) atrial fibrillation

41. The most common cause of myocarditis is

    (A) coxsackie virus
    (B) *Staphylococcus aureus*
    (C) human immunodeficiency virus (HIV)
    (D) lyme disease

42. A late systolic murmur that may be preceded by a systolic click describes this valvular abnormality

    (A) aortic stenosis
    (B) mitral valve prolapse
    (C) aortic regurgitation
    (D) mitral valve stenosis

43. A murmur detected in both systole and diastole is most likely associated with

    (A) atrial myxoma
    (B) patent ductus arteriosus
    (C) mitral regurgitation
    (D) aortic regurgitation

44. A young woman who is otherwise healthy comes to the ED very anxious, complaining of a severe headache and diaphoresis. She has no history of tobacco use or family history of atherosclerosis. She was found to be hypertensive with a blood pressure of 170/109 mm Hg while her heart rate was noted to be 122. Based on this presentation, what is the most likely diagnosis?

   (A) pheochromocytoma
   (B) acute coronary syndrome
   (C) aortic dissection
   (D) epilepsy

DIRECTIONS (Questions 45 through 48): This section consists of lettered headings followed by a set of numbered words or phrases. For each numbered word or phrase, select the ONE lettered heading that is most closely associated with it. Each lettered heading may be selected once, more than once, or not at all.

Questions 45 through 48

Indicate which congenital defects have cyanotic or acyanotic presentations.

   (A) cyanotic
   (B) acyanotic
   (C) both could occur

45. congenital aortic stenosis

46. complete transposition of the great arteries

47. tetralogy of Fallot

48. atrial septal defects

DIRECTIONS (Questions 49 through 90): Select the ONE lettered answer or completion that is BEST in each case.

Questions 49 through 90

49. Which patient population is most associated with the development of varicose veins?

   (A) men
   (B) women
   (C) those with a history of deep venous thrombosis
   (D) those with a history of lymphedema

50. A patient who has been found to have a fixed split of the second heart sound may have which of the following conditions?

   (A) pulmonary embolus
   (B) increased pulmonary vascular resistance
   (C) pulmonary valve stenosis
   (D) atrial septal defect

51. A 53-year-old male who is of relatively good health except his history of tobacco use is brought to the emergency department complaining of severe substernal chest pain that radiates to his back. The pain began when he felt "a ripping sensation." He called 911 immediately. After arriving in the ED, he was placed on the monitor. His blood pressure was recorded at 190/128. Based on this history, what is his most likely diagnosis?

   (A) acute coronary syndrome
   (B) mitral valve stenosis
   (C) cardiogenic shock
   (D) aortic dissection

52. An 81-year-old female with a 10-year history of well-controlled atrial fibrillation complains of a 3-day history of fatigue, dyspnea, and a 10-pound weight gain. She denies angina or diaphoresis. Based on this history what would the most likely diagnosis be?

   (A) acute coronary syndrome
   (B) congestive heart failure
   (C) sinus tachycardia
   (D) cardiac tamponade

53. A 66-year-old female with an 11-year history of hypertension takes furosemide for her disease. Recently, she complained of self-limiting pre-syncopal episodes associated with a "few minutes" of palpitations. She went to her primary care provider and he sent her for Holter monitoring. Which cardiac arrhythmia was the practitioner looking for?

   (A) atrial fibrillation
   (B) sinus bradycardia
   (C) sick sinus syndrome
   (D) ventricular tachycardia

54. A 35-year-old female with no past medical history complains of occasional "skipped beats" or palpations. She denies any associated anginal or pre-syncopal symptoms. What is the most likely diagnosis?

    (A) atrial fibrillation
    (B) atrial extrasystoles
    (C) sinus bradycardia
    (D) ventricular tachycardia

55. A 55-year-old diabetic who has a history of tobacco use complains of a sudden onset of severe pain and paresthesias in his right leg. He denies any history of trauma and states he has not had these symptoms before. What is the most likely diagnosis?

    (A) arterial insufficiency
    (B) venous stasis disease
    (C) Raynaud's syndrome
    (D) arterial occlusion

56. Which of the following descriptions are characteristic of venous stasis ulcers?

    (A) painful, erythematous
    (B) painful, purulent
    (C) painless, erythematous
    (D) painless, pallorous

57. An important risk factor associated with primary hypertrophic cardiomyopathy is

    (A) long-standing hypertension
    (B) high dose radiation to the chest wall
    (C) a history of streptococcal infection
    (D) none of the above

58. Orthostatic hypotension is defined as a drop in systolic blood pressure of at least _____ or a drop of diastolic blood pressure of at least _____ within 3 minutes of standing from the sitting position.

    (A) 5 mm Hg; 10 mm Hg
    (B) 10 mm Hg; 20 mm Hg
    (C) 10 mm Hg; 5 mm Hg
    (D) 20 mm Hg; 10 mm Hg

59. What is the least likely etiology of cardiac tamponade?

    (A) malignant effusion
    (B) coronary artery bypass grafting
    (C) uremia
    (D) idiopathic pericarditis

60. A 65-year-old male with a 15-year history of HIV presents to the Emergency Department in florid congestive heart failure. Which class of medication should be given to this patient immediately?

    (A) vasopressors
    (B) beta-blockers
    (C) calcium channel blockers
    (D) diuretics

61. When your patient with congestive heart failure patient, who takes digoxin, develops atrial fibrillation, you decide to add amiodarone to her medication regimen. How should you adjust the dosing of her medications?

    (A) prescribe a larger dose of amiodarone, when you add it to the digoxin regimen
    (B) decrease the dose of digoxin by half, when you add amiodarone
    (C) increase the dose of digoxin by half, when you add amiodarone
    (D) prescribe a smaller dose of amiodarone, when you add it to the digoxin regimen

62. What is the dose of dopamine, which increases the blood flow to the kidneys and is utilized for diuresis purposes?

    (A) 1 to 2 mcg/dL
    (B) 3 to 4 mcg/dL
    (C) 5 to 7 mcg/dL
    (D) 8 to 10 mcg/dL

63. A 55-year-old hypertensive male comes to the office for a routine check after his myocardial infarction. His blood pressure is 145/98. Three years ago you had placed him on hydrochlorothiazide for his essential hypertension. Which medication class might you add first to improve his symptoms and decrease his blood pressure?

    (A) beta-blockers
    (B) calcium channel blockers
    (C) ace inhibitors
    (D) additional diuretics

64. A 50-year-old stockbroker called 911 when he develops severe substernal chest pain. In the ambulance he is given three sublingual nitroglycerin tablets, which improves his pain but does not alleviate it completely. His blood pressure is stable and he is noted to have STT elevations on his ECG. When he arrives to the ED, which medication will you begin while you are evaluating this patient?

    (A) oral angiotension II blocking agents
    (B) IV calcium channel blockers
    (C) nitroprusside drip
    (D) nitroglycerin drip

65. Which of the following medications is the most potent chronotrope?

    (A) isoproternol
    (B) dobutamine
    (C) epinephrine
    (D) norepinephrine

66. A 74-year-old male with benign prostatic hypertrophy has been sent to your cardiology group for management of his essential hypertension. Which class of medication, given his history, might you utilize in this individual?

    (A) beta-blockers
    (B) alpha-blockers
    (C) ACE inhibitors
    (D) angiotension II receptor blockers

67. Which medication must be avoided by patients with angina pectoris?

    (A) atenolol
    (B) lisinopril
    (C) sumatriptan
    (D) atorvastatin

68. Which medication should be used to control the ventricular rate during rapid atrial fibrillation?

    (A) beta-blockers
    (B) digoxin
    (C) warfarin
    (D) nitroglycerin

69. Amiodarone (Cordarone) may cause all of the side effects below except

    (A) thyroid abnormalities
    (B) photosynthesitivity
    (C) liver abnormalities
    (D) kidney failure

70. What is the prophylactic drug of choice used prior to a dental procedure for patients who have mitral valve prolapse with mitral regurgitation?

    (A) amoxicillin 2 g
    (B) erythromycin 1 g
    (C) clindamycin 600 mg
    (D) cephalexin 2 g

71. An example of a class Ic antiarrhythmic medication is

    (A) lidocaine
    (B) procainamide
    (C) amiodarone
    (D) flecainide

72. The Adult Treatment Panel III guidelines recommend screening initially for hyperlipidemia at what age?

    (A) 20 years
    (B) 35 years
    (C) 50 years
    (D) 65 years

73. Risk reduction for cardiovascular events can be achieved by the use of

 (A) antioxidant vitamins
 (B) statins for less than 6 months
 (C) cholesterol absorption inhibitors
 (D) ACE inhibitors

74. Patients who are known to be diabetic are at an increased risk of developing diabetic dyslipidemia and cardiovascular disease. Which of the following would least likely be recommended to your female patient with diabetes who is 60 years old?

 (A) strict control of blood glucose levels
 (B) utilize HMG-CoA reductase inhibitor therapy
 (C) begin estrogen/progestin combination therapy
 (D) utilize ACE inhibitors to control her hypertension

75. Patients are identified as having metabolic syndrome when they have all but one of the following risk factors?

 (A) blood pressure greater than 130/85
 (B) fasting blood sugar greater than 125 mg/dL
 (C) triglyceride level of greater than 150 mg/dL
 (D) waist circumference of greater than 35 inches in women and 40 inches in men

76. You have been asked to counsel your patient with a history of severe congestive heart failure in how to avoid the precipitating causes of this disease. What would you tell her about her sodium intake?

 (A) ask her to maintain a 1-g sodium diet
 (B) ask her to maintain a 2-g sodium diet
 (C) ask her to maintain a 4-g sodium diet
 (D) She does not need to worry about her sodium intake.

77. Secondary prevention of a ST elevation myocardial infarction should include all but which of the following measures

 (A) beta-blockade
 (B) ACE inhibition
 (C) calcium channel blockers
 (D) aspirin

78. A patient arrives in the ED with ST elevation in leads II, III, and AVF. The patient is hemodynamically stable. What measure should you use to limit the size of infarction in this patient?

 (A) non-steroidal anti-inflammatory medication
 (B) glucocorticoids
 (C) calcium channel blockers
 (D) fibrinolytic agents

79. Which of the following measurements change in patients with a dilated cardiomyopathy?

 (A) mean arterial pressure
 (B) pulse pressure
 (C) cardiac output
 (D) wall tension

80. An increase in which factor is most likely to increase the preload?

 (A) arterial vascular tone
 (B) stroke volume
 (C) heart rate
 (D) intravascular volume

81. During the first half of pregnancy the cardiac output increases. Which of the following factors is responsible for this change?

 (A) increases in blood volume
 (B) increases in mean arterial pressure
 (C) increases in systemic vascular resistance
 (D) decrease in heart rate

82. In order to maintain cardiac output in a patient with heart failure, neurohumoral mechanisms must be activated. Which of the following events begins this cascade?

(A) increased norepinephrine release

(B) increased afterload

(C) increased sodium retention

(D) increased atrial natriuretic peptide

83. Cardiac tamponade is potentially life threatening. What is the mechanism by which the effusion impedes stroke volume?

(A) direct compression increases end diastolic volume

(B) increased pressure in pericardium decreases coronary blood flow

(C) increased pressure decreases sinus rhythm

(D) compression of inferior vena cava decreases preload

84. Diastolic dysfunction is characterized by

(A) increased systemic vascular resistance

(B) decreased ventricular compliance

(C) decreased stroke volume

(D) decreased afterload

85. Patients with atrial fibrillation may not tolerate this rhythm well due to the loss of the synchronized atrial contraction. The explanation for this is

(A) the period of diastolic filling of the atrium is shortened

(B) the contribution of atrial contraction to left ventricular filling is 40% at rest

(C) the venous return to the heart increases

(D) the contribution of atrial contraction to ventricular filling is lost

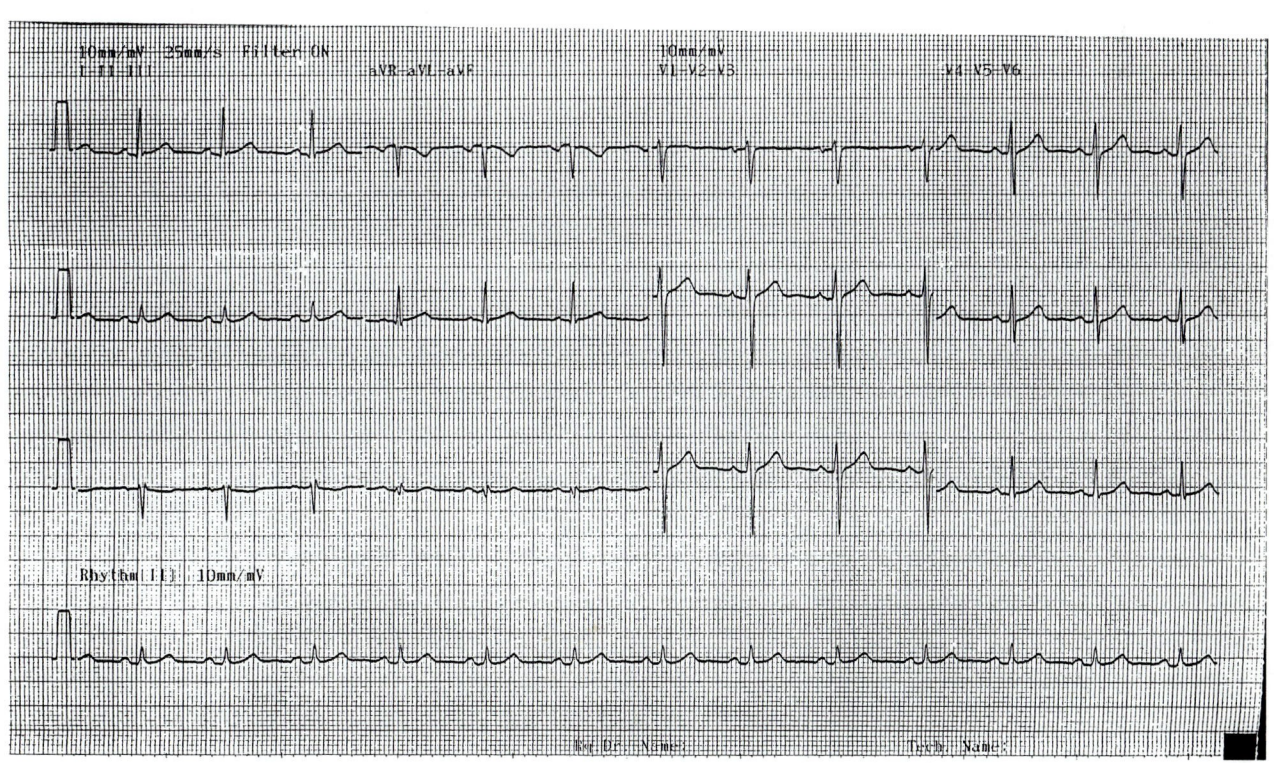

Fig. 2–1. ECG A.

86. The fall in right atrial pressure during inspiration is associated with

   (A) an increase in right atrial and ventricular preloads
   (B) a decrease in right atrial and ventricular preloads
   (C) no change in the right atrial and ventricular preloads
   (D) an initial decrease in the pressures with a rebound

87. Arterial baroreceptors are found in all of the following locations except

   (A) right and left atria
   (B) aortic arch
   (C) pulmonary veins
   (D) external jugular vein

88. Which tissue type has the lowest conduction speed in the myocardium?

   (A) SA node
   (B) Bundle of His
   (C) Purkinje system
   (D) ventricular muscle

89. A 44-year old female with a history of diabetes presents to the emergency department complaining of "indigestion." She has an ECG in the triage area. What is your diagnosis? (Refer to Fig. 2–1.)

   (A) normal sinus rhythm
   (B) atrial fibrillation
   (C) tachycardia
   (D) nodal rhythm

90. A 35-year old male comes to the ED complaining of palpitations. What is the abnormality noted in this ECG?

   (Refer to Fig. 2–2.)

   (A) bradycardia
   (B) premature ventricular contractions
   (C) bundle branch block
   (D) atrial fibrillation

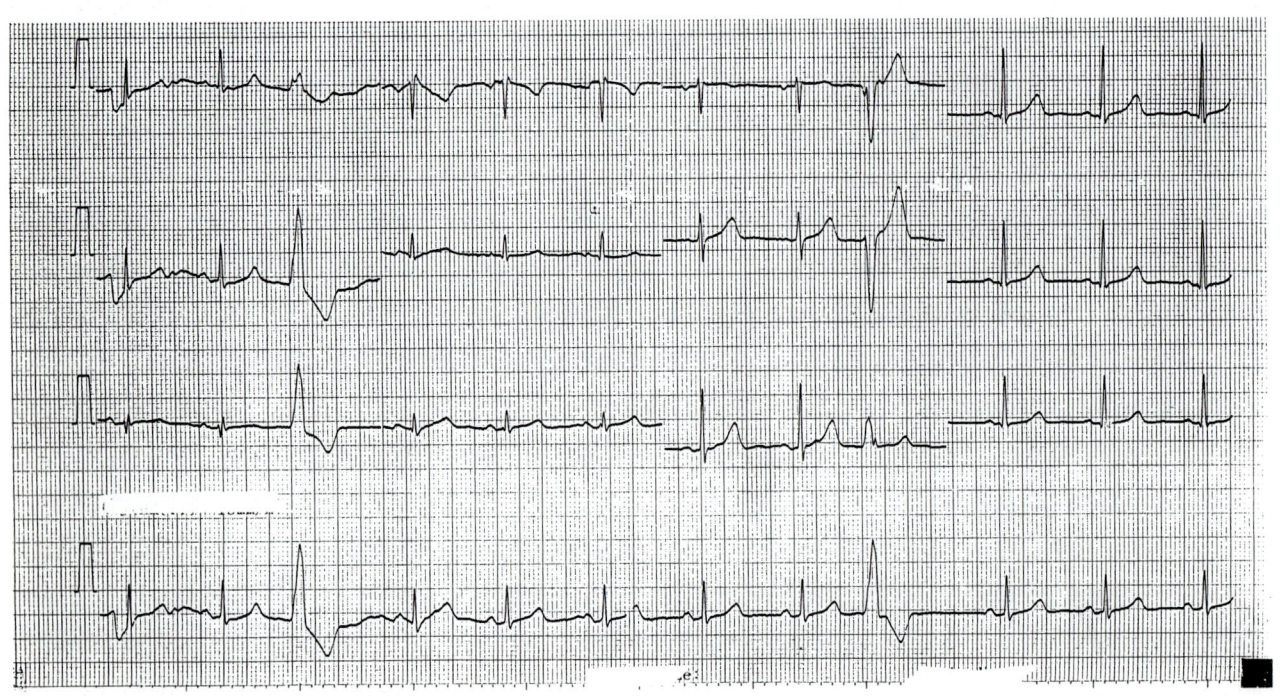

Fig. 2–2. ECG C.

Answers and Explanations

1. **(C)** The American College of Cardiology recommendations for permanent pacing include symptomatic third degree heart block. First degree AV block is not an indication for a pacemaker. Mobitz Type I heart block generally does not progress to complete heart block, so it is unlikely to require permanent pacing. Heart rates of greater than 120 may require pacing if they are associated with sustained pause-dependent ventricular tachycardia or if pharmacological therapy is ineffective. (*Kasper et al, 2005, pp. 1337, 1340*)

2. **(B)** These devices have been known to discharge in the absence of ventricular tachycardia or other sustained arrhythmias. The newer devises tend to have a pause built in to avoid discharge. Pacemaker syndrome is defined as fatigue, dizziness, syncope, and pulsations in the neck. This condition may be associated with hemodynamic instability as well. Pericarditis is not a complication seen in patients with pacemakers or ICDs. Bronchospasm is a side effect of sotalol, which is a therapy for ventricular arrhythmias. (*Kasper et al, 2005, pp. 1341, 1357*)

3. **(A)** Coronary artery perforation is extremely rare in patients undergoing balloon angioplasty without instrumentation. The rate of this complication in patients who have had extensive atherectomy is one percent. When this complication occurs, the patient may develop a hemopericardium, which will require pericardiocentesis. (*Kasper et al, 2005, p. 1462*)

4. **(C)** According to the Duke database, patients would benefit more from CABG if they have proximal LAD lesions, triple vessel disease, or double vessel disease with diabetes. (*Kasper et al, 2005, p. 1443*)

5. **(A)** Patients who are under the age of 65 years are generally good candidates for a mechanical valve replacement. Bioprostheses deteriorate over time so that while anticoagulation is not required with this type of prosthesis the revision of these prostheses is very high over time. Nearly half of all replacements will need to be revised within 15 years. Patients who are older than 65 should be screened to determine what their life span may be, and whether the inherent risk of anticoagulation is worth the benefit of a longer prosthetic reliability. (*Kasper et al, 2005, p. 1402*)

6. **(C)** Evidence suggests that aspirin in a patient with acute ischemia is beneficial. There is no need to get further tests to confirm this patient's condition until they get to the hospital. Time delay should be minimized. Verapamil in acute ischemia is not indicated. (*Kasper et al, 2005, pp. 1438–1441, 1453*)

7. **(D)** Active internal bleeding precludes the use of thrombolytic medications due to the risks associated with hemorrhagic shock. Patients with severe sustained hypertension (greater than systolic of 180 or diastolic of greater than 110) should not be given thrombolytic medications. Patients who are elderly

may be at a higher risk for hemorrhagic complications, but to date, the evidence suggests that the benefits for thrombolysis generally outweigh the risks. Patients who have active peptic ulcer disease are at a relative risk for complications with this class of medications but the risk: benefit ratio must be discussed. (*Kasper et al, 2005, pp. 1453–1454*)

8. **(C)** The INR range recommended for patients with a mechanical valve replacement is 2.5 to 3.5. Prophylaxis of thrombotic events may require an INR of less than 2.0. Generally, patients who require anticoagulation for other reasons are monitored to maintain an INR of 2.0 to 3.0. Patients with an INR greater than 3.0 are at a high risk of developing warfarin-associated bleeding. (*Kasper et al, 2005, p. 690; Way and Doherty 2003, p. 429*)

9. **(A)** An aneurysm that is 5.5 cm in size requires surgical intervention. Patients who have an aneurysm between 4 and 5 cm require surgical intervention but only if their co-morbidities are low. (*Kasper et al, 2005, p. 1483*)

10. **(D)** A patient with a history of sustained ventricular tachycardia has an improved survival with coronary revascularization. The mortality rates of CABG are less than 1% overall. Factors that increase the morbidity and mortality of the procedure include those listed above as well as a surgeon's lack of operative experience. (*Kasper et al, 2005, p. 1443*)

11. **(A)** Streptokinase should not be given to patients who have received it before since they may acquire streptococcal antibody levels sufficient to neutralize its activity. The other medications listed are not associated with this outcome. (*Kasper et al, 2005, p. 690*)

12. **(B)** Pentoxifylline is the only medication that has been shown to improve the exercise tolerance in patients with PVD, by decreasing blood viscosity and increasing the red blood cell flexibility. Papaverine, calcium channel blockers and alpha-adrenergic blockers, while known for the vasodilatory effects, have been shown to be ineffective in improving tissue oxygenation in patients with PVD. (*Kasper et al, 2005, pp. 1486–1487*)

13. **(B)** Ascending aorta dissections are associated with an extremely high mortality rate. Emergent surgical correction is required. Even with surgical intervention in the hospital mortality rate is up to 25%. Patients with descending aortic dissections (Type B) and hemodynamically stable may be treated with conservative therapy and should be followed every 6 months with serial CT scans. Additionally, both patients with Type A and Type B dissections benefit from intravenous beta blockade as well as intravenous nitroprusside. (*Way and Doherty, 2003, pp. 432–433*)

14. **(D)** Patients with no previous history and a diastolic pressure of 100 mm Hg should be treated with diuretics. If there is evidence of previous history of hypertension or evidence of end-organ damage, treatment should begin at lower diastolic levels. (*Leveno et al, 2002, p. 356*)

15. **(B)** Patients with all of these conditions may be diaphoretic and complaining of dyspnea. Hypotension in acute coronary syndrome occurs when the right coronary artery is affected. Acute coronary syndromes do not usually present with systolic murmurs and the ECG changes include ST segment changes. Patients who have severe heart failure will have similar symptoms but also have pulsus alternans and pulmonary rales. Finally, patients with pulmonary embolus may have hemodynamic changes but usually have a low PaO_2 and a normal $PaCO_2$. ECG may show right axis deviation in a pulmonary embolus as well. (*Kasper et al, 2005, pp. 1370–1371, 1377–1378*)

16. **(C)** This patient likely has renovascular disease, which is responsible for her secondary hypertension. Patients with renovascular stenosis have decreased blood flow to one kidney. This ischemic state initiates renin release, which increases the vascular tone in the remaining normal renal artery. Essential hypertension usually responds to medication and is more likely to be diagnosed in a patient who is

older. Secondary hypertension is associated with pheochromocytoma, but these patients generally have headaches, palpitations, anxiety attacks, and hyperglycemia as well. Pheochromocytomas are not associated with an abdominal bruit. Isolated systolic hypertension is defined as a systolic pressure greater than 140 mm Hg but a diastolic blood pressure of less than 90 mm Hg. (*Kasper et al, 2005, pp. 1467–1470; Way and Doherty, 2003, p. 802*)

17. **(A)** Patients who complain of occipital headaches that are relieved by mid-day are experiencing severe essential hypertension unless there is a secondary cause identified. Secondary hypertension related to primary aldosteronism is also associated with polyuria, polydipsia, and muscle weakness. Patients who are hypertensive as a result of Cushing's disease complain of weight gain and emotional lability. Patients with accelerated hypertension are noted to have high pressures with evidence of vascular damage on fundoscopic evaluation. (*Kasper et al, 2005, pp. 1468–1469*)

18. **(D)** Tricuspid regurgitation is associated with a holosystolic soft murmur heard best at left sternal border. Aortic stenosis is associated with a paradoxical split of S2, a murmur that is loudest mid systole and is heard best at the base of the heart. Severe disease also is associated with a murmur, which can be heard near the carotid arteries. The murmur of mitral regurgitation is heard best at the apex and radiates to the axilla. The Valsalva maneuver reduces it. Mitral stenosis is associated with an opening snap, which is followed by a low-pitched rumbling murmur in diastole. (*Kasper et al, 2005, pp. 1391–1411*)

19. **(C)** Varicose veins develop when individuals spend a prolonged amount of time on their feet. Lymphedema is a condition also associated with calf heaviness and edema but the symptoms do not resolve spontaneously. Deep venous thrombosis edema is usually unilateral, may be associated with calf tenderness or a palpable cord, and does not resolve on its own. Intermittent claudication is not associated with peripheral edema generally and

while the pain is resolved with rest, walking exacerbates the pain. (*Kasper et al, 2005, pp. 1491–1494*)

20. **(D)** Malignant melanoma is the most common tumor responsible for metastasis to the heart. Lymphomas, prostate cancer, and leukemias also metastasize to the heart but less frequently than melanoma. Patients present with dyspnea, pericarditis, and tamponade symptoms and/or tachyarrhythmias. (*Kasper et al, 2005, p. 1422*)

21. **(B)** Pain relieved with rest, that occurs in the buttock and thigh with exercise, is likely Leriche syndrome. Spinal stenosis pain is often relieved improved with ambulation or moving in to a different position. Patients with myalgias generally complain of associated symptoms such as muscle spasm. Patients with popliteal disease complain of intermittent claudication of their calf rather than of their thigh. (*Kasper et al, 2005, pp. 138, 1486*)

22. **(C)** Anterior infarctions are characterized by ST elevation in I, AVL, and chest leads. Inferior wall myocardial infarction is consistent with elevations in II, III, and AVF. Lateral wall and posterior infarctions have a loss of depolarization, which may be noted simply by increases in the R-wave amplitude in V1 and V2. (*Kasper et al, 2005, p. 1317*)

23. **(A)** Patients with chronic venous insufficiency note occasional pain with prolonged standing, edema, hyperpigmentation, dermatitis, and erythema. Patients with arterial insufficiency complain of claudication and they are found to have decreased pulses, distal hair loss, thick nails, and pallor. Patients with diabetes that is well controlled may have no symptoms in the lower extremities. Peripheral neuropathies are not associated with pigmentation changes or edema although ulcers may develop if the patient has lost their proprioception. (*Kasper et al, 2005, pp. 1486, 1493*)

24. **(B)** Thromboangiitis obliterans or Buergers disease is an inflammatory disease affecting the small and medium arteries of the distal

extremities. It is seen most commonly in Asian males under the age of 40 years. Little is known about the etiology although one of the risk factors appears to be smoking. Venous insufficiency is most commonly seen in the lower extremities and while associated with ulcers, there are other exam findings noted. Raynaud's phenomenon is most commonly seen in women between the age of 20 and 40 years, who complain of severe pain in one or two digits usually of the hand. Acute arterial thrombosis is not a chronic condition, and so the presentation will be different for acute arterial occlusion. (*Kasper et al, 2005, pp. 1488–1492*)

25. **(D)** Prinzmetal's angina occurs in younger patients at rest, with no preceding angina. It is associated with ECG changes and is thought to be related to transient coronary vasospasm rather than atherosclerosis. A squeezing chest pressure that is crescendo-decrescendo in nature, which lasts from 2 to 5 minutes, characterizes stable angina. It is often exacerbated with exertion. Unstable angina is angina noted in an individual with coronary artery disease who notes severe, new onset pain at rest lasting greater than 10 minutes that is crescendo in character. It may be associated with ECG changes as well. Acute coronary syndrome is usually seen in older patients who have a history of anginal symptoms. (*Kasper et al, 2005, p. 1448*)

26. **(A)** Atrial myxoma is the most common primary cardiac tumor overall. Rhabdomyomas and fibromas are the most common tumor in infants and children. Hemangiomas are small intracardiac tumors that generally affect the AV conduction and may cause sudden death. (*Kasper et al, 2005, p. 1421*)

27. **(D)** Pericarditis occurs in about two-thirds of patients with lupus. It generally follows a benign course. Patients with lupus also may develop valvular endocardial lesions. It is less common for patients to develop acute coronary syndrome, dissection or congestive heart failure although these complications are seen in patients with anti-phospholipid syndromes. (*Kasper et al, 2005, p. 1424*)

28. **(B)** Patients with hypothyroidism will complain of fatigue, dyspnea when pleural effusions are present, and deny changes in their weight. The bradycardia and prolonged QT interval also should help distinguish this condition from others. Diabetes patients often have ST changes and evidence of silent ischemia on their ECG. Sinus bradycardia does not usually occur in these patients. Both pheochromocytoma and hyperthyroidism are associated with tachycardia. (*Kasper et al, 2005, pp. 1422–1424*)

29. **(B)** Peaked T waves are the first electrocardiographic changes seen in hyperkalemia. Late changes associated with higher morbidities and mortalities and potassium levels higher than 7.0 meg/L include prolonged PR interval and QRS duration, atrioventricular conduction delays and loss of the P wave. Prominent U waves are associated with hypokalemia and anti-arrythmic medication toxicity. (*Kasper et al, 2005, pp. 262, 1314*)

30. **(A)** The most common location of an aortic aneurysm is the distal aorta. Aneurysms in other locations are less common. (*Way and Doherty, 2003, p. 829*)

31. **(B)** The diagnosis of mild to moderate congestive heart failure is made using the clinical signs and symptoms and an echocardiogram to determine the underlying etiology of the heart failure. An arterial blood gas in this patient may show a slight decrease in her PaO_2; however, since she is not in acute distress and her pulse oximetry on room air is 92%, this test is not critically important at this time. Dobutamine stress tests are used to assess the myocardial perfusion and function. CBC and troponin levels may help elucidate the related causes of congestive heart failure but an echocardiogram is needed to document the severity of the systolic or diastolic dysfunction. (*Kasper et al, 2005, pp. 1370, 1436*)

32. **(B)** Electrophysiology studies are used to evaluate the excitability of the myocardium and to reproduce the ventricular tachycardia. Repeating the ECG in the face of documented ventricular tachycardia on Holter monitor and

evidence of multifocal PVCs in unnecessary. Dobutamine stress tests are used to access the myocardial perfusion and function. Transesophageal echocardiography is used most commonly to evaluate the aorta for evidence of dissection, to elucidate evidence of atrial clots and to assess for evidence of valvular vegetations. (*Kasper et al, 2005, pp. 1322, 1350–1352, 1436*)

33. **(A)** Prominent U waves are noted on ECG when there are ventricular repolarization abnormalities, which are associated with hypokalemia or anti-arrhythmic medications. Very prominent U waves are related to the development of torsades de pointes. Hypocalcemia prolongs the QT interval. Build up of procainamide metabolite N-acetylprocainamide (NAPA) is associated with QT interval prolongation. Hypothermia is associated with J-point elevation. (*Kasper et al, 2005, pp. 17, 1314, 1318*)

34. **(C)** Troponin levels are useful in the diagnosis of acute coronary syndrome because this amino acid does not exist in skeletal muscle. Troponins have a high sensitivity and specificity for acute coronary syndromes. The enzyme levels rise after 6 hours and peak at 12 hours. Abnormalities in arterial blood gases exist for many reasons but are not sensitive or specific to acute coronary syndromes. CPK enzymes vary in their specificity due to the distribution of these enzymes in other parts of the body. CPK release can occur from the myocardium as well as skeletal muscle. AST and ALT may be elevated but these are not specific markers for acute coronary syndrome. (*Tintinalli et al, 2004, p. 338; Kasper et al, 2005, p. 1450*)

35. **(C)** This troponin level is considered normal. If one suspects the individual is suffering from acute coronary syndrome, serial samples must be obtained to confirm the diagnosis. Additional testing of a normal level is required to evaluate the potential serum markers of ischemia longitudinally. A normal troponin level does not aid in making the diagnosis of angina. (*Tintinalli et al, 2004, p. 338*)

36. **(B)** This patient is suffering from pericarditis. Pericarditis is diagnosed using the Doppler echocardiography. Holter monitor should be used to aid in the diagnosis of arrhythmias and to work up syncope. Cardiac catheterization is generally used to evaluate individual coronary arteries and cardiac function. Electrocardiographic stress tests are used to screen for coronary artery disease in an ambulatory patient who is complaining of chest discomfort. (*Kasper et al, 2005, p. 1419*)

37. **(C)** The ECG changes in myocarditis specifically associated with Chagas' disease, present with right bundle branch block and left hemiblock. Acute coronary syndrome is associated with ECG changes that most commonly include ST elevation or depression and Q waves. Hypotension is not associated with ECG changes by itself. Endocarditis is generally diagnosed using echocardiography and blood cultures. (*Kasper et al, 2005, pp. 735, 1413, 1444*)

38. **(D)** The most likely diagnosis in this patient is infective endocarditis. Evaluation of the blood flow and the functional status of the myocardium can be evaluated with either transthoracic or transesophageal echocardiogram. However, vegetations can be detected with more sensitivity and specificity using the transesophageal echocardiogram. Holter monitors and cardiac catheterization do not detect valvular lesions or vegetations. (*Kasper et al, 2005, pp. 734–735*)

39. **(A)** Widened mediastinum is associated with aortic dissection. Pneumothorax and consolidation are not seen with this condition. Pleural effusion may occur with a dissection but it is usually an effusion on the left side. (*Kasper et al, 2005, p. 1484*)

40. **(A)** Right ventricular hypertrophy is associated with tetralogy of Fallot. This condition is characterized by a malaligned ventricular septal defect and obstruction of the right ventricle outflow tract. Right axis deviation with an rSr' pattern is associated with an ostium secundum defect. Left ventricular hypertrophy is associated with coarctation of the aorta. Atrial fibrillation is associated with Epstein's anomaly and atrial septal defects. (*Kasper et al, 2005, pp. 1385–1389*)

41. **(A)** The most common cause of myocarditis is the Coxsackie B virus. The most common bacterial agent related to myocarditis is diphtheria, not *Staphylococcus aureus*. Diphtheria is a very rare cause of myocarditis. Both HIV and Borrelia infection can cause myocarditis but these infections are less common than the Coxsackie virus. (*Kasper et al, 2005, p. 1413*)

42. **(B)** Mitral valve prolapse is characterized by midsystolic click and a late systolic murmur. The murmur associated with aortic stenosis is a midsystolic murmur also known as a systolic ejection murmur. Aortic regurgitation is characterized by a high-pitched decrescendo murmur in early diastole. Mitral valve stenosis is associated with a low-pitched mid-diastolic murmur. (*Kasper et al, 2005, pp. 1309–1310*)

43. **(B)** Patent ductus arteriosus is the known cause of a murmur continuous murmur, unless the patient has pulmonary hypertension. Patients with atrial myxoma may have a mid-diastolic or presystolic murmur. Mitral and aortic regurgitation are associated with either systolic or diastolic murmurs. (*Kasper et al, 2005, pp. 1310–1311*)

44. **(A)** Pheochromocytoma is associated with a sudden onset of hypertension, tachycardia, and other findings consistent with catecholamine stimulation. Autonomic epilepsy may present in the same way but patients generally complain of an aura. This patient is not complaining of chest pain and so it is unlikely that the patient has either ACS or dissection. (*Kasper et al, 2005, p. 2150*)

45. **(B)** Congenital aortic stenosis is an acyanotic congenital heart disease without a shunt. Malformations that cause obstruction to left ventricular outflow include congenital valvular aortic stenosis, subaortic stenosis, supravalvular aortic stenosis, and hypertrophic obstructive cardiomyopathy. (*Kasper et al, 2005, p. 138*)

46. **(A)** Complete transposition of the great arteries is a cyanotic congenital heart disease with increased pulmonary blood flow. The aorta arises from the right ventricle to the right of and anterior to the pulmonary artery, which emerges from the left ventricle. This causes two parallel and separate circulations and some communication must exist between them after birth if life is to be sustained. Most patients have an inter-atrial communication, two-thirds have a patent ductus arteriosus, and about one-third have an associated ventricular septal defect. This defect accounts for 10% of cyanotic heart disease. (*Kasper et al, 2005, p. 1388*)

47. **(A)** Tetralogy of Fallot is a cyanotic congenital heart disease with decreased pulmonary blood flow. The resistance of blood flow from the ventricles into the aorta and into the pulmonary vessels plays a major role in determining the hemodynamic and clinical picture. The severity of obstruction to right ventricular outflow is of fundamental significance. With severe obstruction, the pulmonary blood flow is reduced markedly, and a large volume of desaturated systemic venous blood is shunted from right to left across the ventricular septal defect. Severe cyanosis and erythrocytosis occur. Symptoms and effects of systemic hypoxemia are prominent. (*Kasper et al, 2005, p. 1389*).

48. **(B)** Atrial septal defects are an example of acyanotic congenital heart disease with a left-to-right shunt. The amount of left-to-right shunt through an atrial septal defect depends on the defect size, the diastolic properties of both ventricles, and the relative impedance in the pulmonary and systemic circulations. The shunt causes diastolic overload of the right ventricle and increased pulmonary blood flow. (*Kasper et al, 2005, p. 1385*)

49. **(B)** Women are two to three times more likely to develop varicosities of their lower extremities. Patients who develop secondary varicosities may have a history of deep venous insufficiency. Patients with lymphedema generally have a different physical presentation, which is inconsistent with varicose veins. Lymphedema does not increase one's risk of developing varicosities. (*Kasper et al, 2005, p. 1493*)

50. **(D)** Physiologic splitting of the second heart sounds occur in inspiration as the aortic and pulmonic valves close at different times. Fixed splitting of the S2 heart sound is heard in

patients with atrial septal defects. Patients with pulmonary embolus and pulmonary valve stenosis have split that is prolonged and is noted in expiration. Patients with increased pulmonary vascular resistance have a narrowing of the second heart sound split. (*Kasper et al, 2005, p. 1307*)

51. **(D)** The differential diagnosis includes acute coronary syndrome. However, if the patient is hypertensive, a tobacco user, and complains of a severe pain that radiates to the back, the patient most likely is experiencing an aortic dissection. Mild mitral stenosis may be asymptomatic but moderate stenosis is associated with dyspnea on exertion and cough. Cardiogenic shock is characterized by hypotension and chest pain. (*Kasper et al, 2005, pp. 1390, 1612–1614*)

52. **(B)** Congestive heart failure is associated with fatigue, dyspnea, and sudden weight gain. Myocardial infarction may be a precipitating case for her congestive heart failure but would generally present in a manner suggestive of ischemia. Sinus tachycardia is unlikely since this patient has had long-standing atrial fibrillation. Cardiac tamponade is a possibility; however, generally while there is fatigue and dyspnea, patients with this condition do not experience such a sudden change in their weight. (*Kasper et al, 2005, p. 1301*)

53. **(D)** Ventricular tachycardia is associated with bursts of tachycardia and pre-syncope. Patients who are taking diuretics that are not potassium sparing may develop hypokalemia as a result of the medication. This deficit predisposes patients to ventricular arrhythmias. Atrial fibrillation is generally characterized by a sustained irregular rhythm. Sinus bradycardia is a slow regular rhythm and is associated with abrupt syncopal episodes rather than pre-syncope. Sick sinus syndrome is associated with heart rates that are slow, normal, fast and are associated with sinus pauses. (*Kasper et al, 2005, pp. 81, 128*)

54. **(B)** This patient is experiencing palpitations. She does not have atrial fibrillation or sinus bradycardia because her symptoms are transient. Atrial fibrillation is characterized by sustained irregular rhythm. Sinus bradycardia is characterized by a slow, often regular rhythm, while ventricular tachycardia is characterized by sustained bursts of rapid heart rate. Ventricular tachycardia usually presents with pre-syncopal symptoms. (*Kasper et al, 2005, p. 81*)

55. **(D)** The pain associated with arterial occlusion occurs as a sudden onset of severe pain and associated paresthesias. Arterial insufficiency is characterized by intermittent claudication, pain at rest, and it generally has a gradual onset. Venous insufficiency presents with edema that is relieved with leg elevation. Venous stasis ulcers are large, painless ulcerations. Patients with Raynaud's syndrome complain of pallor, rubor, limb coldness, and paresthesias and pain. The cycles of vasoconstrictions responsible for these symptoms are often triggered by exposure to stress or cold environments. (*Way and Doherty, 2003, pp. 815, 825, 843, 883*)

56. **(C)** Ulcerations associated with venous stasis disease are painless, while ulcerations associated with peripheral arterial insufficiency are painful. With severe arterial disease, thickened nails, hair loss, pallor with elevation of the extremity, and dependent rubor are common findings. The skin changes with venous disease may include erythema and hyperpigmentation. (*Way and Doherty, 2003, pp. 818, 883*)

57. **(D)** Hypertrophic cardiomyopathy is defined as a somewhat disorganized pattern of hypertrophy in a non-dilated chamber, with no obvious etiologic cause. Patients with a history of hypertension or aortic stenosis have secondary hypertrophic cardiomyopathy. Patients who have had high dose radiation to the mediastinum may develop pericarditis. (*Kasper et al, 2005, pp. 1410, 1414*)

58. **(D)** Orthostatic hypotension, which may occur for many reasons, is related to autonomic nervous system abnormalities or intravascular volume deficits. Orthostasis is defined as a drop in the systolic pressure of greater than 20 mm Hg or a drop in the diastolic pressure of greater than 10 mm Hg. When the drop in pressure is related to neurogenic causes, the compensatory change in the pulse rate is not seen. (*Kasper et al, 2005, p. 2430*)

59. (B) Often innocent pericardial effusions are noted after bypass surgery. However, unless there is profound bleeding and inadequate drainage capacity of the chest tube, it is unlikely to cause tamponade. The three remaining etiologies are the most common causes. (*Kasper et al, 2005, p. 1416*)

60. (D) The treatment of congestive heart failure includes preventive measures, control of excess fluid, and enhancement of myocardial contractility. Diuretics should be used to decrease the fluid overload. ACE inhibitors, beta-blockers, and sympathomimetic agents are important adjuncts to emergent treatment. Calcium channel blockers have no role in the treatment of congestive heart failure. (*Kasper et al, 2005, pp. 1373–1375*)

61. (B) Amiodarone increases the serum levels of digoxin, so one must decrease the dose of digoxin to avoid toxicity in this instance. This effect is also seen with the addition of quinidine and verapamil. (*Kasper et al, 2005, p. 1375*)

62. (A) At low doses, dopamine dilates the renal and mesenteric blood vessels. This dose is also known as "renal dose dopamine." This dose can be used to facilitate diuresis in heart failure. (*Kasper et al, 2005, p. 1375*)

63. (A) For a patient who has underlying cardiac disease, beta-blockers have been shown to decrease morbidity and mortality in patients with hypertension. If the patient's hypertension remains recalcitrant, ACE inhibitors may help if the patient has left ventricular dysfunction. Calcium channel blockers and additional diuretics have not been shown to improve the survival of patients who are hypertensive and have known cardiac disease. (*Kasper et al, 2005, p. 1479*)

64. (D) Nitroglycerin is indicated in this patient. It will both improve the myocardial oxygen availability but its vasodilatory effects and the myocardial oxygen demand. Medications by mouth are not indicated at this time. Nitroprusside will decrease the systemic vascular resistance and decrease the blood pressure. It is not indicated in this acute stage because of its potent hypotensive effects. Calcium channel blockers do not have a role in the therapy of an acute myocardial infarction. (*Kasper et al, 2005, p. 1452*)

65. (A) Isoproternol has the most significant increase in heart rate due to its beta-1 and beta-2 activities. Dobutamine may increase the heart rate slightly but has less of a chronotropic effect. Epinephrine increases the heart rate more than both dobutamine and norepinephrine but less than isoproterenol. (*Tintinalli et al, 2004, pp. 210–214*)

66. (B) Alpha-blockers are effective as antihypertensive agents as are the other classes of medications listed. Alpha-1 blockers prevent urinary retention in patients with benign prostatic hypertrophy. (*Tintinalli et al, 2004, pp. 403–404*)

67. (C) Sumatriptan prescribed for migraine and cluster headaches must be avoided in patients with angina pectoris due to its stimulant properties and its ability to aggravate coronary insufficiency. Atenolol allows for beta-adrenergic blockade of receptors on vascular and cardiac muscle cells. This results in sympatholytic action, controlling heart rate, blood pressure, and cardiac contractility. Angiotensin-converting enzyme inhibitors are indicated if there is left ventricular dysfunction. Atorvastatin is an appropriate medication and may improve the control of hypercholesterolemia.

68. (A) Beta-blockers should be used to control the ventricular rate in rapid atrial fibrillation. While digoxin will slow the ventricular rate, it is no longer the drug of choice. Warfarin is used for anticoagulation and the prevention of clot formation that is a risk with the occurrence of atrial fibrillation. There is not a clear need for nitroglycerin at the time of this rhythm, but if there is associated ischemia, it may be appropriate and feasible to use nitroglycerin. (*Kasper et al, 2005, p. 1345*)

69. (D) Major side effects of amiodarone are photosensitivity, thyroid, CNS, and liver abnormalities. (*Kasper et al, 2005, pp. 303, 1842, 2119*)

70. **(A)** The drug of choice for oral endocarditis prophylaxis when MVP is present with associated mitral regurgitation is amoxicillin 2 gm po 1 hour prior to a dental procedure. If the patient is allergic to penicillin, then clindamycin 600 mg po 1 hour prior to dental procedures may be used. Prophylaxis is not necessary for mitral valve prolapse without mitral regurgitation. (*Kasper et al, 2005, p. 739*)

71. **(D)** Flecainide is a class Ic antiarrhythmic. Class Ic medications are indicated for life-threatening ventricular tachycardia or fibrillation. They may also be used in refractory supraventricular tachycardia. (*Kasper et al, 2005, p. 1346*)

72. **(A)** The Expert Panel on Detection, Evaluation and Treatment of High Blood Cholesterol recommends initial screening of all patients over the age of 20 years. It is then recommended that depending on the patient's risk factors, intervention may be required as well. (*Kasper et al, 2005, p. 1430*)

73. **(D)** The use of ACE inhibitors has been shown to reduce the risk of stroke and heart failure as well as coronary artery disease. While oxidation plays a role in the formation of foam cells, use of anti-oxidant vitamins have not been shown to reduce cardiovascular events. The use of statins will decrease cardiovascular events, however, not until they have been used for at least 6 months. The use of cholesterol absorption inhibitors has not yet been shown to be effective in reducing cardiovascular events. (*Kasper et al, 2005, p. 1431*)

74. **(C)** Microvascular complications of diabetes can be reduced by strict glucose controls. The VA HDL Intervention Trial demonstrated a decreased stroke and cardiovascular events occurred when gemfibrozil was given to patients. The Women's Health Initiative study concludes that there was no reduction in coronary events with the use of estrogen/progestin tablets. ACE inhibition has been shown to decrease coronary events in diabetics. (*Kasper et al, 2005, p. 1432*)

75. **(B)** Metabolic syndrome is characterized by all of the following except fasting blood sugar greater than 125 mg/dL. In order to rule out metabolic syndrome, the fasting blood sugar should be less than 110 mg/DL. (*Kasper et al, 2005, p. 1432*)

76. **(A)** For patients with a history of heart failure, sodium excess can have an adverse effect on the patient's fluid homeostasis. Patients should restrict their sodium intake to 1 gm. (*Kasper et al, 2005, p. 1368*)

77. **(C)** Calcium channel blockers have been shown to increase mortality in patients who have had a previous myocardial infarction. However, beta-blocker, ACE inhibitors and aspirin have been shown to improve the morbidity and mortality rates in patients who have had a myocardial infarction. (*Kasper et al, 2005, p. 1459*)

78. **(D)** Fibrinolytic agents should be initiated within 30 minutes of presentation if there are no contraindications. NSAIDS and glucocorticoids have not been helpful to reduce the size of infarction and are known to impair infarct healing. Calcium channel blockers are not indicated in the treatment of myocardial infarction. (*Kasper et al, 2005, pp. 1452–1453*)

79. **(D)** Laplace's law dictates that the transmural pressure is equal to the vessel wall tension divided by the vessel radius. When the radius of the myocardium is dilated, the heart must generate more wall tension in order to maintain the same systemic pressure. Initially, the mean arterial pressure will not change as the heart tries to compensate for the change in its radius. The pulse pressure, which is defined as the difference between the systolic and diastolic pressures, is not impacted initially. The cardiac output initially will be maintained when the dilated heart increases its wall tension. (*Ganong, 2005, pp. 586–590*)

80. **(D)** Preload is defined as the ventricular end-diastolic volume. Factors that increase the ventricular end-diastolic volume include an increase in the intravascular volume. Arterial vascular tone increases the blood pressure but does not affect the venous return to the heart directly. Increases in the stroke volume will

increase the cardiac output. The heart rate does not increase the ventricular end-diastolic volume. In fact, if the heart rate increases, it provides less time for ventricular filling so that it may decrease the ventricular end-diastolic volume. (*Kasper et al, 2005, pp. 1361–1363*)

81. **(A)** Women have up to a 50% increase in their blood volume during pregnancy. The mean arterial pressure in pregnant women generally stays the same or decreases. The cardiac output increases within the first months of pregnancy as a result a concomitant decrease in their systemic vascular resistance and an increase in their heart rate. (*Leveno et al, 2002, p. 20*)

82. **(A)** The compensation for the fall in cardiac output in patients with heart failure occurs with the release of norepinephrine. Norepinephrine will support the myocardial contractility but on a long term basis causes an increase in the afterload. When the cardiac output is no longer maintained, there is an activation of the renin–angiotensin system, which further increases the sodium retention and afterload. (*Kasper et al, 2005, pp. 1362–1364*)

83. **(D)** Compression caused by cardiac tamponade decreases the preload, which is an important component of stroke volume. Direct compression prevents inflow of blood to the heart muscle, which will decrease the end-diastolic volume. While tamponade does increase the pressure in the heart muscle itself, stroke volume is the amount of blood that is ejected with each contraction. The increased intracardiac pressure associated with tamponade effects the patient's cardiac output. Tamponade has no intrinsic effect on the heart rate. (*Kasper et al, 2005, pp. 1415–1416; Ganong, 2005, p. 571*)

84. **(B)** Diastolic dysfunction affects stroke volume by decreasing it. This is true of systolic dysfunction as well. The distinction between the two is that the increase in intrapericardial pressure and the increased stiffness of the ventricle decreases the end diastolic volumes. (*Ganong, 2005, p. 573*)

85. **(D)** The loss of atrial contraction in atrial fibrillation, decreases the ventricular filling. The volume gained by atrial systole is generally noted to be up to 20% of the overall end-diastolic volume. For patients with hypertrophy or other underlying cardiac disease, the loss of this additional volume may have a profound effect on their cardiac output. (*Kasper et al, 2005, p. 1363; Ganong, 2005, p. 573*)

86. **(A)** Inspiration makes the negative pressure in the intrathoracic cavity more negative. This increases the thoracic blood volume and increases venous return to the heart. Valsalva maneuvers, positive pressure ventilation, and excessive coughing increase the intrathoracic pressure that decreases venous return. (*Kasper et al, 2005, p. 1363*)

87. **(D)** Baroreceptors are stretch receptors found in the walls of the heart and blood vessels. They are also noted in the carotid sinus, the atria, and the pulmonary veins. (*Ganong, 2005, p. 605*)

88. **(C)** The purkinje system has a conduction rate of 4 m/s while the other types of cardiac tissue have between 0.05 and 1.0 m/s rates. The SA and AV nodes are known to have the fastest rates of conduction in the myocardium. (*Ganong, 2005, p. 549*)

89. **(A)** This patient has normal sinus rhythm. Atrial fibrillation is characterized by the absence of P waves. Tachycardia exists when the heart rate is greater than 100. Nodal rhythm is characterized by heart rates in the 40s. (*Ferry, 2001, pp. 65, 122–125*)

90. **(B)** Premature ventricular contractions are generally isolated widened QRS beats followed by a compensatory pause seen here. The patients heart rate is greater than 60, so there he does not have bradycardi (A). Bundle branch block is characterized by a wide QRS complex well visualized throughout most of the precordial leads. (*Ferry, 2001, pp. 46, 65, 185*)

REFERENCES

Kasper DL. Way, LW, Dohert, GM, Leveno, KJ, Tintinalli, JE, Ganong, WF, Ferry, DR, *Harrison's Principles of Internal Medicine*, 16th ed. New York: McGraw Hill; 2005.

Way and Doherty, *Current Surgical Diagnosis and Treatment*, 11th ed. New York: McGraw Hill; 2003.

Leveno et al, *Williams Manual of Obstetrics*, 21st ed. New York: McGraw Hill; 2002.

Tintinalli et al, *Emergency Medicine A Comprehensive Study Guide*, 6th ed. New York: McGraw Hill; 2004.

Ganong, *Review of Medical Physiology*, 22nd ed. New York: McGraw Hill; 2005.

Ferry, *Basic Electrocardiography in Ten Days*, 1st ed. New York: McGraw Hill; 2001.

CHAPTER 3

Dermatology
Questions

Michelle DiBaise, MPAS, PA-C

DIRECTIONS (Questions 1 through 36): Each of the numbered items or incomplete statements in this section is followed by answers or by completions of the statement. Select the ONE lettered answer or completion that is BEST in each case.

Questions 1 through 36

1. Erythema with scale-forming yellowish plaques on the eyebrows, nasolabial folds, glabella, and presternal area best describes (see Fig. 3–1)

   (A) bacterial folliculitis
   (B) allergic contact dermatitis
   (C) rosacea
   (D) seborrheic dermatitis

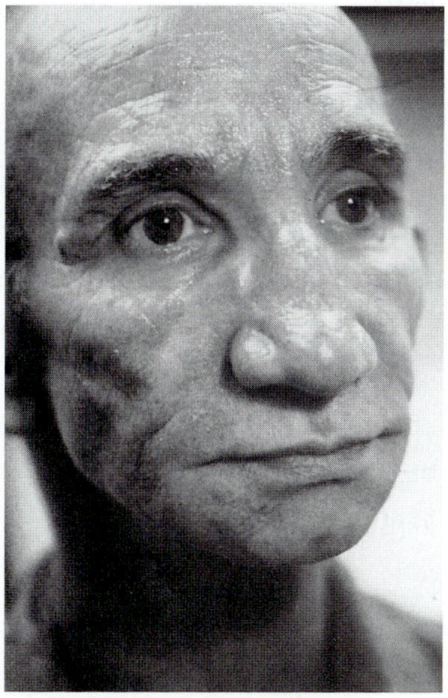

2. A 36-year-old patient reporting sudden hair loss is found to have a round, well-circumscribed 3-cm area of alopecia on the parietal scalp area with exclamation point hairs. The most likely diagnosis is

   (A) anagen effluvium
   (B) androgenetic alopecia
   (C) alopecia areata
   (D) tinea capitis

3. A Tzanck smear demonstrating multinucleated giant cells indicates which of the following conditions? (Fig. 3–2)

   (A) scabies
   (B) tinea versicolor
   (C) impetigo
   (D) herpes simplex

Fig. 3–1. Courtesy of Jack Cohen, D.O.

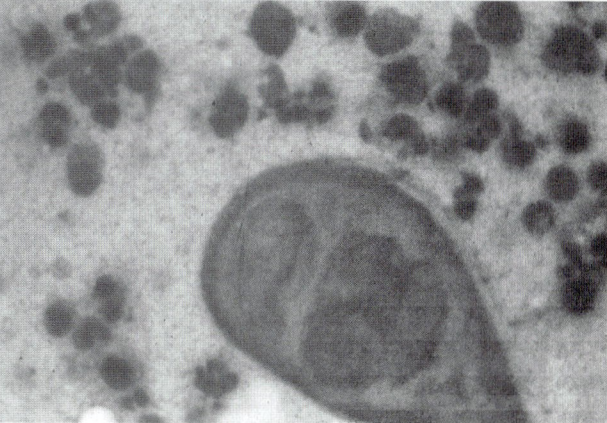

Fig. **3–2**. Positive Tzanck smear with arrow indicating giant multinucleated cell. (Photo courtesy of William H. Fenn.) From Rodney M (ed). Primary Care for Physician Assistants, 2nd ed. McGraw-Hill, Inc., 2001, with permission.

4. An acute eruption of violaceous, pruritic, polygonal, shiny, flat-topped papules involving the flexor surfaces is suggestive of which of the following?

   (A) lichen planus
   (B) pityriasis rosea
   (C) psoriasis
   (D) seborrheic dermatitis

5. Arthropod bites that typically reveal a central blue color of impending necrosis with a surrounding white area of vasospasm and a peripheral red halo of inflammation are associated with

   (A) scabies
   (B) black widow spiders
   (C) brown recluse spiders
   (D) deer ticks

6. Linear, pruritic, vesicles with underlying erythema on the hands, arms and legs best describes

   (A) impetigo
   (B) varicella
   (C) rhus dermatitis
   (D) herpes simplex virus

7. The condition manifesting as velvety, hyperpigmented, papillomatous lesions of the neck, axillae and groin, associated with insulin resistance, is known as

   (A) verruca vulgaris
   (B) acanthosis nigricans
   (C) hidradenitis suppurativa
   (D) seborrheic keratoses

8. A patient known to have allergic rhinitis and asthma presents with chronic pruritic inflammatory lesions of the flexor surfaces, wrists, and dorsal areas of the feet. The lesions are excoriated, lichenified with crusted patches and plaques. The most likely diagnosis is

   (A) nummular eczema
   (B) psoriasis
   (C) seborrheic dermatitis
   (D) atopic dermatitis

9. Which of the following diseases can affect the skin, nails, and joints?

   (A) erythema nodosum
   (B) psoriasis
   (C) pityriasis rosea
   (D) lichen planus

10. Using the "rule of nines" to calculate body surface area, what would the percentage of burned area be in an adult patient with second-degree burns involving the entire right arm, the anterior chest and abdomen, and the entire right leg?

    (A) 27
    (B) 36
    (C) 45
    (D) 52

11. A 65-year-old patient presents with a 4-week history of dark red pruritic urticarial plaques on the flexor surfaces. The plaques begin developing tense bullae on the surface. This clinical presentation is most suggestive of

    (A) bullous pemphigoid
    (B) bullous impetigo
    (C) pemphigus vulgaris
    (D) dermatitis herpetiformis

12. Mupirocin (Bactroban) ointment is indicated for the treatment of a localized case of

    (A) impetigo
    (B) atopic dermatitis
    (C) tinea pedis
    (D) cellulitis

13. Organ transplant recipients have a significantly increased risk for developing (see Fig. 3–3)

    (A) squamous cell carcinoma
    (B) erythema multiforme
    (C) bullous pemphigoid
    (D) pseudomonas folliculitis

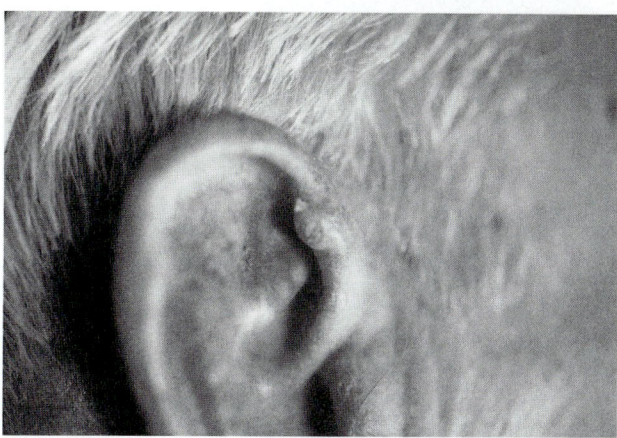

Fig. 3–3. Courtesy of Jack Cohen, D.O.

14. A predisposing condition for cellulitis of the lower extremity is

(A) onychomycosis

(B) tinea pedis

(C) verruca plantaris

(D) erythema nodosum

15. A patient being treated for acne reports symptoms of headaches and blurred vision. Which of the following agents is most likely responsible?

(A) minocycline (Minocin)

(B) erythromycin (E-Mycin)

(C) trimethoprim-sulfamethoxazole (Septra DS)

(D) tretinoin (Retin-A)

16. A 12-year-old female presents with complaints of pruritis of the scalp for 2 weeks that started at the occiput and post-auricular areas, but has now spread. Based on Fig. 3–4, the most likely diagnosis is

(A) psoriasis

(B) seborrheic dermatitis

(C) pediculosis capitis

(D) tinea amiantacea

17. A 22-year-old patient presents with multiple, flat, round light brown lesions measuring 1 to 5 mm in diameter as noted in Fig. 3–5. Several are noted to form a linear pattern. The most likely diagnosis is

(A) lichen planus

(B) verruca plana

(C) seborrheic keratoses

(D) syringomas

18. A nursing home patient with a history of diabetes develops an indurated, painful crusted ulcer with surrounding erythema on the anterior shin as seen in Fig. 3–6. The most likely diagnosis is

(A) ecthyma

(B) porphyria cutanea tarda

(C) decubitus ulcer

(D) bullous pemphigoid

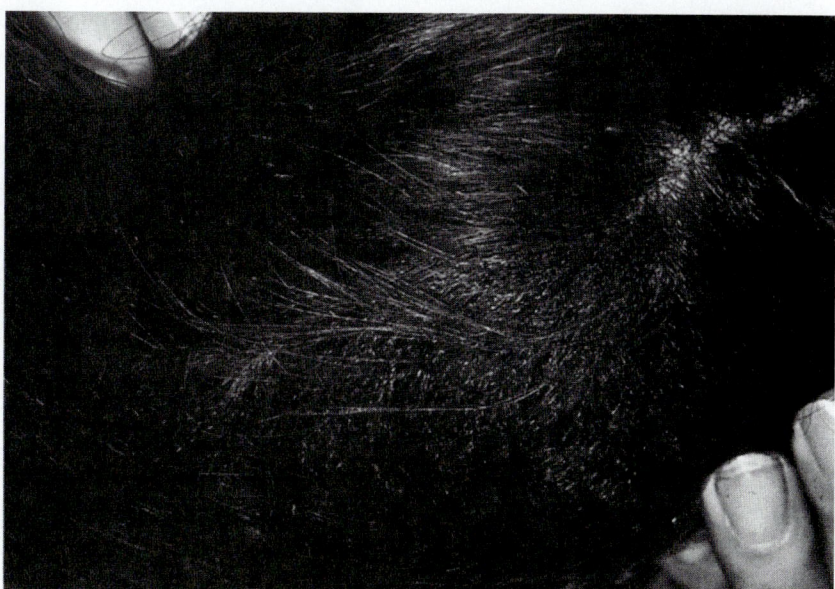

Fig. 3–4. From Fitzpatrick, Johnson, Wolff, et al. Dermatology in General Medicine, 4th ed. McGraw-Hill, Inc., 1993, with permission.

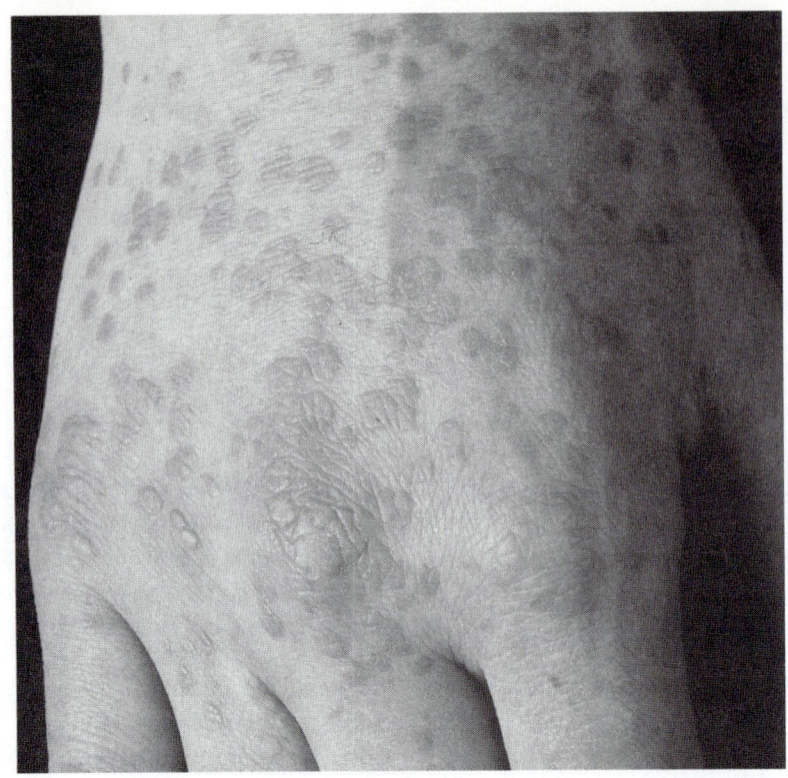

Fig. 3–5. From Fitzpatrick, Johnson, Wolff, et al. Color Atlas and Synopsis of Clinical Dermatology, 3rd ed. McGraw-Hill, Inc., 1997, with permission.

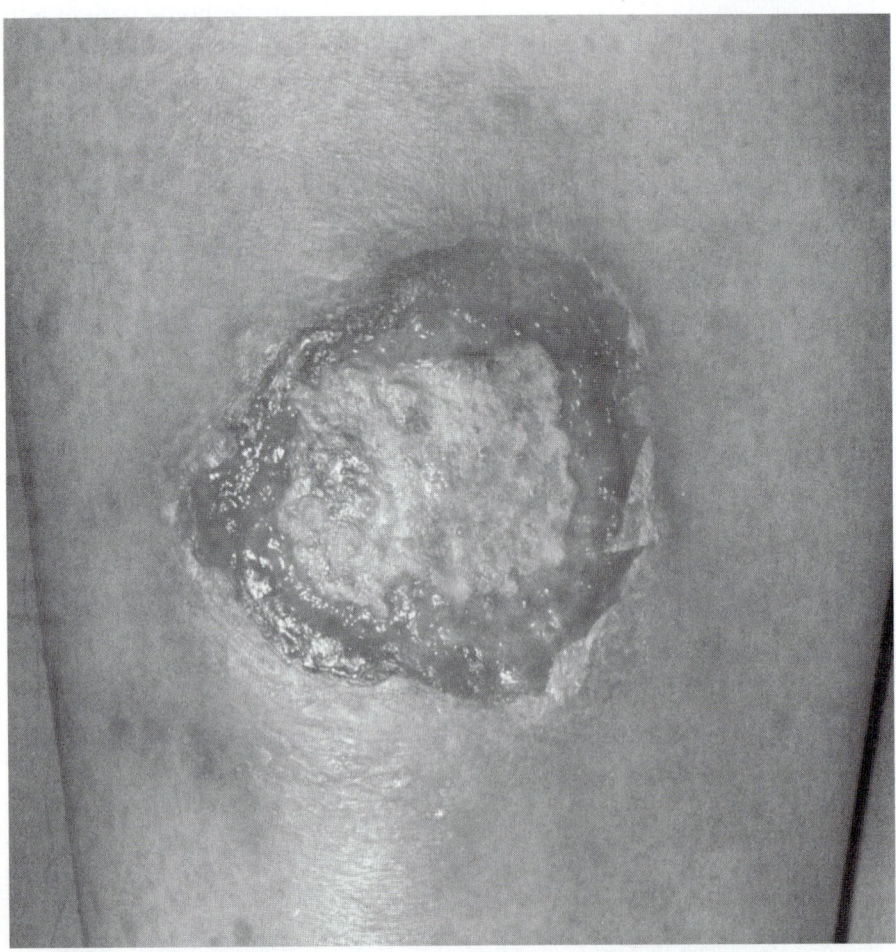

Fig. 3–6. From Fitzpatrick, Johnson, Wolff, et al. Color Atlas and Synopsis of Clinical Dermatology, 3rd ed. McGraw-Hill, Inc., 1997, with permission.

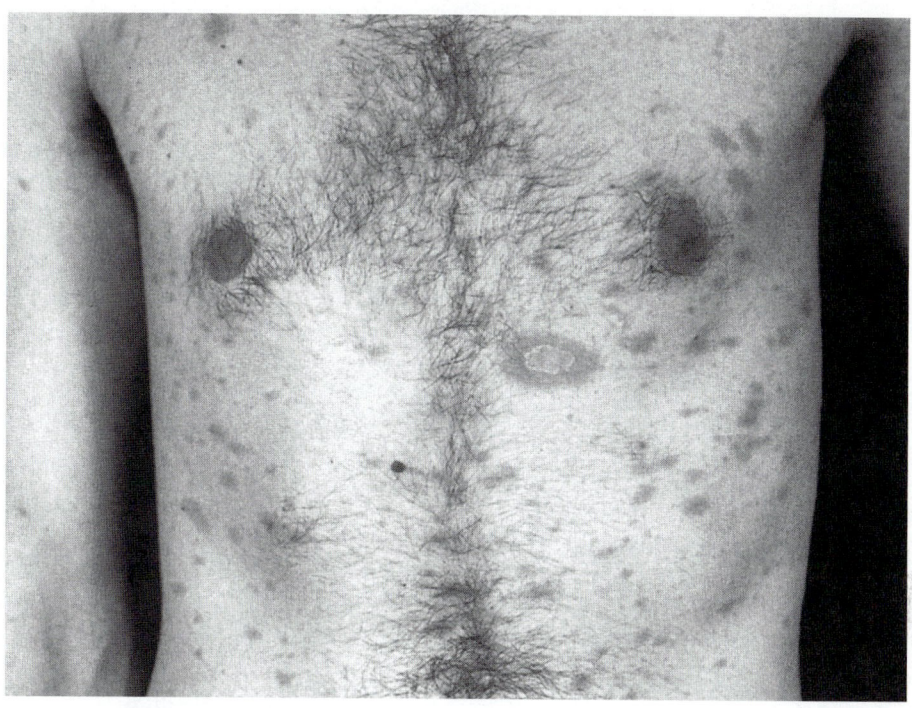

Fig. 3–7. From Fitzpatrick, Johnson, Wolff, et al. Color Atlas and Synopsis of Clinical Dermatology, 3rd ed. McGraw-Hill, Inc., 1997, with permission.

19. Perifollicular purpura, corkscrew hairs and gingival bleeding are most likely due to what deficiency?

   (A) vitamin A
   (B) vitamin B_{12}
   (C) vitamin C
   (D) vitamin K

20. A 19-year-old presents with the minimally pruritic rash seen in Fig. 3–7. The lesion on the left chest was the first to appear followed a week later by the remaining lesions. The most likely diagnosis is

   (A) tinea corporis
   (B) scabies
   (C) nummular eczema
   (D) pityriasis rosea

21. A 7-year-old white female presents to family practice to clear up a rash that has come and gone for a number of years, but now wants to wear a strapless dress to prom. The lesions are discrete, hyperpigmented, velvety lesions on the chest, shoulders, and upper back. The most likely diagnosis is

   (A) acanthosis nigricans
   (B) tinea versicolor
   (C) ephelides
   (D) melasma

22. A 45-year-old African American female presents with an indurated, reddish-orange lesion on her cheek and is found to have an elevated angiotensin converting enzyme level. The most important diagnostic test to order is

   (A) an erythrocyte sedimentation rate
   (B) a complete blood count
   (C) an electrocardiogram
   (D) a chest x-ray

23. The best treatment for a 4-mm lesion that is asymmetrical, black and red, on the left forearm and came up rapidly in the past 6 months, would be to

(A) have the patient observe the lesion every month for changes

(B) see the provider every 6 months to photograph for changes

(C) remove the lesion with a vascular laser

(D) completely excise the lesion as soon as possible

24. A patient with recurrent erythema multiforme minor lesions approximately every month should be treated prophylactically with

(A) oral steroids

(B) acyclovir

(C) dapsone

(D) oral terbenifine

25. Painful, erythematous, indurated nodules on the lower extremities of a female on an oral contraceptive pill is most likely

(A) erythema nodosum

(B) erythema multiforme

(C) erythema annulare centrifigum

(D) erythema chronica migrans

26. Thickening of the epidermis secondary to scratching best describes

(A) lichen striatus

(B) lichen planus

(C) lichen simplex chronicus

(D) lichen nitidus

27. Onycholysis with oil spots is pathognomonic for

(A) liver disease

(B) tinea unguium

(C) eczema

(D) psoriasis

28. One to two millimeter, dome-shaped, umbilicated, waxy papules best describes

(A) varicella

(B) molluscum contagiosum

(C) basal cell carcinoma

(D) impetigo

29. Folliculitis under occlusion of the bathing suit is most likely secondary to

(A) *Staphylococcus aureus*

(B) *Candida albicans*

(C) group A β-hemolytic streptococcus

(D) *Pseudomonas aeruginosa*

30. Pink lesions on the distal extremities and face that rapidly depigment best describes

(A) vitiligo

(B) pityriasis alba

(C) guttate psoriasis

(D) contact dermatitis

31. Which of the following would NOT be used to treat a 5-cm plaque of Bowen's disease (squamous cell carcinoma in situ) on the lower leg

(A) topical imiquimod

(B) topical 5-fluorouracil

(C) intralesional steroids

(D) surgical excision

32. A 1-cm pearly papule with central ulceration and telangiectasias on the left temple of a 67-year-old male is most likely

(A) rosacea

(B) basal cell carcinoma

(C) ecthyma

(D) sebaceous gland hyperplasia

33. Comedonal acne is best treated with

(A) benzoyl peroxide

(B) topical antibiotics

(C) oral antibiotics

(D) topical retinoids

34. Acquired ichthyosis is NOT usually associated with

(A) HIV

(B) lymphoma

(C) CREST syndrome

(D) sarcoidosis

35. Which of the following does NOT exacerbate the flushing of rosacea?

(A) cigarette smoking

(B) stress

(C) caffeine

(D) spicy foods

36. The causative organism of erythema chronica migrans is

(A) *Treponema pallidum*

(B) *Borrelia burgdorferi*

(C) *Bartonella henselae*

(D) *Rickettsia rickettsii*

Answers and Explanations

1. **(D)** This is a classic distribution pattern for seborrheic dermatitis, a common, chronic inflammatory dermatitis associated with Pityrosporum ovale as well as genetic and environmental factors. Bacterial folliculitis presents as dome-shaped pustules with small erythematous halos arising in the center of hair follicles. Allergic contact dermatitis is characterized by vesicles, edema, erythema, and pruritus. Rosacea presents as eruptions of erythema, telangiectasias, pustules, and papules localized to the face. (*Habif, 2004, pp. 84, 198, 245, 279*)

2. **(C)** Alopecia areata is an autoimmune process presenting as localized, well-circumscribed loss of hair in oval or round patterns without visible evidence of inflammation, most commonly on the scalp with exclamation point hairs at the periphery of alopecia. Anagen effluvium is diffuse hair loss involving the entire scalp and is commonly caused by drugs or chemotherapy. Androgenetic alopecia is progressive balding secondary to genetic predisposition and the influence of androgen and typically spares the parietal region. Tinea capitis is uncommon in adults, and it has "black dots" in the area of alopecia from broken off hairs with scale and possibly inflammation and adenopathy. (*Habif, 2004, pp. 427, 842, 843, 855*)

3. **(D)** The Tzanck smear is a microscopic exam of cells obtained from the base of vesicles and bullae for multinucleated giant cells seen in herpes simplex, herpes zoster, and varicella. Scabies is diagnosed with a scabies prep, a microscopic exam for mites, scybala (fecal pellets), or eggs. Tinea versicolor is a dermatophyte infection diagnosed with a potassium hydroxide (K^1OH^2) test looking for hyphae and spores in a classic spaghetti-and-meatballs pattern. Impetigo is caused by streptococci and/or staphylococci typically diagnosed by the clinical presentation, but culture and sensitivity tests can isolate the causative organism(s). (*Habif, 2004, pp. 272, 350, 453, 502; Moser, 2001, p. 82*)

4. **(A)** Lichen planus is an inflammatory reaction pattern of unknown etiology, with characteristic "five P" clinical features: pruritic, planar (flat), polyangular/polygonal, purple papules. Pityriasis rosea is typically confined to the trunk, beginning with a single red oval plaque that is followed by a number of similar smaller plaques with spontaneous resolution in 4 to 8 weeks. Psoriasis is a papulosquamous disease commonly presenting as scaly plaques involving the elbows, knees, and scalp. Seborrheic dermatitis is a common, chronic inflammatory disease commonly seen on the scalp and scalp margins, eyebrows, nasolabial folds, and presternal areas. (*Habif, 2004, pp. 209, 242, 246, 250*)

5. **(C)** Brown recluse (*Loxoscelidae recluses*) spider bites in fatty areas such as thighs and buttocks can become necrotic within 4 hours, with a rapidly expanding blue-gray halo

around the puncture site surrounded by a white area of vasospasm and a peripheral red halo of inflammation. Scabies (*Sarcoptes scabiei*) lesions are pleomorphic and often vesicular, pustular, or excoriated with linear, curved, or S-shaped burrows. Black widow (*Latrodectus mactans*) bites result in slight swelling with small red fang marks. Deer tick (*Ixodes dammini*) lesions can present as a small papule with a slowly enlarging ring (erythema migrans), a bluish-red nodule (Borrelia lymphocytoma), or an atrophic plaque (acrodermatitis chronica atrophicans). (*Habif, 2004, pp. 497, 512, 514, 517*)

6. **(C)** Rhus dermatitis occurs most commonly on areas at risk of contact with the plants, hands, arms, and legs. They form linear pruritic vesicles caused by the resin of the plant being dragged by scratching. Impetigo may or may not be pruritic, but occurs mainly on the face (nose and mouth). Varicella is pruritic, not linear, and predominantly noted on the trunk. Herpes simplex virus, generally more painful than pruritic, occurs either around the lips and nose or on the genitalia. (*Habif, 2004, pp. 88, 267, 381, 389; Moser, 2001, pp. 82, 89*)

7. **(B)** Acanthosis nigricans is commonly associated with obesity, insulin resistance, and diabetes mellitus. Verruca vulgaris lesions can occasionally be hyperpigmented and are frequently papillomatous, but there is no association with insulin resistance. Hidradenitis suppurativa results in deep dermal inflammation with large painful abscesses in the axillae, anogenital region, and female inframammary folds. Seborrheic keratoses are common, benign, generally brown, may be smooth or papillomatous and may appear throughout the entire body, face and scalp. They are not associated with insulin resistance. (*Habif, 2004, pp. 202, 368, 698, 900*)

8. **(D)** Atopic dermatitis often occurs in association with a family or personal history of atopy, to include allergic rhinitis, asthma, and eczema. It is characterized as the "itch that rashes," and is associated with dry skin, icthyosis vulgaris, keratosis pilaris, sensitivity to wool, and hyperlinear palmar creases. Pso-

riasis is a papulosquamous disease commonly presenting as scaly plaques involving the elbows, knees, and scalp. Nummular eczema presents as chronic, coin-shaped plaques with small papules and vesicles on an erythematous base, typically seen on the lower legs of older males in winter months. Seborrheic dermatitis presents as erythema with yellowish scale-forming plaques on the eyebrows, nasolabial folds, glabella, and presternal area of the chest. (*Fitzpatrick, 1997, pp. 54, 68, 76; Habif, 2004, pp. 54, 105, 209, 242*)

9. **(B)** In addition to erythematous scaly papules and plaques, psoriasis may present with nail pitting and onycholysis. Psoriatic arthritis occurs in 5% to 8% of those affected with psoriasis. Erythema nodosum is an inflammatory nodular pattern of panniculitis typically involving only the lower extremities. Pityriasis rosea is an epidermal papulosquamous disorder typically confined to the trunk, with no nail or joint involvement. Lichen planus is an inflammatory reaction pattern with mucous membrane and cutaneous lesions and no associated joint involvement. (*Habif, 2004, pp. 219–220, 246, 250, 635*)

10. **(C)** The anterior chest and abdomen are 18%, each leg is 18%, and each arm is 9%, for a total of 45% body surface area. (*Niederhuber, p. 187*)

11. **(A)** Bullous pemphigoid is a subepidermal blistering disease presenting on the flexor surfaces of elderly patients. A hallmark is the presence of tense bullae overlying erythematous plaques. Bullous impetigo is a superficial skin infection caused by streptococci and/or staphylococci, typically distributed on the face and distal extremities in children and adolescents. Pemphigus vulgaris presents as multiple flaccid blisters from one to several centimeters in diameter, often involving the oral mucosa and skin from the neck to the knees. Dermatitis herpetiformis is a glutensensitive enteropathy presenting with severe pruritus and clustered herpetiform grouped vesicles on the elbows, knees, sacrum, nuchal area, shoulders, and buttocks. (*Habif, 2004, pp. 268, 554, 559–564, 567–569*)

12. **(A)** Mupirocin is the first topical antibiotic approved for the treatment of impetigo. Atopic dermatitis is typically treated with topical steroid preparations. Tinea pedis is a dermatophyte infection treated with antifungals. Cellulitis typically requires treatment with oral or parenteral antibiotics. (*Habif, 2004, pp. 122, 272, 273, 415*)

13. **(A)** Immunosuppressive agents required following organ transplant greatly increase the risk for developing squamous cell carcinoma. Erythema multiforme, a reaction pattern of idiopathic, drug, and infectious origin, is unrelated to organ transplant immunosuppression, as is bullous pemphigoid, an autoimmune subepidermal blistering disease. Pseudomonas folliculitis is an acute skin infection that follows exposure to contaminated water and is also known as "hot tub folliculitis." (*Habif, 2004, pp. 290, 567–569, 626, 746*)

14. **(B)** Fungal infection of the interdigital spaces can result in breaks in the dermal barrier, permitting bacterial entry through the skin, and requires careful exam of the feet in lower extremity cellulitis. Onychomycosis typically involves the nail plate and not the surrounding soft tissue. Plantar warts (verruca plantaris) are isolated to weight-bearing plantar surfaces. Erythema nodosum, a hypersensitivity reaction to a variety of antigenic stimuli, typically presents as erythematous nodules over the anterior shin area, and is not associated with the development of cellulitis. (*Habif, 2004, pp. 274, 374, 635, 874*)

15. **(A)** These are classic symptoms of pseudotumor cerebri, a known complication of minocycline. Side effects of erythromycin typically include nausea, vomiting, diarrhea, and abdominal pain and cramps. Trimethoprim-sulfamethoxazole side effects include Stevens– Johnson syndrome, agranulocytosis, and pseudomembranous colitis. Tretinoin side effects include skin irritation with localized erythema and scaling. (*Physician's Desk Reference, pp. 438, 1525, 2177, 2655*)

16. **(C)** Pediculosis capitis (head lice) begins most commonly at the occiput and post-auricular area where grayish-white, oval-shaped nits are seen adhered to the hair shaft. Psoriasis presents with well-demarcated, erythematous plaques with silvery-white scale. Seborrheic dermatitis presents with diffuse erythema with greasy yellow scale throughout the scalp. Tinea amiantacea appears as plates of yellowish-white scale that firmly adheres to the scalp and binds to the hair shaft ranging in length from 2 to 10 cm. (*Habif, 2004, pp. 209, 242, 243, 506; Moser, 2001, pp. 61, 98, 101*)

17. **(B)** Flat warts or verruca plana are light-brown or flesh-colored papules ranging from 1 to 5 mm in diameter. Because the virus spreads with scratching or shaving, a linear pattern forms. Lichen planus are pruritic, planar (flat), polyangular/polygonal, purple papules, generally seen on the volar aspects of the wrist and forearm as opposed to the dorsum. Seborrheic keratoses range from 2 mm to 3 cm and can be tan, brown, or black in color, can appear on the dorsum of the hands, but do not form a linear pattern secondary to trauma. Syringomas are small firm yellowish-white papules that occur on the lower eyelids, forehead, chest, and abdomen. (*Habif, 2004, pp. 250, 373, 698, 721; Moser, 2001, p. 86*)

18. **(A)** Ecthyma is caused by group A β-hemolytic streptococcus and seen most commonly in diabetics, elderly, and alcoholic patients and is usually found on the lower extremities. Porphyria cutanea tarda is caused by a combination of genetic predisposition and alcohol abuse or hepatitis C infection and presents with vesicles, scarring, and milia on sun-exposed surfaces, most commonly the dorsum of the hands. Decubitus ulcers occur from pressure over bony prominences (i.e., the sacrum, ischial tuberosities, iliac crest, heels, elbows, knees, malleoli, and scapula) in bed-ridden patients. Bullous pemphigoid is an autoimmune disease that presents with multiple tense bulla that can rupture or ulcerate most commonly on the lower abdomen, groin and flexural areas on the arms and legs. (*Fitzpatrick, 1999, pp. 1542; Habif, 2004, pp. 568, 675; Moser, 2001, p. 91*)

19. **(C)** Scurvy (vitamin C deficiency) presents with petechiae around the hair follicles, corkscrew hairs and gingival bleeding. Vitamin A deficiency presents with phrynoderma or "toad-skin," which is perifollicular hyperkeratosis, in addition to keratomalacia. Vitamin B_{12} deficiency or pernicious anemia is associated with vitiligo, alopecia areata, and premature graying of the hair. Vitamin K deficiency leads to clotting abnormalities and the presence of purpura, but will not have corkscrew hairs present. (*Fitzpatrick, 1999, pp. 1730–1736*)

20. **(D)** Pityriasis rosea starts with the herald patch and then 7 to 10 days later smaller ovoid lesions with inverse collarette of scale erupt following the skin lines in a Christmas tree pattern. Tinea corporis has a leading scale edge unlike Pityriasis rosea, which has a trailing scale. The lesions do not follow the skin lines. A KOH will help confirm a diagnosis of tinea. Scabies presents with burrows at the edge of vesicles or papules and excoriations in the interdigital webspaces, axilla, groin, breasts, buttocks, wrist, and waistband area. Nummular eczema presents as chronic, coin-shaped plaques with small papules and vesicles on an erythematous base, typically seen on the lower legs of older males in winter months. (*Habif, 2004, pp. 54, 246, 420, 500; Moser, 2001, pp. 64, 97, 104*)

21. **(B)** Tinea versicolor comes and goes, but tends to flare in hot and humid weather. The lesions are hyper- or hypopigmented, velvety, in a collar distribution and the lesions do not tan. Acanthosis nigricans does not come and go and is a velvety, thickened brown plaque located in the axilla and back of the neck. Ephelides or freckles are small, red or light brown macules that are promoted by sun-exposure and fade in the winter, but do not go away. Melasma is an area of hyperpigmentation, generally on the face that gets darker in the sun and fades in the winter, but does not go away. It is most common in women particularly those on oral contraceptive pills or who are pregnant. (*Habif, 2004, pp. 451, 691, 692, 900; Moser, 2001, p. 105*)

22. **(D)** Sarcoidosis is commonly seen in middle-aged, African American females and the lesions are reddish-orange to purple indurated nodules and plaques with a predilection for the central face and elevated angiotensin converting enzyme levels in up to 60% of all patients with sarcoidosis. Sarcoid affects many organs but most commonly the lungs and eyes, therefore a chest x-ray looking for pulmonary infiltrates and an ophthalmology exam are necessary diagnostic steps. (*Fitzpatrick, 1999, pp. 2099–2105*)

23. **(D)** Based on the ABCDE criteria this lesion fails in four categories; Asymmetrical, irregular Borders, two Colors particularly black and red, which are ominous, and rapid Enlargement or Elevation. It is under 6 mm in Diameter. However, this lesion is highly suspicious for a melanoma and should be excised as soon as possible for diagnosis. (*Habif, 2004, pp. 786–788; Moser, 2001, p. 94*)

24. **(B)** Recurrent erythema multiforme is most commonly due to recurrent herpes simplex virus outbreaks. Prophylactic treatment with Acyclovir or related compund should suppress future herpes simplex virus outbreaks, and therefore, future erythema multiforme recurrences. (*Habif, 2004, pp. 626–629; Moser, 2001, p. 78*)

25. **(A)** Erythema nodosum presents with painful nodules generally on the lower extremities. The most common causes are oral contraceptive use, sarcoidosis and Behçets. Erythema multiforme is usually due to herpes simplex virus infection or a drug reaction, but the lesions are targetoid in appearance. Erythema annulare centrifigum presents as one or more urticarial-type papules that enlarge to form indurated ringed lesions, that may herald an internal malignancy. Erythema chronica migrans is the rash associated with Lyme disease and is usually a solitary ringed lesion at the site of the tick bite. (*Fitzpatrick, 1999, pp. 1149–1150; Habif, 2004, pp. 517, 626–629, 635; Moser, 2001, pp. 78, 79*)

26. **(C)** Lichen simplex chronicus is the name for lichenification that occurs secondary to scratching. Lichen striatus presents as tiny 1- to 2-mm, flat-topped, scaly erythematous papules, in a linear configuration along

Blaschko's lines, most commonly occurring on the limbs, and less frequently on the trunk, face, neck, or buttocks. Lichen planus are purple, polygonal, planar papules. Lichen nitidus are multiple, discrete smooth, flat papules that are flesh-colored and can appear throughout the body. (*Fitzpatrick, 1999, pp. 577–580, 878; Habif, 2004, pp. 54, 250*)

27. **(D)** Nail disease in psoriasis presents with onycholysis and a yellowish-brown discoloration under the nail plate resembling oil spots. Nail pitting can also be seen, but nail pits are also noted in eczema. Liver disease can present with Terry's nails where the nail bed is white with a normal distal band (cirrhosis) or in the case of Wilson's disease, azure (blue) lunulae. Tinea unguium presents as thickened, yellow, crumbly nails. (*Habif, 2004, pp. 869–870, 885–887*)

28. **(B)** Molluscum contagiosum are 1- to 2-mm, dome-shaped, umbilicated waxy papules. Varicella starts as erythematous papules that progress to vesicles, then pustules that umbilicate and crust in crops. Basal cell carcinoma can have central ulceration, but are not waxy lesions and generally are larger than 1 to 2 mm. In addition, they usually have telangiectasias on the lesion that are not seen in molluscum. Impetigo begins as vesicles or bulla that umbilicate and then rapidly becomes a honey-colored crust. (*Habif, 2004, pp. 267, 379, 389, 724; Moser, 2001, pp. 68, 89, 95*)

29. **(D)** Hot tub folliculitis occurs under areas of occlusion of the bathing suit and is usually due to improperly cleaned hot tubs caused by *Pseudomonas aeruginosa. Staphylococcus aureus* tends to occur in areas of trauma, such as shaving with a predilection of the beard area in men and the legs in women. Group A β-hemolytic streptococcus does not generally cause a folliculitis. It tends to cause impetiginization of open skin areas. Candida albicans folliculitis is seen in febrile bed-ridden patients generally on the back due to occlusion. (*Fitzpatrick, 1999, pp. 2194–2203, 2363; Habif, 2004, pp. 279, 290*)

30. **(A)** Vitiligo presents as pink lesions that depigment on the acral extremities and central

face (periorbital and perioral areas). Pityriasis alba is hypopigmentation secondary to an inflammatory rash of eczema. Guttate psoriasis are pink-red teardrop lesions of psoriasis, but do not depigment. Contact dermatitis presents as erythematous areas that on resolution can leave post-inflammatory hypopigmentation but not depigmentation. (*Habif, 2004, pp. 81, 212, 684, 689*)

31. **(C)** Intralesional steroids are of no benefit in the treatment of squamous cell carcinoma in situ. The other three modalities have all been used with varying success. (*Habif, 2004, p. 748*)

32. **(B)** Basal cell carcinoma is most commonly found on the sun-exposed areas of the face (temples, nose, cheeks), behind the ears in men, and upper back/shoulders. They generally appear in the 5th and 6th decades of life, and are noted to have central ulceration and telangiectasias. Rosacea is adult acne characterized by papules, pustules, a notable absence of comedones and flushing that can lead to permanent telangiectasia formation of the central face. Ecthyma is caused by group A β-hemolytic streptococcus and seen most commonly in diabetics, elderly and alcoholic patients and is usually found on the lower extremities. Sebaceous gland hyperplasia are enlarged oil glands, approximately 2 to 4 mm, yellowish-white, with telangiectasias and generally more than one are noted on the forehead, nose and cheeks, but rarely, if ever, get as large as 1cm. (*Habif, 2004, pp. 198, 272, 720, 724*)

33. **(D)** The four treatment areas for acne include: decrease sebum production, normalize abnormal desquamation of follicular epithelium, inhibit *Propionibacterium acnes* proliferation and colonization, and reduce the inflammatory response. Topical retinoids normalize follicular desquamation which is the key factor in comedonal production. They also reduce the inflammatory response preventing the development of papules and pustules. Benzoyl peroxide, topical and oral antibiotics have a weak effect on comedones and follicular desquamation, but rather all three work to inhibit *P. acnes* proliferation and colonization as well as re-

ducing the inflammatory response. (*Gollnick et al, 2003, pp. S1–S38*)

34. **(C)** HIV infection, lymphoma, sarcoidosis, and thyroid disease are all associated with the development of acquired ichthyosis, a sudden appearance of tile-like scales, usually of the lower extremities, but possibly throughout the entire body. CREST is not associated with the development of acquired ichthyosis, but rather sclerodermatous skin, which demonstrates hypo- and hyperpigmentation, shiny, taut skin with decreased mobility. (*Fitzpatrick, 1999, pp. 2194–2203, 2363; Habif, 2004, pp. 613–617, 894*)

35. **(A)** Cigarette smoking is a vasoconstrictor, so will not exacerbate flushing, whereas the others are vasodilators and will increase the flushing associated with rosacea. (*Fitzpatrick, 1999, pp. 1986–1991*)

36. **(B)** Borrelia burgdorferi is the causative organism of Lyme disease of which erythema chronica migrans is the distintive rash. Treponema pallidum is the causative organism of syphilis. Bartonella henselae is the causative organism of cat scratch disease, bacillary angiomatosis and bacillary peliosis hepatitis.

Rickettsia rickettsii is the causative organism of Rocky Mountain Spotted Fever. (*Habif, 2004, pp. 315, 516, 517, 528*)

REFERENCES

Freedberg IM, Eisen AZ, Wolff K, et al (eds), *Fitzpatrick's Dermatology in General Medicine*, 5th ed. New York: McGraw-Hill; 1999.

Fitzpatrick TB, Johnson RA, Wolff K, Polano MK, Suurmond D (eds), *Color Atlas and Synopsis of Clinical Dermatology*, 3rd ed. New York: McGraw-Hill; 1997.

Gollnick H, Cunliffe W, Berson D, et al. Management of acne: a report from a Global Alliance to Improve Outcomes in Acne. *J Am Acad Dermatol* 2003; 49 (Suppl 1):S1–S38.

Habif TP. *Clinical Dermatology: A Color Guide to Diagnosis and Therapy*, 4th ed. Philadelphia: Mosby; 2004.

Moser RL (ed), *Primary Care for Physician Assistants, Clinical Practice Guidelines*, 2nd ed. New York: McGraw-Hill; 2001

Niederhuber JE (ed), *Fundamentals of Surgery*. Stamford: Appleton & Lange; 1998.

Physicians' Desk Reference, 54th ed. Montvale, NJ; 2000.

CHAPTER 4

Endocrinology
Questions

Christina M. Robohm, MS, PA-C, and Susan Symington, MPAS, PA-C

DIRECTIONS (Questions 1 through 5): This section consists of lettered headings followed by a set of numbered words or phrases. For each numbered word or phrase, select the ONE lettered heading that is most closely associated with it. Each lettered heading may be selected once, more than once, or not at all.

Questions 1 through 5

Match the following hormones with the sites where they are produced.

(A) posterior pituitary
(B) anterior pituitary
(C) hypothalamus

1. antidiuretic hormone (ADH)

2. growth hormone (GH)

3. oxytocin

4. corticotropin-releasing factor (CRF)

5. thyroid-stimulating hormone (TSH)

DIRECTIONS (Questions 6 through 50): Select the ONE lettered answer or completion that is BEST in each case.

Questions 6 through 50

6. A 43-year-old obese male presents for a health maintenance visit. On physical exam, it is noted that his waist circumference is 106 cm and blood pressure is 148/92. Which of the following fasting laboratory levels would suggest a diagnosis of metabolic syndrome (syndrome X) in this patient?

   (A) HDL of 45 mg/dL
   (B) LDL of 180 mg/dL
   (C) triglyceride of 190 mg/dL
   (D) glucose of 100 mg/dL

7. A 36-year-old woman (see Fig. 4–1) presents to the office complaining of weight loss and a feeling of "nervousness." During the last several weeks, she also complains she is losing hair. Exam reveals a diffusely enlarged, firm, nontender thyroid gland with an audible bruit. Her eyes have marked proptosis and lid retraction. Her TSH is very low; her free and total thyroid hormone levels are elevated. What is the most likely pathophysiology of this patient's disease?

   (A) subacute thyroiditis
   (B) Hashimoto thyroiditis
   (C) Graves' disease
   (D) multinodular goiter
   (E) Cushing's disease

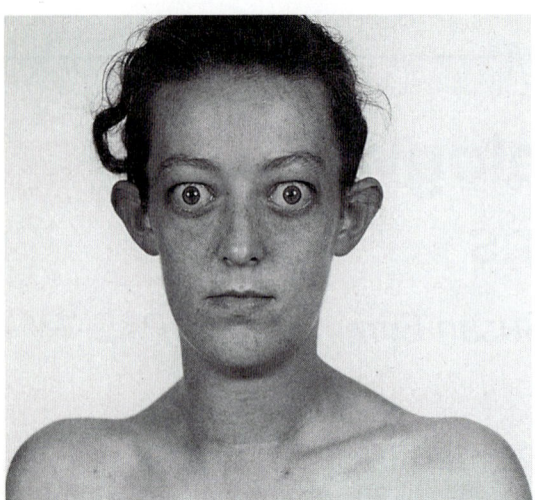

Fig. 4–1. Reprinted from Kasper DL, Braunwald E, et al. *Harrison's Online: Harrison's Principles of Internal Medicine*, 16th ed. Figure 320-6A, Copyright 2006 with permission from McGraw-Hill, Inc.

8. An 8-year-old boy develops type 1 diabetes. He is following up in the office one year after his diagnosis for a complete physical exam. The child's mom is asking what referrals and/or tests are required at this time as she wants him monitored closely for any complications related to the diabetes. Which of the following is recommended at this time?

   (A) ophthalmology referral
   (B) urine microalbumin
   (C) podiatry referral
   (D) TSH

9. A 67-year-old man is admitted with pneumonia and a fractured hip. Therapy includes bed rest, administration of antibiotics, and subcutaneous heparin. Several days into his hospitalization, he develops hyponatremia and abdominal pain. What is the most likely etiology of his new symptoms?

   (A) Graves' disease
   (B) Cushing's syndrome
   (C) Addison's disease
   (D) toxic goiter
   (E) pheochromocytoma

10. A 67-year-old female with type 2 diabetes is being treated for dyslipidemia. What is the target LDL goal for this patient?

    (A) < 100 mg/dL
    (B) < 120 mg/dL
    (C) < 130 mg/dL
    (D) < 160 mg/dL

11. A 44-year-old man has been drinking large quantities of water, up to 12 L per day, for the last week. In addition, he has been passing large quantities of urine. Upon physical exam, there are no remarkable findings except for increased capillary refill time and tacky mucous membranes. Laboratory results show sodium 166 mmol/L, potassium 4.2 mmol/L, chloride 123 mmol/L, and bicarbonate 27 mmol/L. His fasting serum glucose is 80 mg/dL and creatinine 1.2 mg/dL. His serum osmolality is 343 mOsm/kg. Which of the following hormone deficiencies is most likely present in this patient?

    (A) prolactin
    (B) oxytocin
    (C) insulin
    (D) GH
    (E) antidiuretic hormone

12. A 42-year-old woman has experienced recent weight gain, heavy periods, fatigue, cold intolerance, and constipation. She has a rough voice, and her rate of speech is slow. Physical exam is significant for an enlarged thyroid, slow reflexes, and the presence of brittle and coarse hair. She denies any history of bipolar disease or treatment with lithium. Lab tests show an elevated TSH and low free T4. What is the most appropriate treatment for this patient?

    (A) propylthiouracil (PTU)
    (B) levothyroxine
    (C) surgical resection
    (D) radioiodide ablation

13. A 22-year-old man (see Fig. 4–2-left hand) is being evaluated for extremity enlargement unlike anyone in his family. Over the past 2 years, he has noticed that his rings no longer fit and his feet are so wide that he cannot find shoes to fit. He has always been tall for his age, >95th percentile throughout his teenage years. He has very coarse facial features, macroglossia, and a very deep voice. What is the most likely cause of this patient's condition?

   (A) adrenal neoplasm

   (B) multinodular goiter

   (C) pituitary macroadenoma

   (D) Rathke's cleft cyst

   (E) testicular neoplasm

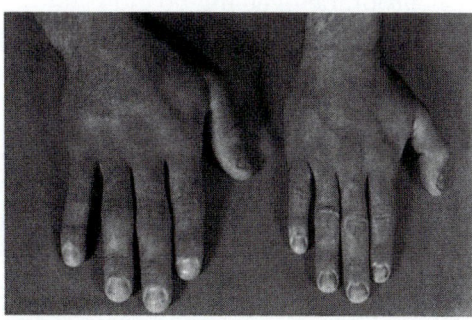

Fig. 4–2. Reprinted from Gagel R and McCutcheon IE. *N Engl J Med* 1999; 324:524, with permission from NEJM. Massachusetts Medical Society.

14. Which of the following is considered 24-hour long acting insulin and is given once in the evening?

    (A) ultralente

    (B) NPH

    (C) lispro

    (D) glargine

15. A 49-year-old man presents to the office complaining of general malaise with muscle aches, anorexia, fever, and severe pain over his anterior neck radiating to his ears. He states that he was ill about 2 weeks ago with a sore throat, but it resolved within a few days. On palpation, the thyroid gland is enlarged and tender. His labs show a high T4 level and increased erythrocyte sedimentation rate (ESR). What is the most appropriate therapy for this patient's disease?

    (A) thyroxin therapy

    (B) PTU therapy

    (C) radioiodine ablation

    (D) surgery

    (E) supportive therapy only

16. A 65-year-old male with type 2 diabetes, presents with complaints of abdominal bloating after meals. For the past 2 months, he has noticed an increase in anorexia and nausea. This week he vomited twice several hours after eating. The KUB does not show any sign of a small bowel obstruction. He denies any heartburn, hematemesis, hematochezia, or melena. Which of the following would be the best treatment for his symptoms?

    (A) ranitidine

    (B) omeprazole

    (C) cisapride

    (D) metoclopramide

17. Which of the following is the most likely cause of hypercalcemia in an ambulatory patient?

    (A) parathyroid adenoma

    (B) renal insufficiency

    (C) malabsorption

    (D) multiple myeloma

18. A 45-year-old female presents with weight gain, fatigue, dry skin, and oligomenorrhea. On physical exam the patient has a palpable thyroid mass over the right lobe. An ultrasound evaluation of the thyroid shows diffuse heterogeneous enlargement of the gland. Which of the following is the most likely diagnosis?

    (A) multinodular goiter

    (B) thyroid carcinoma

    (C) thyroid adenoma

    (D) Hashimoto's thyroiditis

19. Sulfonylureas stimulate the release of insulin from pancreatic B cells. Which of the following sulfonylureas has the highest insulinotropic potency?

   (A) chlorpropamide
   (B) glipizide
   (C) glyburide
   (D) tolbutamide

20. A 29-year-old woman presents to the office with complaints of poor sleep, irritability, and nervousness. She appears anxious and restless. You note tachycardia and edematous skin change on the dorsum of the lower legs and feet. She has exophthalmos and a diffusely enlarged thyroid gland on exam. Which of the following findings should you expect on further evaluation?

   (A) low levels of free T4 level
   (B) high levels of TSH
   (C) low uptake on radioiodide nuclear scan
   (D) high levels of thyroid-stimulating antibodies

21. When treating the dyslipidemia associated with type 2 diabetes, which of the following is the drug class of choice?

   (A) bile acid sequestrants
   (B) fibrate
   (C) fiber supplements
   (D) HMG CoA reductase inhibitors
   (E) nicotinic acid derivatives

22. A 43-year-old woman presents to the emergency department complaining of weakness, abdominal pain, fever, nausea, and vomiting. On evaluation, she is found to have a blood pressure of 82/54, increased serum potassium, decreased serum sodium, and an increased BUN. A cosyntropin stimulation test is unsuccessful. What is the most appropriate immediate treatment for this patient?

   (A) acetaminophen, 500 mg by mouth
   (B) hydrocortisone, 300 mg IV
   (C) flagyl, 500 mg IV
   (D) propranol HCl, 40 mg by mouth
   (E) levothyroxine, 200 μg by mouth

23. Following an intravenous pyelogram to rule out a renal calculi, a diabetic patient develops oliguria, nausea and vomiting and an altered sensorium. Which of the following is the most likely cause for this patient's symptoms?

   (A) metformin
   (B) glimepiride
   (C) glyburide
   (D) tolbutamide

24. A patient develops Graves' disease at 25 weeks gestation. Which of the following is the most appropriate treatment?

   (A) PTU 100 mg po tid
   (B) methimazole 10 to 30 mg po qd
   (C) propranolol 80 mg po qid
   (D) radioactive iodine therapy (RAI, 131I)
   (E) levothyroxine 0.1 mg po qd

25. A 75-year-old man with type 2 diabetes presents to the emergency room with a 2-day history of confusion and lethargy. On physical exam there is notable dehydration, tachycardia, and confused mental state. Serum sodium, potassium, magnesium, and chloride are normal. The arterial blood gases are normal and serum ketones are negative. The abnormal laboratory findings are as follows:

Normal reference range*		
Glucose	700 (mg/dL)	70–110 (mg/dL)
Osmolality	380 (mOsm/kg)	280–300 (mOsm/kg)

   *Data from Ferri, *Practical Guide to the Care of the Medical Patient*, 5th ed. Philadelphia, PA: W.B. Saunders, 2001.

   Given this information, what is the most likely diagnosis?

   (A) diabetic ketoacidosis
   (B) hyperglycemic hyperosmolar state
   (C) hypoglycemia
   (D) dehydration

26. Which of the following oral agents used to treat type 2 diabetes mellitus is effective in lowering fasting blood glucose levels and postprandial hyperglycemia without causing hypoglycemia?

    (A) glyburide
    (B) metformin
    (C) repaglinide
    (D) troglitazone

27. A 23-year-old type 1 diabetic has been having difficulty sleeping at night. Usually around 3 AM the patient will wake up feeling sweaty, nauseated, and tachycardic. For the past two evenings the patient has recorded blood glucose levels of 40 and 45, respectively. The 7 AM blood sugar levels have been 200 and 220, respectively. What advice is the best for this patient?

    (A) stop eating a bedtime snack
    (B) increase the evening regular insulin dosage
    (C) decrease the evening intermediate insulin dosage
    (D) exercise before going to bed at night

28. A 16-year-old boy complains he is the shortest boy in his class. He has a normal past medical history, and although he was always a bit small for age, he has really noticed that he has fallen behind his peers in the last 2 years. He is Tanner stage 3, and is at the 5th percentile for height. His father reports that he began puberty at age 14 and completed his growth in college at age 19; he is now 6 feet, 2 inches tall. His mother began her pubertal development at age 10 and had her first menstrual period at age 13; her height is 5 feet, 4 inches. What is the most important in the initial workup of this patient?

    (A) radiograph of left hand and wrist
    (B) measurement of somatomedin C
    (C) liver function studies
    (D) measurement of serum GH
    (E) chromosomal analysis

29. A 52-year-old woman presents to the office complaining of fatigue, weight loss, heat intolerance, and difficulty concentrating for the last several weeks. In addition, she has had bouts of diarrhea and heavy periods. Which of the following pharmacological agents most likely responsible for these symptoms?

    (A) amiodarone
    (B) digoxin
    (C) procainamide
    (D) propranolol
    (E) verapamil

30. A 34-year-old man presents to the office complaining of frequent urination progressively worsening for the last 3 weeks. He is having enuresis and nocturia approximately four times per week. He has been thirsty and drinking more fluids during this time and complains of some fatigue. His physical exam is unremarkable. His initial lab results are as follows:

    Urinalysis: specific gravity 1.001, otherwise normal
    24 hour urine: output >50 mL/kg per day; osmolality <300 mOsm/kg
    Fasting plasma glucose: 98 mg/dL
    Fasting insulin: 24 μU/L (6–35)

    What is the most likely cause of this patient's symptoms?

    (A) type 2 diabetes mellitus
    (B) syndrome X
    (C) diabetes insipidus
    (D) pituitary adenoma
    (E) urinary tract infection

31. You are treating a healthy 50-year-old man with no cardiac risk factors. This patient has no other medical conditions and takes no medications. His fasting lipid panel from last week demonstrates the following:

    TC — 245 mg/dL
    LDL — 155 mg/dL
    HDL — 160 mg/dL

    What is the LDL goal for this patient?

    (A) < 100 mg/dL
    (B) < 120 mg/dL
    (C) < 130 mg/dL
    (D) < 160 mg/dL
    (E) < 190 mg/dL

32. A 47-year-old woman presents to the office with increased blood pressure, bradycardia, constipation, muscle cramps, and weight gain. What is the best initial laboratory workup for this patient?

    (A) TSH level
    (B) T3 and T4
    (C) free T4 and TSH
    (D) serum thyroglobin
    (E) RAI uptake and thyroid scan

33. A 31-year-old woman is being evaluated for irregular, infrequent periods. On further questioning, she complains of headaches, fatigue, and breast discharge. She takes only occasional ibuprofen. Which of the following labs would most likely be elevated in this patient?

    (A) BUN & creatinine
    (B) luteinizing hormone (LH) and FSH (follicle-stimulating hormone)
    (C) oxytocin
    (D) prolactin
    (E) TSH

34. A 65-year-old type 2 diabetic female presents to the office with constipation, weakness, and light-headedness when standing. The patient has been taking milk of magnesia four times daily for the past two weeks without much relief in the constipation. When reviewing the chart, it is noted that the patient has significant renal insufficiency related to the diabetes. What is the most likely laboratory abnormality?

    (A) hypophosphatemia
    (B) hypokalemia
    (C) hypermagnesemia
    (D) hypercalcemia

35. Which of the following medications requires monitoring of liver function tests every 2 months for the first year of usage and periodically thereafter?

    (A) rosiglitazone
    (B) glyburide
    (C) metformin
    (D) acarbose

36. A patient develops a case of hypopituitarism with no known cause. Which of the following serum levels is pertinent to finding the etiology?

    (A) calcium
    (B) copper
    (C) ferritin
    (D) magnesium

37. A 15-year-old female with type 1 diabetes is at home lying on the couch watching television. She becomes drowsy, shaky, weak, and sweaty. Her blood sugar is noted to be 45 mg/dL. Her mother administers 4 ounces of orange juice and rechecks her blood sugar 10 min later. Her blood sugar is 50 mg/dL. What would be the best choice to give her now?

    (A) peanut butter and jelly sandwich
    (B) cola beverage
    (C) crackers and cheese
    (D) banana or other fruit

38. Which of the following drugs can cause syndrome of inappropriate antidiuretic hormone (SIADH)?

    (A) carbamazepine
    (B) colesevelam
    (C) glyburide
    (D) lithium carbonate
    (E) metoprolol

39. A 30-year-old patient presents 2 months post-thyroidectomy. The patient has had symptoms of increased irritability, muscle spasms, and hair loss for the past month. On physical exam there is a positive Chovstek's sign. Which of the following is the most likely diagnosis?

(A) hypothyroidism
(B) hypopituitarism
(C) hypoparathyroidism
(D) hypogonadism

40. A 45-year-old patient presents 2 days postoperatively a partial thyroidectomy. She has been experiencing vomiting with diarrhea. On physical exam, temperature is 101°F and there is noted jaundice. Her heart rate is irregularly, irregular with a rate of 200. What would be the most appropriate pharmacological intervention?

(A) radioactive iodine (131I)
(B) propranolol 80 mg
(C) PTU 600 mg
(D) iopanoic acid 500 mg

41. A 40-year-old obese woman presents for her annual physical exam. A fasting blood glucose level drawn with her routine laboratory test is 130 mg/dL. In order to confirm the diagnosis of diabetes mellitus, what would be the most appropriate next step?

(A) glycated hemoglobin
(B) 3-hour glucose tolerance test
(C) repeat fasting blood glucose
(D) insulin level

42. A 38-year-old male presents to the emergency department experiencing a severe headache and heart palpitations. He appears to be perspiring heavily and anxious. On exam, he is tachycardic and blood pressure is 158/102. His urine catacholamines are increased. If imaging is performed on this patient, where would a mass lesion most likely be found?

(A) pituitary gland
(B) liver
(C) adrenal gland
(D) testicle
(E) kidney

43. A 28-year-old female is being treated for hypothyroidism with 200 μg of levothyroxine daily. At a periodic dosage reassessment, her TSH was suppressed at 0.08 mU/L and she is symptomatic. What is the appropriate course of action?

(A) increase her levothyroxine dose
(B) decrease her levothyroxine dose
(C) no change to her levothyroxine dose
(D) change her medication to PTU

44. A 35-year-old man presents with difficulty concentrating, easy bruisability, and increased headaches for the past 6 months. He says his arms and legs feel weak. On exam, his blood pressure is 160/100, he has a "buffalo hump," and striae on the abdomen. When examining the patient for an ectopic cause of his symptoms, which of the following would be the most likely area to find the source?

(A) abdomen
(B) pelvis
(C) neck
(D) chest

45. A 38-year-old man presents to the office following a health fair screening of his cholesterol because he was told that it is high. He watches his diet, plays tennis, exercises three to five times a week, and appears in good physical condition. He is a nonsmoker, and has no family history of cardiovascular disease. His blood pressure today is 106/72. His lipid profile is total cholesterol 202 mg/dL, HDL 65 mg/dL, LDL 128 mg/dL, and triglycerides 145 mg/dL. Following a review of this patient's profile, which of the following would you recommend?

(A) prescribe gemfibrozil
(B) prescribe HMG CoA reductase inhibitor
(C) prescribe low-dose niacin and slowly increase to achieve 3 g daily
(D) give diet education and continued exercise program

46. A 65-year-old woman presents to the office with decreased hearing and pain over her sternum, pelvis, and her right tibial tubercle. On x-ray, the involved bones are expanded and denser than normal. Her serum calcium and phosphorus are normal, but serum alkaline phosphatase is markedly elevated. Which of the following would be appropriate initial treatment for this patient?

    (A) ibuprofen 600 mg by mouth every 6 hours
    (B) indomethacin 25 mg by mouth three times daily
    (C) meclizine 25 mg by mouth three times daily
    (D) methotrexate 7.5 mg by mouth daily
    (E) tiludronate 400 mg by mouth daily

47. An 8-year-old boy is being evaluated for short stature. His mother reports that he has begun to gain a bit of weight over the last year, has little or no energy, sleeps more than normal, and complains of being cold all of the time. His growth curve demonstrates that he has fallen from the 50th percentile for height to the 5th percentile for height, but his weight has increased to the 90th percentile for height. On physical exam, he is obese, has immature facies, thin hair, and slow reflexes. Based on these clinical symptoms, what is the most likely test to diagnose this child's condition?

    (A) Epstein-Barr virus titers
    (B) thyroid function tests
    (C) IGF-1
    (D) bone age
    (E) somatomedin C level

48. You are treating a 60-year-old man with a history of angina. He has been on the therapeutic lifestyle change (TLC) diet for 12 weeks (with solid effort). This patient has no other medical conditions and takes nitroglycerine as needed and daily enteric-coated aspirin. His fasting lipid panel from last week demonstrates the following:

    total cholesterol – 295 mg/dL
    low density lipoproteins – 145mg/dL
    high density lipoproteins – 48 mg/dL

    What is the most appropriate treatment at this time?

    (A) prescribe colestipol
    (B) prescribe ezetimibe
    (C) prescribe lovastatin
    (D) prescribe niacin
    (E) no pharmacological treatment

49. A 30-year-old woman presents to the office with polyuria, fatigue, and a chronic white vaginal discharge with vaginal pruritis. The discharge has been off and on for the past 6 months with recurrent treatment failures. Which of the following is the most likely diagnosis?

    (A) type 1 diabetes mellitus
    (B) type 2 diabetes mellitus
    (C) hyperthyroidism
    (D) hypothyroidism
    (E) diabetes insipidus

50. Which of the following medications increases both the secretion of prolactin and GH?

    (A) amantadine HCL (Symmetrel)
    (B) bromocriptine (Parlodel)
    (C) apomorphine HCL (Apokyn)
    (D) estradiol (Estrace)

Answers and Explanations

1. **(A); 2. (B); 3. (A); 4. (C); 5. (B)** The anterior pituitary produces the following six major hormones: prolactin, GH, adrenocorticotropin-releasing hormone (ACTH), LH, FSH, and TSH. Two posterior pituitary hormones are oxytocin and antidiuretic hormone. Known hypothalamic hormones include corticotrophin- releasing hormone, thyrotropin-releasing hormone, GH releasing hormone, somatostatin, gonadotropin releasing hormone, and dopamine. (*Kasper et al, 2004, pp. 2019–2024*)

6. **(C)** Metabolic syndrome is found in approximately 25% of Americans. It is defined as three of more of the following findings: waist circumference of >102 cm in men or >88 cm in women; serum triglyceride level of at least 150 mg/dL, HDL level of <40 mg/dL in men or <50 mg/dL in women; blood pressure of at least 130/85 mm Hg; and serum glucose level of at least 110 mg/dL. (*Tierney et al, 2004, p. 1213*)

7. **(C)** This patient is suffering from Graves' disease. Her symptoms are consistent with a hyperthyroid state. Based upon her physical exam, Graves' disease is the most likely diagnosis due to the specific associated eye findings of thyroid-associated ophthalmopathy. The lab findings of low TSH and elevated free and total thyroid hormone levels are also consistent with the diagnosis. (*Kasper et al, 2004, pp. 2069–2073*)

8. **(D)** Since this child was diagnosed 1 year prior the likelihood of retinopathy, nephropathy, or neuropathies are highly unlikely. Other endocrinopathies are more likely to be found and therefore a TSH is recommended annually. (*Hay et al, 2005, p. 983*)

9. **(C)** This patient likely has Addison's disease, a disorder caused by destruction or dysfunction of the adrenal cortices. Addison's disease can present with numerous signs and symptoms, including hypotension, abdominal pain, hyperkalemia, and weakness. The patient is at risk for Addison's due to administration of heparin, which can cause an adrenal infarct or hemorrhage. (*Tierney et al, 2004, pp. 1129–1130*)

10. **(A)** Type 2 diabetes mellitus is a coronary heart disease risk equivalent condition. The LDL goal for these patients is <100 mg/dL. (*Tierney et al, 2004, pp. 1203–1209*)

11. **(E)** This patient's symptoms and labs are consistent with diabetes insipidus. This condition results from a deficiency of antidiuretic hormone causing polyuria and polydipsia. (*Tierney et al, 2004, pp. 1077–1079*)

12. **(B)** This patient's signs and symptoms are consistent with hypothyroidism. Treatment of choice is levothyroxine which is partially converted in the body to T3. Significant increases are seen within 1 to 2 weeks with maximum levels reached in 3 to 4 weeks. (*Tierney et al, 2004, pp. 1098–1101*)

13. **(C)** This patient's signs and symptoms are consistent with acromegaly, which is caused

by an increased secretion of GH. These are almost always caused by pituitary macroadenomas. The tumors may be locally invasive into the cavernous sinus but are typically not malignant. (*Tierney et al, 2004, pp. 1079–1081*)

14. **(D)** Insulin glargine is a form of insulin that lasts for up to 24 hours and is routinely given once daily at bedtime. (*Tierney et al, 2004, p. 1182*)

15. **(E)** This is subacute, painful thyroiditis. This is a self-limiting disorder that at most requires symptomatic therapy. In mild cases, analgesics are sufficient. Prednisone may bring more relief if needed. (*Kasper et al, 2004, p. 2074*)

16. **(D)** This patient has signs and symptoms of diabetic gastroparesis. Smaller meals that are more frequent and also high in fiber and low in fat sometimes improve symptoms. The best choice of the medications listed is metoclopramide 10 mg prior to each meal. This helps facilitate gastric emptying. H2 blockers (ranitidine) and proton pump inhibitors (omeprazole) do not improve gastric emptying. Cisapride is generally not available in the United States due to its side-effect profile and can only be prescribed in special circumstances. (*Kasper et al, 2004, p. 2166*)

17. **(A)** The most common cause of hypercalcemia in an ambulatory patient is a primary hyperparathyroid condition. These include parathyroid adenomas and parathyroid malignancies. Both of these account for 90% of the causes of hypercalcemia. Renal insufficiency, malabsorption, and multiple myeloma are all causes of elevated calcium but they are all secondary causes. (*Tierney et al, 2004, pp. 850, 851*)

18. **(D)** Hashimoto's thyroiditis is an autoimmune disorder of the thyroid gland. This condition causes hypothyroidism. On physical exam a goiter may be palpated. In order to distinguish this from other conditions laboratory and diagnostic studies should be done. When an ultrasound is performed, it will show diffuse heterogeneous enlargement of the gland

and not a solitary or multinodular gland. (*Kasper et al, 2004, pp. 2110–2111*)

19. **(B)** The newer sulfonylurea agents bind more specifically to the pancreatic B cells. Therefore, glyburide has a high affinity for specific receptors on the surface of the pancreatic B cells. (*Tierney et al, 2004, pp. 1169, 1170*)

20. **(D)** This patient's signs and symptoms are consistent with Graves' disease. The pathogenesis of Graves' disease involves the formation of autoantibodies that bind to TSH receptors causing the gland to hyperfunction. The disease is often associated with a personal or family history of autoimmune disorders. (*Kasper et al, 2004, pp. 2069–2073*)

21. **(D)** HMG CoA reductase inhibitors (statins) are the preferred initial choice for treatment of dyslipidemia in diabetic patients. (*Tierney et al, 2004, pp. 1211–1213*)

22. **(B)** This patient's symptoms are consistent with Addisonian crisis. Immediate treatment with 100 to 300 mg of IV hydrocortisone is indicated. (*Tierney et al, 2004, pp. 1128–1129*)

23. **(A)** Metformin is the most likely cause of acute renal failure following the administration of any radiocontrast agent. (*Tierney et al, 2004, pp. 1173*)

24. **(A)** In nonpregnant patients PTU and methimazole are the drugs of choice for the management of Graves' disease. During pregnancy PTU has a lower incidence of crossing the placental barrier than methimazole. It also is excreted into breast milk to a lesser degree than methimazole. Propranolol will help with the symptoms of Graves' but not treat it. It can also cause low birth rate in the infant. RAI is contraindicated in pregnancy. Levothyroxine will worsen a Graves' patient's hyperthyroidism. (*Goldman et al, 2003, pp. 1398–1401*)

25. **(B)** A hypergylcemic hyperosmolar state is characterized by dehydration, significant hyperglycemia, and an elevated serum osmolality with an insignifcant or negative ketosis.

Because of the lack of ketosis, the patient may present with a gradual onset of symptoms and it can go unnoticed until the dehydration becomes more severe than in ketoacidosis. (*Tierney et al, 2004, pp. 1194–1195*)

26. **(B)** Metformin is considered a "euglycemic" or "antihyperglycemic" drug because it does not cause a hypoglycemic reaction at therapeutic levels. (*Tierney et al, 2004, p. 1173*)

27. **(C)** The patient has described the Somogyi effect. This effect occurs because the patient is receiving too much intermediate insulin at dinnertime. Either the intermediate insulin dosage can be shifted to a lower dosage at bedtime or the patient can eat a larger snack at bedtime. (*Tierney et al, 2004, p. 1183*)

28. **(A)** This patient is presenting with short stature. The initial step in evaluation of this patient is to determine if between normal variants or pathological conditions affecting growth. The study to help determine this is a bone age, which is done by bone radiograph of the left wrist and hand. The growth plates are compared with age norms to determine a relative bone age. (*Hay et al, 2005, pp. 963–970*)

29. **(A)** Amiodarone is type II antiarrhythmic agent that is structurally similar to thyroid hormone. It may inhibit deiodinase activity, and its metabolites function as weak antagonist of thyroid hormone action. The drug may have multiple effects on thyroid function including hyper or hypothyroidism in certain populations. (*Kasper et al, 2004, pp. 2075–2076*)

30. **(C)** This patient's symptoms and labs are consistent with diabetes insipidus. This patient needs further evaluation to determine which type of diabetes insipidus is present prior to beginning treatment. (*Kasper et al, 2004, pp. 2055–2057*)

31. **(D)** Recommendations of the National Cholesterol Education Program (NCEP) Adult Treatment Panel III Report states that the LDL goal for patients with 0-1 risk factor to be <160 mg/dL. (*Tierney et al, 2004, p. 1209*)

32. **(C)** This patient is displaying symptoms of hypothyroidism. The most appropriate tests to differentiate the cause for this are free T4 and TSH. Serum T3 is not a sensitive test for hypothyroidism. (*Tierney et al, 2004, pp. 1098–1099*)

33. **(D)** This patient's symptoms are consistent with a pituitary adenoma. Prolactinomas account for about half of all functioning pituitary tumors and may secrete PRL, GH, and ACTH. (*Kasper et al, 2004, pp. 2038–2040*)

34. **(C)** Hypermagnesemia can occur when a patient with renal insufficiency ingests drugs containing magnesium. Physical exam findings include muscle weakness and neurological changes such as confusion and decreased deep tendon reflexes. Serum phosphate and potassium are usually elevated and serum calcium levels are low. (*Tierney et al, 2004, p. 856*)

35. **(A)** Rosiglitazone is in the thiazolidinediones class of drugs. The first medication produced in this class was troglitazone and it was removed from the market due to liver failure and deaths related to its usage. None of the newer drugs in this class have shown to be hepatotoxic but the FDA has recommended that even with a mildly elevated ALT, caution should be used when starting a patient on one of these agents. (*Tierney et al, 2004, p. 1175*)

36. **(C)** The correct answer is a ferritin level. Hemochromatosis is the most likely cause of hypopituitarism when there is no other known cause. (*Tierney et al, 2004, p. 1075*)

37. **(B)** The best choice of food for her is a liquid. Since it has been 10 min and her blood sugar remains below 60 mg/dL it is recommended that she receive liquids. Once the blood sugar is over 60, solid foods can be given. (*Hay et al, 2005, p. 983*)

38. **(A)** Of all the drugs listed carbamazepine is the only one known to potentially cause SIADH. Lithium carbonate can cause diabetes insipidus. The other drugs listed do not cause SIADH. (*Tierney et al, 2004, p. 841*)

39. (C) Hypoparathyroidism commonly presents following thyroidectomy surgery. This patient has classic signs and symptoms of a low calcium and hypoparathyroidism. Chovestek's sign is a physical exam finding that is positive after tapping in front of the ear in the facial nerve region. When doing this, the muscle contracts. When the calcium is low this occurs. Hypothyroidism can occur following a thyroidectomy but the symptoms are not the same. (*Tierney et al, 2004, p. 1114*)

40. (C) This patient is in a thyrotoxic crisis or thyroid storm. She needs to be admitted for monitoring and supportive care. The initial treatment would be PTU 600 mg loading dose followed by 200 to 300 mg every 6 hours given either by an NG or rectally. (*Kasper et al, 2004, p. 2117*)

41. (C) Diabetes mellitus is confirmed by a fasting serum glucose >126 mg/dL on more than one occasion. Repeating a fasting serum glucose would be the next best step to confirm diabetes in this patient. (*Tierney et al, 2004, p. 1157*)

42. (C) Pheochromocytomas produce, store and secrete catecholamines. They are usually derived from the adrenal medulla, although they may be found in other locations. (*Tierney et al, 2004, pp. 1138–1139*)

43. (B) It is important to perform regular periodic dosage reassessments for patients with hypothyroidism. Suppressed TSH levels (<0.1 mU/L) may indicate over-replacement with levothyroxine. The dosage should be reduced. (*Tierney et al, 2004, p. 1101*)

44. (D) Glucocorticoid excess secondary to pituitary ACTH hypersecretion is called Cushing's syndrome. Cushing's syndrome has numerous etiologies. More than 90% of ectopic secreting tumors are found in the chest and the most common of these is the bronchial carcinoid. (*Goldman et al, 2003, p. 1414*)

45. (D) Analysis using the Framingham criteria places this patient at a 2% 10-year risk. This patient does not need any further treatment at this time. (*Tierney et al, 2004, pp. 1206–1210*)

46. (E) This patient signs and symptoms are consistent with Paget's disease of bone. Biphosphates have become the treatment of choice for this disease. Tiludronate, taken orally for 3 months, is very effective in treatment of this disease. (*Tierney et al, 2004, pp. 1126–1127*)

47. (B) This patient's signs and symptoms are consistent with juvenile hypothyroidism. Growth changes of this disorder include short stature, infantile skeletal proportions, infantile facies, delayed epiphyseal development and retarded dental eruption. Treatment of acquired hypothyroidism does not guarantee predicted adult height. (*Hay et al, 2005, pp. 974–975*)

48. (C) This patient's coronary heart disease risk factors and failed TLC diet warrant pharmacological treatment based on his LDL level. Although there are no absolute guidelines for selection of lipid-modifying medications, an HMG CoA reductase inhibitor is preferred. (*Tierney et al, 2004, pp. 1210–1213*)

49. (B) Polyuria, polydipsia, and fatigue are all findings that can be consistent with both type 1 and type 2 diabetes. Any woman who presents with a chronic vaginal discharge or chronic vaginal pruritis should be screened for type 2 diabetes. (*Tierney et al, 2004, p. 1161*)

50. (D) Estrogen increases both the secretion of prolactin and GH. All of the other medications have an affect on either prolactin or GH but not both. (*DeCherney, et al, 2003, p. 152*)

REFERENCES

DeCherney A, Nathan L. *Current Obstetric & Gynecologic Diagnosis and Treatment*, 9th ed. New York: McGraw-Hill; 2003.

Ferri, F. *Practical Guide to the Care of the Medical Patient*, 5th ed. St. Louis, MS: Mosby; 2001.

Goldman L and Ausiello D. *Cecil Textbook of Medicine*, 22nd ed. Philadephia, PA: W.B. Saunders; 2003.

Hay WW, Levin MJ, Sondheimer JM and Deterding RR. *Current Pediatric Diagnosis and Treatment*, 17th ed. New York: McGraw-Hill; 2005.

Kasper DL, Braunwald E, Fauci A, Hauser S, Longo D and Jameson JL. *Harrison's Principles of Internal Medicine*, 16th ed. New York: McGraw-Hill; 2004.

Tierney LM, McPhee SJ and Papadakis MA. *Current Medical Diagnosis and Treatment, 2005*, 44th ed. New York: McGraw-Hill; 2004.

CHAPTER 5

Gastroenterology
Questions

Nancy Ivansek, MA, PA-C, and Anthony A. Miller, MEd, PA-C

DIRECTIONS: (Questions 1 through 50) Each of the numbered items or incomplete statements is followed by answers or by completions of the statement. Select the ONE lettered answer or completion that is BEST in each case.

Questions 1 through 50

1. Diffuse yellowish pseudomembraneous plaques found on colonoscopy are characteristic of which infectious agent?

    (A) *Clostridium difficile*
    (B) *Shigella*
    (C) *Salmonella*
    (D) *Heliobacter pylori*
    (E) *Yersinia*

2. Patients with chronic gastroesophageal reflux (GERD) are at risk for

    (A) candidal esophagitis
    (B) Zenker's diverticulum
    (C) Barrett's esophagus
    (D) Esophageal varices

3. Hepatitis D infection requires coinfection with

    (A) hepatitis A
    (B) hepatitis B
    (C) hepatitis C
    (D) hepatitis E
    (E) hepatitis G

4. The most common anal–rectal problem affecting patients over the age of 50 is

    (A) infected pilonidal cyst
    (B) fissures
    (C) perirectal abscess
    (D) hemorrhoids
    (E) anorectal carcinoma

5. Predictive factors of duodenal ulcer disease recurrence include

    (A) intensity of symptoms, onset of disease over age 50, and family history of ulcer disease
    (B) hospitalization with initial disease, failure of H_2 blockers to relieve symptoms, and male gender
    (C) cigarette smoking, earlier disease onset (under age 40), and evidence of duodenal scarring or erosions
    (D) female gender, onset of disease over age 60, and a high-fat diet
    (E) female gender, need for more than one medication to control disease

6. Hyperparathyroidism is associated with which of the following causes of acute abdominal pain?

    (A) duodenal ulcers
    (B) cholelithiasis
    (C) small bowel obstruction
    (D) acute pancreatitis
    (E) diverticulitis

7. Which of the following conditions is associated with perifollicular hemorrhages, ecchymoses of legs, bleeding gums, loose teeth, and gastrointestinal (GI) bleeding?

   (A) Peutz–Jeghers syndrome
   (B) Rendu–Osler–Weber
   (C) scurvy
   (D) neurofibromatosis
   (E) Blue-Rubber-Bleb Nevus

8. A patient has chronic hepatitis C infection; which of the following medical conditions would be considered a contraindication to starting a patient with chronic hepatitis C infection on interferon?

   (A) hypertension
   (B) hyperlipedemia
   (C) diabetes
   (D) migraine headaches
   (E) lupus

9. Which of the following syndromes is characterized by melanin spots on the lips, buccal mucosa, and tongue along with bleeding polypoid lesions in the small intestines?

   (A) Peutz–Jeghers syndrome
   (B) Rendu–Osler–Weber
   (C) blue-rubber-bleb nevus
   (D) neurofibromatosis
   (E) scurvy

10. Smoking, a high-fat diet and industrial exposure to coal tar products are all risk factors for what type of cancer?

    (A) liver
    (B) duodenal
    (C) stomach
    (D) pancreatic
    (E) gall bladder

11. A middle-aged female who is not taking any medications, has elevated cholestatic liver enzymes, does not drink alcohol and does not complain of abdominal pain. She has not had any previous biliary tract surgery. She is most likely to have which of the following medical conditions

    (A) primary biliary cirrhosis
    (B) pancreatitis
    (C) cholecystitis
    (D) fatty liver
    (E) primary sclerosing cholangitis

12. The most common cause of parasitic gastroenteritis in the United States is

    (A) *Cryptosporidium parvum*
    (B) *Giardia lamblia*
    (C) *Isospora belli*
    (D) *Entamoeba histolytica*
    (E) *Enterobius vermicularis* (pinworm)

13. *Y. enterocolica*, Rotavirus, and Norwalk agent are most likely to cause diarrhea during which season of the year?

    (A) Summer
    (B) Autumn
    (C) Winter
    (D) Spring
    (E) no seasonal variation

14. A patient has had problems with prolonged diarrhea. Stool cultures grow out cryptosporidium. It is important to

    (A) test the patient for HIV
    (B) check family members for the organism
    (C) perform a colonoscopy
    (D) perform blood cultures
    (E) isolate the patient

15. Which of the following best describes hepatitis C (HCV)?

    (A) the incubation period is 14 days to 6 months

    (B) hepatitis C and D infections must be acquired simultaneously

    (C) less likely than hepatitis B to cause chronic hepatitis

    (D) a DNA virus with simlarities to rotovirus

    (E) insidious onset but the symptoms are usually debilitating

16. A patient presents with weakness, myalgias, nausea, vomiting, distorted taste, abdominal pain, and diarrhea. She is also salivating a great deal. She recently had dinner at an oyster bar. The patient's problems are most likely to be caused by ingestion of which of the following agents?

    (A) cadmium

    (B) hepatitis A virus

    (C) salmonella

    (D) zinc

    (E) Giardia

17. CT findings consistent with acute diverticulitis include

    (A) pericolic and regional lymphadenopathy

    (B) a large asymmetrical or eccentrically placed mass

    (C) diverticula, soft tissue inflammation of the pericolic fat and colon wall thickening

    (D) thinning of the colon wall

18. The Dietary Guidelines for Americians 2005 recommends 2 to 3 servings of protein per day. A 3 oz serving of lean meat is about the size of a

    (A) checkbook

    (B) deck of cards

    (C) paperback book

    (D) matchbook

    (E) legal envelope

19. More than 50% of cases of pill-induced esophogitis result from the use of which of the following agents?

    (A) augmentum

    (B) ibuprophin

    (C) tetracyline

    (D) multivitamins

    (E) ciprofloxin

20. The most common malignant tumor of the esophagus in the African American male population is

    (A) adenocarcinoma

    (B) leiomyoma

    (C) small cell carcinoma

    (D) squamous cell carcinoma

    (E) granular cell tumor

21. In Western society, diverticulosis most often occurs in which portion of the colon?

    (A) transverse

    (B) sigmoid

    (C) descending

    (D) ascending

    (E) equally common in all parts of the colon

22. Which of the following best describes hepatitis D?

    (A) the incubation period is similar to that for hepatitis A

    (B) hepatitis B and D infections cannot be acquired simultaneously

    (C) there are no clinical laboratory test available for testing for hepatitis D

    (D) the clinical course of hepatitis D is similar of that of hepatitis A

    (E) hepatitis D is being recognized with increasing frequency in the United States

23. Sibutramine (Meridia) is currently recommended by the National Institutes of Health for the Treatment of obesity. Using Body Mass Index (BMI) figures, which group would fall into the appropriate treatment category?

    (A) BMI of 15
    (B) BMI of 20
    (C) BMI of 25
    (D) BMI of 27
    (E) BMI of 30

24. The examiner must listen for at least how many minutes before stating that the bowel sounds are absent if they are not initially audible?

    (A) 1
    (B) 2
    (C) 3
    (D) 4
    (E) 5

25. Which of the following statements concerning gastroesophageal reflux (GERD) is NOT true?

    (A) may cause asthma or chronic cough
    (B) behavioral interventions include weight loss and eating smaller meals
    (C) mild to moderate symptoms are treated with H_2-receptor agonists (e.g. ranitidine or cimetidine) or proton pump inhibitors
    (D) barium esophagography is recommended for most patients

26. In addition to discontinuation of drinking alcohol, what else is recommended for the treatment of alcoholic cirrhosis?

    (A) 1 mg of folic acid per day and supportive measures for iron and electrolyte deficiencies
    (B) high-dose glucocorticoid steroid therapy
    (C) portacaval shunting procedure
    (D) high-dose glucocorticoid and interferon therapy
    (E) D-penicillamine therapy

27. An endoscopy should be performed if a patient does not respond or does not adequately respond to proton pump inhibitors (PPIs) after how many month(s)?

    (A) 24
    (B) 12
    (C) 6
    (D) 3
    (E) 1

28. A syndrome characterized by marked hypergastrinemia, gastric hypersecretion, and peptic ulceration, as well as an associated gastrin-producing tumor in the pancreas, is known as?

    (A) insulinoma
    (B) cystadenocarcinoma
    (C) Verner–Morrison
    (D) Zollinger–Ellison
    (E) glucagonoma

29. A 62-year-old male presents to the emergency room complaining of colicky abdominal pain, nausea, and vomiting. The abdomen is distended. There is tympany, and decreased bowel sounds are noted on exam. A large, tender irreducible hernia is found in the right groin. The correct diagnosis is

    (A) indirect inguinal hernia
    (B) direct inguinal hernia
    (C) incarcerated hernia
    (D) strangulated hernia
    (E) ventral hernia

30. What is the most common drug to cause acute liver failure?

    (A) alcohol
    (B) ketoconazole
    (C) lisinopril
    (D) acetaminophen
    (E) methotrexate

31. Which of the following is the most specfic test for diagnosing celiac sprue?

    (A) checking stool for steatorrhea
    (B) barrium enema
    (C) intestinal biopsy
    (D) reticulin antibodies
    (E) food challenge

32. Mrs. Jones was found to have colorectal cancer. Her colonoscopy was negative preoperatively. Her surgery was felt to be curative. She should have subsequent surveillance exams every

    (A) 1 year
    (B) 2 years
    (C) 3 years
    (D) 5 years
    (E) 10 years

33. A mucosal tear of the gastroesophageal junction is known as

    (A) Boerhaave's syndrome
    (B) Plummer–Vinson
    (C) Paterson–Kelly
    (D) Mallory–Weiss
    (E) fissure

34. In contrast to the 2000 edition, the Dietery Guidelines for Americans 2005 recommends

    (A) discouraging the consumption of dairy products
    (B) consuming nearly double the previous amount of fruits and vegtables
    (C) following a high-protein diet
    (D) 30 minutes of exercise each day to lose weight
    (E) follow the serving recommendations of the food pyramid and not counting calories

35. The treatment of choice for diarrhea caused by Giardia is

    (A) erythromycin
    (B) tetracycline
    (C) quinolones
    (D) metronidazole
    (E) ampicillin

36. The incubation period for hepatitis B is

    (A) 3 to 10 days
    (B) 10 to 30 days
    (C) 3 to 180 days
    (D) 30 to 90 days
    (E) 90 to 180 days

37. Having a patient stand straight kneed then raise from the flat foot, up on to their toes and drop down on to their heels, is a test used to evaluate patients with abdominal pain. It is known as

    (A) rebound tenderness
    (B) Blumberg sign
    (C) Markle sign
    (D) succussion splash
    (E) Kernig's sign

38. Which of the following factors places an individual at risk for squamous cell cancer of the esophogus?

    (A) tobacco smoking
    (B) lye ingestion
    (C) achalasia
    (D) excessive alcohol ingestion
    (E) GERD

39. Pellagra is the result of what vitamin deficiency?

    (A) thiamine
    (B) vitamin K
    (C) riboflavin
    (D) niacin
    (E) pyridoxine

40. An elderly patient is brought in to the ER complaining of incontinence of liquid "like tea water" stool. He is complaining of rectal pressure and lower abdominal pain. The pain is cramping in quality and the patient's abdomen is "bloated." Digital rectal exam reveals hard stool in the rectum. Which of the following should be selected as the initial treatment for this patient?

    (A) passing a nasogastric tube
    (B) soapsuds enema
    (C) milk of magnesia
    (D) administration of opiate analgesics for pain
    (E) manual disimpaction

41. The best diagnostic modality to diagnose gallstones is

    (A) CT scan of the abdomen
    (B) ultrasound of the abdomen
    (C) oral cholecystogram
    (D) KUB
    (E) positron emission tomography (PET) scan

42. Cullen's sign is associated with

    (A) diastasis recti
    (B) umbilical calculi
    (C) umbilical fistula
    (D) umbilical hernia
    (E) retroperitneal bleeding

43. Which of the following descriptions most accurately describes heartburn?

    (A) mechanical sensation that something is coming up the esophogus
    (B) discomfort between the umbilicus any xiphoid
    (C) crushing chest pain that radiates to the neck
    (D) a constant anterior chest discomfort

44. Common GI symptoms of hypercalcemia include

    (A) diarrhea
    (B) abdominal bloating
    (C) constipation
    (D) greasy stools
    (E) reflux

45. Which of the following vitamins helps increase the absorption of calcium in the GI tract?

    (A) A
    (B) B
    (C) C
    (D) D
    (E) E

46. Risk factors that remain important clues in the diagnosis of *C. difficile* include

    (A) patients of advanced age and comordid conditions such as diabetes
    (B) diabetes with a history of antibiotic use within the past year
    (C) travel to Third World nations
    (D) antibiotic use or a hospital stay within the past 3 months
    (E) attending a daycare or preschool center

47. The 2005 Dietary Guidelines for Americans recommends sensible and moderate alcohol intake for those who choose to drink, which translates to

    (A) 1 drink per month for women and 2 drinks per month for men
    (B) 1 drink a week for women and 2 drinks per week for men
    (C) 1 drink per day for women and 2 drinks per day for men
    (D) 5 drinks per day for both men and women
    (E) current guidelines suggest abstaining from alcohol completely

48. A 45-year-old patient presents with a pruritic papulovesicular rash on her extensor surfaces of the arms and legs, trunk and neck. A diagnosis of dermatitis herpetiformis is made. Which GI disorder is associated with this rash?

(A) irritable bowel syndrome

(B) celiac disease

(C) pancreatitis

(D) diverticulosis

(E) chronic hepatitis

49. Which of the following clinical profiles is consistent with a diagnosis of Whipple's disease?

(A) 40-year-old female, RUQ severe pain related to fatty food ingestion and vomiting

(B) older female, LLQ pain and mass, and fever

(C) 50-year-old male, fever, arthritis, and malabsorption

(D) 20-year-old male, abdominal cramps, frequent bloody diarrhea and anemia

50. Which of the following is more likely to be associated with ulcerative colitis versus Crohn's disease?

(A) more common in smokers

(B) small bowel involvement

(C) associated with perianal disease

(D) bloody diarrhea

Answers and Explanations

1. **(A)** All of the infectious agents listed may result in the presence of inflammatory changes on colonoscopy. *C. difficile* is the organism that will produce diffuse yellowish pseudomembranous plaques on colonoscopy exam. (*Schiller, 2006, p. 295*)

2. **(C)** Patients with chronic GERD are at risk for Barrett's esophagus which is a metaplasia linked to chronic reflux-induced injury to the squamous epithelium. It may lead to esophageal adenocarcinoma. Therefore screening endoscopy may be recommended. Candidal esophagitis is likely to be found in immunosuppressed patients, uncontrolled diabetics and those being treated with systemic steroids or antibiotics. A Zenker's diverticulum is a protrusion of the pharyngeal mucosa that develops at pharyngoesophageal junction. Symptoms include dysphagia and regurgitation. It is not a complication of GERD. Esophageal varices develop in patients secondary to portal hypertension. They are associated with cirrhosis and may result in serious upper gastrointestinal bleeding. (*Tierney et al, 2006, pp. 565–575*)

3. **(B)** Hepatitis D appears to be a virus infecting a virus. It is a defective RNA virus that can only exist in the presence of hepatitis B. When there is coinfection, the illness produced is more severe than an infection with hepatitis B alone. (*Stoller et al, 2002, p. 672*)

4. **(D)** Hemorrhoids are the most common anal-rectal problem and affect about half of patients over the age of 50. An infected pilonidal cyst or sinus is most common in males between the ages of 16 to 30. Perirectal abscess and fissures may be more problematic in patients with Crohn's disease or immunodeficiency states. Anal-rectal carcinoma is by far a less prevalent anal-rectal problem than hemorrhoids. (*Goroll et al, 1995, p. 373*)

5. **(C)** A risk index has been developed to predict the likelihood of ulcer reoccurrence. Cigarette smoking, alcohol intake, early onset of disease (less than age 40), repeated duodenal ulcers, and endoscopic evidence of duodenal scarring or erosions were additive factors in the prediction of duodenal ulcer recurrence. (*Stoller et al, 2002, p. 731*)

6. **(D)** Hyperparathyroidism can cause acute pancreatitis. It can also disrupt calcium metabolism and cause nephrolithiasis but not cholelithiasis. Acute pancreatitis presents with acute abdominal pain, and other causes of abdominal pain must be kept in the differential and ruled out. (*Hutton, 2005, p. 32*)

7. **(C)** Scurvy is caused by the lack of dietary vitamin C. It will cause perifollicular hemorrhages, ecchymoses of the legs, bleeding gums, loose teeth, and GI bleeding. Melanin spots on the lips, buccal mucosa, and tongue with bleeding polypoid lesions in the small intestines is referred to as Peutz–Jeghers syndrome. Rendu–Osler–Weber is associated with telangectagias on the face and buccal

mucosa and similar lesions in the GI tract. Neurofibromatosis is associated with café au late pigmentation, pedunculated fibromas, and fibromas in the GI tract that may bleed. Rubber-Bleb Nevus syndrome is associated with cavernous hemangiomas of the skin and similar lesion in the small intestines. (*LeBlond et al, 2004, pp. 607–608*)

8. **(E)** Interferon is contraindicated in patients with autoimmune disease. Interferon is also contraindicated in patients with major depressive disorders, cytopenia, hyperthyroidism and renal transplantation. Patients who consume large amounts of ethanol, use injectable drugs or are noncompliant should not be entered into interferon treatment programs. (*Bosker and Thatcher, 2004, p. 202*)

9. **(A)** Melanin spots on the lips, buccal mucosa, and tongue and bleeding polypoid lesions in the small intestines are characteristics of Peutz–Jeghers syndrome. Rendu–Osler–Weber is associated with telangectagias on the face and buccal mucosa and similair lesions in the GI tract. Blue-Rubber-Bleb Nevus syndrome is associated with cavernous hemangiomas of the skin and similar lesion in the small intestestines. Neurofibromatosis is associated with café au late pigmentation with pedunculated fibromas and fibromas in the GI tract that may bleed. (*LeBlond et al, 2004, pp. 607–608*)

10. **(D)** Smoking, a high fat diet and exposure to coal tar products as well as a history of chronic pancreatitis are all risk factors for pancreatic cancer. (*Stoller et al, 2002, p. 706*)

11. **(A)** Primary bilary cirrhosis affects females over the age of 30. Most cases are found when bloodwork is being done for other reasons. Many patients do not have pain, which is more common in cholecystitis or pancreatitis. Primary scelorosing cholangitis is more likely to occur in a patient with known inflammatory bowel disease. (*Stoller et al, 2002, pp. 679–681*)

12. **(B)** *Giardia* is the most common cause of parasitic gastroenteritis in the Unitied States. *Entamoeba histolytica* rarely causes diarrhea in the United States. Both *Cryptosporidium parvum*

and *Isoporabelli* can cause diarrhea in immunocompromised patients. Pinworms will often cause problems with perirectal itching. (*Bosker and Thatcher, 2004, p. 1153*)

13. **(C)** Rotovirus, Norwalk agent, and *Y. enterocolitica* diarrhea are most frequent in Winter months. Enteroviral infections occur more frequently in the Autumn and *C. jejuni*, Salmonella, and *E. coli* occur most commonly in the summer months. (*Bosker and Thatcher, 2004, p. 1148*)

14. **(A)** Cryptosporidium may be indicative of an underlying autoimmune problem. Patients who culture positive, should be checked for HIV. Rarely do patients with intact immune systems have problems with this organism, so checking family members would not be useful. Isolation also is not indicated. Blood cultures and colonoscopy study would not offer increased information with this diagnosis. (*Weinstock and Neides, 2003, p. 62*)

15. **(A)** Hepatitis C is an RNA virus that is similar to flaviviruses. The incubation period is 14 days to 6 months. It is more likely than hepatitis B to become chronic. Coinfection with hepatitis D occurs with hepatitis B, not hepatitis C. (*Stoller et al, 2002, p. 673*)

16. **(A)** Cadmium may be found in seafood as well as grains and peanuts. Ingestion will cause myalgias, bloating, nausea, vomiting, abdominal pain, diarrhea as well as increased salivation. The onset of symptoms is rather rapid; within hours as compared to infections with hepatitis A and Salmonella. The problem is self limiting and the symptoms will abate gradually over hours. Symptoms associated with hepatitis C are rather insidious and do not have such a sudden onset. (*Bosker and Thatcher, 2004, p. 1182*)

17. **(C)** CT findings consistant with diverticulitis include diverticula, soft tissue infiltration of the pericolic fat, colon wall thickening, and pericolic abcesses. In immunosuppressed patients, findings may include intraperitoneal and extraperitoneal gases without fluid or abcess formation. Pericolic and regional

lymphadenopathy along with asymmetrical or eccentrically placed masses are typical of colon cancer. (*Wu and Baker, 2005, p. 624*)

18. **(B)** A deck of cards or a bar of soap is a good way to help a person visualize a 3 oz portion size of lean meat. A match box would be about the size of a 1 oz serving and a thin paperbook would represent an 8 oz serving of lean meat. (*Blackburn and Waltman, 2005, p. 612*)

19. **(C)** More than 50% of cases of pill-induced esophogitis result from tetracyline derivatives. Other commonly prescribed medications causing esophegeal injury include: slow release of potassium chloride, iron sulfate, quinine sulfate, alendronate sodium, and nonsteroidal antiinflammatory drugs. (*Stoller et al, 2002, p. 717*)

20. **(D)** Males are more likely than women to get esophageal cancer. The most common esophageal malignancy in the African American population is squamous cell carcinoma. Risk factors include excessive alcohol and tobacco use. Adenocarcinoma is more common in whites and is thought to be a complication of chronic gastroesophageal reflux. Benign tumors such as leiomyomas are rare. (*Tierney et al, 2006, pp. 573–579*)

21. **(B)** Diverticulosis may arise anywhere in the large intestine, from the cecum to the end of the sigmoid colon. In Western societies, diverticula most often occur in the sigmoid colon where there is greatest interluminal pressure. (*Wu and Baker, 2005, p. 620*)

22. **(E)** Hepatitis D is being recognized with increasing frequency in the United States. It has an incubation period similar to that of hepatitis B. A diagnosis of hepatitis D is made by demonstrating the appearance of the antibody to hepatitis D or anti-HDV. Hepatitis D, or delta hepatitis, is caused by defective RNA and requires the coinfection with hepatitis B to support its replication. Transmission is primarily by sexual contact. (*Tierney et al, 2006, p. 654*)

23. **(E)** Patients with a BMI of 30 or more, would be appropriate for the use of sibutramine (Meridia) for the treatment of their obesity. If a patient has a BMI of 27 and other obesity related risk factors, they would also be an appropriate candidate for use of Meridia. A patient with a BMI of 15 is considered to be under weight. A BMI of 20 is considered to be normal. A BMI of 25, places a patient in an overweight category, but they are not yet considered obese. (*Bosker and Thatcher, 2004, pp. 1216–1217*)

24. **(E)** Bowel sounds may be sparse or soft, so it is important to listen for a full 5 minutes before declaring bowel sounds absent. (*LeBlond et al, 2004, p. 516*)

25. **(D)** Barium esophagography has a limited role in the diagnostic management of patients with GERD. It may be used in patients with severe dysphagia to evaluate the degree of stricture. Asthma, chronic cough, chronic laryngitis, sore throat and atypical chest pain are increasingly being recognized as atypical manifestations of GERD and reflux may be a causative or exacerbating factor. Behavioral interventions such as those mentioned above (B) as well as avoiding bending after meals have a role in the management of GERD as do the H_2-receptor agonists and proton pump inhibitors. (*Tierney et al, 2006, pp. 565–569*)

26. **(A)** Alcoholic cirrhosis requires complete abstinence from further alcoholic intake because prognosis is markedly worsened if one continues to drink. Attention to good nutrition as well as daily multiple vitamin supplementations, which include 1 mg of folic acid and a correction of iron deficiency or electrolyte deficiency, is important. Supportive measures may also be necessary. The search continues for agents that may halt hepatitic fibrosis and promote hepatocyte regeneration. Glucocorticoid steroids and portacoval shunting have failed to demonstrate any improvement in survival rates. Liver transplantation has proven to be a viable option in individuals who have become completely abstinent. Wilson's disease, not alcoholic cirrhosis, is treated with D-penicillamine and chronic active hepatitis may benefit from corticosteroid therapy or interferon-alpha therapy, but it is not

indicated for the treatment of alcoholic cirrhosis. (*Stoller et al, 2002, p. 669*)

27. **(E)** Endoscopy is indicated in patients who either do not respond or do not adequately respond to PPIs at the standard doses after 4 weeks. (*Rao et al, 2005, p. 6*)

28. **(D)** Zollinger–Ellison syndrome is characterized by marked hypergastrinemia and gastric hypersecretion, as well as peptic ulcerations. There is usually an associated gastrin-producing tumor of the pancreas with cells of the nonbeta type. Usually the tumors are in other sites, particularly in the duodenal wall. An insulinoma is a rare islet cell tumor with insulin hypersecretion. A cystadenocarcinoma is a rare pancreatic tumor that arises as a malignant degeneration of a mucous cystoadenoma and presents as upper abdominal pain and a palpable abdominal mass. Verner–Morrison syndrome is associated with non-beta islet cell tumors and endocrine neoplasias. Glucagonoma is a pancreatic alpha cell glucagon-secreting tumor that is very rare but similar to other islet cell tumors. (*LeBlond et al, 2004, pp. 587–589*)

29. **(D)** A strangulated hernia is an irreducible one in which the blood supply to the entrapped bowel loop has been compromised, resulting in small bowel obstruction and infarction. Patients present with colicky abdominal pain, nausea, and vomiting and show signs of small bowel obstruction with distention, tympany, and hyperperistalsis. An irreducible or incarcerated hernia does not necessarily mean the hernia is strangulated. A ventral hernia is a hernia located along the abdominal wall. An indirect inguinal hernia accounts for one half of all hernias in adults; it passes through the internal abdominal inguinal ring along the spermatic cord through the inguinal canal and exits through the external inguinal canal. A direct inguinal hernia passes through the posterior inguinal wall medial to the inferior epigastric vessel through Hesselbach's triangle. (*Bosker and Thatcher, 2004, p. 1501*)

30. **(D)** All of the drugs listed can cause acute liver failure. Drug intoxication, especially with acetaminophen taken in a suicide attempt is the most common cause of acute liver failure. (*Stoller et al, 2002, pp. 691–692*)

31. **(C)** Intestinal biopsy is the most specific test in establishing the diagnosis of celiac sprue. Patients with celiac sprue will experience diarrhea but not steatorrhea. Serologic testing for retculin antibodies is often helpful in screening patients with atypical symptoms or asymptomatic relatives. (*Stoller et al, 2002, pp. 764–765*)

32. **(C)** In patients with colorectal cancer who undergo curative surgery, a repeat colonoscopy should be performed in 3 years. If that study is normal, the schedule should be changed to every 5 years. (*Stoller et al, 2002, p. 741*)

33. **(D)** A mucosal tear of the gastroesophageal junction is known as a Mallory Weiss tear. Paterson–Kelly and (also known as Plummer–Vinson) is a congenital syndrome associated with anemia and webbing of the esophagus. Boerhaave's syndrome is a rare life-threatening problem characterized by a full thickness tear of the esophageal wall. (*Stoller et al, 2002, p. 721*)

34. **(B)** The 2005 dietary guidelines have recommended consuming nearly double the amount of fruits and vegetables as previously recommended. Dairy recommendation is for 2 to 3 servings per day. A balanced diet that counts calories and not the proportion of carbohydrate, fat or protein is recommended. For weight loss, the guidelines recommend 60 to 90 minutes of exercise per day. (*Blackburn and Waltman, 2005, pp. 609–613*)

35. **(D)** The treatment of choice for diarrhea caused by *Giardia* is metronidazole 250 to 750 mg p.o. three times per day. Erythromycin can be used to treat campylobacter. Doxycycline or tetracycline can be used to treat cholera. Quinolones can also be use to treat cholera and shigellosis. (*Weinstock and Neides, 2003, p. 62*)

36. **(C)** The incubation period for hepatitis B is 3 to 180 days. (*Weinstock and Neides, 2003, p. 60*)

37. **(C)** Markle sign is also known as the jar sign and it may prove superior to rebound tenderness as

a localizing sign of peritoneal irritation, especially in the pelvis. It is performed by having the patient go from standing on their toes to dropping quickly down to their heels. When they hit the floor, the location of their abdominal pain should be noted. Blumberg sign is another name for rebound tenderness. It is illicited by pressing the fingers gently into the abdomen then suddenly withdrawing them. The pain will worsen in a certain area when the fingers are taken away. Succession splash refers to air and fluid in the stomach and bowel moving and making audible splashing noise. Kernig's sign is a test for spinal cord irritation. (*LeBlond et al, 2004, pp. 548, 551*)

38. **(D)** Of the factors listed, excessive alcohol ingestion, places an individual at increased risk for squamous cell cancer of the esophogus. (*Cooper and Pappes, 2004, p. 132*)

39. **(D)** Niacin deficiency is known as pellagra. It is rare in the United States and is most often a complication of alcoholism or malabsorption syndrome. Clinical signs of pellagra are known as the 3 D's—dermatitis, diarrhea, and dementia. (*Tierney et al, 2006, pp. 1273–1274*)

40. **(E)** Mechanical bowel obstruction in the rectum does not usually respond to oral laxatives. Soapsuds enemas are also ineffective because the contents cannot be retained. A nasogastric tube would not be used for an obstruction in the distal colon/rectum. One would avoid opiates in fecal impactions and other constipation problems because they tend to be more constipating. This patient needs to be disimpacted. (*Tierney et al, 2006, p. 544*)

41. **(B)** Ultrasound has replaced oral cholecystograms as the test of choice for diagnosing cholelithiasis. CT is useful in the evaluation of the acute abdomen but the sensitivity for viewing the gallstones is poor. KUB is also not a sensitive study for cholelithiasis. PET scan studies are expensive and are not a routine imaging study used for abdominal pain. (*Cooper and Pappes, 2004, p. 132*)

42. **(E)** A faint blue coloration may occur as a result of retroperitoneal bleeding. This is known as Cullen's sign. Diastasis recti occurs when the rectus muscles lack a normal fibrous band that attaches them at the midline. An umbilical calculus is usually the result of poor hygiene. An umbilical hernia will occur when a weakness occurs in the abdominal wall in the area of the umbilicus and a fistula in that area can tract from various organs causing discharge from the umbilicus. (*LeBlond et al, 2004, p. 547*)

43. **(A)** Heartburn is best described in two ways: a burning discomfort centered in the chest that radiates in an upward direction and a mechanical sensation that something is coming up the esophagus. Heartburn is not consistently below the xiphoid and it usually does not spread across the chest, to the neck or to the extremities. It is not associated with activity, nor is it constant in nature. (*Rao et al, 2005, pp. 1, 2*)

44. **(C)** Common GI symptoms associated with hypercalcemia include nausea, vomiting, abdominal pain, constipation, fever, and anorexia. Hypercalcemia with weight loss and anorexia, fever, and lethargy is highly suggestive of a malignancy (*Hutton, 2005, p. 32*)

45. **(D)** Vitamin D increases the absorption of calcium and phosphorus in the GI tract and induces osteoclast activity, which causes an overall increase in serum calcium levels. (*Hutton, 2005, p. 32*)

46. **(D)** Risk factors for the development of *C. difficile* include the use of antibiotics within the past 3 months as well as a hospital or nursing home stay within the past 3 months. Contact with someone who has been hospitalized or in a nursing home in the past 3 months is also a risk factor for *C. difficile* infection (*Schiller, 2006, p. 294*)

47. **(C)** The Dietary Guidelines for America 2005 recommend that those who choose to drink alcoholic beverages should do so in moderation. The guidelines suggest moderation is no more than 1 drink per day for women and 2 drinks per day for men. (*Blackburn and Waltman, 2005, p. 617*)

48. (B) Nearly all patients presenting with dermatitis herpetiformis have histological evidence of celiac disease even if it is not clinically apparent. Less than 10% of patients with celiac disease will also have this dermatologic disorder. Dermatitis herpetiformis is not associated with the other disorders. (*Tierney et al, 2006, p. 602*)

49. (C) Whipple's disease typically occurs in white men in their 4th to 6th decades. It is characterized by seronegative arthritis, fever, lympadenopathy, weight loss, malabsorption, and diarrhea. Whipple's disease is caused by the *Tropheryma whippelii* organism and is diagnosed by polymerase chain reaction (PCR) or endoscopic biopsy of the duodenum. (*Tierney et al, 2006, pp. 603–604*)

50. **(D)** Ulcerative colitis (UC) is an idiopathic inflammatory condition that primarily effects the distal portions of the colon. It is more common in nonsmokers and former smokers and is characterized by bloody diarrhea, lower abdominal cramps, and feacle urgency but the presentation is highly variable and dependent on the severity of disease. It is diagnosed by sigmoidoscopy. Crohn's disease primarily involves the small bowel (terminal ileum) and the proximal ascending colon. It is more common in smokers. Crohn's disease may be associated with perianal disorders (e.g., fistulas), oral ulcers, or other extraintestinal manifestations. The clinical picture is variable but includes intermittent episodes of fever, nonbloody diarrhea, and RLQ pain. (*Tierney et al, 2006, pp. 620–630*)

REFERENCES

Blackburn GL, Waltman BA. Physician's guide to the new 2005 dietary guidelines: How best to counsel patients. *Cleveland Clinic Journal of Medicine* 2005; 72 (7):609–617.

Bosker G, Thatcher S. *Textbook of Primary and Acute Care Medicine.* Atlanta: Thomson American Health Consultants; 2004.

Cooper JAD, Pappes PG. *Cecil's Review of General Internal Medicine.* Philadelphia: Saunders; 2004.

Goroll AH, May LA, Mulley AG. *Primary Care Medicine: Office Evaluation and Management of the Adult Patient.* Philadelphia: Lippincott; 1995.

Hutton E. Evaluation and management of hypercalcemia. *JAAPA* 2005; 18 (6):30–35.

LeBlond RF, DeGowin RL, Brown DD. DeGowin's *Diagnostic Examinination: A Complete Guide to Assessment, Examination and Differential Diagnosis.* New York: McGraw-Hill; 2004.

Rao G, Davis, RH Peura, DA Wright WL. Heartburn Issues in Patient Management. *The Journal of Family Practice (Special Edition)* June 2005; 1–6.

Schiller LR, Clostridium difficile-associated diarrhea: Coming soon to a practice near you. *Consultant* 2006; 46 (3):294–296.

Stoller JK, Muzaffar,A, Longworth DL. *The Cleveland Clinic Intensive Review of Internal Medicine.* Philadelphia: Lippincott; 2002.

Tierney LM, McPhee SJ, Papadakis, M. *2006 Current Medical Diagnosis and Treatment,* 45th ed. New York: McGraw-Hill; 2006.

Weinstock MB, Neides, DM. *The Resident's Guide to Ambulatory Care.* Columbus: Anadem; 2003.

Wu JS, Baker ME. Recognizing and managing acute diverticulitis for the internist. *Cleveland Clinic Journal of Medicine* 2005; 72 (7):620–626.

CHAPTER 6

Hematology/Oncology
Questions

Maura Polansky, MS, PA-C, and Katherine Kennon, MS, PA-C

DIRECTIONS (Questions 1 through 6): Each of the numbered items or incomplete statements in this section is followed by answers or by completions of the statement. select the ONE lettered answer or completion that is BEST in each case.

Questions 1 through 6

1. A 32-year-old African American asymptomatic woman presents to her gynecologist's office for a physical exam. She has no prior medical history. She mentions that she has recently become engaged and that she is aware that her fiancée's family has suffered from sickle cell disease, although he is "healthy." They are planning a honeymoon to the mountains. Which of the following issues would be most appropriate to discuss?

    (A) the risk of infertility for her husband, if he carries the sickle cell gene

    (B) reassure her of the low risk of illness for her children, given her and her future husband's lack of apparent sickle cell disease

    (C) offer to refer her for genetic counseling

    (D) advise against travel to high altitude regions for her husband

    (E) counsel regarding the increased risk of sexually transmitted infections for those with sickle cell trait

2. Which of the following is true of iron deficiency anemia?

    (A) is most commonly due to acute blood loss

    (B) does not frequently occur from the typical American diet

    (C) often occurs in pregnancy due to increased RBC destruction

    (D) should be confirmed by bone marrow aspiration

    (E) requires treatment with long-term iron replacement, typically greater than one year

3. Which of the following are consistent with lead poisoning?

    (A) profound anemia

    (B) severe complaints of mild and persistent muscle weakness

    (C) acute difficulty concentrating, after exposure

    (D) basophilic stippling

    (E) treatment with chelating agent is always required

4. A 48-year-old previously healthy, African American man presents to his local emergency center with acute onset of dyspnea on exertion while mowing the grass. He has no past medical history. Laboratory studies reveal a WBC 6.1, Hgb 5.8, Hct 20.1, mean corpuscle volume (MCV) 68, and platelet (Plt) count 254,000. What diagnosis is most likely the cause of his symptoms?

(A) sickle cell anemia

(B) thalassemia

(C) iron deficiency

(D) hemolytic anemia

(E) TTP

5. Which of the following is true of macrocytic anemias?

(A) causes include poor absorption of vitamin B_{12} in the stomach due to prior gastrectomy

(B) Schilling's test is used to diagnose folate deficiency

(C) folate supplementation should be started empirically to prevent worsening anemia, while further studies are being performed

(D) when associated with loss of taste and atrophy of the tongue mucosa, it suggests vitamin B_{12} deficiency

(E) strict vegetarians are at risk of folate deficiency and may need chronic supplementation

6. One day, while covering the internal medicine floor, you evaluate a patient who was admitted for pneumonia. Upon reviewing the routine laboratory studies ordered for that day, you note that the patient has developed an anemia. The chemistry profile reveals a total bilirubin of 2.6 with an elevated LDH. Potential causes of the anemia and hyperbilirubinemia may include all of the following EXCEPT

(A) malaria

(B) drug use

(C) folate deficiency

(D) recent blood transfusion

(E) disseminated intravascular coagulopathy (DIC)

DIRECTIONS (Questions 7 through 12): Each question in this section consists of five lettered headings followed by several numbered words or phrases. For each word or phrase, choose the ONE lettered heading that is closely associated with it. Each lettered heading may be selected once, more than once, or not at all.

Questions 7 through 12

Match common toxicities of anticancer therapy with the appropriate treatment.

(A) secondary malignancy

(B) peripheral neuropathy

(C) cardiomyopathy

(D) pulmonary fibrosis

(E) DIC

7. cisplatin

8. adriamycin

9. tamoxifen

10. external beam irradiation

11. vincristine

12. bleomycin

DIRECTIONS (Question 13 through 17): Each of the numbered items or incomplete statements in this section is followed by answers or by completions of the statement. Select the ONE lettered answer or completion that is BEST in each case.

Question 13 through 17

13. Which tumor marker may be used in the screening of patients for cancer?

(A) prostatic acid phosphate

(B) carcinoembryonic antigen

(C) cancer antigen 125

(D) alpha-fetoprotein

(E) beta-human chorionic gonadotropin

14. Thalassemia

    (A) is a rare cause of normocytic, nor-mochronic anemia

    (B) is most common in those of European descent

    (C) may result in few problems, except during stress states

    (D) may be diagnosed by peripheral smear

    (E) may be an acquired or hereditary disease

15. A 76-year-old woman presents to the ER after experiencing severe pain in the left hip, worse upon standing or walking. She denies any falls or trauma precipitating the pain. Physical exam reveals enlarged suboccipital and cervical lymph nodes. Electrophoresis studies were positive for serum IgM. Subsequent urinalysis was positive for Bence-Jones proteins. Which of the following would NOT be expected in this patient, given the probable diagnosis?

    (A) hypercalcemia

    (B) anemia

    (C) renal failure

    (D) splenomegaly

    (E) fever

16. A 16-year-old female presented with an enlarged lymph node at the back of her neck. After an ultrasound of the lymph node, she was told that it was "benign." However, another node appeared in the same general region and it was mildly tender. Upon questioning, she stated she does have cats but does not remember being scratched prior to the first enlarged lymph node. The patient was placed on tetracycline without resolution. Her hematocrit is 31.8 and WBC is 152.4 with a differential of 26% neutrophils (normal 48% to 55%), 69% lymphocytes (normal 7% to 33%), 3% monocytes (normal 2% to 7%), 1% eosinophils (normal 1% to 4%), 1% basophils (normal 0% to 1%). Given the patient's age and presentation, the probable diagnosis is

    (A) cat-scratch disease

    (B) chronic myelogenous leukemia (CML)

    (C) chronic lymphocytic leukemia (CLL)

    (D) aplastic anemia

    (E) acute lymphocytic leukemia (ALL)

17. A 62-year-old woman presents to your clinic for a routine physical exam. She notes that her energy has recently declined, which she attributes to her age. Her history is significant for being treated for non-Hodgkins lymphoma at age 49, manifested by axillary adenopathy. On the last visit to her oncologist, she was reassured that the disease had been cured. On exam no adenopathy, hepatomegaly, or splenomegaly is noted. Laboratory studies are remarkable for Hgb 9.1, MCV 85, WBC 3.2, and Plt count 120,000. What is the next diagnostic evaluation that should be arranged?

    (A) CT scan of the chest

    (B) biopsy of an axillary lymph node

    (C) serum for B_{12} and folate

    (D) exploratory laparotomy

    (E) bone marrow aspiration and biopsy

DIRECTIONS (Questions 18 through 40): Each of the numbered items or incomplete statements in this section is followed by answers or by completions of the statement. Select the ONE lettered answer or completion that is BEST in each case.

Questions 18 through 40

18. All of the following are true regarding DIC, EXCEPT

    (A) it may be referred to as a consumptive coagulopathy

    (B) complications include life threatening bleeding

    (C) it frequently causes both micro- and macrothrombosis

    (D) heparin may be used in the treatment

    (E) use of fresh frozen plasma (FFP) and platelets is contraindicated

19. Anticipated complications of external beam irradiation may include all of the following EXCEPT

    (A) myelosuppression
    (B) infection
    (C) fatigue
    (D) worsening bone pain during treatment of bone metastasis
    (E) delayed wound healing

20. Choose the correct statement regarding the condition known as Christmas disease.
    (A) is a deficiency of factor XI
    (B) is similar to factor VIII deficiency and may be treated with factor VIII concentrates
    (C) may result in both easy bleeding and clotting
    (D) another name for this disease is Hemophilia A
    (E) is a x-linked recessive disease, affecting primarily males

21. A 44-year-old 80-kg Caucasian male presents to the emergency room with slurred speech and right arm numbness for 1 hour. He has a history of a similar episode 6 months prior, without residual effect. He also had an MI at age 40 and DVT of the right leg with no history of hypertension or diabetes. Which of the following should be included in his work-up?

    (A) myelogram
    (B) lupus anticoagulant
    (C) hemoglobin electrophoresis
    (D) platelet function assay

22. Causes of hemolytic anemia include all of the following EXCEPT

    (A) blood transfusion reaction
    (B) lead poisoning
    (C) thrombotic thrombocytopenic purpura
    (D) sickle cell anemia
    (E) DIC

23. A 28-year-old female presented to her PCP for her annual exam reporting that she had noticed recently that when she took her normal dose of two aspirin for menstrual cramps, she subsequently experienced a small amount of nose bleeding. She was concerned because she had been told that her family had "problems with bleeding." She was found to have a prolonged bleeding time and a reduced level of VIII antigen. Considering the patient's age, the most appropriate initial tests would include

    (A) plasma von Willebrand's factor (vWF) concentration
    (B) factor VIII:C level
    (C) factor IX coagulant activity
    (D) vitamin K level

24. Splenomegaly is identified on exam of an unconscious man brought in the emergency room after a motor vehicle accident. No history is available. What additional finding on exam may be of most importance in determining the cause of the splenomegaly?

    (A) absence of hepatomegaly
    (B) absence of spider angiomas
    (C) presence of bruising
    (D) pallor
    (E) lymphadenopathy

25. In which situation below would you most consider referring a patient for genetic counseling?

    (A) personal history of breast cancer at age 52
    (B) family history of a mother with primary brain tumor at age 3
    (C) family history with maternal grandmother with breast cancer at age 52, maternal grandfather with prostate cancer diagnosed at age 78, and paternal grandfather with lung cancer diagnosed at age 64
    (D) family history of a sister with colon cancer at age 29
    (E) personal history of several skin cancers and 3 prior colonic polyps, now with colon cancer at age 58

26. Heparin induced thrombocytopenia

    (A) typically occurs within 24 hours of first exposure to heparin

    (B) is more common with low molecular weight heparin

    (C) is frequently associated with severe bleeding complications

    (D) is treated with steroids, which may allow for continuation of heparin when medically necessary

    (E) can result in complications, such as pulmonary embolus

27. When encountering a patient with petechiae noted on physical exam

    (A) a platelet or Plt count of 204,000 suggests evolving thrombocytopenia as the cause

    (B) a platelet or Plt count of 204,00 in a patient on clopidogrel (Plavix) suggests this agent is not therapeutic in its antiplatelet effect

    (C) with a Plt count of 45,000, a bleeding time should be performed

    (D) hepatic dysfunction should be in the differential diagnosis

    (E) suspected overdose of coumadin should be considered, in those on that agent

28. A 40-year-old woman presents to her primary care provider for an annual evaluation. Routine laboratory studies include a CBC with a hemoglobin of 11.2 (nl 12–14) and MCV 84 (nl 82–98). Due to the low hemoglobin the patient is asked to return to the lab for additional studies. These include to following:

Serum iron 57 (nl 49–181)	Ferritin 193 (nl 22–322)
TIBC 545 (nl 250–450)	Folate 40.4 (nl 1.5–22)
B12 260 (nl 211–911)	Reticulocyte count 0.9 (0.5–1.5)

The results suggest that the low hemoglobin is caused by

    (A) normal variant in hemoglobin level

    (B) anemia of chronic disease

    (C) pernicious anemia

    (D) iron deficiency anemia

    (E) sickle cell trait

29. A 33-year-old man presents after passing out at the gym. His wife states he had been feeling OK, but had recently experienced some gingival bleeding while brushing his teeth. There is no past medical history in this previously healthy young man. The only medication he uses is a nonsteroidal anti-inflammatory agent. On exam, he is slightly pale; otherwise the exam is completely normal. His blood counts are as follows: hemoglobin 5.2, hematocrit 15.6, MCV 90, platelets 20,000, and white blood cell count 1.3 with a normal differential. What is the most likely diagnosis?

    (A) Hodgkin's disease

    (B) aplastic anemia

    (C) CLL

    (D) brain tumor

    (E) idiopathic thrombocytopenic purpura

30. What is the most frequent cause of anemia in cancer patients?

    (A) iron deficiency

    (B) intrinsic factor deficiency

    (C) inadequate erythropoietin

    (D) pernicious anemia

    (E) hemolysis

31. If a patient with history of active malignancy presents to your emergency while undergoing chemotherapy with fever, what is the most important diagnostic tests to order?

    (A) chest radiology

    (B) blood culture

    (C) bone marrow aspirate

    (D) complete blood count

    (E) urine analysis

32. A 52-year-old man presents complaining of early satiety and mild fatigue for the last 5 months. He has no other complaints and no significant medical history, other than a tonsillectomy at age 6 and well-controlled hypertension. On exam, there is no lymphadenopathy or hepatomegaly, but his spleen is palpable. A blood smear shows a hemoglobin 13.9, hematocrit 42.0, platelets 580,000, and a white blood cell count of 85,000 with some immature cells but only 1% blasts. A bone marrow done the next day shows a hypercellular sample with essentially a normal differential, and again, only 1% blasts. Chromosome analysis shows presence of the Philadelphia chromosome (t(9;22)). What is the most likely diagnosis?

    (A) ALL
    (B) acute myelogenous leukemia (AML)
    (C) CML
    (D) CLL
    (E) Burkitt's lymphoma

33. A 33-year-old woman presents complaining of profound fatigue for the past 6 weeks, necessitating her quitting her job. She looks pale and is tachycardic at 110 bpm, but otherwise her exam is normal. A blood smear shows a hemoglobin 4.5, hematocrit 13.4, platelets 19,000, and white blood cell count 3.1 with 21% blasts that have Auer rods. The most likely diagnosis is

    (A) Hodgkin's disease
    (B) non-Hodgkin's lymphoma
    (C) CML
    (D) acute leukemia
    (E) hemolytic anemia

34. On routine exam of a young man entering college, supraclavicular lymphadenopathy is noted. The patient denies any pain on palpation. Which of the following specific symptoms does not support your suspected diagnosis?

    (A) hoarseness
    (B) fever
    (C) pruritus
    (D) abdominal pain
    (E) early satiety

35. A 55-year-old African American male recently presented to the clinic with severe back pain, constipation, and confusion. Laboratory studies revealed anemia, hypercalcemia, and renal failure. Plain radiographs revealed a pathological fracture involving T5-T6 vertebrae. Lytic lesions were also present in the skull and fifth rib. What is the most likely diagnosis?

    (A) vitamin D deficiency
    (B) primary hyperparathyroidism
    (C) multiple myeloma
    (D) large cell lymphoma
    (E) Paget's disease of bone

36. A 25-year-old female presented with reddish purple spots on the upper and lower extremities. She had no complaints other than menorrhagia. Blood work was Hgb 11.2, WBC 8.2 with normal differential, platelets 32,000. No blast cells were present. What is the most likely diagnosis?

    (A) acute leukemia
    (B) idiopathic thrombocytopenia purpura
    (C) Sweets syndrome
    (D) aplastic anemia
    (E) DIC

37. Which of the following are true regarding Vitamin K deficiencies?

    (A) may result in abnormal platelet function
    (B) are most commonly due to inadequate intake in the US
    (C) should be suspected in patients with prolongation of the PTT
    (D) typically requires treatment with FFP
    (E) occurs in primary biliary cirrhosis

38. Decreased platelets may be observed in all of the following conditions EXCEPT

    (A) hypersplenism
    (B) DIC
    (C) Henoch-Schonlein disease
    (D) essential thrombocytosis
    (E) alcoholism

39. A patient presents for a routine evaluation. A CBC reveals a Hgb of 10.1 with a MCV 72. Ferritin, serum iron, TIBC, and iron saturation studies are all normal. A reticulocyte count is 2.3. Which test would be most appropriate to perform?

(A) hemoglobin electrophrosis
(B) Schilling test
(C) bone marrow biopsy
(D) guiaic
(E) direct and indirect Coombs test

40. Which of the following is an incorrect statement regarding Hodgkin's disease?

(A) there is a bimodal age distribution
(B) lymphadenopathy results in severe pain
(C) patient's typically experience fever, severe night sweats and weight loss
(D) diagnostic malignant cells present in this disease are the Reed-Sternberg cells
(E) Ann Arbor Stage III involves lymph node regions on both sides of the diaphragm

Answers and Explanations

1. **(C)** Sickle cell disease (hemoglobin S disease) is an autosomal dominant hemoglobinopathy. The homozygous form (SS), sickle cell anemia, results in sickling of erythrocytes, occurring when oxygen levels decrease at the tissue level. This results in impedance of blood flow to organs. Hemolysis often accompanies these abnormal erythrocytes. Although sexual and growth maturation are often delayed, most patients with the disease are fertile. Sickle cell crises are often precipitated by infection and those with sickle cell disease are at increased risk of infections from encapsulated organisms.

   Given the apparent good health of this woman's finacee, he likely does not have sickle cell disease but may carry the trait. Those heterogenous (AS) for the gene are referred to as having sickle cell trait. The risk of carrying the trait is approximately 8% for those of African decent in the US. Therefore, those with family histories of the disease likely carry the trait and genetic testing should be offered before childbearing. Given the strong family history of this man and the woman being of African decent, testing should be offered as they both may carry the gene. Those with sickle cell trait are typically asymptomatic with mild or absent anemia. Although sickle cell crises may occur at high altitudes for those with the disease, sickle cell crises are rare in those who are only carriers. The risk of sexually transmitted diseases is not increased for those with the trait or disease. (*Besa et al, 1992, pp. 127–133*)

2. **(B)** Iron deficiency anemia is most commonly due to chronic blood loss. In the United States, dietary deficiency is uncommon (except during pregnancy) and should not be presumed unless potential sources of blood loss have been excluded. However, dietary deficiency often occurs in pregnancy due to increased production of erythrocytes. Supplementation during pregnancy is routinely recommended. In mild to moderate iron deficiency, the reticulocyte count is mildly elevated although the corrected reticulocyte count is usually low. Low reticulocyte counts are seen in more severe forms of the disease. Elevated TIBC and low levels of iron, ferritin, and transferritin in the setting of microcytic anemia confirm the diagnosis. Although diminished iron stores are noted on bone marrow aspiration, this is not routinely needed to confirm the diagnosis. Once the diagnosis of iron deficiency anemia is made, the underlying cause must be found and treated. Iron replacement may be needed in moderate to severe cases and is typically accomplished within 3 to 6 months. Once iron stores have been replaced, iron supplementation should be stopped to prevent iron toxicity or mask further blood loss. (*Besa et al, 1992, pp. 62–66; Simon and Miller, 2004, pp. 403–430*)

3. **(D)** Lead poisoning is a common occurrence, usually resulting in a mild anemia. Patients often have vague complaints including fatigue, abdominal pain, difficulties with concentration, and muscle weakness. The most common severe complication of the disease is

the development of episodic paralytic ileus. Mild anemia and the presence of basophilic stippling are often seen. Lead levels should be checked in anyone presenting with these complaints and at risk, including children and adults with an occupational/environmental exposure. Primary treatment is to remove the source of lead. Chelating agents may be needed for those who are symptomatic or with very high levels. (*Simon and Miller, 2004, pp. 403–430*).

4. **(C)** Anemia may be the result of a wide variety of causes. Once a patient is found to be anemic, the next step is determining the underlying etiology. Anemia may be divided into microcytic, normocytic, and macrocytic based on the MCV of the erythrocytes. Once this has been determined, the differential diagnosis may be narrowed and appropriate adjuvant tests can be ordered. Microcytic anemia is most commonly seen in the presence of iron deficiency. Thalassemia will also result in a microcytic anemia but is less common in the United States. Both lead poisoning and anemia of chronic illness may result in a mildly lower MCV, but a normocytosis is more commonly seen. In addition, patients with chronic illnesses often have more than one contributing factors for their anemia and therefore the MCV may be low, high, or normal. In a previously healthy individual with severe microcytic anemia, and with normal WBC and Plt count, iron deficiency should be suspected. (*Simon and Miller, 2004, pp. 403–430*)

5. **(D)** Vitamin B_{12} and folate deficiencies are the common forms of macrocytic anemia. Vitamin B_{12} is found in animal products and is generally available in typical American diets. Intrinsic factor is secreted in the stomach to allow absorption of B_{12} in the small intestine. Those with prior gastrectomy are at high risk of B_{12} deficiency anemia and therefore commonly need monthly replacement. B_{12} deficiency results in neurologic injury and atrophy of the tongue along with loss of taste sensation. Schilling's test may be used to determine the cause of B_{12} deficiency. A 24-hour urine sample is collected after radiolabeled cyanocobalamin is taken orally. If absorbed

normally, at least 7% of the isotope will be excreted in the urine. If less than 7% is excreted, the cause of malabsorption will be determined by administering intrinsic factor along with oral cyanocobalamin. If an intrinsic factor deficiency exists, this will correct the B_{12} deficiency. If the deficiency is not corrected, the problem is due to poor absorption in the small bowel. The Shilling's test is not commonly used in the United States, having been largely replaced by serum B_{12} level direct measurement. Folate (folic acid) is found in vegetables, and deficiencies are more commonly seen in the United States. It is important to confirm the cause of macrocytic anemia prior to beginning folate replacement. Folate supplementation in a patient deficient in B_{12} may help to correct the anemia but will mask B_{12} deficiency and could result in permanent neurologic impairment. (*Besa et al, 1992, pp. 84–91*)

6. **(C)** Anemia associated with hyperbilirubinemia and elevated LDH suggests hemolytic anemia. There are many causes of hemolytic anemia. In hospitalized patients, the differential may include DIC, idiopathic thrombocytopenia purpura, thrombotic thrombocytopenia purpura, drug reactions, and blood incompatibility. Drug reactions may also develop in the setting of G-6-P deficiency. Although malaria is not commonly seen in this country, some regions do report cases. In addition, frequent travel and immigration necessitate consideration of additional infectious causes of illness when evaluating patients. Folate deficiency does not result in hemolysis and therefore elevated bilirubin and LDH would not be expected. (*Besa et al, 1992, pp. 95–110*)

7. **(B); 8. (C); 9. (A); 10. (A); 11. (B); 12. (D)** Anticancer therapy often results in complications that may be mild to severe, acute, and chronic. Many chemotherapeutic agents share similar side effects including alopecia, nausea, vomiting, diarrhea, mucositis, fatigue, and myelosuppresion. The frequency and severity of these common toxicities vary with each drug and dosage. Cisplatin is also known to cause renal impairment and neuropathy (including

auditory dysfunction at high doses). Adriamycin may result in acute and (more commonly) chronic cardiac toxicity. Varying dosing schedules and limiting total dose exposure have been shown to reduce this risk. Tamoxifen use has been shown to increase the risk of uterine malignancies. Although this risk remains relatively low, it must be considered and discussed with patients when considering its use in treatment and prevention of malignancy. External beam irradiation is commonly associated with myelosuppression and local toxicities to the surrounding tissue, depending on the site treated. Secondary malignancies may occur following radiation therapy to including sarcomas, breast, thyroid, and uterine cancer. Vincristine is commonly associated with peripheral neuropathy, which is frequently dose limiting. Bleomycin is most known for its long-term pulmonary toxic effects. (*Pillot et al, 2004, pp. 117–122; Kasper et al, 2005, pp. 471–474, 477, 488*)

13. **(D)** Tumor markers are biochemical abnormalities, which are often elevated in particular malignancies. They are typically measured in the blood, but may sometimes be analyzed in urine or tumor tissue. Tumor markers are often present at low levels in healthy individuals and may occasionally be elevated in nonmalignant conditions. Although tumor markers are often quite helpful in monitoring patients with known cancer, they are rarely sensitive enough to allow for screening of the disease. Prostate specific antigen (PSA) is the most commonly used tumor marker for cancer screening (eg, prostate cancer). Prostatic acid phosphate may be elevated in prostate cancers, particularly when metastatic disease is present, but is much less sensitive than PSA and should not be used for screening. Carcinoembryonic antigen (CEA) may be elevated in a variety of malignancies, most commonly colon cancer, while cancer antigen 125 (CA 125) may be elevated in ovarian cancer. Unfortunately, neither CEA nor CA 125 are sensitive enough for cancer screening. Alpha feta protein is recommended in screening for hepatocellular carcinoma in those considered at increased risk, including those with chronic hepatitis B and C and those with cirrhosis

from all causes. (*Simon and Miller, 2004, pp. 153–192; Kasper et al, pp. 438–39 and 533–535*)

14. **(C)** Thalassemia is a group of genetic disorders affecting one or more of the subunits of the hemoglobin chain resulting in a microcytic, hypochromic anemia. It is most common in those of African descent. Presentation may occur early or later in life, depending on the affected subunit and number of genetic abnormalities involved. The most common form (Thalassemia minor) results in only mild disease, often going undiagnosed and requiring no treatment, other forms are life threatening. Diagnosis is made by Hb electrophoresis, which should be ordered when the disease is suspected. (*Simon and Miller, 2004, pp. 403–430*)

15. **(D)** This patient has multiple myeloma, confirmed by serum electrophoresis. Multiple myeloma is a malignancy of plasma cells arising from a single clone. These plasma cells secrete immunoglobin, resulting in a clone spike on electrophoresis. Plasma cells proliferate bones resulting in osteolytic lesions. Bone pain and fracture as well as hypercalcemia are the most common findings. Associated infiltration of the bone marrow results in anemia, neutropenia, and thrombocytopenia. Splenomegaly does not occur with multiple myeloma. (*Pillot et al, 2004, pp. 98–102*)

16. **(E)** ALL is the most common childhood leukemia. Although most patients present with symptoms such as fatigue, frank bleeding, or shortness of breath, others may present with more subtle complaints. The presence of a significant leukocytosis with associated lymphocytosis suggests this as a possible diagnosis. Bone marrow biopsy is necessary to confirm the diagnosis. (*Simon and Miller, 2004, pp. 403–430*)

17. **(E)** In patients with histories of malignancy, recurrent disease should always be suspected, particularly in the first 5 years after treatment. A variety of tests may be performed to evaluate for possible recurrence. However, in a patient who is now 14 years since her treatment, with no other signs or symptoms to suggest

recurrent disease, this is less likely. Complications of treatment may also develop over time and myelodysplasic syndrome should be considered in a patient with prior chemotherapy or radiation therapy. In patients with pancytopenia, bone marrow biopsy is necessary to evaluate for and confirm the diagnosis of myelodysplasia, as progression to acute leukemia may also result. (*Pillot et al, 2004, pp. 60–64*)

18. **(E)** DIC is a systemic disorder resulting from abnormal and excessive activation of the clotting cascade. The result is both excessive bleeding and clotting, often resulting in organ damage such as renal impairment. Treatment of the underlying cause is the most important consideration. The condition may be life threatening and rapid treatment of the underlying disease is critical for survival. Use of replacement factors such as platelets, FFP, and cryoprecipitate should be used if needed; however, they could result in worsening organ damage because of increased clotting. Heparin is sometimes used for treatment of the disease with the goal to reduce thrombosis formation; however, heparin therapy remains controversial since it also has the potential of worsening bleeding. (*Besa et al, 1992, pp. 241–253*)

19. **(D)** External beam irradiation is a common modality of anticancer therapy. In previous years, it had been used to treat benign conditions including thyroid disorders and acne. Complications may include local damage to tissues/organs, including delayed wound healing, fatigue, and myelosuppression with the associated risk of infection. Radiation therapy is often used to palliate pain for patients with metastatic disease to the bone. It may produce relief of pain within a few days of initiation of treatment. Worsening bone pain is not expected but may signal a complication of the disease, such as a pathologic fracture. (*Kasper et al, 2005, pp. 486–488*)

20. **(E)** Christmas disease, also known as hemophilia B and factor IX (not factor XI) hemophilia, is a hereditary bleeding disorder. Abnormal thrombosis does not occur. It is managed with factor IX concentrates or FFP. It is necessary to distinguish between hemophilia A from B, since both diseases present similarly, but require appropriate factor replacement. (*Simon and Miller, 2004, pp. 403–430*)

21. **(B)** This patient's history suggests some form of coagulopathy, resulting in an increased incidence of thrombotic events. Although a myelogram may be helpful in evaluating peripheral neuropathy, in the setting of concurrent slurred speech, a central cause should be suspected. Hemoglobin electrophoresis is used in evaluation of hemoglobinopathies, such as sickle cell disease. Although sickle cell disease may result in microthrombotic events, macrothrombotic events such as DVT would not occur. Sickle cell disease occurs most commonly in those of African decent and should be diagnosed earlier in life. Platelet function assays are helpful in the evaluation of platelet functional defects. With the clinical information, there is no sign of any chronic platelet abnormalities. Lupus anticoagulant, an antibody against phospholipids, may occur in autoimmune diseases and results in increased thrombotic events. (*Besa et al, 1992, pp. 223–235*)

22. **(B)** Hemolysis may occur in a variety of settings and is associated with both acute and chronic illness. Distinguishing intravascular and extravascular hemolysis will assist in determining the underlying cause. Testing for hemoglobinemia and hemoglobinuria will make this distinction. Causes of intravascular hemolysis include transfusion reactions, malaria and mechanical heart valves. Extravascular hemolysis may occur with drugs such as antibiotics and antimalarial agents, DIC, TTP, and sickle cell anemia. Lead poisoning results in inhibition of heme synthesis and injury to red cell membranes, resulting in a mild to moderate microcytic anemia. It is not typically associated with hemolysis. (*Simon and Miller, 2004, pp. 403–430*)

23. **(A)** von Willebrand's factor is found in both plasma and platelets. Deficiencies may manifest with variable degrees of easy bleeding.

von Willebrand's disease is the most common inherited bleeding disorder and should be considered first in someone with abnormal bleeding. Factor VIII:C level should be measured in evaluation for hemophilia A, while factor IX results in hemophilia B. Vitamin K deficiencies typically occur in those with chronic disease and would be unlikely in an otherwise healthy young woman. (*Besa et al, 1992, pp. 223–235*)

24. **(E)** Splenomegaly may be caused from a variety of illnesses including infectious, oncologic, and inflammatory. Splenomegaly frequently is a result of hepatic parenchymal or veno-occlusive disease and patients presenting with unexplained splenomegaly should be examined for the presents of findings to suggest portal hypertension. The lack of hepatomegaly or spider angiomas makes this less likely. Bruising and pallor may be noted in patients with associated thrombocytopenia and anemia, although in a patient involved in a MVA, these would both be expected. Lymphadenopathy however suggests possible infectious or malignant causes of splenomegaly in this patient. The distribution, size and feel of enlarged lymph nodes may also help in narrowing the differential diagnosis. (*Kasper et al, 2005, pp. 345–348; Besa et al, 1992, pp. 11–25*)

25. **(D)** Genetic testing has become increasingly available for a variety of genetic mutations, although there is much work to be done in this field. As cancer is now the number one cause of death in the U.S. prior to the age of 85, virtually all patients will have some family history of the disease. Personal and family histories, which may raise concern for a possible hereditary disease, include multiple family members with malignancy and the diagnosis of malignancy at a young age (i.e., younger than expected for the particular disease). Consideration of genetic susceptibility is most important when screening tests for the disease are available and when risk reduction strategies are available. For these patients, referral to a genetics counselor should be considered. A first degree family member with colon cancer at <30 years of age, may result

from an inherited predisposition for colon cancer and other malignancies. Since colon cancer can be prevented by polypectomy or diagnosed early by carefully screening, diagnosing a genetic disorder may be of particular benefit to a family member of such a patient (*Kasper et al, 2005, pp. 386–391, 446–450*)

26. **(E)** Heparin induced thrombocytopenia (HIT) is an immune-mediated disease resulting in the formation of immune complex binding of platelets, which results in typically mild to moderate thrombocytopenia. These platelet complexes can result in thrombotic complications. HIT may occur after prior exposure to heparin and typically develops within the first few days following exposure. It is more common with unfractionated heparin, as opposed to low molecular weight heparin. Management is primarily withdrawal of the agent and further exposure to heparin is contraindicated. (*Pillot et al, 2004, pp. 49–59*)

27. **(D)** Petchiae is a sign of thrombocytopenia or platelet dysfunction. It does not typically occur with other disorders of the coagulation cascade. It would not be expected in patient who receive excess coumadin, in the absence of a platelet abnormality. Antiplatelet medications affect platelet function but should not result in thrombocytopenia. Platelet function may be evaluated by performing a bleeding time. In patients with a normal platelet or Plt count and petchiae on exam, this test should be ordered.

A variety of conditions may result in thrombocytopenia, including immune, infectious, oncologic, and hepatic or splenic dysfunction. (*Besa et al, 1992, pp. 257–268*)

28. **(D)** In the presence of a mild anemia and normocytosis, consideration of a variety of causes must be considered to include iron, vitamin B_{12}, and folate deficiencies. Although this patient has a normal serum iron and ferritin level, her total iron binding capacity is mildly elevated. Once the iron saturation level (nl <15%) is calculated (iron (100/TIBC), one sees that the patient's labs do reflect an

iron deficiency. Appropriate evaluation for the underlying cause of iron deficiency should be pursued. (*Besa et al, 1992, pp. 59–73*)

29. **(B)** Profound pancytopenia, with a normocytic anemia and few signs or symptoms (except for bleeding), is characteristic for aplastic anemia. A bone marrow aspiration and biopsy must be done to confirm—it will be hypocellular. This is a typical presentation of aplastic anemia, in this case, probably caused by chronic medication use. Management includes discontinuation of the offending drugs, providing supportive care (transfusions, rapid treatment of any infection), and close observation to determine if the marrow recovers spontaneously. If it does not, then therapeutic intervention is needed. Hodgkin's disease does not usually present in this manner, and often the blood smear is normal, except in advanced disease when the bone marrow is affected. CLL may present in a similar manner; however, the white blood cell count must be elevated for the diagnosis of CLL to be made, with an absolute lymphocytosis of >10,000/mL. CLL is rare in this age group. Significant anemia and leukopenia are extremely rare in idiopathic thrombocytopenic purpura (ITP), with presentations typically acute in onset, and patients manifest bleeding, with or without splenomegaly. (*Simon and Miller, 2004, pp. 403–430*)

30. **(C)** Anemia in cancer patients is quite common. Patients may have acute or chronic bleeding, malabsorption of iron, B_{12} or folate or even hemolysis. However, the most common cause is anemia of chronic illness, with low or ineffective erythropoietin hormone. Erythropoietin therapy may be beneficial in the treatment of these patients anemia, but careful evaluation of other potential causes is essential prior to beginning therapy (*Besa et al, 1992, pp. 51–57*)

31. **(D)** When cancer patients undergoing chemotherapy develop fever, neutropenic infection must be considered. Prompt medical attention is critical in reducing mortality from neutropenic fever. These patients should undergo careful evaluation for possible sources of infection. However, for many patients, an infectious source may not be identified. Prompt treatment with broad-spectrum antibiotics is critical for all patients with neutropenic infection, regardless of an identifiable source. Therefore, patients with fever need initial evaluation with a CBC to determine if neutropenia does or does not exist. If the patient is found to be non-neutropenic, more directed treatment of possibly infectious causes should be provided. (*Pillot et al, 2004, pp. 255–261*)

32. **(C)** The myeloproliferative disorder CML is the most likely diagnosis here. Early satiety is a common manifestation of splenomegaly; fatigue is a general complaint with a single cause often never found (other than the disease). Causes of leukemias are rarely identified, although radiation is considered a cause of some leukemias, of which CML is one. Often, splenomegaly is the only physical finding in a newly diagnosed CML patient. An elevated white blood cell count might be the only abnormality on a blood smear. If there were more blasts (>30%), this would be correctly diagnosed as an acute leukemia. Bone marrow analysis is necessary for diagnosis. The Philadelphia chromosome is characteristic of CML, although it also occurs in approximately 25% of ALL patients. The presence of the Philadelphia chromosome in AML is exceedingly rare. CLL is a lymphoproliferative disorder; the Philadelphia chromosome abnormality does not occur in CLL or in Burkitt's lymphoma. Typical chromosomal translocations in Burkitt's lymphoma are t(8;14) and t(8;22). (*Simon and Miller, 2004, pp. 403–430*)

33. **(D)** Auer rods are pathognomonic of acute leukemia, especially AML. This presentation is typical for AML. Lymphomas do not present with profound pancytopenias. CML could be in the differential; however, the high number of blasts rules out the chronic phase of CML. There would be no thrombocytopenia and no blasts (definitely no Auer rods) if hemolytic anemia was the cause of this woman's fatigue. Therefore, acute leukemia is the most likely diagnosis. Auer rods are eosinophilic

needle-like inclusions in the cytoplasm, seen in AML. Hodgkins and Non-Hodgkins lymphomas can present with anemia but rarely are abnormal Pltss counts involved nor are Auer rods present. CML and CLL usually presents with high counts but no Auer rods. (*Simon and Miller, 2004, pp. 403–430*)

34. **(A)** Non-tender adenopathy in an otherwise healthy appearing patient is suspicious for lymphoma. Hodgkin's lymphoma has a bimodal age distribution with the first peak in the 20s. The presence of B symptoms (weight loss, fatigue, fevers) and pruritis should raise your clinical suspicion, although many patients are asymptomatic. Early satiety and abdominal pain often occur in the presence of splenomegaly, which is present with advancing stages of lymphoma. Hoarseness may occur with some upper respiratory diseases but would not be expected in a patient with lymphoma. (*Simon and Miller, 2004, pp. 403–430*)

35. **(C)** Multiple myeloma is a clonal malignancy of the plasma cells. It is seen more commonly in African Americans and typically presents with bone pain. Radiographs reveal the presence of osteolytic lesions commonly found in the axial skeleton, skull, long bones, spine, and ribs. A variety of other conditions may result in bone pain. Vitamin D deficiency, due to inadequate sun exposure, malnutrition or malabsorption, can also be associated with bone pain as well as proximal muscle weakness. Primary hyperparathyroidism is associated with an adenoma of the parathyroid gland resulting in increased PTH levels and hypercalcemia. Large cell lymphoma is a type of non-Hodgkins lymphoma that presents with painless adenopathy and be associated with B symptoms of fever, night sweats, or unintentional weight loss. Less commonly, it can affect the lymphatic system, the central nervous system, or any organ including the bone. Paget's disease is often asymptomatic, but may produce bone pain usually of the skull, femur, tibia, pelvis, or humerus. In this patient, the presence of anemia, hypercalcemia and renal failure, suggest multiple myeloma as the cause of his bone pain. (*Simon and Miller, 2004, pp. 403–430*)

36. **(B)** Idiopathic thrombocytopenia purpura is an acquired disease, often presenting in young, otherwise healthy, patients. As the name implies, no known cause is identified in this condition of isolated thrombocytopenia. Due to the resulting bleeding, such as menorrhagia, patients may have associated anemia. In conditions such as DIC, acute leukemia, aplastic anemia or Sweets syndrome (a rare cutaneous form of myelodysplasic syndrome) other symptoms or laboratory abnormalities would be expected. (*Simon and Miller, 2004, pp. 403–430*)

37. **(E)** Vitamin K is a fat-soluble vitamin that is stored in the liver. It is critical in the clotting casade and deficiencies result in prolongation of the prothrombin time. With severe or prolonged deficiencies, prolongation of the PTT may also occur. Deficiencies may occur from dietary deficiencies, malabsorption and most commonly, chronic liver disease, such as cirrhosis. Treatment is with parenteral administration of vitamin K, with monthly injections in those with chronic deficiencies. FFP may be needed if patients have active hemorrhage. (*Kasper et al, 2005, pp. 409, 683*)

38. **(D)** A variety of conditions may result in thrombocytopenia. These include DIC (due to consumption of platelets during abnormal clotting), hypersplenism resulting in sequestration of platelets and Henoch Schonlein Purpura (a systemic vasculitis with typical manifestations of palpable purpura, abdominal pain, and hematuria). Alcoholism may result in cirrhosis, particularly in the presence of hepatitis C or other chronic liver disease. Cirrhosis results in portal hypertension, splenomegaly, and thrombocytopenia. Essential thrombocytosis is a rare myeloproliferative disorder that is identified by an elevated Plt count caused by abnormal proliferation of megakaryocytes in the bone marrow. Increased risk of thrombosis is therefore a complication and may occur in small veins such as the mesenteric, hepatic, or portal venous system (*Kasper et al, 2005, pp. 341, 2010–2011*)

39. **(A)** Microcytic anemia is most commonly caused by iron deficiency. However, thalassemia and lead poisoning may also result

in microcytosis. In patients with normal iron studies, including iron saturation levels, consideration of these differential diagnoses is necessary. Although thalassemia is not common, it may be found in patient with microcytic anemia by serum electrophoresis. (*Besa et al, 1992, pp. 59–73, 115–122*)

40. **(B)** Hodgkin's disease is a group of cancers. They are usually characterized by Reed-Sternberg cells, which are necessary, but NOT sufficient for a diagnosis of Hodgkin's disease. Patients typically experience fever, severe night sweats, and weight loss. The Ann Arbor staging system is as follows: Stage I–one lymph node region involved, Stage II–involvement of two lymph node areas on one side of the diaphragm, Stage III–lymph node regions involved on both sides of the diaphragm, Stage IV–disseminated disease with liver or bone marrow involvement. Generally patients do not complain of severe pain with the lymph nodes but can complain of discomfort if the lymph nodes are "bulky." (*Simon and Miller, 2004, pp. 403–430*)

REFERENCES

Simon AF, Miller AA (eds). *Appleton & Lange Outline Review for the Physician Assistant Examination*, 2nd ed. New York: McGraw-Hill; 2004 (Chapters 7 and 14).

Pillot G, et al (ed). *The Washington Manual Hematology and Oncology Subspecialty Consult*. Philadelphia: Lippincott Williams & Wilkins; 2004 (Chapters 8, 17, 19, and 26).

Kasper DL, et al (eds). *Harrison's Principles of Internal Medicine*, 16th ed. New York: McGraw-Hill; 2005 (Chapters 53, 54, 58, 61, 67, 68, 70, 71, 102, and 306).

Besa, EC, et al (eds). *The National Medical Series for Independent Study: Hematology*. Philadelphia: Lippincott Williams & Wilkins; 1992 (Chapters 2, 4–9, 14–16).

CHAPTER 7

HIV-AIDS
Questions

Rebecca Lovell Scott, PhD, PA-C

DIRECTIONS (Questions 1 through 30): Each of the numbered items in this section is followed by possible answers. Select the ONE lettered answer that is BEST in each case.

Questions 1 through 30

1. The two major risk factors for HIV infection in American women are intravenous drug use and which of the following?
   - (A) history of blood transfusion
   - (B) needle stick injuries
   - (C) pelvic inflammatory disease
   - (D) sexual contact with an infected male
   - (E) use of oral contraceptives

2. Of the following sexual practices, which poses the greatest risk of HIV transmission when practiced with an infected partner but without use of a reliable barrier method of prophylaxis?
   - (A) insertive anal intercourse
   - (B) insertive vaginal intercourse
   - (C) receptive anal intercourse
   - (D) receptive fellatio with ejaculation
   - (E) receptive vaginal intercourse

3. Which of the following patients, if HIV negative, meets the Centers for Disease Control and Prevention case definition for AIDS?
   - (A) 29-year-old male with pulmonary tuberculosis
   - (B) 32-year-old male with Kaposi's sarcoma
   - (C) 35-year-old female with invasive cervical cancer
   - (D) 36-year-old male with recurrent *Salmonella septicemia*
   - (E) 40-year-old female with recurrent pneumonia

4. A 28-year-old man has a positive HIV ELISA and Western Blot, but has never had an opportunistic infection. Of the following laboratory parameters, which, if present, is consistent with a diagnosis of AIDS in this man?
   - (A) CD4 lymphocyte count of 175/mL
   - (B) HHV-8 titer 1:160
   - (C) HSV-2 titer of 1:80
   - (D) platelet count of 10,000/mL
   - (D) total white blood cell count of 1500/mL

5. A 35-year-old patient with AIDS has had unintended weight loss of nearly 30 pounds over the past 6 months. This loss has been primarily in muscle mass. He has little appetite, but no nausea, diarrhea, or evidence of oral candidiasis. He reports interest in resuming his former weight-training regimen. Which of the following is the most appropriate pharmacologic agent to help him gain weight?
   - (A) dronabinol
   - (B) megestrol acetate
   - (C) odansetron
   - (D) prochlorperazine
   - (E) testosterone enanthate

6. A 42-year-old man who is HIV positive develops fever of 38.8°C, mild nonproductive cough, and shortness of breath. He takes no medications other than a multivitamin tablet, does not smoke cigarettes, or use alcohol or illicit drugs. Of the following findings on diagnostic studies, which is most consistent with a diagnosis of *Pneumocystic jiroveci* pneumonia in this man?
    (A) apical infiltrates on chest radiography
    (B) bronchiolar consolidation on CT scan
    (C) CD4 count of 300 cells/mL
    (D) PO2 of 54 mm Hg
    (E) serum LDH level of 54 units/L

7. A 33-year-old man with HIV disease is brought in by his partner for evaluation of altered mental status. The partner has noticed waxing and waning periods of confusion throughout the day, difficulty in performing tasks such as balancing a checkbook, and deterioration of handwriting. The patient reports no fever or headache. What is the most likely diagnosis?
    (A) AIDS dementia complex
    (B) central nervous system lymphoma
    (C) cryptococcal meningitis
    (D) progressive multifocal leukoencephalopathy (PML)
    (E) toxoplasmosis

8. A 38-year-old man with HIV disease has had fever and a severe generalized headache for the past several hours. On examination he is alert and oriented, and gives a coherent history that is corroborated by his partner. He has no papilledema or meningismus. What is the most likely diagnosis?
    (A) AIDS dementia complex
    (B) central nervous system lymphoma
    (C) cryptococcal meningitis
    (D) progressive multifocal leukoencephalopathy
    (E) toxoplasmosis

9. Which of the following findings on diagnostic testing most strongly suggests a diagnosis of toxoplasmosis in an HIV-infected patient?
    (A) multiple lesions on MRI of the head
    (B) negative culture of spinal fluid
    (C) nonenhancing white matter lesions without mass effect
    (D) positive serologic test for toxoplasma
    (E) single contrast-enhancing lesion on CT of the head

10. A 42-year-old man with AIDS has had gradual onset of "my feet always going to sleep on me." This tingling and burning keeps him awake much of the night and he "can't cope much longer" because of the sleep deprivation. He drinks no alcohol nor does he use any illicit drugs. His physical examination reveals no gross motor or sensory deficits. His thyroid function tests and vitamin B_{12} levels are within normal limits and syphilis screening is negative. Of the following, what is the recommended initial therapy?
    (A) didanosine
    (B) gabapentin
    (C) ibuprofen
    (D) recombinant nerve growth factor
    (E) stavudine

11. A 28-year-old man who is HIV positive has developed white lesions on the lateral aspects of his tongue. While not painful, they bother him for cosmetic reasons. On examination, these lesions are raised and appear corrugated. They adhere to the tongue when gently scraped with a tongue depressor. What is the most likely cause of these lesions?
    (A) *Candida albicans* infection
    (B) Epstein-Barr virus infection
    (C) herpes simplex virus infection
    (D) iron deficiency
    (E) vitamin B_{12} deficiency

12. At what point should an HIV-infected individual receive prophylaxis against *Pneumocystis jiroveci* pneumonia?

(A) as soon as the individual tests positive for HIV

(B) when the CD4 count is less than 500 cells/mL

(C) when the CD4 count is less than 200 cells/mL

(D) when the CD4 count is less than 75 cells/mL

(E) when the CD4 count is less than 50 cells/mL

13. A physician assistant student suffers a needle-stick injury while caring for an HIV-positive patient whose viral load is currently undetectable. Of the following, which is the most appropriate management for the student?

(A) drug treatment based on results of HIV testing performed immediately and at 6 weeks, 3 months, and 6 months

(B) administration of zidovudine and lamivudine until results of baseline testing are received

(C) administration of zidovudine and lamivudine for 4 weeks

(D) administration of zidovudine, lamivudine, and indinavir for 4 weeks

14. A surgical physician assistant suffers a deep puncture wound during surgery on an HIV-positive patient. The patient, who is on a multidrug regimen, has a viral load of 120,000 copies. Which of the following drugs is contraindicated for the physician assistant due to its potential for hepatotoxicity in the setting of HIV prophylaxis?

(A) abacavir

(B) indinavir

(C) lamivudine

(D) nevirapine

(E) zidovudine

15. A 24-year-old woman with HIV is diagnosed with *Mycobacterium avium* complex infection. She is started on a treatment regimen of clarithromycin with ethambutol. She needs to be educated that which of the following is a potential complication of this therapy?

(A) anemia

(B) azotemia

(C) methemoglobinemia

(D) mucositis

(E) optic neuritis

16. Which one of the following tests should be used to monitor success of antiretroviral therapy in a patient with HIV?

(A) absolute CD4 lymphocyte count

(B) CD4 lymphocyte percentage

(C) HIV enzyme-linked immunosorbent assay

(D) serum viral load

(E) Western blot

17. An HIV-positive man develops elevated cholesterol and triglycerides while taking an antiretroviral cocktail that includes two nucleoside analogs and a protease inhibitor. Which of the following cholesterol-lowering therapies is contraindicated in this patient due to its interactions with protease inhibitors?

(A) atorvastatin

(B) gemfibrozil

(C) lovastatin

(D) pravastatin

18. A 29-year-old man who is taking combination antiretroviral therapy develops severe right-sided flank pain and dysuria. He is also nauseated, which he attributes to the severity of the pain. He is unable to sit still and paces about the examination room. Dipstick urine is remarkable for 3+ hematuria. Which of the following drugs is most likely to be responsible for this clinical picture?

(A) delavirdine

(B) didanosine

(C) indinavir

(D) nelfinavir

(E) stavudine

19. A 26-year-old African-American man with HIV disease has a CD4 lymphocyte percentage of 12%. Prior to beginning prophylactic therapy for *Pneumocystis jiroveci* pneumonia, which of the following drugs requires testing for G6PD deficiency?

(A) aerosolized pentamidine

(B) atovaquone

(C) dapsone

(D) trimethoprim-sulfamethoxazole

20. A 25-year-old gravida 1 woman who is HIV positive arrives at the hospital in early labor. Membranes are intact and the cervix is 50% effaced and 3 to 4 cm dilated. Fetal heart rate is 150 beats/min. Which of the following procedures is contraindicated during labor?

(A) amniotomy

(B) augmentation of labor with oxytocin

(C) external monitoring

(D) operative delivery

(E) use of fetal scalp electrodes

21. A 25-year-old woman with HIV disease delivers a 6-pound infant at 39 and 1/2 weeks' gestation. She received three-drug prophylaxis during her pregnancy. Of the following, what is the most appropriate course of action regarding the infant?

(A) continue combination therapy for 1 to 2 weeks

(B) indefinite therapy with zidovudine alone

(C) no additional prophylaxis is needed

(D) treat only if two separate HIV-PCR tests are positive

22. An infant is born to an HIV-positive mother. A positive HIV ELISA or Western blot test performed on the infant's blood reflects the maternal antibodies rather than the baby's own until approximately what age?

(A) 6 weeks

(B) 12 weeks

(C) 6 months

(D) 10 months

(E) 3 years

23. An 6-month-old infant whose mother is HIV positive develops a flu-like illness. HIV testing shows 5000 viral copies/mL. What is the most appropriate course of action for this infant?

(A) begin three-drug antiretroviral therapy immediately

(B) initiate zidovudine therapy once the symptoms have resolved

(C) treat only the symptoms at this time

(D) treat when an opportunistic infection develops

(E) treat when viral load is >100,000 copies/mL

24. At how many months of age should an asymptomatic HIV-positive infant receive her first measles—mumps—rubella (MMR) vaccine?

(A) 12

(B) 15

(C) 18

(D) 24

(E) 60

25. A 4-week-old baby whose mother is HIV positive is started on *Pneumocystis* prophylaxis with trimethoprim-sulfamethoxazole (TMP-SMX). Two weeks later the TMP-SMX is discontinued when she develops a rash over much of her body. What is the most appropriate next step regarding prophylaxis?

(A) administer monthly intravenous immune globulin instead

(B) discontinue prophylaxis unless the CD4 count drops below 500/mL

(C) reintroduce TMP-SMX when the rash resolves

(D) substitute dapsone or atovaquone for TMP-SMX

26. A 3-year-old boy who is HIV positive begins preschool. He is toilet trained and is not known to bite other children or have any open skin lesions. What is the most effective means of preventing transmission to the other children in his class?
    (A) having the child use a separate toilet
    (B) excluding the child from activities likely to cause sweating
    (C) reminding the staff to use blood precautions with all children
    (D) requiring the child to stay home if he has gastrointestinal symptoms
    (E) using disposable plates and flatware for this child

27. The risk of vertical transmission of HIV seems to be proportional to which of the following parameters?
    (A) CD4 count
    (B) CD4 percentage
    (C) number of other children with HIV disease
    (D) number of opportunistic infections
    (E) viral load

28. What is the most common tumor associated with pediatric HIV infection?
    (A) astrocytoma
    (B) Kaposi's sarcoma
    (C) leiomyosarcoma
    (D) non-Hodgkin's lymphoma

29. A 29-year-old man who is HIV positive has developed dark purple papular nonblanching lesions between the toes of his right foot. He has no other symptoms. Careful examination shows that this is the only area of involvement. His CD4 count is 150 cells/mL. Of the following, what is the most appropriate treatment?
    (A) alpha interferon
    (B) chemotherapy with daunorubicin, bleomycin, and vinblastine
    (C) intralesional vinblastine
    (D) liposomal doxorubicin
    (E) radiation

30. A 28-year-old woman has recently been diagnosed with HIV disease. She has no evidence of opportunistic infection and her CD4 count is >200. She has had Pap smears every year for the past 5 years and they have all been normal. In how many months should she have another Pap and pelvic examination?
    (A) 3
    (B) 6
    (C) 12
    (D) 24
    (E) 36

Answers and Explanations

1. **(D)** The major risk factors for HIV infection in American women are intravenous drug use and heterosexual contact with an infected partner. Thanks to universal blood donor screening using the HIV ELISA, antigen, and viral load testing, the risk for any person contracting HIV from a screened unit of blood is only 1:1,000,000. The risk for any person following a needle-stick injury is about 1:300 with deeper sticks, hollow bore needles, visible blood on the needle, and advanced stage of disease in the source increasing the risk. HIV infection puts a woman at increased risk for gynecologic complications such as pelvic inflammatory disease. Unlike the use of latex condoms, the use of oral contraceptives does not protect against HIV transmission, but is not, per se, a risk factor for HIV disease. (*Katz et al, 2005, pp. 1275–1276*)

2. **(C)** In unprotected intercourse with an infected partner, receptive anal intercourse carries a risk of HIV transmission between 1:100 and 1:30. Insertive anal intercourse, receptive vaginal intercourse, and fellatio with ejaculation each carry a risk of about 1:1000. Insertive vaginal intercourse carries a risk of 1:10,000. (*Katz et al, 2005, p. 1276*)

3. **(B)** The Centers for Disease Control and Prevention AIDS case definition includes the following diseases that, with or without laboratory evidence of HIV infection, constitute a definitive diagnosis of AIDS: candidiasis of the esophagus, trachea, bronchi, or lungs; extrapulmonary cryptococcosis; cryptosporidiosis with diarrhea persisting more than 1 month; cytomegalovirus disease of an organ other than liver, spleen, or lymph nodes; herpes simplex virus infection causing a mucocutaneous ulcer that persists longer than 1 month or causing bronchitis, pneumonitis, or esophagitis; Kaposi's sarcoma in a patient younger than 60; lymphoma of the brain in a patient younger than 60; disseminated *Mycobacterium avium* complex or *Mycobacterium kansasii* disease; *Pneumocystis carinii* pneumonia; progressive multifocal leukoencephalopathy; or toxoplasmosis of the brain. Other conditions in the case definition require laboratory evidence of HIV infection. (*Katz et al, 2005, p. 1275*)

4. **(A)** Persons with a CD-4 count less than 200/mL or a CD-4 percentage below 14% are now included in the Centers for Disease Control and Prevention category of "definitive AIDS diagnoses with laboratory evidence of HIV infection." Persons with HIV-AIDS may have positive herpes titers or depressed platelet or white cell counts, but these are not diagnostic of AIDS in the absence of symptoms. (*Katz et al, 2005, pp. 1274–1275*)

5. **(E)** Anabolic steroids, most commonly testosterone enanthate or cypionate, increase lean body mass in AIDS patients, particularly those who do weight training. Dronabinol, an antiemetic, and megestrol acetate, a progestational agent, are used to increase appetite and

assist in weight gain, but have little effect on lean muscle mass. Odansetron and prochlorperazine are both used to treat weight loss caused by nausea of unclear origin in AIDS patients and are given prior to meals. (*Katz et al, 2005, pp. 1278–1279*)

6. **(D)** Severe hypoxemia is a common finding in *Pneumocystis* pneumonia even when symptoms are not severe. The characteristic chest radiograph findings are diffuse or perihilar infiltrates. Apical infiltrates are more likely to be seen in patients who have been receiving aerosolized pentamadine prophylaxis. High resolution chest CT scanning would most likely demonstrate interstitial lung disease. This pneumonia is rare unless the CD4 count is less than 250. An elevated LDH is found in about 95% of patients. (*Katz et al, 2005, p. 1279*)

7. **(A)** AIDS dementia complex is the most common cause of mental status changes in patients with HIV disease. The deterioration of handwriting is often an early manifestation. Difficulty in performing cognitive tasks and diminished motor speed are typical, as is the waxing and waning of manifestations of dementia. Patients with central nervous system lymphoma and toxoplasmosis present with headache, focal neurologic deficits, seizures, and/or altered mental status. Patients with cryptococcal meningitis have, most typically, headache and fever, but fewer than 20% have meningismus. They also usually have normal mental status. Patients with PML have primarily focal neurologic deficits such as aphasia, hemiparesis, and cortical blindness. (*Katz et al, 2005, p. 1281*)

8. **(C)** Patients with cryptococcal meningitis have, most typically, headache and fever, but fewer than 20% have meningismus. They also usually have normal mental status. AIDS dementia complex is characterized by difficulty in performing cognitive tasks, diminished motor speed, and waxing and waning of manifestations of dementia. Patients with central nervous system lymphoma and toxoplasmosis present with headache, focal neurologic deficits, seizures, and/or altered mental status. Patients with progressive multifocal leukoencephalopathy have primarily focal neurologic deficits such as aphasia, hemiparesis, and cortical blindness. (*Katz et al, 2005, p. 1281*)

9. **(A)** Toxoplasmosis most typically appears as multiple contrast-enhancing lesions on CT scan. When CT scanning reveals a single lesion, an MRI, because of its greater sensitivity, may reveal multiple lesions. The presumptive diagnosis may be made on the characteristic appearance of lesions on CT or MRI. A positive serologic test for toxoplasma does not confirm a diagnosis of toxoplasmosis, because many HIV-positive patients will have detectable titers. Nonenhancing white matter lesions of the brain without mass effect are characteristic of progressive multifocal leukoencephalopathy. (*Katz et al, 2005, p. 1281*)

10. **(B)** It is not unusual for persons with HIV infection to develop peripheral neuropathies. Recommended initial treatment is gabapentin, which provides symptomatic relief for neuropathic pain. Since this is not an inflammatory process, ibuprofen is not indicated. Recombinant nerve growth factor has been shown to reduce pain in a randomized study; however, this is not available outside of the research setting. Didanosine and stavudine are the most common causes of peripheral neuropathy (*Katz et al, 2005, p. 1282*)

11. **(B)** The lesions described are hairy leukoplakia, caused by the Epstein-Barr virus. *Candida* usually causes uncomfortable lesions that may be either removable white plaques or red friable plaques. Herpes simplex virus causes painful ulcerations. Both iron and vitamin B_{12} deficiencies can cause pain. The tongue appears smooth and beefy. (*Katz et al, 2005, p. 1282*)

12. **(C)** Health maintenance for individuals who first test positive for HIV should include purified protein derivative testing, pneumococcal vaccine administration, and aggressive search for evidence of syphilis. Earlier recommendations were for beginning antiretroviral therapy when the CD4 counts dropped below 500 cells/mL, but this has been changed. Persons

with HIV who are symptomatic are treated, as are those who are asymptomatic and who have a CD4 count less than 200 cells/mL. *Pneumocystis* pneumonia prophylaxis should be initiated when the CD4 count is less than 200 cells/mL. When the CD4 count falls below 75 cells/mL, the provider should initiate *Mycobacterium avium* complex prophylaxis. Cytomegalovirus prophylaxis is recommended with CD4 counts less than 50 cells/mL. (*Katz et al, 2005, p. 1287*)

13. **(C)** After a needle-stick injury, a health-care worker should have baseline testing with follow-up testing at 6 weeks, 3 months, and 6 months. Risk of seroconversion is approximately 1:300. Administration of antiviral therapy decreases this risk by 79%, so the worker should be offered treatment with zidovudine and lamivudine as soon as possible after the injury, for a total of 4 weeks. However, workers with a high-risk exposure (source patient with advanced disease, a viral load >50,000, or with resistant organisms) should have a protease inhibitor added to the prophylactic regimen. (*Katz et al, 2005, p. 1289*)

14. **(D)** Nevirapine should be avoided for HIV prophylaxis as reports have linked it to hepatotoxicity in the prophylactic setting. Abacavir may cause rash and fever, indinavir kidney stones, lamivudine rash and peripheral neuropathy, and zidovudine anemia, neutropenia, nausea, malaise, headache, insomnia, and myopathy. (*Katz et al, 2005, p. 1289*)

15. **(E)** Optic neuritis is associated with the use of ethambutol. Anemia is associated with many of the drugs used to treat AIDS-related opportunistic infections, including trimethoprim-sulfamethoxazole, pentamidine, amphotericin B, ganciclovir, and valgancyclovir. Amphotericin B is associated with azotemia, trimethoprim with methemoglobinemia. Trimetrexate can cause mucositis. (*Katz et al, 2005, p. 1291*)

16. **(D)** As the goal of antiretroviral therapy is to suppress viral replication, the most appropriate test for monitoring therapy is the viral load in the serum. The CD4 count and percentage are useful in deciding when to initiate prophylaxis for opportunistic infections. The ELISA and Western Blot tests are used to diagnose HIV infection. (*Katz et al, 2005, p. 1295*)

17. **(C)** Lovastatin and simvastatin should be avoided in patients taking protease inhibitors because of drug interactions. In general, patients should be started on atorvastatin or pravastain. Gemfibrozil is used for patients who have very high triglyceride levels that do not respond to dietary modification. (*Katz et al, 2005, p. 1297*)

18. **(C)** A common side effect of indinavir is the development of kidney stones. Delavirdine is associated with rash; didanosine is associated with peripheral neruopathy, pancreatitis, dry mouth, and hepatitis. Diarrhea is the most common side effect of nelfinavir; peripheral neuropathy, hepatitis, and pancreatitis are the side effects of stavudine. (*Katz et al, 2005, p. 1297*)

19. **(C)** Patients with G6PD deficiency are at increased risk for developing hemolytic anemia if treated with dapsone. In all patients, adverse effects associated with dapsone include anemia, nausea, and methemoglobinemia. Risks associated with aerosolized pentamidine include bronchospasm and, rarely, pancreatitis. Those associated with trimethoprim-sulfamethoxazole include rash, neutropenia, hepatitis, and Stevens-Johnson syndrome. Atovaquone is used only in those patients who cannot tolerate the other treatments. Adverse effects include rash, nausea, vomiting, diarrhea, fever, and abnormal liver function. (*Katz et al, 2005, p. 1301*)

20. **(E)** Use of fetal scalp electrodes and scalp sampling is contraindicated in the HIV-positive woman because it increases the risk of vertical transmission of the human immunodeficiency virus to the infant. While ruptured membranes for more than 4 hours is associated with increased risk of vertical transmission, amniotomy per se is not contraindicated. Augmentation of labor, external monitoring, and operative delivery are not contraindicated

and, in fact, may be indicated in specific instances for the well-being of the infant and/or mother. (*Ainbinder and Ramin, 2003, p. 747*)

21. **(A)** Zidovidine or other antiretroviral prophylaxis during pregnancy with additional prophylaxis for the infant during the first 1 to 2 weeks of life decreases vertical transmission to less than 1%. No evidence exists to show that indefinite zidovudine therapy is useful. If the infant is HIV positive, as shown by two separate HIV-PCR tests, HIV cultures, or HIV antigen tests, treatment should commence according to current guidelines. (*McFarland, 2003, p. 1145*)

22. **(D)** The median age at which infants no longer show the maternal antibody is 10 months. By 18 months they all do. HIV ELISA and Western blot are not appropriate for testing pediatric patients until after that age. Appropriate tests for infants include HIV culture, HIV polymerase chain reaction, and HIV antigen (p24). (*McFarland, 2003, p. 1142*)

23. **(A)** Young infants are at higher risk for disease progression than older children. Therefore, the consensus is that antiretroviral therapy should be initiated as soon as the diagnosis of HIV disease is confirmed. In older children, clinical or immunological status or viral load is used to determine the initiation of therapy. (*McFarland, 2003, p. 1146*)

24. **(A)** HIV-positive children should receive most standard pediatric vaccines at the usually scheduled times. However, the measles–mumps–rubella (MMR) vaccine should be given at 12 months rather than the usual 15, with a booster 1 month later. The risk of measles is considered greater than the risk of the vaccine in children who are not symptomatic. However, titers decrease over time and with increased immunodeficiency, so an immunized infant who is exposed to measles should receive immune globulin. (*McFarland, 2003, p. 1148*)

25. **(D)** Centers for Disease Control and Prevention recommendations are that babies of HIV-positive mothers receive prophylaxis against infection with *Pneumocystis jiroveci* pneumonia because this infection has its highest incidence during the first year of life. Prophylactic treatment should be continued until 12 months of age if the infant becomes HIV positive, but may be discontinued at 3 to 4 months if testing is negative. Appropriate agents include trimethoprim-sulfamethoxazole, dapsone, atovaquone, or pentamidine. Monthly immune globulin is effective in reducing other bacterial infections and hospitalizations in babies not receiving *Pneumocystis jiroveci* pneumonia prophylaxis. (*McFarland, 2003, p. 1148*)

26. **(C)** The HIV-positive child who is well should receive the same treatment as other children. Unless contaminated with gross blood, other body fluids (saliva, tears, urine, stool) are not contagious. All schools and daycares should have written policies and training regarding precautions to prevent blood-borne illness. (*McFarland, 2003, p. 1150*)

27. **(E)** Viral load seems to be most closely associated with vertical transmission. Women who have more than 1000 viral copies/mL should be offered early operative delivery. (*Ainbinder and Ramin, 2003, p. 747*)

28. **(D)** Non-Hodgkins lymphoma in extranodal sites such as bone, liver, lungs, or gastrointestinal tract is the most common tumor seen in children with HIV infection. The incidence of leiomyosarcoma is increased in these children, but it is not the most common tumor. Kaposi's sarcoma rarely occurs in children. There is no increased incidence of astrocytoma in children with HIV disease. (*McFarland, 2003, p. 1144*)

29. **(C)** Kaposi's sarcoma that is in a limited area of the skin may be treated with intralesional vinblastine or by simply observing it over time. Liposomal doxorubicin and alpha interferon are used for extensive or aggressive skin disease, while combination chemotherapy is used for visceral disease. (*Katz et al, 2005, p. 1292*)

30. **(B)** Semiannual Pap smears are recommended for all HIV-infected women. Quarterly Paps

are appropriate for any woman in the first year following treatment for human papilloma virus infection. For women with no risk factors, annual Paps are recommended during the reproductive years. Some groups recommend alternate or every third year Pap testing following three normal annual smears in a low-risk woman. (*Katz et al, 2005, p. 1288*)

REFERENCES

Ainbinder, SW, Ramin, SM. Sexually transmitted diseases and pelvic infections. In DeCherney, AH, Nathan, L (eds), *Current Obstetric and Gynecologic Diagnosis and Treatment*, 9th ed. New York: McGraw-Hill; 2003.

Katz, MH, Hollander, H. HIV Infection. In Tierney LM, McPhee SJ, Papadakis MA (eds), *Current Medical Diagnosis and Treatment*, 44th ed. New York: McGraw-Hill; 2005.

McFarland, EJ. Human immunodeficiency virus (HIV) infection. In Hay WW, Hayward AR, Levin MJ, Sondheimer JM (eds), *Current Pediatric Diagnosis and Treatment*, 16th ed. New York: MGraw-Hill; 2003.

CHAPTER 8

Infectious Disease
Questions

Brenda Kaminski, MPH, PA-C

DIRECTIONS (Questions 1 through 25): Each of the numbered items or incomplete statements in this section is followed by answers or by completion of the statement. Select the ONE lettered answer or completion that is BEST in each case.

Questions 1 through 25

1. The most common cause of community-acquired bacterial pneumonia in the United States is

    (A) *Streptococcus pyogenes*
    (B) *Streptococcus pneumoniae*
    (C) *Legionella pneumophila*
    (D) *Staphylococcus aureus*
    (E) *Haemophilus influenzae*

2. Which of the following purified protein derivative (PPD)-tested patients should receive antituberculosis prophylaxis?

    (A) PPD of 13 mm in a person with no risk factors
    (B) PPD of 8 mm in a foreign-born person from a country with a high prevalence of tuberculosis
    (C) PPD of 3 mm in an HIV-positive person
    (D) PPD of 6 mm in a Native American person
    (E) PPD of 12 mm in an inmate at a correctional institution

3. A patient with no history of treatment for primary syphilis presents with symptoms and signs consistent with secondary syphilis. During your workup on this patient, you would expect to find all of the following EXCEPT

    (A) generalized lymphadenopathy
    (B) condyloma lata
    (C) elevated alkaline phosphatase
    (D) generalized maculopapular rash
    (E) superficial painless gummas

4. Community-acquired endocarditis in non-intravenous drug users is most likely to be caused by alpha-hemolytic streptococci or members of the HACEK group of organisms. Which of the following is NOT a member of the HACEK group?

    (A) *Histoplasma*
    (B) *Actinobacillus*
    (C) *Cardiobacterium*
    (D) *Eikenella*
    (E) *Kingella*

5. A 30-year-old male presents to the office for follow-up on an endoscopically diagnosed gastric ulcer. At endoscopy, he was found to have a *Helicobacter pylori* infection and now he has completed appropriate therapy. He has another refill available on the proton-pump inhibitor. He is currently asymptomatic. What is the most appropriate follow-up on the infection?

(A) because he is asymptomatic, no further testing is required

(B) check urea breath test or fecal antigen today

(C) repeat endoscopy with histologic testing for *H. pylori*

(D) check *H. pylori* serology today

(E) collect stool specimen for culture

6. An adult male, not previously vaccinated for rabies, presents to the emergency room after being bitten by an aggressive stray dog. The dog was captured, and declared "probably rabid" by a local veterinarian. Which of the following treatment options should you select for this patient?

(A) administer human rabies immune globulin only

(B) administer equine rabies antiserum only

(C) administer human rabies immune globulin and equine rabies antiserum

(D) administer human rabies immune globulin and equine rabies antiserum and human diploid cell rabies vaccine

(E) administer human rabies immune globulin and human diploid cell rabies vaccine

7. An otherwise healthy, immunocompetent health-care worker converts to a positive PPD. Which of the following drugs is recommended for this person?

(A) rifampin

(B) pyrazinamide

(C) ethambutol

(D) streptomycin

(E) isoniazid

8. Which of the following is NOT true concerning childhood vaccinations?

(A) Hepatitis B vaccine may be given to infants within 12 hours of birth

(B) the first two doses of inactivated oral polio vaccine (OPV) should be followed by two doses of inactivated polio vaccine (IPV)

(C) the second dose of measles–mumps–rubella (MMR) vaccine is recommended at 4 to 6 years of age

(D) combined diphtheria and tetanus toxoids and acellular pertussis vaccine is the preferred combination for all doses in the initial vaccination series

(E) the *Haemophilus influenzae* type b (Hib) conjugate vaccination series should begin at 2 months of age

9. In the treatment of peptic ulcer disease (PUD) of infectious etiology, which of the following drug combinations will provide the most efficacious therapy?

(A) metronidazole and omeprazole

(B) bismuth subsalicylate and omeprazole and sucralfate

(C) amoxicillin and bismuth subsalicylate and antacid

(D) omeprazole and amoxicillin and clarithromycin

(E) clarithromycin and metronidazole and sucralfate

10. An adult with a high risk for bacterial endocarditis is scheduled for a dental extraction. The patient has a history of penicillin allergy. Which of the following is an appropriate oral prophylactic drug to give this patient?

(A) amoxicillin

(B) vancomycin

(C) clindamycin

(D) doxycycline

(E) gentamicin

11. Which of the following is NOT true of pinworm infections?

    (A) usually presents in pediatric patients
    (B) primary symptom is perianal itching
    (C) diagnosis often made with "scotch-tape" test
    (D) entire household should be treated with metronidazole
    (E) may be responsible for recurrent urinary tract infections in girls

12. Septic arthritis in adults younger than 30 years is usually caused by

    (A) *Neisseria gonorrhea*
    (B) *Staphylococcus aureus*
    (C) *Pseudomonas aeruginosa*
    (D) *Streptococcus pyogenes*
    (E) *Salmonella* species

13. A 30-year-old female presents with 2 weeks of arthralgias, migrating from distal to proximal joints. It began with increased warmth and erythema in her right ankle and left knee. She has a low-grade fever and reports a history of sore throat and swollen glands about 1 month ago. Antistreptolysin O titer is positive. The most likely explanation for her joint pain is

    (A) new-onset rheumatoid arthritis
    (B) rheumatic fever
    (C) gonococcal arthritis
    (D) Gram-positive septic arthritis
    (E) osteoarthritis

14. In the humoral defense system, which class of antibody is the body's first-line response to infection?

    (A) IgA
    (B) complement
    (C) IgM
    (D) IgG
    (E) IgE

15. The gold standard for diagnosis of tuberculosis is

    (A) chest x-ray
    (B) PPD skin test
    (C) sputum stain for acid-fast bacilli
    (D) sputum culture and sensitivity
    (E) clinical symptoms of fever, night sweats, and hemoptysis

16. A sexually active 19-year-old female presents with clusters of painful vesicles on an erythematous base on the vulva and cervix, accompanied by temperature of 100°F and mild malaise. She reports a history of a similar outbreak last month, which resolved in 10 days. Microscopic exam of cells from the basement of a blister treated with Giemsa stain is likely to reveal

    (A) multinucleated giant cells
    (B) Gram-positive cocci in clusters
    (C) Gram-positive cocci in chains
    (D) Gram-negative rods
    (E) hyphae and buds

17. All of the following are common findings in the cerebrospinal fluid of a patient with acute bacterial meningitis EXCEPT

    (A) glucose <40 mg/dL
    (B) 100 to 10,000 WBC/dL
    (C) protein >100 mg/dL
    (D) elevated C-reactive protein
    (E) >10,000 RBC/dL

18. Which of the following characteristics is most helpful in distinguishing *Mycoplasma pneumoniae* as the etiologic agent in community-acquired pneumonia from other bacteria and viruses?

    (A) mycoplasma has an incubation period that averages 28 days compared to weeks for most viruses
    (B) mycoplasma is more common in the elderly
    (C) sputum Gram stain often shows increased WBCs with little or no bacteria
    (D) sputum culture is the gold standard for diagnosis
    (E) mycoplasma often follows exposure to cockroach infestation

19. Which of the following treatments is first-line therapy for sputum culture-positive Legionnaire's pneumonia in an immunocompetent patient?

    (A) ampicillin/sulbactam
    (B) erythromycin
    (C) ceftriaxone
    (D) vancomycin
    (E) clindamycin

20. Which of the following is NOT a complication of untreated streptococcal pharyngitis?

    (A) glomerulonephritis
    (B) scarlet fever
    (C) suppurative head and neck infection
    (D) toxic shock syndrome
    (E) septic arthritis

21. Koplik's spots are a differentiating diagnostic feature of which of the following viral exanthems?

    (A) rubella
    (B) rubeola
    (C) varicella
    (D) parvovirus
    (E) Kawasaki disease

22. A 16-year-old female presents to the office complaining of very sore throat, swollen lymph nodes, fever, and general malaise. Exam reveals temperature 102.2°F, enlarged exudative tonsils, tender cervical lymphadenopathy, and borderline enlarged spleen. Rapid strep screen is positive. All of the following antibiotics are appropriate EXCEPT

    (A) erythromycin
    (B) azithromycin
    (C) penicillin
    (D) cefprozil
    (E) amoxicillin

23. Which of the following statements about poliomyelitis is FALSE?

    (A) poliomyelitis has been effectively eradicated in the Western hemisphere
    (B) oral live-attenuated vaccine is recommended in the United States for primary vaccination at 2 months, 4 months, 6 months, and 4 to 6 years
    (C) complications include urinary tract infection, pneumonia, pulmonary edema, and myocarditis
    (D) adults should be immunized when traveling to endemic nations
    (E) bulbar poliomyelitis may affect respiratory and vasomotor function and is fatal in up to 50% of cases

24. Which of the following viruses is rodent-borne and the cause of hemorrhagic fever and a pulmonary syndrome, which begins with a fever and may rapidly progress to shock and adult respiratory distress syndrome?

    (A) human T-cell lymphotropic virus (HTLV)
    (B) flavivirus
    (C) hantavirus
    (D) filovirus
    (E) coronavirus

25. A 5-year-old male is brought in by his mother with low-grade fever, headache, maculopapular rash on back and abdomen, and a fiery red rash on both cheeks. The most likely etiologic agent is

    (A) varicella
    (B) humanherpes 6 virus
    (C) parvovirus
    (D) Coxsackie virus
    (E) poxvirus

DIRECTIONS (Questions 26 through 29): Each group of items in this section consists of lettered headings followed by a set of numbered words or phrases. For each numbered phrase, select the lettered disease that is most closely associated with the description.

Questions 26 through 29

Match the following clinical presentations with the appropriate etiology:

    (A) Lyme disease

    (B) Rocky Mountain spotted fever

    (C) erlichiosis

    (D) Q fever

26. associated with erythema chronicum migrans rash

27. has no insect vector but often follows exposure to sheep, cattle, or goats

28. microcolonies grow in hematopoietic cells, forming inclusions seen with Giemsa stain

29. maculopapular rash begin on the wrists and ankles

DIRECTIONS (Questions 30 through 40): Each of the numbered items or incomplete statements in this section is followed by answers or by completion of the statement. Select the ONE lettered answer or completion that is BEST in each case.

Questions 30 through 40

30. Which of the following is NOT a contraindication for influenza immunization?

    (A) hypersensitivity to chicken eggs

    (B) concomitant warfarin therapy

    (C) Guillain—Barré syndrome

    (D) thrombocytopenia

    (E) acute febrile illness

31. Severe acute respiratory syndrome (SARS) is an atypical pneumonia caused by

    (A) West Nile virus

    (B) flavivirus

    (C) coronavirus

    (D) hantavirus

    (E) respiratory syncytial virus

32. A 4-year-old male presents with 5 days of fever, conjunctivitis, strawberry tongue, red lips, and injected throat. He has large, swollen, slightly tender lymph nodes in his neck and a peeling rash in the palms and soles. The most likely cause is

    (A) Kawasaki syndrome

    (B) respiratory syncytial virus

    (C) Coxsackie virus

    (D) Fifth's disease

    (E) mycoplasma

33. A 25-year-old female presents not feeling well 1 week after returning from a trip to central Africa. She has had steadily increasing fever, abdominal distention, and diarrhea. She also has rashes on her abdomen, chest, and back, which are characterized by 3-mm pink papules, which blanch with pressure. Heart rate is 60 beats/min. Blood culture is positive but final identification is pending. Most likely diagnosis is

    (A) typhoid fever

    (B) yellow fever

    (C) malaria

    (D) hepatitis

    (E) shigellosis

34. The etiology of plague is the *Yersinia pestis* bacterium. In a patient with high fever, malaise, and severe myalgias, which of the following additional pieces of history would raise the index of suspicion for plague?

    (A) history of tick bite in the northeastern United States
    (B) exposure to wild rats in Southern California
    (C) history of drinking stream water while hiking in the Appalachian mountains
    (D) history of raising sheep in Wyoming
    (E) exposure to exotic birds in upper Midwest

35. A 14-year-old girl presents 1 week after her hand was bitten by the neighbor's cat. In the first 3 days after the bite she developed a shallow ulcer at the bite site. Because her parents knew the cat was up to date on shots, they treated the ulcer with topical antibiotics and did not seek medical care. Now the patient has low-grade fever, headache, and feels tired. Axillary nodes on the affected side are swollen. The ulcer on the hand is nearly healed. Indicated therapy includes

    (A) doxycycline 100 mg bid × 21 days
    (B) augmentin 500 mg po bid × 10 days
    (C) azithromycin 500 mg po qd × 7 days
    (D) acyclovir 400 mg po bid × 10 days
    (E) no therapy required

36. Which of the following statements about *Lymphogranuloma venereum* is FALSE?

    (A) the initial genital lesion often goes unnoticed
    (B) it is transmitted through intercourse or contact with infected exudates
    (C) must be differentiated from syphilis and herpes simplex
    (D) therapy is single dose Rocephin 250 mg IM
    (E) proctitis is another common manifestation

37. A 27-year-old female presents with 3 days of fever, chills, headache, and a deep dry cough. She has been working at a pet store for the past month and thinks that one of the parakeets that came in 10 days ago may be sick. On exam, she has dullness to percussion of the right lung base and right-sided rales. The most likely diagnosis is

    (A) sarcoidosis
    (B) tularemia
    (C) psittacosis
    (D) brucellosis
    (E) listeriosis

38. A 35-year-old forest ranger presents with a rash on his back. It started 4 days ago as a red maculopapular lesion about 2 cm in diameter. Now it is 14 cm in diameter with an area of central clearing. In addition to the rash, he has had a headache, fever, chills, and muscle aches. The most likely diagnosis is

    (A) cellulitis
    (B) wasp sting
    (C) Rocky Mountain spotted fever
    (D) poison ivy
    (E) Lyme disease

39. All of the following are consistent with the clinical presentation of *Giardia lamblia* infection EXCEPT

    (A) abdominal distention and cramps
    (B) greasy stools
    (C) bloody diarrhea
    (D) history of camping and drinking from streams
    (E) malabsorption and weight loss

40. Pregnant women should avoid contact with cat feces because of the potential harmful sequelae of congenital transmission of

    (A) toxoplasmosis
    (B) schistosomiasis
    (C) leishmaniasis
    (D) brucellosis
    (E) echinococcosis

DIRECTIONS (Questions 41 through 45): Each group of items in this section consists of lettered headings followed by a set of numbered words or phrases. For each numbered phrase, select the lettered disease that is most closely associated with the description.

Questions 41 through 45

Match the following diagnoses with the most likely etiologic agent. Each answer may be used only once.

- (A) *Moraxella catarrhalis*
- (B) *Escherichia coli*
- (C) *Staphylococcus aureus*
- (D) *Pneumococcus*
- (E) *Campylobacter*

41. septic arthritis

42. otitis media

43. gastroenteritis

44. meningitis

45. pyelonephritis

DIRECTIONS (Questions 46 through 50): Each of the numbered items or incomplete statements in this section is followed by answers or by completion of the statement. Select the ONE lettered answer or completion that is BEST in each case.

Questions 46 through 50

46. Which of the following is the appropriate treatment for acute *Clostridium tetani* infection?

- (A) tetanus immune globulin, tetanus toxoid, and metronidazole
- (B) tetanus immune globulin and penicillin
- (C) tetanus toxoid and penicillin
- (D) tetanus immune globulin, tetanus toxoid, and penicillin
- (E) tetanus immune globulin and tetanus toxoid

47. A 73-year-old male is hospitalized for a prolonged period because his prostate surgery was complicated by pneumonia. After 10 days of broad-spectrum antibiotics, he develops fever, leukocytosis, and dysentery. Colonoscopy reveals pseudomembranes in his colon. Stool cultures are pending. The most likely etiology for his diarrhea is

- (A) Norwalk virus
- (B) *Clostridium difficile*
- (C) *Clostridium perfringens*
- (D) Enterobacteriaciae
- (E) *Pseudomonas aeruginosa*

48. Which of the following findings does NOT support a diagnosis of osteomyelitis?

- (A) lytic lesions on x-ray
- (B) periosteal elevation and thickening on x-ray
- (C) decreased radionuclide uptake on bone scan
- (D) vertebral cortical destruction
- (E) bone edema on MRI

49. All of the following distinguish smallpox from chickenpox EXCEPT

- (A) the distribution of the rash is primarily the face and extremities in smallpox
- (B) fever occurs at the same time as skin eruption in smallpox
- (C) all the lesions are at the same stage in smallpox
- (D) the palms and soles are involved in smallpox
- (E) the first lesions appear on the buccal mucosa in smallpox

50. Which of the following forms of anthrax is most common?

- (A) inhalational
- (B) hematogenous
- (C) cutaneous
- (D) gastrointestinal
- (E) congenital

Answers and Explanations

1. **(B)** Pneumococcal pneumonia, caused by *Streptococcus pneumoniae*, is the most commonly occurring pneumonia worldwide. In the United States, it is the leading cause of community-acquired bacterial pneumonia, affecting over a half million people annually. Pneumococcal vaccine confers excellent protection against the most common serotypes that cause the disease. (*Tierney et al, 2005, pp. 244–250*)

2. **(E)** Recommendations by the Advisory Committee for the Elimination of Tuberculosis indicate that the following high-risk groups should receive preventive chemotherapy if their tuberculin skin test (PPD) is >10 mm:

   1. foreign-born persons from high-prevalence countries
   2. medically underserved, low-income populations, including high-risk racial or ethnic minority populations
   3. residents of facilities for long-term care (e.g., correctional facilities, nursing homes) (*Tierney et al, 2005, p. 256*)

3. **(E)** Secondary syphilis generally manifests itself a month or two after appearance of the primary chancre. Patients will complain of headache, fever, sore throat, and malaise and will exhibit generalized lymphadenopathy along with a maculopapular rash that begins at the sides of the trunk and later spreads over the rest of the body. The skin lesions may coalesce in warm moist areas, such as the perineum, and form large, flat-topped, pale papules termed *condyloma lata*. Elevated alkaline phosphatase is common in secondary syphilis. Formation of granulomatous nodules (*gummas*) is not a feature of secondary disease, but rather is the hallmark of tertiary syphilis. (*Tierney et al, 2005, pp. 1398–1399*)

4. **(A)** The HACEK group of microorganisms must be considered in any case of community-acquired endocarditis. Although not as frequently involved as alpha-hemolytic streptococci in cases of endocarditis, they constitute an important group of pathogens capable of producing serious cardiac complications. The HACEK group is composed of species of *Haemophilus*, *Actinobacillus*, *Cardiobacterium*, *Eikenella*, and *Kingella*. *Histoplasma* species are fungi not commonly implicated with endocarditis and are not members of the HACEK group. (*Tierney et al, 2005, pp. 1365–1370*)

5. **(D)** *Helicobacter pylori* is a spiral, Gram-negative rod that resides in the gastric mucosa, where it causes PUD. It may be diagnosed by rapid urease test or by histology when endoscopy is performed. Noninvasive *H. pylori* testing options include the urease breath test, fecal antigen testing, and serology. Serological and fecal antigen tests are the most cost-effective methods. All three noninvasive tests have sensitivities and specificities greater than 90%. Proton-pump inhibitor therapy should be discontinued 1 to 2 weeks prior to the fecal antigen or

breath tests because they may increase the number of false negatives. In this case, serology is the least invasive, most cost-effective, and least likely to be invalidated by the proton-pump inhibitor therapy. (*Tierney et al, 2005, pp. 566–569*)

6. **(E)** Transmission of rabies to this patient must be seriously considered, and postexposure immunization should begin immediately by the administration of human rabies immune globulin (HRIG; 40 units/kg). About half the HRIG should be infiltrated around the bite wound, and the remainder injected intramuscularly. Human diploid cell rabies vaccine (HDCV) should also be given (1 mL IM in the deltoid), and again on days 3, 7, 14, and 28. HDCV should be delivered in a different syringe and administered at a different site than HRIG. (*Tierney et al, 2005, pp. 1322–1324*)

7. **(E)** The drug of choice for prophylaxis of tuberculosis is isoniazid (INH), given at a daily dose of 300 mg/day for 6 to 12 months (children: 10 to 14 mg/kg/day). The major risk of INH prophylaxis is drug-induced hepatitis, especially in the elderly. Therefore, periodic monitoring of liver function tests during the course of INH treatment is recommended for persons aged 35 and older. Minor transferase elevations (up to three times normal) are not indications to discontinue therapy. (*Tierney et al, 2005, pp. 256–258*)

8. **(B)** The Advisory Committee on Immunization Practices (ACIP), the American Academy of Pediatrics (AAP), and the American Academy of Family Practice (AAFP) recently approved a revised schedule for recommended childhood vaccinations. The schedule covers recommendations for administration of the following vaccines: hepatitis B (HepB), diphtheria/tetanus/pertussis (DtaP), *Haemophilus influenzae* type b (Hib), poliovirus (IPV and OPV), measles/mumps/rubella (MMR), and varicella zoster (Var). Two poliovirus vaccines are currently available: inactivated polio vaccine (IPV) and oral polio vaccine (OPV). Current recommendations are to use the IPV for all four doses. (*Tierney et al, 2005, pp. 1260–1266*)

9. **(D)** Combination therapy is recommended for eradication of *Helicobacter pylori*–associated PUD. Administration of a proton-pump inhibitor (omeprazole or lansoprazole) and two antibiotics (clarithromycin and either amoxicillin or metronidazole) achieves eradication rates of over 85%. However, emerging resistance of *H. pylori* to metronidazole makes amoxicillin preferable for combination therapy. Regimens using bismuth compounds required higher dosing and linkage with antibiotics, plus a proton-pump inhibitor, to enhance efficacy. Also, bismuth regimens are associated with a higher incidence of side effects than proton-pump inhibitor regimens. Antacids and sucralfate are outmoded as primary therapy for PUD. (*Tierney et al, 2005, pp. 568–573*)

10. **(C)** The American Heart Association recommends that patients who are at moderate to high risk for bacterial endocarditis receive antibiotic prophylaxis prior to undergoing oral/dental, respiratory tract, or esophageal procedures. Amoxicillin 2.0 g orally 1 hour before the procedure is the standard regimen. Patients who have a history of amoxicillin/penicillin allergy may be given clindamycin, azithromycin, or clarithromycin. For adults, clarithromycin is given at a dose of 600 mg po 1 hour before the procedure. Clarithromycin for children is dosed at 20 mg/kg, given 1 hour before the procedure. (*Tierney et al, 2005, pp. 1365–1370*)

11. **(D)** The entire household should be treated to avoid reinfection, but metronidazole is not the drug of choice. Pinworms are often treated with mebendazole or albendazole in single-dose therapy. Therapy should be repeated in 2 weeks because it is not effective against eggs. Pinworms are most commonly found in pediatric patients. The adult pinworm crawls out of the anus at night to lay eggs, resulting in intense itching. Resultant scratching leads to contaminated fingernails and autoreinfection or spread to other contacts. Pinworms may move into the vagina or urethra in girls as well, which explains why pinworm treatment sometimes brings resolution to recurrent bladder infections in pediatric females. Diagnosis is

often made by applying transparent tape to the perianal area in the morning prior to bathing and then applying to a slide with a drop of xylene. The ova are usually seen under the microscope. (*Hay et al, 2005, p. 1267*)

12. **(A)** In patients younger than 30 years, gonococcus is the most common cause of septic arthritis. When all patients are considered, *Staphylococcus aureus* is the most common cause. Patients with prevalent joint disease and intravenous drug users are especially susceptible to *Staphylococcus*. *Pseudomonas* is also a common cause of septic arthritis in intravenous drug users. *Salmonella* is not a common cause of joint infection. (*Andreoli et al, 2004, p. 895*)

13. **(B)** Rheumatic fever is an immune-mediated process occurring in response to prior infection with Group A *Streptococcus*. The arthritis often moves from joint to joint in an asymmetrical pattern. In some cases there may be cardiac symptoms, skin rash (erythema marginatum), and subcutaneous nodules. Antistreptolysin O titer is often positive. It is important to quickly diagnose rheumatic fever because it requires long-term prophylaxis against *Streptococcus*. (*Andreoli et al, 2004, p. 895*)

14. **(C)** IgM is the body's first-line response to infection. The most prevalent immune globulin in the bloodstream is IgG. IgG is important to phagocytosis of the invading pathogen and is responsible for transplacental immunity. IgA is found in mucosal surfaces (e.g., oral mucosa) and is responsible for secretory immunity. IgE is present in allergy and also antihelminthic immunity. (*Andreoli et al, 2004, pp. 804–805*)

15. **(D)** Chest x-ray is an important part of diagnosis with apical shadowing as a typical finding. Cavitations are also a possibility, particularly in more advanced or reactivated pulmonary tuberculosis. Acid-fast stains are still used in some laboratories. Acid-fast bacilli on microscopic exam combined with exam and x-ray findings are highly suggestive but it is not specific. Other types of *Mycobac-*

terium in sputum will yield the same results. A positive PPD skin test demonstrates an exposure to tuberculosis but is not diagnostic of active infection. Culture and sensitivity are the gold standard though they may require 3 to 6 weeks to complete. (*Goldman and Ausiello, 2004, p. 1896*)

16. **(A)** The clinical presentation is consistent with herpes simplex II. The appropriate microscopic study is a Tzanck smear, prepared by staining cells from the floor of a vesicle using Papanicolau, Giemsa, or Wright methods. The Tzanck smear will show multinucleated giant cells. It has a sensitivity of 60% to 70% and as a result should be confirmed by viral culture. Gram-positive cocci are consistent with staphylococcal or streptococcal infection and Gram-negative rods are usually enteric pathogens. Hyphae and buds are seen on KOH prep with candidal infection. (*Goldman and Ausiello, 2004, p. 1990*)

17. **(E)** Elevated WBCs, protein, and glucose <40 mg/dL are all common findings in the cerebrospinal fluid (CSF) of patients with acute bacterial meningitis. In addition, they may have an elevated C-reactive protein. RBCs are not a normal part of the CSF. They may be found in the first tube drawn, resulting from a traumatic lumbar puncture. In that case, the number of RBCs should decrease in each of the subsequent tubes. Culture and sensitivity of the CSF are also important to identify the etiologic agent and direct antibiotic therapy. (*Goldman and Ausiello, 2004, pp. 1812–1813*)

18. **(C)** The incubation period for mycoplasma is actually longer than that of most viruses (weeks vs. days). Mycoplasma is much more common in adolescents and young adults than in the elderly. Sputum culture will grow mycoplasma but it is of limited clinical utility because the mycoplasma organism persists in the sputum for months after the illness has resolved. Exposure to insects is associated with Q fever or tularemia, rather than mycoplasma. Sputum gram stain can be helpful because it will show the WBCs consistent with an inflammatory process but very few or no bacteria. The WBCs are predominantly

polymorphonuclear cells or lymphocytes. (*Goldman and Ausiello, 2004, pp. 1770–1773*)

19. **(B)** First-line therapy for legionella pneumonia in the immunocompetent host is erythromycin 500 mg – 1 g IV qid or 500 mg po qid for 14 to 21 days. Another option for first-line therapy is doxycycline 200 mg IV or po once daily for 14 to 21 days. Alternatives include levofloxacin 500 mg IV or po qd for 7 to 10 days or azithromycin 500 mg IV or po qd for 3 days. Severe infection or treatment in the immunocompromised patient is levofloxacin or azithromycin. (*Goldman and Ausiello, 2004, p. 1781*)

20. **(E)** Possible complications of streptococcal pharyngitis include scarlet fever, bacteremia, suppurative head and neck infections, streptococcal toxic shock syndrome, poststreptococcal glomerulonephritis, and rheumatic fever. The strain of *Streptococcus* may determine which complication is most likely. The pharyngitis usually resolves in 3 to 4 days regardless of treatment. The reason to encourage completion of a course of antibiotic with good efficacy against strep is to prevent the above complications. Septic arthritis does not present as a result of prior pharyngitis. (*Goldman and Ausiello, 2004, p. 1784*)

21. **(B)** Koplik's spots, white lesions on the buccal mucosa, are characteristic of rubeola. The rash in rubeola usually presents as a red-brown rash starting with the head and moving caudally. It follows a 3- to 4-day prodrome consisting of fever, nasal drainage, conjunctivitis, and cough. Varicella may also present with mucosal lesions but they are vesicular on an erythematous base. Parvovirus, rubella, and Kawasaki disease generally do not have mucosal involvement. (*Tierney et al, 2005, p. 1310*)

22. **(E)** Penicillin is still the first-line therapy of choice for acute streptococcal pharyngitis. All of the others also have reasonable strep coverage. This patient, however, appears to have a concommitment infectious mononucleosis. Amoxicillin and ampicillin have been found to cause a rash when used to treat streptococcal pharyngitis in patients who also have mononucleosis. (*Tierney et al, 2005, p. 1313*)

23. **(B)** The inactivated (Salk) parenteral vaccine is now used for routine immunization in developed countries because of a concern that the oral vaccine will induce poliomyelitis. Due to the ongoing efforts of the WHO's Polio Eradication Campaign and ministries of health around the world, polio has been eradicated from the Western Hemisphere and is now limited to five nations in Africa in addition to Pakistan and India. For this reason, individuals traveling to developing nations should check with the Centers for Disease Control and Prevention for the latest information on endemic areas and recommendations on immunizations. (*Tierney et al, 2005, pp. 1320–1321*)

24. **(C)** Hantavirus has a rodent vector and usually manifests in either hemorrhagic fever or hantavirus pulmonary syndrome, which can be fatal. In the United States, outbreaks are usually in the southwest. There have been 300 cases since 1993. HTLV is a lymphotropic oncovirus associated with lymphoma. Dengue and yellow fever are both caused by flaviviridae, which is carried by mosquitoes. Filoviruses cause Ebola fever and Marburg fever. The vector is unknown. Coronavirus is the etiologic agent in severe acute respiratory syndrome. During the 2002–2003 epidemic that began in Southeast Asia, it was postulated that it was carried by the masked palm civet. (*Tierney et al, 2005, pp. 1328–1336*)

25. **(C)** The clinical presentation is consistent with *Erythema infectiosum*, Fifth's disease. Treatment is symptomatic. It is usually self-limited with excellent prognosis. Etiology is parvovirus. Varicella is the cause of chickenpox, which usually presents with progressive development of fluid-filled vesicles on an erythematous base. It can now be prevented by varicella vaccine. HHV-6 is the cause of exanthema subitum, which occurs primarily in toddlers and is the most common cause of febrile seizures in infants. Hand, foot, and mouth disease is caused by Coxsackie virus. There are nine different poxviruses with pre-

sentations including variola, molluscum contagiosum, monkey pox, and vaccinia. (*Tierney et al, 2005, pp. 1315, 1338–1339*)

26. **(A)** Lyme disease is a tick-borne illness that is characterized by a raised red rash beginning 1 week after tick bite. The rash borders advance over several days and central clearing occurs. 10% to 20% of patients do not develop a rash. (*Tierney et al, 2005, pp. 1406–1407*)

27. **(D)** Q fever has a worldwide distribution and is one rickettsial disease with no known insect vector. Presentation typically includes acute or chronic fever with significant headache, cough, abdominal pain, and prostration. It often follows exposure to cattle, goats, or sheep. (*Tierney et al, 2005, pp. 1348–1349*)

28. **(C)** Ehrlichiosis may present as human monocytic or human granulocytic. They are both tick-born, with dogs, rodents, deer, and sheep as possible reservoirs. Microcolonies of ehrlichiosis grow in hematopoietic cells, forming inclusions seen with Giemsa stain. (*Tierney et al, 2005, p. 1347*)

29. **(B)** RMSF begins with a prodrome of fever, chills, headache, myalgias, and restlessness. It occasionally progresses to delirium and coma. The characteristic rash begins 3 to 6 days into the illness. It begins on the hands and wrist and moves to the trunk. It may also be petechial. (*Tierney et al, 2005, p. 1346*)

30. **(B)** Influenza vaccine is an important adjunct to clinical and public health practice. The vaccine is produced from different components and is recommended yearly in the fall for adults older than 50 years, people with chronic heart or lung disease, nursing home residents, and health-care workers. It is contraindicated in those with hypersensitivity to the vaccine or eggs, in patients with Guillain—Barré syndrome, low platelets, or fever. Patients on steroids or warfarin are able to take it if they have no other contraindication. (*Tierney et al, 2005, p. 1335*)

31. **(C)** SARS was first identified in 2003 in Guangdong province in China. It appears to be transmitted when mucus membranes are contacted by respiratory droplets or fomites. SARS has been identified in people of all ages. It has an incubation period of less than 1 week, and presents with symptoms consistent with atypical pneumonia, including fever, cough, dyspnea, headache, sore throat, myalgias and, in some, watery diarrhea. Rales and rhonchi may be heard on physical exam. None of the symptoms or physical exam findings are diagnostic. Several laboratory studies may return abnormal results including decreased WBCs and platelets. Liver functions and coagulation studies may also be abnormal. Arterial oxygen saturation is often low. Chest CT may show ground-glass opacifications. The etiologic organism is the coronavirus. (*Tierney et al, 2005, pp. 1336–1337*)

32. **(A)** Kawasaki syndrome occurs throughout the world, primarily in children. It is thought to be infectious but the etiologic agent has never been isolated. The syndrome is composed of fever and four of five of the following symptoms: bilateral conjunctivitis, some type of mucous membrane change, a peripheral extremity change, transverse grooves on the nails, a polymorphous rash, and cervical lymph nodes >1.5 cm. It can be complicated by arteritis. Treatment may include aspirin, immune globulin, plasmapheresis, or corticosteroids. (*Tierney et al, 2005, p. 1349*)

33. **(A)** Typhoid fever is caused by *Salmonella typhus*. It is contracted by contaminated food or water. There are several endemic areas throughout Africa. Symptoms and signs may be nonspecific but often include blanchable, pink, papular rash over the trunk, and fever that increases in stepwise fashion. Blood culture is positive in 80% of cases in the first week. Abdominal symptoms may include distention and constipation, initially, followed by diarrhea and possibly, splenomegaly. Prevention is accomplished by multidose oral or single-dose vaccine. (*Tierney et al, 2005, pp. 1375–1376*)

34. **(B)** Plague is transmitted by direct contact with wild rodents or fleabites by fleas that have bitten the rodents. Droplet transmission is also possible with exposure to an infected

human host. Symptoms include high fever, increased heart rate, malaise, and headache. There may be signs of meningitis in addition to axillary, cervical, and inguinal adenopathy. Lymph nodes are very swollen and may drain purulent material. Central nervous system changes can progress to coma, and in "black plague," purpura is visible on the skin. Blood and aspirate cultures confirm the diagnosis. Treatment is with streptomycin or gentamycin. *Yersinia pestis* must also be considered as a possible agent of bioterrorism. (*Tierney et al, 2005, p. 1381*)

35. **(E)** The history and course of illness are consistent with cat-scratch fever. It is caused by infection with *Bartonella henselae*. Cat scratch or bite transmits it to humans. Clinical course usually begins with papule or ulcer at the site within a few days of the bite. Fever, headache, and malaise develop 7 to 21 days later. Lymph drainage of the site may result in swollen, tender, and/or suppurative nodes. Clinical diagnosis is the norm but special cultures or biopsy is possible. The symptoms usually resolve spontaneously with no specific therapy required. Complications may include encephalitis or disseminated disease in immunocompromised patients. (*Tierney et al, 2005, p. 1384*)

36. **(D)** Lymphogranuloma venereum is caused by *Chlamydia trachomatis*. Clinical course begins with a genital lesion that may be vesicular or ulcerative. It may be overlooked by the patient and is followed up to a month later by inguinal buboes. These swollen, tender nodes often progress to fused lesions with draining sinus tracts. In women and homosexual men, proctitis and rectal stricture are also common. Transmission may occur with intercourse or exposure to the drainage from the buboes. Treatment is doxycycline 100 mg po bid or erythromycin 500 mg po qid for 3 weeks. (*Tierney et al, 2005, p. 1391*)

37. **(C)** The key piece of history in this question is the new exposure to parakeets. The symptoms and signs, including atypical pneumonia, are consistent with psittacosis but are not pathognomonic. Sarcoidosis is an illness of unknown cause. Listeriosis has been linked to exposures to contaminated food, particularly dairy products and hot dogs. Brucellosis can be caused by exposure to hogs, cattle, or goats. Tularemia is associated with contact with rabbits, other rodents, and biting arthropods. (*Tierney et al, 2005, p. 1392*)

38. **(E)** The description of the rash is consistent with the erythema chronicum migrans rash of Lyme disease. Lyme disease is caused by the spirochete, *Borrelia burgdorferi*, which is transmitted by tick bite. The course of Lyme disease usually involves progression through three stages. In stage 1, 80% to 90% of patients develop the rash, usually within a week of a tick bite. The rash begins with a maculopapular red lesion at the site. Over several days, the lesion can become much larger and develop centrally clearing. It is often described as looking like a bull's-eye. In addition to the rash, half of the patients will develop fever, chills, and myalgias. Stage 1 symptoms usually resolve within a month without treatment. Stage 2 is characterized by disseminated symptoms, generally involving the skin, central nervous system, and musculoskeletal system. Symptoms may include headaches, stiff neck, and joint pains. Arrhythmias and heart block are also possible. Bell's palsy, personality changes, forgetfulness, peripheral neuropathy, and conjunctivitis can all manifest in stage 2 as well. Months to years after the bite, untreated patients can develop stage 3 symptoms, including arthritis and synovitis and permanent disability. Further neurologic symptoms may develop, along with a diffuse fasciitis. Treatment for Lyme disease is doxycycline 100 mg po bid for 3 to 4 weeks in stage 1. Central nervous system involvement requires intravenous therapy. Alternative antibiotics are amoxicillin or cefuroxime. (*Tierney et al, 2005, pp. 1406–1411*)

39. **(C)** *Giardia lamblia* infection occurs worldwide and often is an asymptomatic infection. For the symptomatic, presenting complaints usually include acute or chronic diarrhea of variable severity. The stools are large, greasy, and malodorous. Diarrhea is often associated with abdominal pain and cramps, as well as excess flatus and fatigue. Malabsorption of some proteins, vitamins A and B_{12}, and disaccharides

can also occur. When malabsorption occurs, it is associated with weight loss. *Giardia*-infected stools do not contain blood or pus. Diagnosis is made by examining stools for ova and parasites or by immunoassay. Immunoassay has sensitivity and specificity greater than 90%. Because of the variable number of parasites passed in the stool daily, ova and parasites exams should be checked on three specimens collected over 6 days. Treatment is with tinidazole, metronidazole, quinacrine, or furazolidone. Retreatment is common because none of the therapies is 100% effective. Tinidazole is single dose but not available in the United States. Metronidazole is commonly used (off-label) at a dose of 250 mg po tid for 5 to 7 days. Because *Giardia* can be transmitted by person-to-person contact in addition to oral—anal sexual contact and through contaminated food and water, treatment is recommended for asymptomatic carriers. (*Tierney et al, 2005, p. 1428–1430*)

40. **(A)** Cats are the definitive host for the parasite, *Toxoplasma gondii*. It can exist in three forms but it is the oocyst that is found in cat feces. These oocysts can remain infective in soil for years. Human infections are frequently asymptomatic. In an otherwise healthy individual, symptoms resemble infectious mononucleosis. They may include swollen lymph nodes, malaise, arthralgias, headache, sore throat, and rash. Up to 1% of women have been found to be infected during pregnancy. Fetal effects are more severe if maternal infection occurs in the first trimester. Less than 15% of births among infected mothers result in severe brain or eye damage at birth but more than 85% manifested brain or eye effects later in their lives. Diagnosis can be made with serological tests. Treatment of pregnant women includes spiramycin 750 mg qid for 3 to 4 weeks. Spiramycin does not cross the placenta and so if the fetus is infected, sulfadiazine 1 g qid and pyrimethamine and folinic acid should be added. (*Tierney et al, 2005, pp. 1447–1450*)

41. **(C)** The most likely etiologic agent for septic arthritis is *Staphylococcus aureus* or *Neisseria gonorrheae*. In the acutely ill, hospitalized patient, antibiotic therapy should be started based on the need to cover these organisms. Initial treatment may include ceftriaxone 1 to 2 g IV daily until the definitive organism is cultured and sensitivities are completed. (*Tierney et al, 2005, p. 1504*)

42. **(A)** Otitis media is generally treated on an empirical basis. The three most common organisms cultured from middle ear aspirates include *Streptococcus pneumoniae*, *Haemophilus influenza*, and *Moraxella catarrhalis*. Antibiotic choices are based on that information and regional resistance. First-line therapy is amoxicillin 500 mg tid or trimethoprim-sulfamethoxazole DS po bid for 10 days for adults. Pediatric doses are adjusted for weight. Second-line therapy may include Augmentin or a cephalosporin. (*Tierney et al, 2005, p. 1505*)

43. **(E)** The most common bacterial infectious causes for gastroenteritis are *Salmonella*, *Shigella*, *Entamoeba histolytica*, and *Campylobacter*. Gastroenteritis often has a viral origin, so antibiotic therapy should only be initiated when cultures demonstrate a bacterial etiology. Antiobiotic therapy is not required for gastroenteritis caused by *Salmonella*. Pending sensitivities, *Shigella* is treated with trimethoprim- sulfamethoxazole, ampicillin, or ciprofloxacin. Erythromycin and ciprofloxacin are the appropriate treatments for *Campylobacter*. All of the above therapies are continued for 5 days. *E. histolytica* is treated with metronidazole for 5 to 10 days followed by diiodohydroxyquin for an additional 3 weeks. (*Tierney et al, 2005, pp. 1505–1506*)

44. **(D)** Bacterial meningitis is most often caused by pneumococcal or meningococcal infection. In older patients, *Listeria monocytogenes* and Gram-negative bacilli are also possible. Meningitis in the postoperative setting may be caused by *Staphylococcus aureus* as well. These patients are usually acutely ill and hospitalized, requiring intravenous antibiotic therapy with a cephalosporin and possibly, vancomycin. (*Tierney et al, 2005, p. 1504*)

45. **(B)** The most common etiologic agents for pyelonephritis in the adult outpatient population include *Escherichia coli*, *Klebsiella pneumoniae*, *Proteus* species, and *Staphylococcus*

saprophyticus. First-line therapy includes the fluoroquinolones that concentrate well in the urine (ciprofloxacin, ofloxacin, or levofloxacin). Alternative treatment may include trimethoprim-sulfamethoxazole. (*Tierney et al, 2005, p. 1505*)

46. **(A)** *Clostridial tetani* infection is a vaccine-preventable disease that results in approximately 50 cases/yr in the United States. Even with modern medical resources 1 of 4 or 1 of 5 patients with generalized tetanus dies. Almost all cases occur in individuals who are not properly immunized. Sixty percent of cases occur in older adults for whom immunity has waned. Tetanus presents in different forms including generalized, localized, cephalad, and neonatal. Generalized is the most common and symptoms include mood changes, trismus, diaphoresis, dysphagia, and drooling. Later symptoms include painful flexion and adduction of the arms and pain with extension of the legs. Convulsions and spasms are possible, along with a variety of autonomic symptoms. Treatment includes airway protection, benzodiazepines for muscle spasm, tetanus immune globulin immediately, and three doses of tetanus toxoid given by the standard schedule. Metronidazole has been demonstrated to be the most effective antimicrobial. Labetalol may be used for catecholamine-induced hypertension but the patient must also be monitored for hypotension and bradycardia. (*Goldman and Ausiello, 2004, pp. 1840–1842*)

47. **(B)** Pseudomembranous colitis is caused by the toxin-producing *Clostridium difficile.* It usually presents as fever, elevated WBC count, abdominal pain, and diarrhea (possibly bloody) following antibiotic therapy. It is thought *C. difficile,* which is generally harmless when colonized, overgrows when the normal balance of gut flora is altered by antibiotic use. In addition to making the diagnosis on colonoscopy, *C. difficile* can be cultured or the toxins detected by immunoassay. It can be treated by cessation of antibiotics and fluid replacement but most often an antibiotic targeted at the organism is employed. Metronidazole, oral or intravenous, is usually the first choice. Vancomycin is another option. Recurrence is relatively common (up to 25% of cases) and development of antibiotic-resistant organisms possible. (*Goldman and Ausiello, 2004, pp. 1836–1838*)

48. **(C)** Osteomyelitis is an infection of bone that can occur through three different pathways: "seeding" of bone by bacteria in the bloodstream; traumatic or surgical introduction of bacteria; or spread of bacteria from surrounding tissue. *Staphylococcus aureus* is the most common bacterial cause. In children, osteomyelitis originating from the bloodstream usually affects the long bones whereas, in adults, the vertebrae are more often involved. Diabetic patients with foot ulcers are also at risk, as are trauma victims. Presenting complaints often include fever, chills, and malaise, along with bone pain. Diagnosis is made by culturing the etiologic organism and locating the bone damage with imaging studies including x-ray, MRI, or bone scan. Positive x-ray findings include lytic lesions, periosteal elevation and thickening, and/or vertebral cortical destruction. Bone edema may be seen on MRI and bone scan will show an *increase* in radionuclide uptake. Treatment should be guided by culture and sensitivity reports. Acute osteomyelitis can usually be treated effectively by 4 to 6 weeks of appropriate oral or parenteral antibiotics. (*Goldman and Ausiello, 2004, pp. 1827–1829*)

49. **(B)** Smallpox (variola minor) was eradicated worldwide in 1978. In the past few years, it has returned to the forefront of public health as a potential biological weapon. It has the potential to be effective as a weapon because with worldwide eradication came cessation of vaccination programs, resulting in a large pool of susceptibles around the world. The lesions of smallpox can be differentiated from chickenpox in that the fever of smallpox often precedes the rash by 4 days, the rash begins in the oral mucosa and is concentrated in the face and distal extremities. The rash of smallpox progresses through the same stages as the chickenpox rash but in smallpox all the lesions progress simultaneously. In chickenpox, the skin outbreak occurs in crops. The palms

and soles are involved in smallpox whereas they are usually spared in chickenpox. Smallpox is also more lethal than chickenpox, with up to a 30% mortality rate. (*Andreoli et al, 2004, p. 956*)

50. **(C)**. *Bacillus anthrax* is one of the biological agents that is now being used in acts of terrorism. Anthrax infection manifests in three forms: cutaneous, gastrointestinal, and inhalational. The cutaneous form occurs in 95% of cases. The incubation period can last up to a week. The initial manifestation is papular and evolves over days to an ulcer. The ulcer is surrounded by swelling and redness and eventually becomes an eschar. The eschar falls off in 7 to 14 days. The cutaneous lesions are usually painless. Gastrointestinal anthrax is caused by eating infected meat. It is very uncommon and can be highly lethal. Inhalational anthrax happens when spores are inhaled. The incubation period may be up to 2 months. The symptoms may include fever, fatigue, body aches, chest discomfort, and later, shortness of breath, shock, and death. First-line therapy is ciprofloxacin or doxycycline. Currently, the Centers for Disease Control and Prevention recommends one or two additional antibiotics because of resistance issues. (*Andreoli et al, 2004, pp. 955–956*)

REFERENCES

Andreoli TE, Carpenter CJC, Griggs RC, Loscalzo J (eds). *Cecil Essentials of Medicine*, 6th ed. Philadelphia: WB Saunders; 2004.

Goldman L, Ausiello D (eds). *Cecil Textbook of Medicine*, 22nd ed. Philadelphia: WB Saunders; 2004.

Hay WW, Levin MJ, Sondheimer JM, Deterding RR (eds). *Current Pediatric Diagnosis and Treatment*, 17th ed. New York: McGraw-Hill; 2005.

Tierney LM, McPhee SJ, Papadakis MA (eds). *Current Medical Diagnosis and Treatment*, 44th ed. New York: Lange McGraw Hill; 2005.

Nephrology
Questions

Carla J. Moschella, PA-C, MS, RD

DIRECTIONS (Questions 1 through 45): Each of the numbered items or incomplete statements in this section is followed by answers or by completions of the statement. Select the ONE lettered answer or completion that is BEST in each case.

Questions 1 through 45

1. The earliest sign of chronic kidney disease (CKD) is

   (A) microscopic hematuria
   (B) hypertension
   (C) proteinuria
   (D) abnormal creatinine
   (E) hyperkalemia

2. Assuming that a patient has maintained a normal baseline creatinine of 1.0 mg/dL with a normal glomerular filtration rate (GFR) of 100 mL/min, which of the following indicates a more significant change in the GFR?

   (A) increase in creatinine from 1.0 to 2.0 mg/dL
   (B) increase in creatinine from 2.0 to 4.0 mg/dL
   (C) increase in creatinine from 4.0 to 8.0 mg/dL
   (D) increase in creatinine from 8.0 to 16.0 mg/dL
   (E) all represent equal changes in the GFR

3. Which of the following is NOT a complication of CKD?

   (A) anemia
   (B) hyperphosphatemia
   (C) worsening blood pressure control
   (D) osteoporosis
   (E) nephrolithiasis

4. How often should patients with diabetes mellitus be screened for microalbuminuria?

   (A) once a month
   (B) every 3 months
   (C) every 6 months
   (D) once a year
   (E) there is no specific timetable

5. Which of the following urinary findings is suggestive of acute glomerulonephritis?

   (A) red cells and red cell casts
   (B) white cells and white cell casts
   (C) renal tubular epithelial cells
   (D) oval fat bodies
   (E) hyaline casts

6. Which of the following is an absolute indication to initiate dialysis?

   (A) proteinuria >3 g/24 h
   (B) GFR <10 mL/min
   (C) hyperkalemia >5.0 meq/L
   (D) seizures
   (E) hyperphosphatemia >6.5 mg/dL

7. A renal ultrasound would be most beneficial for diagnosing which of the following?

   (A) nephrotic syndrome
   (B) polycystic kidney disease
   (C) glomerulonephritis
   (D) acute tubular necrosis
   (E) lupus nephritis

8. Which of the following types of renal calculi is associated with an infectious cause?

   (A) struvite
   (B) uric acid
   (C) calcium oxalate
   (D) cystine
   (E) calcium phosphate

9. Which of the following is diagnostic of nephrotic syndrome?

   (A) hypoalbuminemia, hypolipidemia, proteinuria >10 g/24 h
   (B) hypoalbuminemia, hyperlipidemia, proteinuria >1 g/24 h
   (C) hypoalbuminemia, hyperlipidemia, proteinuria >2 g/24 h
   (D) hypoalbuminemia, hyperlipidemia, proteinuria >3.5 g/24 h
   (E) normal albumin, hyperlipidemia, proteinuria >10 g/24 h

10. Prolonged, heavy use of nonsteroidal anti-inflammatory drugs (NSAIDs) causes which type of kidney damage?

    (A) glomerular
    (B) tubulointerstitial
    (C) autoimmune
    (D) macrovascular
    (E) NSAIDs do not cause kidney damage

11. A 16-year-old girl is referred for a sports physical. Blood pressure is 170/92 mm Hg. Urinalysis reveals 2+ protein. The girl's mother reports multiple episodes of urinary tract infections (UTIs) throughout childhood that were never investigated. The most likely diagnosis is

    (A) obstructive uropathy
    (B) orthostatic proteinuria
    (C) chronic reflux nephropathy
    (D) nephrotic syndrome
    (E) exercise-induced proteinuria

12. Which of the following best describes the mechanism of action of angiotensin-converting enzyme (ACE) inhibitors in controlling blood pressure and preventing or slowing kidney damage?

    (A) they result in systemic vasodilation
    (B) they increase renal tubular excretion of sodium
    (C) they result in dilation of the efferent arteriole, reducing glomerular pressure
    (D) they block the angiotensin II receptor on the cell membrane
    (E) they reduce production of angiotensinogen, the precursor to angiotensin I

13. In which of the following settings would the use of an ACE inhibitor be contraindicated?

    (A) diabetic nephropathy
    (B) hypertensive nephrosclerosis
    (C) lupus nephritis
    (D) polycystic kidney disease
    (E) significant renal artery stenosis

14. Which of the following is most useful in diagnosing renal artery stenosis?

    (A) magnetic resonance angiography (MRA)
    (B) computerized tomography (CT) scanning
    (C) captopril renal scan
    (D) renal artery biopsy
    (E) intravenous pyelogram (IVP)

15. Abnormal urinary protein excretion is defined as

    (A) >30 mg/24 h
    (B) >150 mg/24 h
    (C) >300 mg/24 h
    (D) >1 g/24 h
    (E) >3.5 g/24 h

16. Which class of medications is useful to treat renal calculi due to hypercalciuria?

    (A) calcium channel blockers
    (B) colchicine
    (C) allopurinol
    (D) citrate
    (E) thiazide diuretics

17. Glucose will spill into the urine when the serum glucose reaches what level?

    (A) >126 mg/dL
    (B) 150 to 175 mg/dL
    (C) 180 to 200 mg/dL
    (D) >250 mg/dL
    (E) >400 mg/dL

18. Which of the following is MOST indicative of UTI?

    (A) positive nitrite on dipstick
    (B) positive leukocyte esterase on dipstick
    (C) 2 to 3 WBCs/HPF on urine dipstick
    (D) urine culture revealing 10,000 to 20,000 colonies of *Lactobacillus*
    (E) positive nitrite and leukocyte esterase on dipstick

19. A unilateral small kidney on ultrasound would suggest which of the following etiologies?

    (A) polycystic kidney disease
    (B) hypertensive nephrosclerosis
    (C) diabetic nephropathy
    (D) renal artery stenosis
    (E) malignancy

20. Which of the following statements about postinfectious glomerulonephritis is TRUE?

    (A) it is an inflammatory immunologic reaction to a streptococcal antigen
    (B) it is a process that will inevitably result in renal failure
    (C) it occurs in 50% of people with a history of streptococcal pharyngitis
    (D) it is a disease that results only from infection with *Streptococcus*
    (E) treatment of the streptococcal infection with antibiotics will prevent its development

21. Which of the following treatments for hyperkalemia works by redistributing potassium from the blood into the cell?

    (A) sodium polystyrene sulfonate p.o.
    (B) insulin and D5W IV
    (C) low potassium diet
    (D) calcium gluconate IV
    (E) hemodialysis

22. Complications associated with hyperkalemia include

    (A) hyperventilation
    (B) nausea and vomiting
    (C) ventricular arrhythmias
    (D) diarrhea
    (E) seizures

23. Which of the following signals a good prognosis for recovery from acute renal failure (ARF)?

    (A) maintenance of normal urine output as creatinine increases
    (B) low blood urea nitrogen level
    (C) the etiology of the ARF is sepsis
    (D) the etiology of the ARF is pregnancy
    (E) aggressive use of furosemide to stimulate urine output

24. Which of the following BEST describes one of the pathophysiologic mechanisms that occurs in prerenal ARF?

    (A) decreased effective circulating volume
    (B) obstruction
    (C) inflammatory reaction in the renal parenchyma
    (D) toxin-induced damage to the glomerulus
    (E) renal artery vasoconstriction

25. A 72-year-old male is transported via ambulance to the emergency department with severe chest pain and shortness of breath. EKG reveals ST-segment elevation in leads II, III, and AVF. While in the emergency department, he loses consciousness and is found to be in ventricular fibrillation. Resuscitation is successful, and a pulse is restored within 3 minutes. He is taken to the cardiac catheterization lab, where he undergoes two-vessel stenting. Two days later his creatinine has increased from a baseline of 1.1 mg/dL to 2.2 mg/dL. The next day the creatinine is 3.9 mg/dL. Fractional excretion of sodium is ordered. You would expect this to be

(A) <1

(B) >1

(C) unchanged from baseline

(D) undetectable

(E) equal to the serum creatinine level

26. In ARF, the serum creatinine level tends to increase at what rate per day?

(A) 0.5 to 1.0 mg/dL

(B) 1 to 2 mg/dL

(C) 2 to 3 mg/dL

(D) 3 to 4 mg/dL

(E) 4 to 5 mg/dL

27. Which of the following would NOT be considered part of the initial screening process for CKD?

(A) 24-hour urine collection

(B) blood pressure measurement

(C) serum creatinine level

(D) spot urine protein measurement

(E) obtaining a history to ascertain presence of risk factors

28. A 32-year-old construction worker presents to the emergency room after being involved in an accident at a job site. His left thigh was pinned under a 100-pound cement block. He is in moderate pain on presentation, and there is swelling and a large ecchymosis over the entire anterior thigh. Urine is rust-colored. Urine dip is positive for blood and protein, negative for glucose, ketones, nitrite, and leukocyte esterase. Urine sediment is negative for cells, organisms, and casts. What is the most likely cause of the positive urine dip for blood?

(A) hemoglobin due to hematoma formation

(B) contamination of the urine sample

(C) myoglobin due to rhabdomyolysis

(D) red cell casts due to glomerulonephritis

(E) UTI

29. Which of the following statements about anemia associated with CKD is TRUE?

(A) p.o. iron and folic acid are the most effective treatments

(B) transfusion of packed red blood cells monthly is the most effective treatment

(C) IM erythropoietin given weekly or biweekly is the most effective treatment

(D) it is due to the inability of the kidney to transform erythropoietin into its physiologically active form

(E) it occurs early in the course of CKD

30. Which of the following best describes the pathophysiologic mechanism of distal renal tubular acidosis?

(A) a defect in the ability of the distal renal tubule to excrete hydrogen ion

(B) a defect in the ability of the distal renal tubule to reabsorb bicarbonate

(C) a defect in the ability of the proximal renal tubule to excrete hydrogen ion

(D) a defect in the ability of the proximal renal tubule to reabsorb bicarbonate

(E) inadequate aldosterone production

31. What is the most common complication of hemodialysis?

(A) hypokalemia

(B) hyperglycemia

(C) hypotension

(D) infection

(E) anemia

32. Most UTIs are caused by

(A) Gram-positive bacteria

(B) *Pseudomonas aeruginosa*

(C) *Staphylococcus aureus*

(D) *Escherichia coli*

(E) *Candida albicans*

33. Of the following organisms, which is most likely to colonize a chronic in-dwelling urinary catheter?

(A) *Escherichia coli*

(B) *Pseudomonas aeruginosa*

(C) *Klebsiella*

(D) *Proteus mirabilis*

(E) *Enterobacter*

34. Which of the following is a potential complication of acute pyelonephritis?

(A) perinephric abscess

(B) renal vein thrombosis

(C) allergic interstitial nephritis

(D) struvite stones

(E) hepatic failure

35. Large numbers of epithelial cells on urine sediment indicate

(A) UTI

(B) acute tubular necrosis

(C) sample contamination

(D) vaginitis in women

(E) prostatitis in men

36. UTIs are classified as complicated or uncomplicated. Which of the following factors is associated with a complicated UTI in a 52-year-old female patient?

(A) patient has hypertension

(B) patient has known renal calculi

(C) patient has a fever

(D) patient is on daily aspirin prophylaxis for coronary artery disease

(E) patient had frequent UTIs as a child but none since age 16

37. Which of the following patients would require the LONGEST antibiotic treatment course for a UTI?

(A) a 32-year-old female with a history of one UTI 3 years ago

(B) a 79-year-old female with a history of renal calculi but no previous history of UTI

(C) an 8-year-old female with no previous history of UTI

(D) a 42-year-old male with no significant past medical history

(E) a 41-year-old female with history of cervical diaphragm use for birth control

38. The most common cause of nephrotic syndrome in children is

(A) post-streptococcal glomerulonephritis

(B) minimal change disease

(C) diabetes mellitus

(D) NSAIDs

(E) polycystic kidney disease

39. You are asked to see a diabetic patient with retinopathy and hypertension. On examination, the patient's blood pressure is 180/90 mm Hg. Urinalysis shows microalbumin of 300 mg/dL. Labs: blood urea nitrogen 22 mg/dL, creatinine 1.5 mg/dL. Which of the following classes of antihypertensive medications would be best to prescribe in this setting?

(A) calcium channel blocker

(B) loop diuretic

(C) alpha blocker

(D) thiazide diuretic

(E) ACE inhibitor

40. Which of the following diuretics is NOT potassium-sparing?

(A) triamterene

(B) amiloride

(C) hydrochlorothiazide

(D) spironolactone

(E) eplerenone

41. When adjusting medication dosing for patients with CKD, which of the following factors is LEAST important?

    (A) blood urea nitrogen level
    (B) serum creatinine level
    (C) age
    (D) weight
    (E) gender

42. The organism responsible for most cases of peritonitis in patients on peritoneal dialysis is

    (A) *Candida albicans*
    (B) *Escherichia coli*
    (C) *Streptococcus*
    (D) *Pseudomonas aeruginosa*
    (E) *Staphylococcus aureus*

43. A patient presents with abrupt onset of edema, azotemia, proteinuria, and cola-colored urine. The MOST likely diagnosis is

    (A) nephrotic syndrome
    (B) minimal change disease
    (C) acute glomerulonephritis
    (D) obstructive uropathy
    (E) renal calculi

44. The most serious consequence of rapid correction of hyponatremia is

    (A) brainstem herniation
    (B) central pontine myelinolysis
    (C) muscle cramps
    (D) hypernatremia
    (E) fluid overload

45. Routine urinalysis done on a 40-year-old female with no significant past medical history reveals 3 to 5 RBCs/HPF. Which of the following additional findings is (are) most suggestive of a nonglomerular source of the hematuria?

    (A) red cell casts
    (B) pyuria
    (C) proteinuria
    (D) new-onset hypertension and edema
    (E) intermittent gross hematuria

DIRECTIONS (Questions 46 through 50): Each group of items in this section consists of lettered headings followed by a set of numbered words or phrases. For each numbered word or phrase, select the ONE lettered heading that is most closely associated with it. Each lettered heading may be selected once, more than once, or not at all.

Questions 46 through 50

Of the acid–base disorders listed as (A) to (E), select a single BEST response to the numbered phrases.

    (A) metabolic acidosis
    (B) respiratory acidosis
    (C) metabolic alkalosis
    (D) respiratory alkalosis
    (E) normal

46. low arterial pH, increased pCO_2, increased bicarbonate

47. high arterial pH, decreased pCO_2, decreased bicarbonate

48. seen in CKD

49. result of excessive diuretic therapy

50. calculation of the anion gap helpful in determining cause of this acid–base disorder

Answers and Explanations

1. **(C)** Injury to the nephron results in excessive protein leak and decreased protein reabsorption from the tubules. This occurs long before the creatinine becomes abnormal and 5 to 10 years before overt proteinuria, detectable by routine dipstick, develops. Persistent proteinuria eventually will result in an abnormal creatinine but, in the case of CKD, years later. Therefore, proteinuria, best assessed by the protein-to-creatinine ratio from a urine specimen, is considered the earliest marker of CKD. Microscopic hematuria can result from many processes, some transient, including infection, malignancy, calculi, acute glomerulonephritis, and IgA nephropathy, and is not, in and of itself, an indicator of permanent kidney damage. Hypertension, if not the cause of the CKD, can occur early in the course of CKD, but proteinuria usually occurs before hypertension develops. Chronic hyperkalemia develops later in the course of CKD, generally when glomerular filtration rate is <30 mL/min. (*NKF-K/DOQI Guidelines, 2002, pp. 48–49*)

2. **(A)** GFR describes the amount of blood passing through the kidneys per minute. Knowing this measurement provides an accurate characterization of kidney function. Because GFR is not usually measured directly (which would require contrast injection and serial measurements of urine output), serum creatinine and creatinine clearance are used as markers of kidney function. There is an inverse relationship between GFR and serum creatinine. In a patient with normal renal function, doubling of the serum creatinine represents a loss of approximately 50% of GFR. Using this information, the loss of GFR can be estimated from changes in the serum creatinine. For example, assume normal creatinine levels of 1.0 mg/dL and normal GFR of 100 mL/min. A doubling of the serum creatinine from 1.0 mg/dL to 2.0 mg/dL represents an approximate reduction in GFR from 100 mL/min to 50 mL/min (50% of GFR has been lost). Each additional doubling of the creatinine decreases the remaining GFR by approximately one half. When renal function is severely impaired, large increases in the creatinine (i.e., 8.0 to 16.0 mg/dL) represent only small decreases in GFR (approximately 12 to 6 mL/min). This example emphasizes the importance of detecting increases in serum creatinine early. However, serum creatinine level does not become abnormal until ~25% of renal function is lost. Therefore, other methods of estimating GFR are more useful in detecting early decreases in GFR. Creatinine clearance, as estimated from the Cockcroft–Gault equation (see Question 41) or 24-hour urine collection, estimates the amount of creatinine being filtered, and is subject to collection error, changes in muscle mass that affect creatinine concentration, and other factors, and overestimates GFR. Increased or decreased creatinine production due to increased muscle catabolism or decreased muscle mass further adds to the insensitivity of using the serum creatinine to estimate GFR. The MDRD (modification of diet in renal disease)

equation incorporates serum creatinine level, age, gender, and race and is the most accurate way to estimate GFR. The equation eliminates the need for a urine sample and can be accessed online at www.kdoqi.org. (*Post and Rose, 2001; Levey, 1999*)

3. **(E)** Anemia develops as the synthesis of erythropoietin declines in the damaged kidneys. Electrolyte abnormalities, such as hyperkalemia, hyperphosphatemia, and hypocalcemia, occur as GFR declines. Blood pressure will worsen as GFR falls and the kidneys begin to lose the ability to autoregulate blood flow. Osteoporosis occurs due to several mechanisms, such as secondary hyperparathyroidism, chronic metabolic acidosis, which results in calcium resorption from bone, and inadequate transformation of vitamin D to its physiologically active form. Nephrolithiasis is not a consequence of CKD. (*NKF-K/DOQI Guidelines, 2002, pp. 63–64*)

4. **(D)** The American Diabetic Association (ADA) recommends checking urine for microalbumin 5 years after the diagnosis is made and once a year thereafter to screen for diabetic nephropathy in patients with Type I diabetes mellitus. For patients with Type II diabetes mellitus, the ADA recommends checking the urine at the time of the diagnosis and yearly thereafter. (*American Diabetic Association, 2005, p. 36*)

5. **(A)** Casts in the urine indicate a pathologic process, with the exception of the presence of the rare hyaline cast (1 to 2/HPF). The acute inflammatory process of glomerulonephritis is characterized by red cells and red cell casts in the urine. White cells and white cell casts occur with an allergic or infectious process, such as acute interstitial nephritis or pyelonephritis, respectively. Renal tubular epithelial cells indicate damage to the renal tubules, as with acute tubular necrosis. Oval fat bodies result from renal tubular cells that have absorbed fats or monocytes and macrophages that have ingested fats. (*McBride, 1998, pp. 100–107*)

6. **(D)** The development of seizures due to uremia is an absolute indication to begin hemodialysis. The waste products of urea metabolism must be removed to abort the seizure activity. Proteinuria is never an indication to begin hemodialysis. Proteinuria is a sign of kidney damage, poses no immediate threat to life (although the underlying process causing it might), and hemodialysis will not correct it. Calculations of GFR are used to assess kidney function, predict when complications of CKD and ESRD (end-stage renal disease) will occur, and guide treatment plan but not to indicate when to initiate hemodialysis. Rather, the decision to initiate renal replacement therapy is a clinical one, based upon clinical assessment of functioning and physical manifestations of ESRD. A potassium level >5.0 meq/L does not represent an immediate threat to the patient and does not mandate the initiation of hemodialysis. Cardiac abnormalities associated with hyperkalemia generally occur at levels >6.5 meq/L, and conservative measures to correct hyperkalemia generally are initiated when the serum level is >5.5 meq/L, although this varies with practice. Hyperphosphatemia is best treated with phosphate binders, such as calcium carbonate and calcium acetate, and a low phosphorus diet. (*Merck Manual, 1992, p. 102*)

7. **(B)** Renal ultrasound is useful for assessing kidney size and thickness of the cortex, and for presence of masses, cysts, obstruction, and hydronephrosis. Intrinsic disease is best assessed by establishing the clinical context, analyzing the urine for protein, cells, and casts, and possibly by doing a biopsy. Loss of cortical thickness is a nonspecific finding, and ultrasound does not establish an etiology. (*Delmez and Windus, 2001, p. 1350; Cronin, 1995, p. 144; Alfrey, 1995, p. 156*)

8. **(A)** Struvite stones form when urea-splitting organisms, such as *Proteus*, *Klebsiella*, *Pseudomonas*, and *Staphylococcus*, are present in the urinary tract. Ammonia is formed when urease breaks down urea. This results in an alkaline urine, which decreases the solubility of struvite, favoring the production of stones. Calcium stones result from hyperabsorption of calcium in the intestine, impaired renal tu-

bular reabsorption of calcium, primary hyper-parathyroidism, intestinal hyperabsorption of oxalate, and hypocitraturia. Uric acid stones are due to hyperuricosuria or a urinary pH <5.5, which causes uric acid to dissociate. They are also the only radiolucent calculi. Cystinuria, an in-born error of metabolism, results in cystine stones. (*Delvecchio and Preminger, 2001, pp. 1373–1376*)

9. **(D)** Nephrotic syndrome is defined as proteinuria >3.5 g/24 h resulting in hypoalbuminemia (<2.5 gm/dL), hyperlipidemia (>250 mg/dL), and edema, probably due to increased renal tubule permeability. Causes include diabetic nephropathy, HIV nephropathy, chronic hepatitis B and C, amyloidosis, systemic lupus erythematosus, constrictive pericarditis, Hodgkin's disease, minimal change disease, and many medications, including phenytoin and NSAIDs. (*Schmitz, 2001; Reikes and Martin, 2001, pp. 1386, 1390–1399; Freidman, 2002, p. 697*)

10. **(B)** Analgesic nephropathy results from long-term use of at least 1 g of analgesics per day. NSAIDs are also one of the most common causes of acute interstitial nephritis. The pathophysiologic mechanism of injury is not certain; however, ischemia of interstitial cells surrounding the tubules due to inhibition of prostaglandin-induced dilation due to the NSAID may be the cause. (*Schmitz, 2001, pp. 1393–1394*)

11. **(C)** Retrograde flow of urine from the bladder damages the renal parenchyma, resulting in chronic reflux nephropathy. If untreated, irreversible damage to the kidneys will occur. Because this is a tubulointerstitial process, the urinalysis will be negative for protein in the early stages of damage. However, if untreated, long-term, glomerular damage will occur and protein will appear in the urine. Hypertension develops as the GFR decreases. (*Schmitz, 2001, p. 1394*)

12. **(C)** ACE inhibitors prevent the conversion of angiotensin I to angiotensin II, thereby interrupting the renin—angiotensin—aldosterone system, which regulates blood pressure. The glomerular efferent arteriole dilates, given the decreased stimulus from angiotensin II to constrict. This lowers pressure in the glomerulus by lowering resistance to outflow. This effectively results in a decrease in GFR, resulting in increased serum creatinine and potassium levels. However, these changes are not necessarily indications to discontinue the ACE inhibitor. Usually, the creatinine increases 0.2 to 0.4 mg/dL and then levels out. Monitoring of the changes to be sure that the hyperkalemia is not worsening or life-threatening and that the patient is not going into acute renal failure is indicated. If none of these things are happening, the ACE inhibitor can, and should, be continued so that the patient derives the beneficial effect of the decline in pressure within the glomerulus, which will slowdown the progression of CKD. (*Alfrey, 1995, p. 158*)

13. **(E)** Among other mechanisms of action, ACE inhibitors interfere with vasoconstriction of the efferent arteriole, thereby decreasing pressure within the glomerulus. If significant blockage is present in the renal artery, blood flow to the glomerulus is already compromised, resulting in lowered glomerular pressure. If pressure within the glomerulus is lowered further due to the vasodilating effect of the ACE inhibitor on the efferent arteriole, blood flow is further compromised. Ischemia, and acute renal failure, can result. (*Harrison's On-line, ch. 267*)

14. **(A)** Magnetic resonance angiography, enhanced with gadolinium, is 90% sensitive and 95% specific for diagnosing renal artery stenosis (RAS). This study has largely replaced the captopril renal scan and contrast-enhanced arteriography in diagnosing RAS. The principle behind the captopril renal scan is that ACE inhibitors lower GFR. In a kidney with already-compromised blood flow due to RAS, administration of the ACE inhibitor further decreases GFR in the affected kidney despite maintenance of adequate plasma volume. GFR in the contralateral kidney remains normal. Subsequent injection of a radionuclide reveals delayed uptake in the compromised kidney. Although arteriography provides the

most definitive diagnosis, it carries its own risks of contrast-induced injury and bleeding. MRA is a low-risk procedure due to its noninvasive nature. There are no accepted indications for renal artery biopsy. IVP is utilized to visualize the anatomical structure of the urinary tract in situations such as urinary tract trauma and outflow obstruction, although increasingly it too is being replaced by noninvasive testing, such as ultrasound, CT scanning, MRI, etc. It remains a useful test to pinpoint the location of a calculus in the urinary tract. (*Pagana and Pagana, 2002, pp. 782–783, 996, 1064; Harrison's On-line, ch. 267; Delmez and Windus, 2001; Delvecchio and Preminger, 2001, pp. 1350, 1376*)

15. **(C)** The normal glomerulus filters a small amount of low-molecular-weight proteins, which are reabsorbed in the tubules, generally at a rate of <150 mg/24 h. However, up to 300 mg/24 h is accepted as normal. High-molecular-weight proteins, i.e. albumin, are not filtered by the normal kidney, and therefore, albumin's appearance in the urine at >30 mg/24 h is considered abnormal. Standard urine dipsticks will react in the presence of all proteins, including glycoproteins, gamma-globulins, Tamm–Horsfall mucoproteins, Bence–Jones proteins, and albumin. However, they generally cannot detect protein until it reaches an excretion level of >200 to 300 mg/24 h. This will produce a urine dipstick reading of 1+ (equivalent to about 30 mg of protein in that sample). Contamination of the urine specimen with blood, semen, pus, vaginal discharge, and mucous can result in false-positive readings. Specific reagent strips designed to detect microalbuminemia, defined as 30 to 300 mg/24 h, have been developed and are the preferred strips to use when testing for early signs of diabetic nephropathy. Expressed another way, a protein level of >300 mg/24 h or a microalbumin level of >30 mg/24 h is defined as abnormal. A random spot urinary albumin-to-creatinine ratio is also a good screening test for early nephropathy, with normal results defined as 17 to 250 mg/g in men and 25 to 355 mg/g in women. (*Delmez and Windus, 2001, p. 1350; Graff, 1983, pp. 27–30; NKF-K/DOQI Guidelines, 2002, p. 21*)

16. **(E)** In patients with hypercalciuria, thiazide diuretics can lower urinary calcium levels, reducing the risk of nephrolithiasis. All patients who present with an episode of nephrolithiasis need a metabolic workup, including blood work to check serum creatinine, parathyroid hormone, calcium, phosphorus, and uric acid, and a 24-hour urine collection to measure pH, total volume, sodium, calcium, oxalate, citrate, cystine, uric acid, etc. (*Coe, 1995, p. 99*)

17. **(C)** Since glucosuria occurs at a serum level much higher than what would be diagnostic for diabetes mellitus, urine testing is not considered an adequate screening tool for diagnosing diabetes mellitus. (*Delmez and Windus, 2001, p. 1347*)

18. **(E)** Nitrite is formed when organisms that produce nitrate reductase, i.e., *Escherichia coli, Klebsiella, Proteus*, and *Enterobacter*, are present in the urine. The enzyme reduces nitrate to nitrite. However, the urine has to be present in the bladder at least 4 hours for this to occur. Leukocyte esterase is produced by various WBCs, including polymorphonuclear neutrophils, monocytes, eosinophils, and basophils. The enzyme can appear in the urine with the presence of any of these WBCs and not just as the result of bacterial infection, although UTI is the most common cause of positive leukocyte esterase in the urine. Other causes are vaginal and perineal contamination. The combination of urinary nitrite and leukocyte esterase has a sensitivity and specificity of 85% and 75%, respectively, and therefore, provides more information than either alone. WBCs can occur in the urine as the result of infection, an inflammatory process, such as interstitial nephritis, or vaginal or perineal contamination, and levels <3 to 5 WBCs/HPF are not considered indicative of infection. Infection is strongly indicated when WBCs reach 4 to 6/HPF. Urine culture is considered positive for infection at >100,000 colonies. (*McBride, 1998, pp. 70–71; Bastani, 2001, p. 1367*)

19. **(D)** Renal artery stenosis causes compromised blood flow to the kidney, resulting in atrophy. Frequently, the contralateral kidney

will hypertrophy in an attempt to compensate for the declining GFR. Polycystic kidney disease results in enlarged kidneys due to growth of multiple cysts. Hypertensive nephrosclerosis and diabetic nephropathy affect both kidneys equally and would result in bilateral, not unilateral, cortical atrophy. Malignancy would not result in atrophy. (*Delmez and Windus, 2001, pp. 1349–1350; Harrison's On-line, ch. 267*)

20. **(A)** Renal biopsies done on patients with postinfectious glomerulonephritis (GN) show deposition of immune complexes and proliferation of inflammatory cells. The most common cause of postinfectious GN is *Streptococcus*, but other organisms can cause it as well. Antibiotic treatment for the underlying infection has no impact on whether or not the patient will develop postinfectious GN since the kidney has already been exposed to the microbial antigen before treatment was initiated. About 25% of those infected with nephritogenic strains will develop postinfectious GN, but not all people are infected with these types of strains. Most patients recover spontaneously, and progression to renal failure is extremely rare. (*Delmez and Windus, 2001, p. 1390*)

21. **(B)** Hyperkalemia can be treated by three mechanisms: antagonizing the effect on the cell membrane, which can be achieved by infusing calcium gluconate 10 to 30 mL of 10% solution IV; redistributing potassium from the blood into the cell, which can be accomplished by infusing sodium bicarbonate 44 to 132 meq IV or regular insulin 10 U along with glucose 50 g; or removing it by giving sodium polystyrene sulfonate (Kayexelate) p.o. or via retention enema or by initiating hemo- or peritoneal dialysis. Insulin acts to drive potassium into the cell but must be given with glucose to avoid significant hypoglycemia. (*Narins et al, 1995, p. 52*)

22. **(C)** Hyperkalemia is defined as serum potassium greater than 5.0 meq/L. EKG changes (tall, peaked T waves and shortening of the QT interval) may start to occur as early as at 5.5 meq/L but generally are not seen until the

serum level reaches ~6.5 meq/L. As the hyperkalemia progresses, the QRS will widen (>6.5 meq/L), the PR interval will be prolonged, and then the P wave will disappear. A sine wave pattern precedes asystole at a serum level of ~10 meq/L. (*Merck Manual, 1992, p. 1002*)

23. **(A)** Maintenance of normal urine output as the serum creatinine level increases—so-called nonoliguric ARF—has a better prognosis for recovery than oliguric ARF. Oliguria is defined as urine output <500 mL/24 h.

Anuria is absence of urine output. A low blood urea nitrogen level does not indicate the degree of renal damage since the blood urea nitrogen level can be affected by other factors, such as an elevated rate of catabolism, dietary protein intake, and gastrointestinal bleeding. Poor outcome is associated with ARF which occurs with sepsis, which can result in multiorgan failure, and pregnancy. Administration of furosemide has not been shown to favorably affect outcome of ARF. (*Alfrey, 1995; August et al, 1995, pp. 147–148, 154, 196; Merck Manual, 1992, p. 1664; Reikes and Martin, 2001, p. 1395*)

24. **(A)** Prerenal ARF is associated with decreased intravascular volume, which occurs with hemorrhage, gastrointestinal losses from vomiting and/or diarrhea, burns, and inadequate distribution of volume due to myocardial failure or hepatorenal syndrome. Other causes include vasodilation from sepsis and anaphylaxis, which results in hypotension and inadequate renal perfusion. Obstruction due to tumor, enlarged prostate, bilateral stones, retroperitoneal fibrosis, etc., results in postrenal ARF. Inflammatory processes, nephrotoxins, and ischemia of blood vessels within the kidney itself are intrinsic causes of ARF. In prerenal ARF, the renal artery would dilate in an attempt to maximize blood flow to maintain adequate perfusion. (*Reikes and Martin, 2001, p. 1396*)

25. **(B)** Intrinsic ARF results in alterations in the kidneys' ability to respond to changes in hemostasis. When the integrity of the kidneys

remains intact, sodium is conserved when GFR declines in an attempt to reestablish volume and perfusion, resulting in a fractional excretion of sodium (FENa) of <1. However, when the glomeruli are injured, the kidneys lose the ability to reabsorb sodium as the GFR decreases, and the FENa will be >1. The etiology of this patient's renal failure is most likely contrast-induced acute tubular necrosis following an ischemic episode, which is intrinsic ARF. (*Reikes and Martin, 2001, p. 1396*)

26. **(B)** In ARF, the serum creatinine increases about 1 to 2 mg/dL per day. (*Merck Manual, 1992, p. 1663*)

27. **(A)** Screening for the presence of chronic kidney disease involves checking a serum creatinine level, checking blood pressure for the presence of hypertension, checking urinary protein for evidence of glomerular injury, and obtaining a history to check for the presence of risk factors, such as hypertension, diabetes mellitus, autoimmune disease, infection, or family history. Initial screening would not include a 24-hour urine collection. This is a cumbersome, inconvenient, more expensive test than the spot urinary protein reading and would not provide additional information. (*NKF-K/DOQI Guidelines, 2002, p. 31*)

28. **(C)** Urine reagent strips test are suffused with an indicator dye that changes color when the dye is oxidized by peroxidase in hemoglobin, thus indicating the presence of blood in the urine. However, myoglobin also has peroxidase activity, and therefore, the indicator for blood on the dipstick will turn positive in the presence of myoglobin without hemoglobin. Myoglobin can appear in the urine as the result of rhabdomyolysis due to crush injuries, surgery, ischemia, hyperthermia, significant exercise, seizures, electric shock, illicit drug use, and muscle-wasting diseases. A positive urine dip for blood, with a negative urinary sediment for red cells, mandates a workup for diseases/injuries resulting in myoglobinuria. (*McBride, 1998, p. 68; Graff, 1983, p. 52*)

29. **(D)** Anemia associated with CKD is the result of inadequate erythropoietin synthesis by the kidneys. This hormone signals the bone marrow to synthesize red blood cells. A deficiency will result in anemia. In the absence of erythropoietin, iron would not be of use since red blood cell synthesis is inadequate. Folic acid would also not be of use and does not play a role in the etiology of this type of anemia. Transfusion is a tempering measure only, used to increase oxygen-carrying capacity in the case of symptomatic ischemia. Anemia due to erythropoietin deficiency generally does not occur until the GFR decreases to <60 mL/min, or approximately 50% of normal. Intramuscular administration of erythropoietin is the only effective treatment to induce red blood cell production. Depending on the formulation used, this can be given once a week or once every two weeks. Sometimes oral iron supplementation is needed to produce adequate hemoglobin for the increased de novo red cell production. (*Guyton and Hall, 1996, pp. 418, 428; NKF-K/DOQI Guidelines, 2002, p. 51*)

30. **(A)** Renal tubular acidosis is classified into subtypes: Type I is characterized by an inability of the distal renal tubule to excrete hydrogen ion. Type II is characterized by overexcretion of HCO_3^- into the urine. Type IV is caused by either aldosterone deficiency or an inability of the distal tubule to respond to aldosterone. (*Merck Manual, 1992, p. 1727; Klahr, 2001, pp. 1353–1354*)

31. **(C)** Hypokalemia can occur rarely as a complication of hemodialysis if excessive potassium is removed during the treatment. Hyperglycemia can result from peritoneal dialysis, since the dialysate contains dextrose. Infection occurs rarely, given meticulous maintenance of sterile technique. Anemia is a result of CKD and can be worsened by hemodialysis if significant bleeding occurs as patients, who have received heparin during the treatment to prevent blood clotting, are removed from hemodialysis. However, hypotension remains the most common complication due to excessive removal of volume during treatment. (*Harrison's On-line, ch. 262*)

32. **(D)** Eighty percent of uncomplicated and 32% of complicated UTIs are caused by *E. coli*.

Other common etiologic agents are the Gram-negative bacteria: *Proteus*, *Klebsiella*, and *Enterobacter*. (*Bastani, 2001, p. 1365*)

33. **(B)** *P. aeruginosa* thrives in moist environments, including urinary catheters. (*Merck Manual, 1992, p. 1711*)

34. **(A)** (*Stoller and Carroll, 2005, p. 910*)

35. **(C)** Squamous epithelial cells line the distal portion of the urethra in men and the entire urethra in women. They appear in the urine due to inadequate cleaning of the external urinary meatus prior to obtaining the sample and indicate that the sample is contaminated. In women, the source is usually vaginal/perineal. Uncircumcised men commonly have squamous epithelial cells in the urine sample. (*McBride, 1998, p. 103*)

36. **(B)** A complicated UTI is defined as one in which there is a risk for renal damage, urosepsis, or abscess formation. Those at risk would be patients with anatomical or functional urinary tract abnormalities; with known presence of calculi; with a urinary stent or catheter; who are pregnant; with history of analgesic abuse; with diabetes mellitus or sickle cell disease; and who are hospitalized or immunosuppressed. Hypertensive patients are not at higher risk for the above-mentioned complications as the result of a UTI. Fever response varies and does not indicate an infection that is worse than one in which no fever is present. Daily low-dose aspirin therapy is not analgesic abuse. Although the patient had frequent UTIs as a child, she has had none in almost 40 years, which does not suggest an anatomical or functional abnormality that would place this patient at higher risk for complications from the UTI. Complicated UTIs require culture-specific antibiotic treatment and a longer course of treatment. (*Bastani, 2001, pp. 1364, 1369–1370*)

37. **(D)** Men and pregnant women require the longest course of treatment for UTI—generally 7 to 10 days. Some advocate single-dose treatment of an uncomplicated UTI, although in practice, this is rare. Most are treated for 3 to 5 days with trimethoprim-sulfamethoxazole (TMP-SMZ) or a fluoroquinolone. Treatment with ampicillin, amoxicillin, and first-generation cephalosporins alone is infrequent given the widespread incidence of resistant organisms, as well as their decreased effectiveness in eliminating vaginal and periurethral colonization compared with TMP-SMZ. Remote history of UTI, history of renal calculi, and UTI in young girls are not indications to prolong antibiotic treatment course. Young, sexually active women are at higher risk for developing UTIs because of the risk of bacterial contamination into an anatomically short urethra, and those who use a diaphragm or spermicides are at highest risk. However, using these types of birth control does not indicate a need for a prolonged antibiotic course. (*Bastani, 2001, pp. 1369–1370*)

38. **(B)** The most common cause of nephrotic syndrome in children is minimal change disease. Diffuse injury to the epithelial cells is the underlying cause, resulting in significant proteinuria, edema, hypoalbuminemia, and hyperlipidemia. It accounts for 80% of cases of nephrotic syndrome in children; however, 20% to 25% of adults over 40 years of age with nephrotic syndrome have minimal change disease. In children, it most commonly occurs between ages 1.5 and 4 years, with a 2:1 predominance in males. Treatment is with corticosteroids for 2 to 4 weeks, dietary sodium restriction, and sometimes diuretics to reduce the edema. Relapse and lack of response to corticosteroids can occur. If the latter occurs, renal biopsy is indicated to rule out other causes of the nephrotic syndrome, such as focal glomerulosclerosis and membranoproliferative glomerulonephritis. (*Merck Manual, 1992, pp. 1692, 1696; Freidman, 2002, pp. 697–698*)

39. **(E)** ACE inhibitors are the drug of choice in this setting. Control of systemic blood pressure can reduce renal vascular damage. In diabetic patients, ACE inhibitors are especially beneficial because of the added effect of reducing intraglomerular pressure and decreasing proteinuria. Current target blood pressure in patients with diabetic nephropathy is

<130/80 mm Hg. Calcium channel blockers and diuretics do not offer renoprotective benefits but may be used to control hypertension. (*Breyer, 1998, pp. 218–219; Shelling, 1999, pp. 88–89; American Diabetic Association, 2005, p. 20; JNC 7 Report, 2003*)

40. **(C)** Triamterene, amiloride, spironolactone, and eplerenone are potassium-sparing diuretics. Triamterene and amiloride act to reduce potassium secretion in the distal tubule. Spironolactone and eplerenone are aldosterone receptor blockers. The thiazide diuretics, including hydrochlorothiazide, block sodium reabsorption in the terminal portion of the loop of Henle and the proximal portion of the distal convoluted tubule. This leads to loss of both sodium and potassium in the urine. (*Ellison, 1998, pp. 115–117; Pitt et al, 2003, p. 1309*)

41. **(A)** Because many drugs are excreted in the urine, knowledge of the renal function is important when dosing medication, especially in patients with abnormal GFR. Drug toxicity or adverse side effects may occur if the drug is dosed improperly. Estimation of the creatinine clearance can help in making the proper drug adjustment for the degree of renal insufficiency. In a steady state (i.e., stable creatinine), the Cockcroft–Gault equation can be used to estimate creatinine clearance. The formula is

$$\text{Creatinine clearance (mL/min)} = \frac{(140 - \text{age}) \times \text{weight (kg)}}{\text{serum creatinine} \times 72}$$

In female patients, the result is multiplied by 0.85 because of smaller muscle mass. Appropriate medication adjustments can be made based on the estimated creatinine clearance. The MDRD equation can also be used to estimate GFR, as described in Question 2. The blood urea nitrogen is not a reliable index, because several factors may alter tubular reabsorption of, or generation of, urea. These include the patient's hydration status, protein intake, and degree of catabolic activity occurring. (*Levey, 1998, p. 23*)

42. **(E)** *S. aureus* is the organism responsible for most cases of peritonitis in patients on peritoneal dialysis. Improper technique by the patient in making catheter connections during dialysis exchanges is the reason for bacterial inoculation in most cases. Abdominal pain, fever, and cloudy dialysis fluid are the presenting symptoms and signs. The enteric bacteria are the second most common organisms causing peritonitis. Peritonitis due to fungus usually requires removal of the peritoneal catheter since it is hard to eradicate the organism. (*Piraino, 1998, p. 418*)

43. **(C)** Acute glomerulonephritis (GN) is associated with sudden onset of microscopic hematuria, proteinuria, and azotemia. Red cell casts in the urine are specific for acute GN and cause the urine to darken, similar to the color of cola. Sodium and water retention occur, causing hypertension and edema. Periorbital edema is common, but edema can be present in the lower extremities as well. Inflammatory lesions in the glomeruli are the underlying pathophysiologic cause. Causes include postinfectious GN, IgA nephropathy, endocarditis, lupus nephritis, cryoglobulinemia associated with hepatitis C, and membranoproliferative glomerulonephritis. Prognosis depends on the specific etiology. Although minimal change disease and nephrotic syndrome cause proteinuria, they do not result in darkened urine. (*Watnick and Morrison, 2005, p. 876*)

44. **(B)** Hyponatremia occurs in about 2% of hospitalized patients and is the most common electrolyte abnormality found in this population. It also occurs in the outpatient setting and is defined as a serum sodium concentration of <130 meq/L. Common causes include dehydration, diarrhea, vomiting, overuse of diuretics, syndrome of inappropriate ADH, postoperative, hypothyroidism, congestive heart failure, liver disease, and pulmonary disease. Rapid correction of hyponatremia can result in severe brain damage, including central pontine myelinolysis. For this reason, the serum sodium concentration in those patients displaying neurological symptoms should be increased by no more than 1 to 2 meq/L/h and no more than 25 to 30 meq/L in the first 2 days. Once neurological symptoms improve, the rate of increase should be decreased to 0.5 to 1 meq/L/h. Rapid correction of hypernatremia can result in cerebral edema. (*Fukagawa et al, 2005, pp. 839, 842, 844*)

45. **(B)** Hematuria from a glomerular source can be distinguished from other sources of hematuria based on history, physical exam, and urinalysis. Red cell casts, proteinuria, new-onset hypertension and edema, and/or intermittent episodes of gross hematuria accompanied by persistent microscopic hematuria are all characteristic of glomerular disease. Pyuria and bacteruria suggest a UTI, which is nonglomerular. Crystals in the urine suggest renal calculi, also a nonglomerular source of hematuria. Some medications, such as warfarin and NSAIDs, can also cause hematuria. Cytology can be obtained if there is reason to suspect bladder or renal cancer. History and physical exam should be focused toward ruling in or ruling out these causes. (*Kashtan, 1998, pp. 36–41; Stoller and Carroll, 2005, p. 906*)

46. **(B)** Respiratory acidosis is the result of decreased alveolar ventilation that leads to hypercapnia. Laboratory findings include low arterial pH, elevated pCO_2, and increased serum bicarbonate levels. Causes include chronic obstructive pulmonary disease, acute respiratory failure, acute opioid overdose, neuromuscular disorders, and airway obstruction. (*Fukagawa et al, 2005, pp. 857, 864; Noble, p. 1357*)

47. **(D)** Respiratory alkalosis occurs when hyperventilation results in hypocapnia. Laboratory findings include elevated arterial pH, low pCO_2, and decreased bicarbonate levels. Hyperventilation syndrome is the most common cause, but other causes may include Gram-negative septicemia, cirrhosis, cerebrovascular accident, pulmonary embolism, pulmonary edema, high altitude, salicylate overdose, pneumonia, and excessive mechanical ventilation. (*Fukagawa et al, 2005, pp. 857, 865*)

48. **(A)** The main mechanism of metabolic acidosis in CKD is the decreased ability of the kidney to excrete hydrogen ion, with retention of acid anions such as PO_4 and SO_4, which re-

sults in a high anion gap. (*Fukagawa et al, 2005, p. 860*)

49. **(C)** Metabolic alkalosis is characterized by an increased HCO_3 level resulting in an elevated arterial pH. Classifying metabolic alkalosis by cause based on its saline-responsiveness (responsive occurs in volume-contracted patients and unresponsive in euvolemic or hypervolemic patients) will lead to treatment plan. In saline-responsive metabolic alkalosis, urinary chloride is low (<10 to 20 meq/L). The most common cause is excessive diuretic therapy, resulting in loss of sodium chloride in the urine and contraction alkalosis. Other causes include large losses of HCl from vomiting or nasogastric suctioning, large intake of alkaline substances such as sodium bicarbonate, sodium citrate, and other antacids, and posthypercapnia. Treatment generally includes administration of normal saline IV and potassium chloride and discontinuation of diuretics or other causative exogenous substances. Saline-unresponsive metabolic alkalosis results in high urinary chloride (>20 meq/L) and is primarily due to hyperaldosteronism and other even more rare syndromes. Treatment is aimed at the underlying cause. Therefore, the volume status of the patient and urine chloride levels need to be determined to treat metabolic alkalosis. (*Fukagawa et al, 2005, pp. 863–864, 892*)

50. **(A)** Various electrolytes (anions and cations) are present in serum, the concentrations of which can be influenced by many factors. The anion gap is the difference between the cations and anions in the extracellular space. A normal gap is 8 to 16 meq/L and is calculated by subtracting the sum of the major anions (chloride and bicarbonate) from the sum of the major cation (sodium). The major unmeasured cations are calcium, magnesium, gamma-globulins, and potassium. The major unmeasured anions are negatively charged albumin, phosphate, sulfate, lactate, and other organic anions. Normal blood pH level is 7.40, which is maintained by removal of CO_2 by the lung and H^+ ion by the kidney. Metabolic acidosis can be categorized as normal anion gap or high anion gap, and calculating the gap can provide information about the cause. Increased anion gap acidosis can be seen in diabetic and alcoholic ketoacidosis, lactic acidosis, GFR <20 mL/min, and salicylate, methanol, and ethylene glycol poisoning. In addition, interference with normal metabolism or accumulation of exogenous organic anions, such as salicylate, methanol, or ethylene glycol poisoning, also results in a normal anion gap acidosis. Gastrointestinal bicarbonate loss, which occurs with large amounts of diarrhea or pancreatic drainage, will also result in a normal anion gap acidosis. Hypoalbuminemia (an unmeasured anion), some antibiotics (carbenicillin is an unmeasured anion, and polymyxin is an unmeasured cation), hypernatremia, or hyponatremia can interfere with accurate anion gap calculations. (*Fukagawa et al, 2005, pp. 856–861*)

REFERENCES

Alfrey AC. Chronic renal disease. In Schrier R (ed), *Manual of Nephrology*, 4th ed. Boston: Little Brown; 1995.

American Diabetic Association. Diabetes Care. *Diabetes Care*. 2005;28:S1–S2.

August P, Katz AI, Lindheimer MD. The patient with kidney disease and hypertension in pregnancy. In Schrier R (ed), *Manual of Nephrology*, 4th ed. Little Brown; 1995.

Bastani B. Urinary tract infections. In Noble J (ed), *Textbook of Primary Care Medicine*, 3rd ed. St. Louis: Mosby; 2001.

Breyer J. Diabetic nephropathy. In Greenberg A, Coffman TM, Cheung AK, Falk RJ, Jennette JC (eds), *Primer on Kidney Diseases*, 2nd ed. San Diego: Academic Press; 1998.

Coe FL. The patient with renal stones. In Schrier R (ed), *Manual of Nephrology*, 4th ed. Boston: Little Brown; 1995.

Cronin RE. The patient with acute azotemia. In Schrier R (ed), *Manual of Nephrology*, 4th ed. Boston: Little Brown; 1995.

Delmez JA, Windus DW. Generalist's guide to diagnostic tests. In Noble J (ed), *Textbook of Primary Care Medicine*, 3rd ed. St. Louis: Mosby; 2001.

Delvecchio FC, Preminger GM. Management of urinary calculi. In Noble J (ed), *Textbook of Primary Care Medicine*, 3rd ed. St. Louis: Mosby; 2001.

Ellison DH. Edema and the clinical use of diuretics. In Greenberg A, Coffman TM, Cheung AK, Falk RJ, Jennette JC (eds), *Primer on Kidney Disease*, 2nd ed. San Diego: Academic Press; 1998.

Freidman A. Nephrology: fluids and electrolytes. In Behrman RE, Kliegman RM (eds), *Nelson Essentials of Pediatrics*, 4th ed. Philadelphia: Saunders; 2002.

Graff L. *A Handbook of Routine Urinalysis*. Philadelphia: Lippincott Williams and Wilkins; 1983.

Greenberg A, Cheung AK, Coffman TM, Falk RJ, Jennette JC. *Primer on Kidney Diseases*. National Kidney Foundation, Academic Press; 1994.

Guyton AC, Hall JE (eds). *Textbook of Medical Physiology*, 9th ed. Philadelphia: Saunders; 1996.

Harrison's On-line, www.accessmedicine.com. From Harrison's Principles of Internal Medicine, 16th ed. New York: McGraw-Hill; 2005.

Kashtan CE. Hematuria. In Greenberg A, Coffman TM, Cheung AK, Falk RJ, Jennette JC (eds), *Primer on Kidney Diseases*, 2nd ed. San Diego: Academic Press; 1998.

NKF-K/DOQI Clinical Practice Guidelines for Chronic Kidney Disease: Executive Summary. New York: National Kidney Foundation; 2002.

Klahr S. Acid–base and fluid and electrolyte disorders. In Noble J (ed), *Textbook of Primary Care Medicine*, 3rd ed. St. Louis: Mosby; 2001.

Levey AS. Clinical evaluation of renal function. In Greenberg A, Coffman TM, Cheung AK, Falk RJ, Jennette JC (eds), *Primer on Kidney Disease*, 2nd ed. San Diego: Academic Press; 1998.

Levey AS. Bosch JP, Lewis JB, Greene T, Rogers N, Roth D. A more accurate method to estimate glomerular filtration rate from serum creatinine: a new prediction equation. *Ann Intern Med*. 1999; 130:461–470.

McBride L. *Textbook of Urinalysis and Body Fluids*. Philadelphia: Lippincott Williams and Wilkins; 1998.

Merck Manual, 16th ed. Merck Research Laboratories; 1992.

Narins RG, Heilig CW, Kupin WL. The patient with hypokalemia or hyperkalemia. In Schrier R (ed), *Manual of Nephrology*, 4th ed. Boston: Little Brown; 1995.

Pagana KD, Pagana TJ. *Mosby's Manual of Diagnostic and Laboratory Tests*, 2nd ed. St. Louis: Mosby; 2002.

Piraino B. Peritoneal dialysis. In Greenberg A, Coffman TM, Cheung AK, Falk RJ, Jennette JC (eds),

Primer on Kidney Disease, 2nd ed. San Diego: Academic Press; 1998.

Pitt B, Remme W, Zannad F, Neaton J, Martinez F, Roniker B, Bittman R, Hurley S, Kleiman, J, Gatlin, M. Eplerenone, a selective aldosterone blocker, in patients with left ventricular dysfunction after myocardial infarction. *NEJM*. 2003;348:1309–1321.

Post TW, Rose BD. Assessment of renal function: plasma creatinine; BUN; and GFR. In Rose BD (ed), *www.uptodate.com*, version 9.1; 2001.

Reikes ST, Martin KJ. Renal failure. In Noble J (ed), *Textbook of Primary Care Medicine*, 3rd ed. St. Louis: Mosby; 2001.

Schmitz PG. Glomerular and tubulointerstitial disease. In Noble J (ed), *Textbook of Primary Care Medicine*, 3rd ed. St. Louis: Mosby; 2001.

The seventh report of the Joint National Committee on Prevention, Detection, Evaluation, and Treatment of High Blood Pressure: the JNC 7 Report. *JAMA*. 2003;289:2560–2572.

Shelling JR. Diabetic nephropathy. In Hricik DE, Sedor JR, Miller T (eds), *Nephrology Secrets*. Philadelphia: Hanley & Belfus; 1999.

Stoller ML, Carroll PR. Urology. In Tierney LM, McPhee SJ, Papadakis MA (eds), *Current Medical Diagnosis and Treatment*, 44th ed. New York: McGraw-Hill; 2005.

Watnick S, Morrison G. Kidney. In Tierney LM, McPhee SJ, Papadakis MA (eds), *Current Medical Diagnosis and Treatment*, 44th ed. New York: McGraw-Hill; 2005.

CHAPTER 10

Neurology
Questions

Bryan Walker, MHS, PA-C, and Mary Hewett, MS, PA-C

DIRECTIONS (Questions 1 through 45): Each of the numbered items or incomplete statements in this section is followed by answers or by completions of the statement. Select the ONE lettered answer or completion that is BEST in each case.

Questions 1 through 45

1. A 6-year-old boy is struck by a car while riding his bicycle. He is reported to be unconscious for 2 minutes following the accident. He is conscious and alert upon arrival to the emergency department, but within 45 minutes he begins to vomit and shortly thereafter he becomes completely unresponsive. Which of the following most likely explains this child's injury?

    (A) acute subdural hematoma
    (B) chronic subdural hematoma
    (C) acute epidural hematoma
    (D) acute traumatic subarachnoid hemorrhage
    (E) grade III concussion

2. Which of the following statements best describes migraine headache?

    (A) usually unilateral, pounding, made worse with physical activity, associated with photophobia and sonophobia, accompanied by nausea and/or vomiting
    (B) usually unilateral, periorbital, stabbing quality of short duration associated with ipsilateral lacrimation and rhinorrhea along with inability to stay still
    (C) usually bilateral, tight in quality, associated with photophobia or sonophobia, sometimes relieved with physical activity
    (D) usually bilateral, boring in quality, associated with blurred vision with no exacerbating or relieving factors
    (E) usually holocephalic, associated with photophobia and described as the "worst headache of my life"

3. A 75-year-old male is involved in a motor vehicle accident and strikes his forehead on the windshield. He complains of neck pain and severe burning in his shoulders and arms. His physical exam reveals weakness of his upper extremities. What type of spinal cord injury does this patient have?

    (A) anterior cord syndrome
    (B) central cord syndrome
    (C) Brown–Séquard syndrome
    (D) complete cord transection
    (E) cauda equina syndrome

4. A 41-year-old female presents to the emergency department complaining of a sudden onset of the "worst headache of my life." A stat CT scan of her head is found to be normal. The next appropriate step in the diagnosis of this patient would be

(A) outpatient MRI of the brain
(B) CBC with differential
(C) injection of imitrex/sumatriptan succinate
(D) lumbar puncture
(E) repeat CT scan in 48 hours

5. A 45-year-old female with a known seizure disorder has been noncompliant with her anticonvulsant medication due to some side effects she has been experiencing. While in your office, she starts convulsing at a frequency that does not allow consciousness. Which of the following is the most appropriate initial drug treatment?

(A) lorazepam
(B) phenytoin
(C) phenobarbital
(D) valproic acid
(E) midazolam

6. While performing a routine history and physical exam on a 70-year-old male, you note a right carotid bruit. He denies any symptoms suggestive of a transient ischemic attack (TIA) or cerebrovascular accident (CVA). A carotid Doppler ultrasound shows a 50% stenosis of the right common carotid artery. The next most appropriate step would be

(A) stat carotid arteriogram
(B) initiate antiplatelet therapy with aspirin
(C) anticoagulate with coumadin
(D) cardiac stress test
(E) carotid endarterectomy

7. A cerebrospinal fluid analysis reveals the following results: opalescent color, increased protein, decreased glucose, and increased WBC (polys). The most likely diagnosis would be

(A) subarachnoid hemorrhage
(B) bacterial meningitis
(C) viral meningitis
(D) multiple sclerosis
(E) encephalitis

8. A 45-year-old male presents to the office with a 24-hour history of right facial droop, slurred speech, and drooling from the right side of his mouth. On exam, the patient is found to have a right facial droop, and he is unable to close his right eye and raise his right eyebrow. The remainder of the physical exam is completely normal. What would be the most appropriate therapy at this time?

(A) prednisone for 1 week and reevaluate in office
(B) stat CT scan of the head and neurology consult to rule out a stroke
(C) obtain Lyme disease titers
(D) aspirin

9. A 30-year-old male presents complaining of back pain radiating down his right leg. On exam, you note that his knee jerk reflex is absent on the right. This finding suggests compression of which spinal nerve root?

(A) L1–L2
(B) L3–L4
(C) S1–S2
(D) T11–T12
(E) C5–C6

10. A 62-year-old obese female presents with progressive numbness and tingling in her feet for the past 3 months. On physical exam, the patient is found to have decreased sensation to pinprick and vibration, absence of ankle reflexes, and difficulty with tandem walking. This patient has a history and physical exam consistent with a peripheral neuropathy. Which is the most likely etiology in her case?

(A) diabetes mellitus
(B) alcoholism
(C) vitamin B_{12} deficiency
(D) spinal cord tumor
(E) rheumatoid arthritis

11. Which of the following is the triad of clinical findings characteristic of normal pressure hydrocephalus?

    (A) gait disturbance, seizures, impaired mental function
    (B) impaired mental function, incontinence, seizures
    (C) gait disturbance, impaired mental function, incontinence
    (D) gait disturbance, incontinence, seizures
    (E) gait disturbance, aphasia, incontinence

12. A 19-year-old female presents to the emergency department complaining of headache. The headaches are generalized and increasing in intensity. They have not responded to over-the counter medications. She complains of approximately 1 week of blurred vision, intermittent diplopia, and vague dizziness. Her previous medical history includes obesity and acne. She takes Accutane and oral contraceptives. She is found to have bilateral papilledema, and visual acuity is 20/30 on physical exam. Suspecting that the patient has an intracranial mass, an MRI of the brain is ordered. The MRI is normal. The next most appropriate step would be

    (A) CT scan of the head
    (B) lumbar puncture
    (C) therapy with high-dose prednisone
    (D) stat cerebral arteriogram
    (E) reassurance and follow-up in the office in 6 months

13. You are asked to evaluate a 12-year-old, left-handed girl for "spells" which she has been experiencing. According to her parents, she was the product of an uncomplicated pregnancy and was a healthy child until last year when she was struck by a drunk driver while walking home from a friend's house. The episodes begin by her complaining of an upset stomach, then she appears confused, turns her head to the left, and raises her left arm in the air. Each episode last for about 30 to 60 seconds, after which she is very tired for another hour. This scenario best describes which type of seizure disorder?

    (A) absence
    (B) tonic-clonic
    (C) simple partial
    (D) complex partial
    (E) pseudoseizures

14. A 65-year-old male presents to the emergency department with an acute ischemic stroke. His CT scan is normal. His blood pressure is 160/100. What is the most appropriate treatment for his hypertension?

    (A) labetalol 20 mg IV
    (B) Procardia 10 mg po
    (C) Nipride drip at 1 mg/kg/min
    (D) oral clonidine
    (E) no antihypertensive should be given at this time

15. A 78-year-old female presents to the office complaining of a constant left-sided headache for 2 months. She has tried various OTC medications without relief. The patient admits to vision loss of her left eye last night for 10 minutes. The patient states that her vision then returned to normal. She denies pain in her eye. On review of systems, she relates several months of muscle aches and weight loss. On physical exam, she is found to have a tender, nonpulsatile superficial temporal artery. Her sedimentation rate is elevated at 90 mm/h. What is the next most appropriate step in the evaluation of this patient?

    (A) stat MRI/MRA of the brain and cranial vessels
    (B) antiplatelet therapy with aspirin
    (C) high-dose prednisone and temporal artery biopsy within 24 hours
    (D) lumbar puncture
    (E) Imitrex injection for her headache

16. The most common intracerebral neoplasm is

    (A) glioma
    (B) meningioma
    (C) lymphoma
    (D) metastasis
    (E) adenoma

17. A 28-year-old male presents with a complaint of new onset headache. The pain awakens him early in the morning and is described as a sharp, lancinating pain around his right eye, which is 9 out of 10. When he looks in the mirror he notices tearing of his right eye as well as redness and a different sized pupil compared to the left. The pain only lasts for a few minutes but can recur later in the morning. This has happened for the past several days. You correctly diagnose him as having cluster headache. Which of the following is the most rapid-acting preventive treatment you can offer him?

(A) sumatriptan via IM injection

(B) dihydroergotamine via IM injection

(C) oxygen at 7 L/min via non-rebreather mask

(D) oral coritcosteroid taper over 2 to 3 weeks

(E) an oral calcium channel blocker such as verapamil

18. An otherwise healthy 16-year-old female presents to your office with a complaint of headache. Reportedly, this is the second time she has experienced such a headache, the last time being last month. The pain builds up over several hours to a 9 out of 10 and can last into the next day. It is holocephalic and throbs when she moves. She has to stop what she is doing to go lay down in a dark and quiet room or she vomits. No over-the-counter medications tried have worked. Her history is consistent with which of the following?

(A) migraine with aura

(B) cluster headache

(C) tension-type headache

(D) migraine without aura

(E) hypnic headache

19. A 20-month-old boy is brought into the emergency department by his parents. They state he has not been feeling well for 2 days and this morning noted he was "shaking all over" and was not responding to commands. This went on for less than 10 minutes and has never happened before. His current rectal temperature is 100.7°F. The seizures are characteristic of

(A) absence seizures

(B) Lennox–Gastaut syndrome

(C) febrile seizures

(D) infantile spasms

(E) juvenile myoclonic epilepsy

20. After a carotid endarterectomy, a patient experienced a unilateral small pupil, mild ptosis with normal response to light and accomodation. This abnormality is called

(A) Adie pupil

(B) Argyll Robertson pupil

(C) Horner's syndrome

(D) Marcus Gunn pupil

(E) light-near dissociation

21. A previously healthy, 27-year-old female experiences an episode of vision loss in her left eye. She states it developed over hours and was like she was "looking through fog." The vision in her right eye was never affected. She denies any paresthesia, weakness, or bladder dysfunction. The sight in her left eye returned after several days but has not returned to baseline. Which of the following is the most likely diagnosis?

(A) diabetic retinopathy

(B) pseudotumor cerebri

(C) amaurosis fugax

(D) multiple sclerosis

(E) carotid artery dissection

22. A 73-year-old male is brought into your office by his adult children with a concern of memory loss. They report their father's memory has been declining since the death of their mother a few months ago but are now concerned because he is loosing weight, sleeping during the daytime, and is not keeping up with current events like he usually does. This type of behavior is most associated with which of the following?

(A) Pick disease

(B) Creutzfeldt–Jakob disease

(C) depression

(D) Alzheimer's disease

(E) vitamin B_{12} deficiency

23. A postural tremor that occurs at rest and may be exacerbated by fear, anxiety, excessive physical activity, or sleep deprivation is consistent with which of the following?

   (A) Wilson's disease
   (B) intention tremor
   (C) asterixis
   (D) physiologic tremor
   (E) hemiballismus

24. Based on a history and physical exam, along with MRI data, you diagnose a patient with multiple sclerosis. Which of the following is generally regarded as appropriate initial treatment?

   (A) beta-interferon
   (B) methylprednisone
   (C) methotrexate
   (D) amantadine
   (E) physical therapy

25. Wernicke's encephalopathy can be a complication of chronic alcoholism. It is caused by which of the following?

   (A) vitamin B_{12} deficiency
   (B) vitamin B_1 deficiency
   (C) cirrhosis
   (D) uremia
   (E) hypoventilation

26. A 62-year-old male presents to the emergency department with aphasia and right lower extremity weakness which started about 4 hours ago. You now notice progressing right upper extremity weakness, worsening right lower extremity weakness, and decreased sensation throughout his right side. This cerebral ischemia is best characterized as

   (A) transient ischemic attack
   (B) stroke in evolution
   (C) completed stroke
   (D) subarachnoid hemorrhage
   (E) global cerebral ischemia

27. A 58-year-old male presents to your office with a complaint of tremor in his right hand. Upon questioning, you discover that the tremor is getting worse and he is having trouble eating with a fork and buttoning his shirt. On your physical exam you notice bradykinesia, rigidity, and a shuffling gait. What is your initial assesment?

   (A) essential tremor
   (B) Wilson's disease
   (C) Huntington's disease
   (D) Parkinson's disease
   (E) progressive supranuclear palsy

28. A 55-year-old right-handed male presents with a 4-hour history of weakness and tingling of his right hand and numbness of the right side of his mouth. Mild difficulty was noted with word finding. His symptoms have improved since onset but have not fully resolved. There is no significant past medical history. Physical exam revealed flat right nasolabial fold, subjective numbness of the right hand, right pronator drift, clumsiness of finger tapping on the right hand, increased deep tendon reflexes on the right, as well as a present Babinski. What is the most likely etiology for this patient's problem?

   (A) migraine headache
   (B) peripheral neuropathy
   (C) syncope
   (D) transient ischemic attack
   (E) seizure

29. A 65-year-old male is brought to the clinic by his family because he has taken to wandering the streets. For the past 6 months he has been increasingly forgetful of names and places. He has become listless and has lost interest in his usual hobbies. Recently his decline has accelerated. This patient is most likely experiencing

   (A) depression
   (B) delerium
   (C) hypothyroidism
   (D) normal pressure hydrocephalus
   (E) Alzheimer dementia

30. A 52-year-old male bus driver presents to the clinic with a chief complaint of intense, shooting pains in his left cheek, each lasting for only a few seconds. He avoids touching certain parts of his face and has started to chew food only on the right side of his mouth because he is afraid he will set off an attack of pain. In between attacks the patient feels well. What is the most likely diagnosis?

    (A) cluster headache
    (B) tension-type headache
    (C) trigeminal neuralgia
    (D) giant cell arteritis
    (E) dental abscess

31. A 22-year-old female, with no previous medical problems, suddenly cried out, fell to the ground, extended her legs, flexed her arms, and jerked her extremities for 30 seconds. There was associated tongue biting and urinary incontinence. She awoke slowly over a 10-minute period and recalled nothing about the episode. She remained lethargic for several hours but the rest of her neurologic exam was normal. What is the most likely etiology for this episode?

    (A) epilepsy
    (B) hyperventilation
    (C) cardiac arrythmia
    (D) seizure
    (E) stroke

32. The diagnosis of multiple sclerosis should be based on which of the following?

    (A) two or more neurologic signs or symptoms that are localized to the brain or spinal cord and are separated in time and space (i.e., different parts of the central nervous system at least 3 months apart)
    (B) an abnormal brain MRI containing periventricular white matter lesions
    (C) cerebrospinal fluid analysis demonstrating increased oligoclonal bands and increased IgG
    (D) remission of symptoms with corticosteroids
    (E) remission of symptoms with interferon therapy

33. A 63-year-old male presents with a 3-year history of slowly progressive incoordination and difficulty in writing. On exam there is masked facies, a 4-Hz resting tremor in the right hand, and mild rigidity of all four extremities, worse on the right. Upon walking the hand tremor increases and there is reduced arm swing. What is the most likely diagnosis?

    (A) diffuse Lewy body disease
    (B) progressive supranuclear palsy
    (C) Guillain–Barré syndrome
    (D) cerebellar astrocytoma
    (E) Parkinson's disease

34. A 22-year-old college student presents to the emergency department with "the worst headache of my life" beginning 3 hours ago. The pain is severe, 10 out of 10, over the right parietal area, continuous and accompanied by right pupil dilatation, right lid ptosis, and difficulty moving the right eye medially. He has no history of headache, trauma, or significant illness. What is the most likely diagnosis?

    (A) migraine headache
    (B) subdural hematoma
    (C) trigeminal neuralgia
    (D) subarachnoid hemorrhage
    (E) Pick disease

35. A 36-year-old auto mechanic presents to the emergency department after hurting his back on the job. While lifting an object, he experienced sudden pain in his lower back with radiation to the right buttock. He was initially treated for muscle strain with a nonsteroidal anti-inflammatory drug (NSAID) after x-rays of his lumbosacral spine demonstrated no pathology. He continued to complain of this low back pain now radiating posterior down his left leg to the mid-thigh. Physical exam is unremarkable. The most likely diagnosis is

    (A) lumbosacral strain
    (B) left S-1 radiculopathy
    (C) cauda equina syndrome
    (D) L5–S1 disc herniation
    (E) lateral femoral cutaneous neuropathy

36. The most common form of multiple sclerosis is

    (A) relapsing-remitting
    (B) congenital
    (C) primary progressive
    (D) secondary progressive
    (E) progrssive-relapsing

37. A 35-year-old female presents with a 4-month history of dysarthria and muscle fatigue. She works as a nurse and at the end of her workday she notices profound difficulty enunciating her words and producing a full smile. These symptoms resolve after rest. On physical exam, you notice ptosis of the left eyelid on prolonged upgaze and progressive dysarthria while speaking. What is the most likely diagnosis?

    (A) multiple sclerosis
    (B) amyotrophic lateral sclerosis
    (C) herpes zoster
    (D) myasthenia gravis
    (E) Guillain–Barré syndrome

38. A 48-year-old female presents with new onset headache which she describes as nonspecific, worse on awakening, intermittent throughout the day but can worsen with bending over or coughing. Her husband reports that she hasn't been herself since the headaches started about 4 to 6 weeks ago. Which of the following tests would be best for determining the etiology of her presenting symptoms?

    (A) noncontrast head CT scan
    (B) lumbar puncture
    (C) contrast enhanced brain MRI
    (D) noncontrast brain MRI
    (E) cerebral angiography

39. An 18-year-old female is transferred to your emergency department from a local college infirmary. She presented yesterday with a complaint of headache but became confused and is now febrile. You notice a petechial rash on physical exam and her cerebrospinal fluid comes back with increased WBCs, increased protein, and decreased glucose. What is the most likely organism responsible for her meningitis?

    (A) *Haemophilus influenzae*
    (B) *Listeria monocytogenes*
    (C) *Neisseria meningitidis*
    (D) *Mycobacterium tuberculosis*
    (E) Coxsackie virus B

40. Huntington's disease is a movement disorder characterized by involuntary writhing of muscle groups. It is characterized by a clincial triad which includes the following:

    (A) progressive dementia, chorea, and a pattern of inheritance
    (B) progressive dementia, tremor, and no pattern of inheritance
    (C) depression, tremor, and no pattern of inheritance
    (D) depression, chorea, and no pattern of inheritance
    (E) depression, chorea, and tremor

41. A 40-year-old male presents to your office with the complaint of tinnitus and vertigo, which is intermittent and does not seem to be affected by position. The episodes can vary in length from minutes to hours and has been occurring over the past week. This has never happened to him before. His neurologic exam is unremarkable except for decreased sensorineural hearing loss in his left ear. This is most consistent with which of the following?

    (A) benign positional vertigo
    (B) Meniere's disease
    (C) otosclerosis
    (D) acute peripheral vestibulopathy
    (E) salicylate toxicity

42. An otherwise healthy 20-year-old male has been given the accurate diagnosis of migraine. His frequency of attack is about 1 per month. He has never experienced adequate relief with any over the counter analgesics. Which of the following would be appropriate to try next?

    (A) verapamil 120 mg qd
    (B) amitriptyline 25 mg q hs
    (C) codeine/acetaminophen 15 mg prn
    (D) rizatriptan 10 mg at onset, may repeat once in 2 hours
    (E) oxygen at 7 L/min inhaled via non-rebreather mask

43. Which of the following is the most common etiology for a subarachnoid hemorrhage?

    (A) trauma
    (B) ruptured aneurysm
    (C) bleeding arteriovenous malformation
    (D) embolic stroke
    (E) primary intracerebral hemorrhage

44. A 34-year-old male presents to your office with the complaint of pain and fatigue in his right wrist. He states that the pain can sometimes wake him up at night and feels as if his thumb is falling asleep. He reports the problem started since he has been writing a chapter for a review book. On physical exam, you note a positive Tinel sign but no response to a Phalen maneuver. While sending him for a nerve conduction study, you tell him the most likely diagnosis is

    (A) ulnar nerve compression
    (B) radial nerve compression
    (C) thoracic outlet syndrome
    (D) median nerve compression
    (E) peroneal nerve compression

45. The physical exam test of placing a vibrating tuning fork in the middle of a patient's forehead to test for sensorineural hearing loss is called

    (A) Rinne
    (B) Tinel
    (C) Dix-Hallpike
    (D) Babinski
    (E) Weber

Answers and Explanations

1. **(C)** This is the classic history of an epidural hematoma. The typical presentation is that of a child who sustains a hard blow to the head and experiences a brief loss of consciousness, followed by a lucid interval, when the child is awake and alert. As the hematoma expands, the patient experiences a headache followed by vomiting, lethargy, and hemiparesis and may progress to coma if left untreated. This injury usually results from a temporal bone fracture with a laceration of the middle meningeal artery or vein and less often a tear in a dural venous sinus. Epidural hematomas are treated with surgical evacuation of the clot and ligation of the bleeding vessel. (*Adams et al, 1997, pp. 885–886*)

2. **(A)** Migraine is a headache which is defined by a pain which is usually unilateral, is pounding or will take on a pounding quality with activity, can be made worse with physical activity, is associated with both light and sound sensitivity, and is associated with nausea and/or vomiting. Cluster headaches are usually unilateral as well but tend to be periorbital and are of shorter duration but greater intensity, often described as a stabbing pain. Additionally, patients may experience ipsilateral autonomic symptoms such as lacrimation, rhinorrhea, and ptosis. Tension-type headaches are mostly due to contraction of cranial and cervical muscles and are described as bilateral, tight or squeezing in nature, and are sometimes relieved by physical activity. Any headache with associated neurologic findings or in which the patient is telling the provider that the pain is different than usual deserves immediate attention. These headaches may be due to increased intracranial pressure as in pseudotumor cerebri or from meningeal irritations as with subarachnoid hemorrhage. (*Aminoff et al, 2005, pp. 85–92; Silberstein et al, 1998, pp. 61–68*)

3. **(B)** The central cord syndrome involves loss of motor function that is more severe in the upper extremities than the lower extremities and more severe in the hands. There is typically hyperesthesia over the shoulders and arms. Urinary retention is common. This injury can be subtle and easily overlooked in the intoxicated patient. (*Adams et al, 1997, p. 1233*)

4. **(D)** The hallmark of a subarachnoid hemorrhage is the very sudden onset of a severe headache. The headache is often described as the "worst headache of my life." A CT scan will detect a subarachnoid hemorrhage in more than 95% of cases. When the history suggests subarachnoid hemorrhage and the CT scan fails to detect bleeding, a lumbar puncture is mandatory. The lumbar puncture will yield bloody cerebrospinal fluid in subarachnoid hemorrhage. (*Adams et al, 1997, pp. 842–845*)

5. **(A)** Status epilepticus, defined as a continuous seizure or repeated seizures in which interval consciousness is not obtained, is a medical emergency if it persists for greater

than 30 minutes. An intravenous infusion of a longer acting benzodiazepine, such as lorazepam, has been shown to be effective in terminating a seizure. This may be followed by a loading dose of phenytoin. If this combination fails, some will use phenobarbital while there have been some reports of using midazolam. (*Adams et al, 1997, pp. 339–340*)

6. **(B)** The patient exhibits an asymptomatic carotid bruit. The most appropriate step would be to initiate antiplatelet therapy with daily aspirin. Arteriography would not be indicated for an asymptomatic carotid bruit. Anticoagulation with Coumadin should be limited to symptomatic bruits manifested as multiple TIAs. Carotid endarterectomy is reserved for carotid stenosis that is greater than 70% in patients who have had recurrent TIAs on medical therapy. It may be necessary in patients with a lesser degree of stenosis when ulcerated plaques are present. Asymptomatic carotid bruits in men are associated with an increased risk of death from ischemic heart disease. Performing a stress test may be appropriate in this patient population. Most deaths in patients with cerebrovascular disease are the result of heart disease. (*Adams et al, 1997, pp. 822–823*)

7. **(B)** The cerebrospinal fluid (CSF) analysis in bacterial meningitis includes a cloudy appearance with a markedly elevated protein and white cell content. The white cells are predominantly polymorphonuclear leukocytes (polys). Bacterial utilization of CSF glucose causes it to be low. Gram stain may or may not be positive for bacteria. The diagnosis of bacterial meningitis requires a culture of the CSF. CSF pressures at the time of the lumbar puncture are elevated in 90% of cases. In viral meningitis, the CSF white count is usually 1000/mL. The cell types are lymphocytes or monocytes, but early in the disease polys may predominate. CSF glucose is normal in viral meningitis and protein is elevated. Gram stain will be negative and the culture will show no growth. The CSF in multiple sclerosis may have a mild lymphocytosis with an increased protein concentration. CSF protein electrophoresis in multiple sclerosis shows discrete bands of IgG called *oligoclonal bands*. These oligoclonal bands are present in 90% of patients with multiple sclerosis. The CSF in subarachnoid hemorrhage is grossly bloody. Because bleeding can be caused by a traumatic puncture, the RBC count should be done on the first and last tubes and the counts compared. In subarachnoid hemorrhage, the RBC count will be the same, whereas in a traumatic lumbar puncture, the RBCs will not be present in the last tube that is collected. The CSF in subarachnoid hemorrhage may reveal xanthochromia. This is a yellow appearance in the centrifuged CSF supernatant caused by the degradation of RBCs in the CSF. The CSF becomes xanthochromic after it has been exposed to blood for several hours. (*Aminoff et al, 2005, p.12*)

8. **(A)** This is a typical presentation of Bell's palsy. Bell's palsy is an idiopathic facial nerve palsy that results in unilateral weakness or paralysis of the facial muscles. This results in facial drooping, slurred speech, drooling, as well as an inability to close the eye and to raise the affected eyebrow. Facial weakness caused by a stroke does not affect the ability to close the affected eye or to move the forehead. This weakness is characteristic of a peripheral seventh nerve palsy. In a stroke, there are often other abnormalities beyond the facial nerve. Bell's palsy is often preceded or accompanied by pain around the ear. It is more common in pregnancy and diabetes. It is believed that starting prednisone within 5 days of the onset of symptoms increases the number of patients who recover completely. The weakness or paralysis is usually maximal between 2 and 5 days. Eighty percent of patients recover in several weeks. In some cases, it may take up to 2 months to resolve. Improvement in facial motor function within the first 5 to 7 days is the most favorable prognostic sign. A CT scan of the head and neurologic consult are not indicated in this patient. Lyme disease would be a rare cause of facial nerve paralysis and is not part of the routine evaluation for it. Aspirin is not indicated, since this is not caused by cerebrovascular disease. (*Aminoff et al, 2005, p. 182*)

9. **(B)** Absence of the knee jerk reflex suggests compression of the L3–L4 spinal nerve root. The four most commonly tested deep tendon reflexes are the Achilles (ankle jerk) reflex, quadriceps (knee jerk) reflex, triceps reflex, and the biceps reflex. The nerve roots that each tests in ascending order are 1 and 2, 3 and 4, 5 and 6 (biceps), and 7 and 8 (triceps). One only needs to remember that the ankle jerk is a sacral nerve root, the knee jerk is a lumbar nerve root, and the biceps and triceps are cervical nerve roots. (*Aminoff et al, 2005, p. 367*)

10. **(A)** Peripheral neuropathy is a syndrome that is manifested by muscle weakness, paresthesias, decreased deep tendon reflexes, and autonomic disturbances most commonly in the hands and feet, such as coldness and sweating. There are many causes of peripheral neuropathy ranging from metabolic conditions to malignant neoplasm, rheumatoid arthritis, and drug and alcohol use. The increase in non-insulin-dependent diabetes mellitus due to obesity in the American population has also increased the incidence of associated disease states. (*Aminoff et al, 2005, pp. 213–214*)

11. **(C)** The classic triad of normal pressure hydrocephalus (NPH) is gait disturbance, dementia, and urinary incontinence. The gait disturbance is the earliest symptom followed by progressive dementia. Urinary incontinence occurs late in the illness. CT scan may show a disproportionate enlargement of the ventricle to the degree of cortical atrophy. The gait disturbance and dementia may be reversible with the placement of a ventriculoatrial or ventriculoperitoneal shunt. NPH may follow a subarachnoid hemorrhage, but in many cases the cause may not be identified. Papilledema is not present in NPH. (*Adams et al, 1997, pp. 631–632*)

12. **(B)** The presence of headache associated with papilledema raises the concern for a brain tumor. The MRI excluded a mass lesion, raising a strong suspicion of pseudotumor cerebri. This is also known as *benign intracranial hypertension*. It is not a benign condition, however, since it causes severe headache and may result in visual loss. It is particularly frequent in obese adolescent girls and young women. The etiology is unknown but may be associated with the use of oral contraceptives, vitamin A, and tetracycline. The presentation consists of headaches caused by an increase in intracranial pressure and blurring of vision. There may be diplopia, but the remainder of the neurologic exam is unremarkable. Papilledema is virtually always part of the presentation. The mental status is normal. The differential diagnosis includes venous sinus thrombosis, sarcoidosis, and tuberculous or carcinomatous meningitis. The last two are excluded by lumbar puncture. An abnormal cerebrospinal fluid is not consistent with pseudotumor cerebri. The diagnosis is made by excluding mass lesions with CT scan or MRI and demonstrating markedly increased intracranial pressure by lumbar puncture. The treatment involves weight loss, diuretics, and steroids. Repeat lumbar punctures to remove cerebrospinal fluid and decrease intracranial pressure are effective. In cases that are unresponsive to these measures, lumbar-peritoneal shunting is effective, as is unilateral optic nerve sheath fenestration. Effective treatment can improve headaches and prevent vision loss. (*Adams et al, 1997, pp. 634–637*)

13. **(D)** Complex partial seizures are usually preceded by some type of sensory aura. This is followed by an impairment of consciousness but not total loss of consciousness along with an involuntary motor activity. The seizure will resolve in about 30 minutes and is followed by a postictal confusion. Simple partial seizures have no alteration of consciousness. Absence and tonic-clonic seizures are generalized seizure disorders in which consciousness is lost. Whereas absence seizures are characterized by staring spells without motor involvement, tonic-clonic seizures involve strong muscle extension and contraction in many major muscle groups. Pseudoseizures are a diagnosis of exclusion. All testing including EEG are normal and the seizures may be a manifestation of an underlying psychiatric disturbance. (*Aminoff et al, 2005, pp. 267–278*)

14. **(E)** Blood pressure is typically elevated at the time of presentation in acute ischemic stroke.

It will decline without medication in the first few hours to days. Aggressively lowering blood pressure in an acute ischemic stroke may decrease the blood flow to the ischemic, but salvageable brain tissue. This potentially salvageable brain tissue is referred to as the *penumbra*. Decreasing blood flow to the ischemic penumbra by acutely lowering blood pressure may result in eventual infarction of this brain tissue. Treatment of previously undiagnosed hypertension should be deferred for several days. Blood pressure should be treated if there are other indications, such as angina or heart failure. Control of blood pressure is appropriate in patients who are receiving tissue plasminogen activator (t-Pa) for their stroke. Blood pressure should be lowered cautiously to a systolic of less than 185 and a diastolic of less than 110. This is thought to decrease the incidence of intracerebral hemorrhage in these patients. (*Aminoff et al, 2005, p. 311; Adams et al, 1997, p. 818*)

15. **(C)** The diagnosis is temporal arteritis. This is an arteritis of the temporal branch of the external carotid artery characterized by unilateral or bilateral headaches that may be localized to a tender temporal artery. The temporal artery may be thickened and tender and may be thrombosed and nonpulsatile late in the disease. Many patients present with malaise and have anemia and a low-grade fever. Fifty percent of patients report generalized muscle aches consistent with polymyalgia rheumatica. The most severe complication of temporal arteritis is blindness resulting from thrombosis of the opthalmic artery. In some cases, this may be preceded by previous episodes of amaurosis fugax before the blindness becomes irreversible. Once blindness occurs in one eye, it may be prevented in the other by initiating treatment. The diagnosis is based on recognizing the clinical picture and obtaining a temporal artery biopsy. Treatment should not be delayed pending the biopsy. Early treatment with prednisone may prevent irreversible blindness. The efficacy of treatment can be measured with serial sedimentation rates. MRI and MRA have no value in establishing the diagnosis of temporal arteritis. Antiplatelet therapy would not be inappropriate,

but is inadequate for this diagnosis. The potentially unilateral headache should not be confused with a migraine for which Imitrex therapy would be appropriate. In addition, lumbar puncture has no role in establishing this diagnosis. (*Adams et al, 1997, pp. 185, 856–857*)

16. **(A)** Gliomas account for nearly 50% of primary brain tumors. The remainder are meningiomas (15%), pituitary tumors (7%), and other tumors. (*Adams et al, 1997, p. 643*)

17. **(D)** Oral corticosteroids started immediately will often force a cluster cycle into remission. Given on a daily basis and tapered over 2 to 3 weeks, they will give other preventive agents, such as verapamil, time to become effective. Sumatriptan, dihydroergotamine, and oxygen are very useful abortive agents but do not work on stopping the cluster cycle. Both sumatriptan and dihydroergotamine have maximum daily doses and may not be used for all attacks during the day as some cluster patients may have multiple attacks throughout the day. (*Silberstein et al, 1998, pp. 118–122*)

18. **(D)** The history is consistent with migraine without aura. Migraine is a headache which is defined by a pain which is usually unilateral, is pounding or will take on a pounding quality with activity, can be made worse with physical activity, is associated with both light and sound sensitivity, and is associated with nausea and/or vomiting. If the headache is preceded by an abnormal sensory experience such as a visual disturbance which lasts no longer than 60 minutes and totally remits, it is classified as a migraine with aura. Cluster headaches are usually unilateral as well but tend to be periorbital and are of shorter duration but greater intensity, often described as a stabbing pain. Additionally, patients may experience ipsilateral autonomic symptoms such as lacrimation, rhinorrhea, and ptosis. Tension-type headaches are mostly due to contraction of cranial and cervical muscles and are described as bilateral, tight or squeezing in nature, and are sometimes relieved by physical activity. Hypnic headaches primarily occur in the elderly and will awaken them

from sleep at the same time every night. (*Aminoff et al, 2005, pp. 85–92; Silberstein et al, 1998, pp. 61–68, 209*)

19. **(C)** Febrile seizures can occur in children under the age of 5 when accompanied by a fever. They are characterized by a brief generalized motor seizure. Absence seizures are generalized seizures characterized by a loss of consciousness without motor involvement typically seen in older children. Lenox–Gastaut syndrome presents in childhood as well but is usually associated with developmental delay and seizures of akinetic and myoclonic nature (refered to as drop attacks). Infantile spasms occur without relation to systemic illness and are massive myoclonic events with bending at the waist. Juvenile myoclonic epilepsy evolves in the teenage years and is characterized by repeated episodes of myoclonic seizure activity. (*Adams et al, 1997, pp. 322–324*)

20. **(C)** Horner's syndrome is defined by a unilateral, small pupil with mild ptosis in which pupilary response to light and accomodation is preserved. It may also be associated with ipsilateral anhydrosis. It is usually caused by some interruption in the oculosympathetic pathway. An Adie pupil is characterized by a unilateral dilated pupil which is sluggish to direct light stimuli. An Argyll Robertson pupil usually affects both eyes, is irregular in shape, and is poorly reactive to light. A Marcus Gunn pupil constricts slower to direct light stimulation than to the consensual stimulation. Light near dissociation is usually bilateral and consists of preserved constriction to accommodation but impared response to light. (*Aminoff et al, 2005, pp. 138–139*)

21. **(D)** Multiple sclerosis is a demylinating disease which is thought to have an autoimmune pathophysiology. The presenting symptoms of multiple sclerosis are highly variable but can include focal weakness, paresthesia, or visual disturbance. Once the patient experiences a set of symptoms, they may improve but will not return to baseline function. The visual loss associated with diabetic retinopathy is usually bilateral. Pseudotumor cerebri is often accompanied by headache and presents as diplopia. Amaurosis fugax is unilateral but will resolve over 10 to 20 minutes and is caused by an embolic source. Carotid artery dissection can also cause unilateral vision loss but is usually total and followed by other, more severe, neurologic deficits. (*Aminoff et al, 2005, pp. 164–167, 293*)

22. **(C)** This patient's symptoms are most consistent with situational depression over the loss of his spouse. Transient memory problems can be a component of depression as a result of decreased attention and interest. Dementia is a progressive impairment of higher cognitive function, and initially, the patient's social graces are preserved. It has many causes, of which Pick disease, Creutzfeld–Jakob disease, and Alzheimer's disease are irreversible. Vitamin B_{12} deficiency can cause reversible form of cognitive impairment, in which the elderly are susceptible, so serum analysis of vitamin B_{12} should be performed in many diagnostic evaluations of dementia in this population. (*Aminoff et al, 2005, pp. 44–51*)

23. **(D)** Physiologic tremor is a postural tremor which may be exacerbated by the factors outlined in this question. Both asterixis and intention tremor are also postural tremors; however, asterixis is seen in the context of metabolic encephalopathy and intention tremor during activity. Wilson's disease occurs with other abnormal cerebellar findings. Hemiballismus is a choreiform movement disorder and not an oscillatory movement. (*Aminoff et al, 2005, pp. 234–236*)

24. **(A)** The goal of the treatment of multiple sclerosis is to reduce the frequency and severity of recurrent attacks. Most data agree that the use of beta-interferons as early as possible in the diagnosis of multiple sclerosis is the treatment of choice for attaining this goal. Corticosteroids may be used to lessen the severity of an acute attack but have not been shown effective in suppressing further attacks. The same is thought for methotrexate. Treatment for the complications of multiple sclerosis as well as healthy lifestyle habits should be encouraged. The use of amantadine and physical

therapy can help with energy and mobility issues. (*Aminoff et al, 2005, pp. 166–167*)

25. **(B)** Wernicke's encephalopathy is due to a dietary deficiency in vitamin B_1. Chronic alcoholics generally are in a state of malnutrition and do not get adequate amounts of thiamine. (*Aminoff et al, 2005, p. 113*)

26. **(B)** During a stroke in evolution, symptoms will worsen or new symptoms will appear. A completed stroke is one in which neurologic symptoms have stablized whereas a transient ischemic attack produces deficits which resolve over time. This patient's symptoms do not match those of an acute subarachnoid hemorrhage. Global cerebral ischemia as seen in sudden cardiac arrest would involve loss of consciousness. (*Aminoff et al, 2005, pp. 286–297*)

27. **(D)** The symptoms of tremor, bradykinesia, and rigidity are classic for Parkinson's disease. Difficulty with activities of daily living will usually prompt a patient to seek medical attention. Essential tremor and Wilson's disease are postural tremors with different characteristics than the tremor seen in Parkinson's disease. Huntington's disease produces choreiform movements and has a much earlier age of onset. Progressive supranuclear palsy is characterized by an ophthalmoplegia in addition to tremor. (*Aminoff et al, 2005, pp. 241–250*)

28. **(D)** Three key features of a transient ischemic attack include sudden onset and complete reversal of symptoms within 24 hours, usually within 15 minutes. The symptoms are usually in the anatomical distribution of a single blood vessel. This patient's history is not suggestive of migraine or syncope. His physical exam findings do not correlate with peripheral neuropathy or seizure. (*Blumenfeld, 2002*)

29. **(E)** This presentation is classic for Alzheimer's dementia. There is a global decrease in mentation, which is chronic yet relatively stable. His symptoms are not fluctuating as are usually seen in delirium. There is no history of urinary incontinence, which would suggest normal pressure hydrocephalus. Depression is a possibility along with his dementia. There are no

other historical or exam findings suggestive of hypothyroidism. (*Samuels, 2003*)

30. **(C)** Trigeminal neuralgia is characterized by sharp, brief pain often described as "shooting, jabbing, electric shock, or stabbing." This history given for cluster headache and tension-type headache is not at all like this patient's. The history for temporal arteritis is generally different but it may be worth getting a sedimentation rate just to be sure. This pain pattern is different than that of a focal dental problem. (*Braunwald, 2004*)

31. **(A)** This event represents a well-demarcated episode effecting some combination of consciousness, motor and/or sensory function consequent to abnormal electrical discharges in the brain. This is consistent with the definition of a seizure. Epilepsy refers to multiple, recurrent seizures. This history is not consistent with hyperventilation, stroke, or cardiac arrhythmia. (*Blumenfeld, 2002*)

32. **(A)** Multiple sclerosis is an idiopathic inflammatory disease of the central nervous system and is characterized pathologically by demyelination and subsequent axonal degeneration. In the absence of a specific immune-based assay, the diagnosis of multiple sclerosis is often difficult to make. The American Academy of Neurology urges providers to document multiple episodes in time and space within the central nervous system before making the diagnosis of multiple sclerosis and starting immunosuppressive therapy. (*Aminoff et al, 2005, pp. 164–167*)

33. **(E)** The four cardinal features of Parkinson's disease are tremor, akinesia (or bradykinesia), rigidity, and postural instability. Parkinson's disease is the most common form of tremor presenting in the fifth or sixth decade of life with initially unilateral symptoms. Pathologic features of Parkinson's disease include loss of pigmented neurons in the substantia nigra and the presense of Lewy bodies. (*Braunwald, 2004*)

34. **(D)** A headache described as "the worst headache of my life" with an acute onset is a

neurosurgical emergency until proven otherwise by a normal head CT, lumbar puncture, and physical exam. Subarachnoid hemorrhage can be caused by trauma, a ruptured intracranial aneurysm, or ruptured arterial venous malformation. It can be associated with hypertension, polycystic kidney disease, or cocaine/amphetamine abuse. (*Samuels, 2003*)

35. **(A)** Low back pain is one of the more common presenting neurologic complaints to a primary care provider. Most acute pain syndromes are benign, self-limiting conditions, with pain arising from myofascial sources. Patients with back pain and normal neurologic exams are unlikely to have any serious underlying pathology and further diagnositc testing is usually unrevealing. (*Braunwald, 2004*)

36. **(A)** Relapsing–remitting multiple sclerosis accounts for approximately 90% of cases. It is characterized by well-defined attacks of neurologic impairment with periods of stability between attacks. (*Hewett, 2003*)

37. **(D)** Myasthenia gravis is an immune-mediated disorder in which there are circulating antibodies against the postsynaptic nicotinic acetylcholine receptors at the neuromuscular junction of skeletal muscle cells. It has a bimodal age-related onset in the second or third decade in women and in the sixth or seventh decade in men. Characteristically, weakness becomes more severe with repeated use of a muscle or during the course of the day. (*Blumenfeld, 2002*)

38. **(C)** This patient has an intracranial mass until proven otherwise. Headaches starting later in life and accompanied by other neurologic or congnitive problems should raise a high suspicion of a tumor. Obtaining a contrast enhanced MRI of the brain will demonstrate an intracranial mass lesion. The contrast will follow blood flow distribution and help in determining possible tumor type. Some lesions are difficult to see without contrast enhancement. MRI scans have a much higher resolution for soft tissue over CT scans and are prefered for looking at brain parenchyma. Prior to the advent of CT and MRI, cerebral angiography

was used to look for intracranial masses. Vascular tumors have characteristic blush patterns, and if a mass effect is present, it will distort the position of the blood vessels. (*Aminoff et al, 2005, pp. 82–83; Lee et al, 1999, pp. 266–270*)

39. **(C)** *Neisseria meningitidis* and *Streptococcus pneumoniae* are the most common etiologic agents for bacterial meningitis in this patient's age group. So much so that many colleges and universities require a vaccine for students who live in dormatories. Her fever and the cerebrospinal fluid values are consistent with a bacterial and not a viral infectious source for the meningeal irritation. (*Aminoff et al, 2005, pp. 20–30*)

40. **(A)** Huntington's disease is characterized by progressive dementia, which may start by subtle changes in cognitive functioning, and by choreiform movements, which may start slightly appearing as restlessness and progressing to expansive, dance-like movements in multiple limbs; and it is an autosomaldominant disorder. (*Aminoff et al, 2005, p. 250; Adams et al, 1997, pp. 1060–1062*)

41. **(B)** Sporadic episodes of vertigo with some degree of sensorineural hearing loss and tinnitus are consistent with Meniere's disease. If the patient is experiencing an attack, one may observe horizontal nystagmus whereas with positional vertigo, reproducing the position will create observable nystagmus. Patients usually will not experience any hearing loss with positional veritgo or a peripheral vestibulopathy. Additionally, patients with acute peripheral vestibulopathy appear ill and experience accompanied emesis. Otosclerosis is accompanied by conductive hearing loss. This patient had no history of high-dose salicylate use. (*Aminoff et al, 2005, pp. 107–112*)

42. **(D)** Rizatriptan, like the other 5-HT receptor agonists, is an extremely effective medication for the acute treatment of migraine. This patient has tried over-the-counter analgesics, which can work for mild forms of migraine, and so the use of a migraine-specific abortive agent is appropriate. Narcotic analgesics

should be avoided not only due to the possibility of dependence but more importantly because they are not as effective as other analgesics for targeting the neurochemical causes of migraine. With a frequency of about 1 attack per month, the use of a preventive agent such as verapamil or amitriptyline is not needed. Oxygen can be useful as an acute treatment for cluster headache but has not been shown to be useful for migraine. (*Aminoff et al, 2005, pp. 88–89; Silberstein et al, 1998, pp. 76–80*)

43.   **(B)** Up to 75% of subarachnoid hemorrhages can be attributed to the rupture of an intracranial aneurysm. Due to cerebrovascular anatomy, the blood is usually confined to the subarachnoid space. Blood from a ruptured arteriovenous malformation can be intraparenchymal and cause focal neurologic symptoms. Trauma is more likely to case epidural or subdural hematoma. (*Aminoff et al, 2005, pp. 74–76*)

44.   **(D)** Median nerve compression can be precipitated by repetitive use of the wrist or hand or by compression of the median nerve within the carpal tunnel at the wrist from inflammation or trauma. Characteristic fatigue and pain, especially at night, may be accompanied by paresthesia in the median nerve distribution. The pain may be reproduced on exam by performing either the Tinel or Phalen maneuver but electrophysiology studies will usually confirm the entrapment. (*Aminoff et al, 2005, pp. 221–222*)

45.   **(E)** The test described is the Weber. Rinne is also used to asses sensorineural hearing loss but is performed by placing a vibrating tuning fork on the mastoid process. Once the patient states the noise is no longer heard, the examiner places the tuning fork by the ipsilateral ear. The patient should still hear the vibratory noise. Tinel is a test for median nerve compression where the examiner taps over the nerve at the wrist to elicit paresthesia. Dix-Hallpike is a maneuver to test for positional vertigo. Babinski is a pathological response to the superficial reflex of the foot, indicating an upper motor neuron lesion. (*Aminoff et al, 2005, p. 103*)

REFERENCES

Adams RD, Victor M, Ropper AH. *Principles of Neurology*, 6th ed. New York: McGraw-Hill; 1997.

Aminoff MJ, Greenberg DA, Simon RP. *Clinical Neurology*, 6th ed. New York: McGraw-Hill; 2005.

Blumenfeld H. *Neuroanatomy through Clinical Cases*, 1st ed. Sunderland: Sinaur Associates; 2002.

Braunwald E. *Harrison's Textbook of Medicine*. New York: McGraw-Hill; 2004.

Hewett M. An overview of multiple sclerosis for the physician assistant. *Physician Assist.* 2003;27:8,15–24.

Lee SH, Rao KC, Zimmerman RA. *Cranial MRI and CT*, 4th ed. New York: McGraw-Hill; 1999.

Samuels, MA. *Hospitalist Neurology*, 1st ed. Boston: Butterworth-Heinemann; 2003.

Silberstein SD, Lipton RB, Goadsby PJ. *Headache in Clinical Practice*, 1st ed. Oxford: Isis Medical Media; 1998.

CHAPTER 11

Internal Medicine: Pulmonology
Questions

Jill Reichman, MPH, PA-C, and Matthew McQuillan, MS, PA-C

DIRECTIONS (Questions 1 through 65): Each of the numbered items or incomplete statements in this section is followed by answers or by completions of the statement. Select the ONE lettered answer or completion that is BEST in each case.

Questions 1 through 65

1. A 19-year-old male college student presents with a 4-day history of fever, headache, sore throat, myalgia, malaise, and a nonproductive cough. On exam you note an erythematous pharynx without exudate. The lung exam is unimpressive. A chest x-ray reveals a right-sided lower-lobe patchy pneumonia.

   Which of the following is the most likely cause?

   (A) *Mycoplasma pneumoniae*
   (B) *Klebsiella pneumoniae*
   (C) *Streptococcus pneumoniae*
   (D) *Staphylococcus aureus*

2. A 40-year-old female presents with the sudden onset of cough productive of blood-speckled sputum, chest pain with cough, shaking chills, high fever, and myalgias for the last 12 hours. On exam she appears acutely ill, is tachypneic, and coughing. Auscultation of the chest reveals rales and chest x-ray reveals unilateral lobar consolidation consistent with pneumonia. Which of the following is the most likely cause?

   (A) *Mycoplasma pneumoniae*
   (B) *Streptococcus pneumoniae*
   (C) *Chlamydia pneumoniae*
   (D) aspiration pneumonia

3. A 3-year-old patient presents with sudden onset of coughing and wheezing which began at the dinner table this evening. Vital signs are pulse 120, respirations 26, temperature 98.6°F. You evaluate the patient and determine that the diagnosis is most likely a partial obstruction secondary to tracheal foreign body. What is the next step in the management of this patient?

   (A) chest physiotherapy
   (B) intubation
   (C) tracheostomy
   (D) bronchoscopy

4. What is the most effective treatment of acute bronchitis in otherwise healthy adults?

   (A) empiric antibiotic therapy
   (B) B_2 agonists
   (C) adequate hydration
   (D) corticosteroid therapy

5. A 32-year-old patient with a 3-week history of fever, malaise, weight loss, joint pain, and dry cough presents to your office. The chest x-ray reveals bilateral hilar adenopathy with no parenchymal abnormalities. You suspect and would like to rule out sarcoidosis. How can the definitive diagnosis be made?

   (A) biopsy of the mediastinal nodes
   (B) perform a bronchoalveolar lavage
   (C) administer an intradermal purified protein derivative
   (D) measure serum angiotensin-converting enzyme

6. What is the most common mode of transmission of the *Mycobacterium tuberculosis* bacteria?

   (A) aerosolized droplets
   (B) blood borne
   (C) transplacental
   (D) transdermal

7. A 65-year-old alcoholic male presents with the acute onset of fever, cough productive of purulent sputum, hemoptysis, chest pain, and shortness of breath. On exam, he is confused and hypotensive. Chest x-ray shows bilateral infiltrates and cavitations. Which of the following is the most likely cause of this pneumonia?

   (A) influenza
   (B) *Mycoplasma pneumoniae*
   (C) *Chlamydia pneumoniae*
   (D) *Klebsiella pneumoniae*

8. What is the drug treatment of choice for *Mycoplasma pneumoniae*?

   (A) penicillin
   (B) erythromycin
   (C) ampicillin
   (D) vancomycin

9. What is the drug treatment of choice for a known case of pneumococcal pneumonia in an area where antibiotic resistance is not a factor?

   (A) dicloxacillin
   (B) gentamycin
   (C) penicillin
   (D) ticarcillin
   (E) vancomycin

10. A 50-year-old male presents with a history of persistent cough, hemoptysis, and weight loss over the past 6 months. He has smoked two packs per day for 30 years and also complains of shoulder and chest pain. On exam he is pale, febrile, and dyspneic upon exertion. The chest x-ray shows hilar adenopathy. What is the most likely diagnosis?

    (A) asthma
    (B) bronchiectasis
    (C) bronchogenic carcinoma
    (D) chronic obstructive pulmonary disease

11. A patient recently diagnosed with tuberculosis is prescribed a treatment regimen that includes isoniazid. Which of the following is a side effect of isoniazid?

    (A) hyperuricemia
    (B) peripheral neuropathy
    (C) red-orange urine
    (D) vestibular toxicity

12. What radiologic finding(s) is/are most suggestive of chronic silicosis?

    (A) eggshell calcification of enlarged hilar lymph nodes
    (B) pneumothorax and atelectasis
    (C) large nodules that appear primarily in the lower lobes
    (D) pleural thickening and plaques

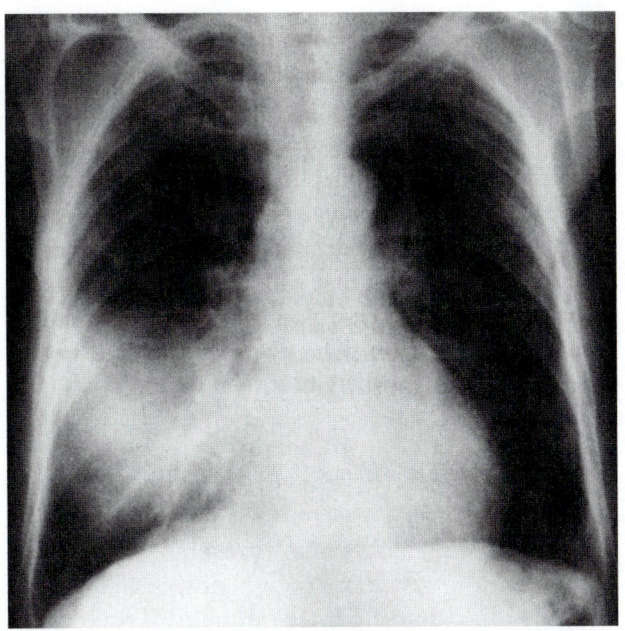

Fig. 11–1. From Novelline R, *Squire's Fundamentals of Radiology*, 5th ed, Harvard University Press, Cambridge, MA, 1999, with permission.

13. The condition shown in Fig. 11–1 is consistent with what physical finding?

(A) vesicular breath sounds

(B) decreased transmitted voice sounds

(C) inspiratory crackles

(D) diffuse hyperresonance

14. Which histological type of lung cancer has the lowest 5-year survival rate?

(A) bronchioalveolar

(B) large cell

(C) small cell

(D) squamous cell

(E) adenocarcinoma

15. What is the current recommended treatment regimen for tuberculosis patients in the United States who are immunocompetent?

(A) three months of isoniazid (INH), rifampin (RIF), and pyrazinamide (PZA) and ethambutol (EMB)

(B) three months of INH and RIF with initial 2 months of PZA and streptomycin (SM)

(C) six months of INH and RIF

(D) six months of INH and RIF with initial 2 months of PZA and SM or EMB

16. A patient with HIV disease is diagnosed with legionella. What is the drug treatment of choice?

(A) cefuroxime

(B) doxycycline

(C) erythromycin

(D) levofloxacin

17. A 19-year-old female, post motor vehicle accident, is hospitalized with a femur fracture. She develops sudden onset of dyspnea, cough, and anxiety with retrosternal chest pain. On exam her pulse is 120, respirations 32, blood pressure 120/80. Chest x-ray shows mild bilateral atelectasis. ECG is normal. What is the most likely diagnosis?

(A) pulmonary thromboembolus

(B) aortic dissection

(C) pneumonia

(D) pneumothorax

18. What imaging study is the "gold standard" used to confirm the diagnosis of deep vein thrombosis?

(A) arteriography

(B) contrast venography

(C) Doppler ultrasound

(D) ventilation perfusion scan

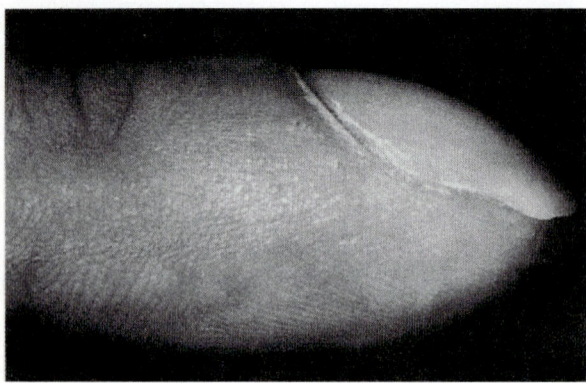

Fig. 11–2. From Bickley LS, Hoekelman RA *Bates' Guide to Physical Examination and History Taking.* 8th ed. Philadelphia, PA; Lippincott Williams & Wilkins; 2003.

19. Figure 11–2 demonstrates a physical finding most often associated with what condition?

   (A) acute dyspnea
   (B) chronic hypoxia
   (C) transient hypercapnia
   (D) chronic hyponatremia

20. What is the mainstay bronchodilator treatment for mild intermittent asthma?

   (A) beta-adrenergic agents
   (B) theophylline
   (C) aminophylline
   (D) antileukotrienes

21. What is the characteristic prodrome of acute pneumonia caused by *Chlamydia*?

   (A) headache and sore throat
   (B) low-grade fever and rash
   (C) sneezing and ear pain
   (D) sudden onset of fever and chills

22. What is considered the primary therapy for patients with pulmonary thromboembolism (PTE)?

   (A) anticoagulation with heparin
   (B) anti-embolization stockings
   (C) insertion of an inferior vena caval filter
   (D) thrombolysis with tissue plasminogen activator (t-Pa)

23. A 79-year-old woman who is 7 days post a total hip replacement complains of sudden onset of dyspnea, cough, and restrosternal chest pain. On exam, she appears anxious with vital signs as follows: pulse 120, respirations 32, blood pressure 138/92. A chest x-ray demonstrates mild bilateral atelectasis and an ECG is normal other than tachycardia. What imaging modality will best confirm the diagnosis?

   (A) arteriography
   (B) contrast venography
   (C) helical CT scan
   (D) ventilation/perfusion scan

24. A 17-year-old woman presents complaining of a nonproductive cough, postnasal drip, and nasal congestion. Examination reveals inflamed nasal turbinates, cobblestoning of the posterior pharynx, and diffuse bilateral end expiratory wheezes. Which lab test will provide the best information to assist in making the diagnosis?

   (A) arterial blood gas
   (B) chest x-ray
   (C) peak flow measurements
   (D) spirometry

25. A 7-year-old boy with a history of asthma presents with nocturnal cough occurring every night along with daily exacerbations of wheezing and shortness of breath. How would his asthma be classified?

   (A) mild intermittent
   (B) mild persistent
   (C) moderate persistent
   (D) severe persistent

26. A 13-year-old girl presents complaining of intermittent episodes of wheezing which occur only when she is exercising. Which of the following medications is most appropriate to prevent her symptoms?

   (A) ipratropium
   (B) fluticasone
   (C) salmeterol
   (D) terbutaline

27. A 35-year-old woman with a history of severe persistent asthma has been treated with inhaled corticosteroids, a long-acting bronchodilator, and prednisone tablets for several years. In order to decrease the severity of side effects of this treatment regimen, which of the following should be prescribed?

   (A) benzodiazepines
   (B) beta-blockers
   (C) folic acid
   (D) vitamin D and calcium

28. A 17-year-old girl with a history of cystic fibrosis presents with a chronic cough productive of copious, foul smelling, purulent sputum. The patient is afebrile and the lung examination reveals crackles at the lung bases bilaterally. What is the most likely diagnosis?

   (A) asthma
   (B) bronchiectasis
   (C) bronchiolitis
   (D) pneumonitis

29. Which of the following disorders of the large bronchioles is characterized by the destruction of bronchial walls?

   (A) asthma
   (B) bronchiectasis
   (C) cystic fibrosis
   (D) pneumonia

30. A 35-year-old man is suspected of having a small right-sided pleural effusion. What imaging modality is most sensitive to detect a small amount of pleural fluid?

   (A) chest CT
   (B) lateral chest film
   (C) left lateral decubitus chest film
   (D) standard upright chest film

31. A 58-year-old man with a history of hypertension and left ventricular hypertrophy presents with shortness of breath. Examination reveals dullness to percussion bilaterally with decreased breath sounds. Pleural fluid is aspirated and analyzed. Which of the following results is consistent with his most likely diagnosis?

   (A) glucose 40 mg/dL
   (B) pH 7.1
   (C) protein 2.9 mg/dL
   (D) WBC <1500/McL

32. A 75-year-old male smoker presents with hemoptysis, weight loss, and chronic cough. Chest film reveals a hilar mass > 5 cm and fluid in the costophrenic sulcus. An analysis of the pleural fluid is completed. Which of the following results is consistent with his most likely diagnosis?

   (A) glucose 40 mg/dL
   (B) pH 7.38
   (C) protein 2.9 g/dL
   (D) WBC 787/McL

33. A 14-year-old healthy male presents to the emergency department complaining of an acute onset of unilateral chest pain and dyspnea that occurred without a precipitating event. Examination reveals unilateral chest expansion, decreased tactile fremitus, and decreased breath sounds. What is the most likely diagnosis?

   (A) atypical pneumonia
   (B) pericarditis
   (C) pulmonary embolus
   (D) spontaneous pneumothorax

34. What are the chest examination findings expected of a patient with a tension pneumothorax?

(A) decreased tactile fremitus; hyperresonant to percussion

(B) increased tactile fremitus; dullness to percussion

(C) decreased tactile fremitus; dullness to percussion

(D) increased tactile fremitus; hyperresonant to percussion

35. Which of the following chest films will best demonstrate a small pneumothorax?

(A) expiratory

(B) lateral decubitus

(C) lordotic

(D) oblique

36. A 65-year-old man presents with a chronic productive cough, dyspnea, and wheeze. Examination reveals cyanosis, distended neck veins, and a prominent epigastric pulsation. What is the most likely diagnosis?

(A) cor pulmonale

(B) chronic bronchitis

(C) emphysema

(D) pneumonia

37. A 4-year-old child is brought to the emergency department with a low-grade fever, barking cough, and respiratory stridor with activity but not at rest. On exam you note the cough and the absence of drooling. What is the most appropriate treatment for this child?

(A) dexamethasone IM

(B) endotracheal intubation and IV antibiotics

(C) inhaled budesonide

(D) nebulized racemic epinephrine

(E) supportive therapy with oral hydration

38. An otherwise healthy 2-year-old is brought to your office in late winter with a low-grade fever, wheezing, and cough. On physical exam you note diffuse wheezing and retractions.

The patient is not having any trouble feeding or swallowing. This is the fifth child you have seen this week with the same symptoms. What is the most likely diagnosis?

(A) bronchiolitis due to respiratory syncytial virus

(B) epiglottitis due to *Haemophilus influenzae* type B

(C) pharyngitis due to Group A *Streptococcus*

(D) pneumonia due to *Mycoplasma pneumoniae*

(E) tracheitis due to *Staphylococcus aureus*

39. What is the most common initial presentation of cystic fibrosis?

(A) congestive heart failure in infancy

(B) failure to thrive in infancy

(C) portal hypertension in early childhood

(D) ulcerative colitis in late childhood

40. Which viral illness is transmitted via the respiratory route by droplet nuclei?

(A) arbovirus

(B) influenza

C) respiratory syncytial virus (RSV)

(D) rhinovirus

(E) severe acute respiratory syndrome (SARS)

41. A 4-year-old child presents with a 2-week history of cough, rhinitis, and sneezing without fever. In the last 2 days the cough has become more severe and is now paroxysmal (10 to 20 forceful coughs at a time). The paroxysms with a loud high-pitched inspiratory sound. The child's history reveals that immunizations were not completed in infancy. What is the most likely diagnosis?

(A) diphtheria

(B) *Haempohilus influenzae* type B

(C) legionella

(D) pertussis

(E) pulmonary tuberculosis

42. What is the treatment of choice for early stage pertussis?

(A) chloramphenicol

(B) erythromycin

(C) isoniazid

(D) supportive treatment only (i.e., fluids, oxygen, and antipyretics)

(E) ceftriaxone

43. Which lab/diagnostic finding is consistent with coal workers pneumoconiosis (CWP)?

(A) CT scan showing predominance of ground-glass abnormality

(B) chest x-ray with eggshell calcifications in hilar lymph nodes

(C) decreased FEV_1

(D) positive antinuclear antibodies

(E) positive rheumatoid factor

44. What is the most appropriate initial treatment of idiopathic pulmonary fibrosis (IPF)?

(A) colchicine in combination with a broad spectrum antibiotic

(B) high-dose steroids in combination with immunomodulator therapy

(C) hospitalization, intubation, and broad spectrum antibiotics

(D) lung transplantation

(E) methotrexate in combination with low-dose corticosteroids

45. A patient diagnosed with lung cancer presents with a 4-cm tumor in the mainstem bronchus. The tumor is not within 2 cm of carina. There is no invasion of the visceral pleura or associated atelectasis. There are no distant metastases or nodal involvement. The TNM descriptor is T2 N0 M0. Given these findings, what is the correct stage of the patient's disease?

(A) 0

(B) 1A

(C) 1B

(D) 11A

(E) 11B

46. A preterm infant (33 weeks) presents at 10 days of age. The mother complains that the infant is experiencing an increasing number of apneic episodes of 20 to 30 seconds associated with cyanosis. After careful history, physical exam, and workup, the decision is made to treat the infant. What is the appropriate treatment for this infant?

(A) corticosteroids alone

(B) corticosteroids in combination with broad spectrum antibiotics

(C) IV glucose and careful electrolyte management

(D) methylxanthines

47. Which epidemiologic characteristic is consistent with cystic fibrosis?

(A) nonpulmonary manifestations most often involve the thyroid

(B) median survival age is now 21 years of age

(C) more common in blacks than whites

(D) most common cause of chronic lung disease in young adults

(E) autosomal dominant disorder

48. A premature infant is born at 32 weeks and after several hours develops rapid shallow respirations at 60/min, grunting retractions, and duskiness of the skin. The chest x-ray reveals fine reticular granularity of the parenchyma and air bronchograms most prominent in the left lower lobe. What is the most likely diagnosis?

(A) hyaline membrane disease

(B) meconium aspiration

(C) tetralogy of Fallot

(D) ventral septal defect

49. A child presents to the office with respiratory symptoms consistent with influenza. What would be most helpful in supporting the diagnosis?

(A) chest x-ray with air bronchograms

(B) elevated WBC

(C) epidemiologic and overall clinical data

(D) history of no influenza immunization

(E) presence of pneumonia

50. What epidemiologic characteristic is consistent with respiratory syncytial virus?

(A) epidemics peak in January through March

(B) incubation period is 14 to 21 days

(C) infection almost universal by 6 months of age in urban settings

(D) spread by fecal-oral transmission

51. Which of the following recommendations for annual influenza immunizations is correct?

(A) healthy children aged 0 to 6 months should be immunized

(B) live attenuated vaccine (nasal spray) is contraindicated in children under 12 years

(C) pregnant women in the second or third trimester should be immunized

(D) two doses of vaccine are recommended for children over 9 years who are receiving vaccine for the first time

52. What antiviral agent is indicated for the treatment of influenza A?

(A) acyclovir

(B) amantadine

(C) famciclovir

(D) lamivudine

(E) vidarabine

53. Imaging of the chest is an essential part of the workup of a patient with suspected occupational interstitial lung disease. What is the most likely diagnosis in a patient with a chest x-ray that reveals a reticular linear pattern with basilar predominance?

(A) asbestosis

(B) coal works pneumoconiosis CWP

(C) silicosis

(D) talcosis

54. Classically, pertussis is an illness which lasts for weeks and is divided into stages. A patient who presents with 5 days of congestion, rhinorrhea, low-grade fever, and sneezing is in what stage?

(A) catarrhal

(B) convalescent

(C) paroxysmal

(D) prodromal

55. What is the name given to chest pain which is described as severe, knife-like and worsened by coughing and/or deep inspiration?

(A) ischemic

(B) neuralgic

(C) pleuritic

(D) visceral

56. What chest x-ray finding is found in noncardiogenic pulmonary edema (acute respiratory distress syndrome)?

(A) air bronchogram

(B) cardiomegaly

(C) flattened diaphragms

(D) Kerley B lines

57. A 7-year-old previously healthy patient presents with acute onset of respiratory distress following ingestion of a piece of candy. Which of the following signs or symptoms is most ominous?

(A) aphonia

(B) cough

(C) drooling

(D) stridor

58. A 55-year-old smoker with lung cancer presents with ptosis and miosis. What is the third clinical finding that comprises this syndrome found in patients with lung cancer?

(A) anhidrosis

(B) pericarditis

(C) pneumonitis

(D) systemic acidosis

59. A 32-year-old African-American woman with a history of erythema nodosum presents with nonspecific complaints such as fatigue and malaise. Based on the fact that she is a smoker with these symptoms, a chest x-ray is ordered which demonstrates bilateral hilar adenopathy. A transbronchial lung biopsy reveals noncaseating granulomas. What is the most likely diagnosis?

(A) bronchogenic carcinoma
(B) mesothelioma
(C) sarcoidosis
(D) tuberculosis

60. A 25-year-old male presents for preadmission testing (PAT) to correct a ventral hernia. The PAT includes a chest x-ray which reveals a single, smooth, calcified, well-defined node of approximately 2 cm in diameter. What is the most appropriate next step in the management of this patient?

(A) obtain a CT scan
(B) obtain old films for comparison
(C) proceed directly to biopsy
(D) watchful waiting

61. A 47-year-old patient with a history of HIV presents with fever, tachypnea, shortness of breath, and a nonproductive cough. Bronchoalveolar lavage reveals *Pneumocystic jiroveci*. What is the treatment of choice?

(A) amoxicillin/clavulanate
(B) azithromycin
(C) doxycycline
(D) trimethoprim-sulfamethoxazole

62. What is considered first-line drug therapy for patients with chronic obstructive pulmonary disease?

(A) corticosteroids
(B) ipratropium bromide
(C) terbutaline
(D) theophylline

63. A 3-year-old child presents to the emergency room with a "seal-like" or barking cough along with rhinorrhea for several days. Examination reveals an afebrile child who exhibits stridor with expiratory wheezing while at rest. What is the recommended treatment?

(A) IM dexamethasone
(B) IM diphenhydramine
(C) nebulized albuterol
(D) nebulized epinephrine

64. In which gender and age group is a spontaneous pneumothorax most likely to occur?

(A) male between 2 and 10 years of age
(B) female between 2 and 10 years of age
(C) male between 20 and 40 years of age
(D) female between 20 and 40 years of age

65. A 32-year-old patient with a history of Wilson's disease is 14 months status post liver transplant. The result of a routine preemployment PPD is induration of 7 mm. What is the recommended management?

(A) no treatment
(B) chest x-ray
(C) isoniazid
(D) isoniazid, rifampin, and pyrazinamide

Answers and Explanations

1. **(A)** Mycoplasma pneumonia often presents after days of constitutional symptoms and a nonproductive cough. Generally, the exam reveals little more than a reddened throat and rarely, bullous myringitis. Diagnosis is often made after the chest x-ray reveals unilateral lower lobe patchy consolidation. (*Goldman and Ausiello, 2004, pp. 1771–1772*)

2. **(B)** Pneumoccocal pneumonia is the most common cause of pneumonia. Classically it presents with the abrupt onset of fever, cough—productive of rusty sputum and pleuritic chest pain. Chest x-ray usually reveals a lobar consolidation. (*Goldman and Ausiello, 2004, pp. 1764–1766; Goroll and Mulley, 2006, pp. 388–392*)

3. **(D)** Patients with obstruction of the trachea typically present with cough, wheezing, dyspnea, and/or cyanosis. In most cases the definitive diagnosis is made by bronchoscopy and treatment can be accomplished at the same time by removal of the object. (*Behrman et al, 2004, p. 1411*)

4. **(C)** Adequate hydration is essential to help clear secretions. In addition, cough suppressants and/or expectorants may be helpful in specific cases. Empiric antibiotic therapy and B_2 agonists are not recommended in otherwise healthy adults. Corticosteroid therapy is not appropriate in the treatment of acute bronchitis. (*Goroll and Mulley, 2006, pp. 393–394*)

5. **(A)** Diagnosis is confirmed by finding well-formed noncaseating granulomas in affected tissues. Because the lung is involved so commonly, the routine chest x-ray is almost always abnormal but cannot be used as the sole criteria. (*Goldman and Ausiello, 2004, pp. 549–550*)

6. **(A)** *Mycobacterium tuberculosis* is most commonly transmitted from a patient with infectious pulmonary tuberculosis to other persons by droplet nuclei, which are aerosolized by coughing, sneezing, or speaking. Crowding in poorly ventilated rooms is one of the most important factors in the transmission of tubercle bacilli, since it increases the intensity of a contact with a case. (*Goldman and Ausiello, 2004, pp. 1894–1895*)

7. **(D)** *Klebsiella pneumoniae* is the most likely cause. It is common, along with other Gram-negative bacilli, in alcoholics and in debilitated patients. It commonly causes the acute onset of cough, chest pain, and shortness of breath. Chest x-ray shows infiltrates; 30% may be bilateral. Cavitations are most likely to be seen in pnuemonias caused by *Klebsiella*. (*Goldman and Ausiello, 2004, pp. 1774–1775; Goroll and Mulley, 2006, pp. 389–392*)

8. **(B)** Erythromycin or tetracycline is the drug of choice in treating *Mycoplasma pneumoniae*. Gastrointestinal intolerance is common with erythromycin. Doxycycline, azithromycin, or clarithromycin may be used as alternatives. (*Goldman and Ausiello, 2004, p. 1773*)

9. **(C)** The pneumoccus is the most common cause of community-acquired pyogenic bacterial pneumonia. Although the prevalence of penicillin-resistant pneumococci is increasing in the United States, in areas where penicillin resistance is not a concern, penicillin remains the drug of choice. On an outpatient basis, amoxicillin is generally used. Penicillin allergic patients may be treated with a macrolide. (*Goldman and Ausiello, 2004, pp. 1767–1769; Goroll and Mulley, 2006, p. 395*)

10. **(C)** The clinical manifestations of bronchogenic carcinoma can vary, and many patients are asymptomatic when the pulmonary lesion is discovered. Cough usually productive of scant sputum is a common symptom; hemoptysis often occurs secondary to ulceration in the pulmonary lesion. Frequently, because of a significant smoking history, patients with carcinoma also have chronic obstructive pulmonary disease and dyspnea upon exertion. Weight loss is also a common complaint of bronchogenic carcinoma, but generally occurs with more extensive disease beyond the time frame that the neoplasm is limited to the lung. Chest pain may be due to pleural involvement, but must also suggest metastatic disease. Pulmonary infections occur distal to the bronchial obstruction and can mask the tumor. Chest x-ray may demonstrate infiltrates, single or multiple nodules. Asthma and chronic obstructive pulmonary disease usually reveal hyperinflation of the lungs and flattened diaphragms. Bronchiectasis shows coarse lung markings and even honeycombing due to the abnormal dilatation of the bronchial tree. (*Goldman and Ausiello, 2004, pp. 1201–1208, Papdakis and McPhee, 2005, p. 198*)

11. **(B)** The two most important adverse effects of isoniazid therapy are hepatotoxicity and peripheral neuropathy. Red-orange urine (and other body fluids) is a common side effect of rifampin and is one easy way to check on a patient's compliance with therapy. Hyperuricemia is a side effect of pyrazinamide, and vestibular toxicity is an adverse effect of streptomycin. (*Goldman and Ausiello, 2004, p. 1899*)

12. **(A)** Eggshell calcification of hilar or mediastinal lymph nodes is characteristic of silicosis. The disease may also be recognized by the presence of small nodules, which appear predominately in the upper lobes. Pneumothorax, atelectasis, and pleural thickening and plaques are not radiologic features of silicosis. (*Goldman and Ausiello, 2004, pp. 536–537*)

13. **(C)** Inspiratory crackles along with bronchial breath sounds, increased tactile fremitus and transmitted voice sounds (the presence of egophony, bronchophony, and/or whispered pectoriloquy), and dullness to percussion over the involved area would be consistent with a consolidated pnuemonia. (*Bickley and Hoekelman, 2003, p. 242*)

14. **(C)** The prognosis for each type of lung cancer varies according to the pathologic stage. However, in general, small cell lung carcinoma has the worst prognosis, with the median survival of 12 to 16 months with 5% to 25% 2-year survival, while patients with extensive disease have a median survival of only 7 to 11 months, with only 1% to 3% surviving 2 years. (*Way and Doherty, 2003, p. 403*)

15. **(D)** The Centers for Disease Control and Prevention currently recommends a minimum of 6 months of INH and RIF with initial 2 months of PZA and SM or EMB for immunocompetent persons. (*Goldman and Ausiello, 2004, p. 1898*)

16. **(D)** The treatment of choice for immunocompromised patients with legionella infection is levofloxacin. An alternative is azithromycin. Erythromycin and doxycycline are acceptable treatments for immunocompetent patients with legionella. Cephalosporins are ineffective for the treatment of legionella (*Goldman and Ausiello, 2004, p. 1781*)

17. **(A)** Pulmonary thromboembolism is most often caused by the embolization of thrombus from the deep veins of the lower extremities. People at risk for pulmonary embolus are those with hypercoagulable states, which may arise from the use of birth control pills, local stasis, immobilization that may be the result of

an accident or illness, fractures, obesity, and congestive heart failure. Signs and symptoms often begin abruptly and include dyspnea, cough, and chest pain (frequently pleuritic in nature). Hemoptysis may occur; tachypnea and tachycardia are common in this illness. A low-grade fever, wheezing, rales, or pleural rub are also signs of pulmonary embolism. (*Goldman and Ausiello, 2004, pp. 560–568*)

18. **(B)** Contrast venography is the imaging study of choice to diagnose a deep vein thrombosis. Doppler ultrasound can be used for screening. Arteriography and V/Q scans would not be appropriate studies. (*Goldman and Ausiello, 2004, p. 478*)

19. **(B)** Digital clubbing is present when the distal phalanx is rounded and bulbous. It accompanies chronic hypoxia associated with conditions such as lung cancer, heart disease, and cirrhosis. (*Bickley and Hoekelman, 2003, p. 110*)

20. **(A)** Beta-adrenergic agents are the mainstay bronchodilator treatment for mild asthma. Theophylline and aminophylline are bronchodilators of moderate potency and are usually reserved for patients with moderate to severe asthma. Antileukotrienes are controller medications not bronchodilators. (*Goldman and Ausiello, 2004, p. 506*)

21. **(A)** Pneumonia caused by *Chlamydia* will have a prodrome similar to mycoplasma pneumonia with headache and sore throat. It is seen often in otherwise healthy adults causing atypical pneumonia or acute bronchitis that is usually self-limited. It accounts for 5% to 15% of community-acquired pneumonia, with higher rates in young adults. Definitive diagnosis is difficult because it requires special tissue culture techniques not routinely performed. (*Goroll and Mulley, 2006, pp. 390–391*)

22. **(D)** Primary therapy consists of clot dissolution with thrombolysis or removal of PTE by embolectomy and is reserved for patients at high risk of death from right heart failure and for those patients at risk of recurrent PTE despite adequate anticoagulation. Anticoagulation with heparin is secondary prevention of

recurrent PTE rather than primary therapy. The use of filters is considered a preventative measure as is the recommended use of antiembolism stockings. (*Goldman and Ausiello, 2004, pp. 564–566*)

23. **(A)** Pulmonary arteriography is the gold standard for the diagnosis of PTE. An intraluminal defect in more than one projection establishes a definitive diagnosis. Contrast venography is the reference standard for the diagnosis for deep vein thrombosis. Helical CT is replacing V/Q scans as the initial diagnostic study for suspected PTE but is less sensitive than pulmonary arteriography. V/Q scans are helpful for screening especially if they are either normal or indicate high probability of PTE. (*Goldman and Ausiello, 2004, p. 564*)

24. **(D)** Evaluation for asthma should include spirometry before and after the administration of a short-acting bronchodilator to determine if airflow obstruction is immediately reversible. Peak expiratory flow meters are designed for home use to assess severity and provide objective data to guide treatment. Arterial blood gases measurement may be normal in mild exacerbations but respiratory alkalosis is also common in severe cases. Chest films may only show hyperinflation and are only indicated if pneumonia or pneumothorax is expected. (*Tierney et al, 2005, p. 225*)

25. **(D)** In this case, the nighttime symptoms and daily exacerbations would classify his asthma as severe persistent. The National Asthma Education and Prevention Program has outlined the classification of severity of chronic asthma, which is useful in directing asthma therapy. The classification is based on the frequency of symptoms, nighttime severity, and peak flow measurements. (*Goldman and Ausiello, 2004, p. 224*)

26. **(C)** Long-acting bronchodilators, such as salmeterol, are indicated for long-term prevention of asthma symptoms and nocturnal symptoms, and for prevention of exercise-induced bronchospasm. It is critical to educate

the patient that this should not be used as a treatment for acute bronchoconstriction. Fluticasone is an inhaled corticosteroid that can be used as part of the treatment strategy for mild persistent, moderate persistent, and severe persistent asthma. Ipratropium is an anticholinergic agent used to reverse vagally mediated bronchospasm but not allergen or exercise-induced bronchospasm. Theophylline is a phosphodiesterase inhibitor which is not recommended for therapy of asthma exacerbations. (*Tierney et al, 2005, p. 228*)

27. **(D)** Concurrent treatment with calcium supplements, vitamin D, and bisphosphonates can be prescribed to prevent steroid-induced bone mineral loss that occurs with long-term use of steroids. Benzodiazepines, folic acid, and bile acid sequestrants are not indicated for patients on long-term steroids. (*Tierney et al, 2005, p. 228*)

28. **(B)** Symptoms of bronchiectasis include chronic cough, purulent sputum, hemoptysis, and recurrent pneumonia. In addition, weight loss, anemia, and other systemic manifestations are common. Cystic fibrosis causes about half of all cases. Asthma can cause cough but is generally characterized as nonproductive and presents with expiratory wheezes. Bronchiolitis is common in infants and children and is most commonly caused by respiratory syncytial virus or adenovirus. Pneumonitis is a general term for inflammation of the lung (alveolitis) and may be the result of an infectious or environmental insult. (*Tierney et al, 2005, p. 241*)

29. **(B)** Bronchiectasis is characterized by permanent, abnormal dilation and destruction of bronchial walls. Asthma is a chronic inflammatory disorder of the airways. Cystic fibrosis causes altered chloride transport and water flux across the apical surface of epithelial cells. Pneumonia is caused by the infiltration of the lower respiratory tract by microorganisms. (*Tierney et al, 2005, p. 241*)

30. **(A)** A chest CT can identify as little as 10 mL of fluid. On the lateral view, at least 75 to 100 mL of pleural fluid must accumulate in the poste-

rior sulcus to be visible. To make fluid in the right side become visible, the patient must be in the right lateral decubitus position. The frontal view requires at least 175 to 200 mL must be present. (*Tierney et al, 2005, p. 298*)

31. **(C)** The patient is most likely in congestive heart failure, which would result in a transudative effusion. Pleural findings consistent with a transudate include glucose $\geq$50 mg/dL; pH $\geq$7.2; protein $\leq$3.0 g/dL; WBCs $\leq$1000 McL. (*Ayala and Spellberg, 2003, p. 21*)

32. **(A)** The patient most likely has carcinoma, which would result in an exudative effusion. Pleural findings consistent with an exudate include glucose <50 mg/dL; pH <7.2; protein >3.0 g/dL; WBCs >1000 McL. (*Ayala and Spellberg, 2003, p. 21*)

33. **(D)** These findings are most consistent with a spontaneous pneumothorax, which is primarily found in tall, thin males between the ages of 10 and 30. Pericarditis is an acute inflammatory process of the pericardium due to either an infectious process or systemic disease, neoplasm, radiation, drug toxicity, or other processes. The clinical presentation includes chest pain, which is relieved by leaning forward. Pulmonary embolus presents as acute onset of chest pain with tachycardia. Breath sounds are usually normal and fremitus is symmetrical. (*Papdakis and McPhee, 2005, p. 768*)

34. **(A)** Due to the accumulation of air in the pleural space, fremitus on the affected side will be decreased and percussion will be hyperresonant. (Tierney et al, 2005, p. 299)

35. **(A)** Small pneumothoraces may only be seen on an expiratory film. Other findings include a visceral pleural line on a chest film and a "deep sulcus sign" on a supine film. (*Papdakis and McPhee, 2005, p. 768*)

36. **(A)** Cor pulmonale is right ventricular hypertrophy and failure resulting from pulmonary disease. It is most commonly caused by chronic obstructive pulmonary disease, which is this patient's underlying disorder precipitating the failure. While the other three

diagnoses may have similar symptoms, none of them would present with distended neck veins and prominent epigastric pulsations. (*Tierney et al, 2005, p. 397*)

37. **(E)** Viral croup is the most likely diagnosis in the patient. It is most often caused by parainfluenza virus. This patient displays mild symptoms: low-grade fever, cough, and stridor only with activity. In this case the most appropriate treatment is supportive. If this patient was more seriously ill and had stridor at rest, other treatment including inhaled, oral or IM steroids, and/or epinephrine would be appropriate. Intubation is reserved for the most severe patients with impending respiratory failure. The use of IV antibiotics is inappropriate in a viral illness. (*Hay et al, 2005, pp. 513–514*)

38. **(A)** Bronchiolitis due to respiratory syncytial virus is the best answer. Respiratory syncytial virus peaks in late winter and is common in young children. It is often a diagnosis made based on symptoms, particularly during an outbreak. Epiglottitis presents more acutely with sudden onset of fever, dysphagia, drooling, and cyanosis. Tracheitis is also more severe; patients develop high fever, toxicity, and upper airway obstruction. Pneumonia due to mycoplasma is not usually seen in this age group; generally patients with mycoplasma are over 5 years old. Pharyngitis generally presents with sore throat and fever; cough and wheezing are not part of the clinical presentation. (*Hay et al, 2005, pp. 515, 535, 1138–1140*)

39. **(B)** Fifty percent of patients with cystic fibrosis present in infancy with failure to thrive with respiratory compromise. The age of presentation may be variable from infancy into adulthood. Portal hypertension is a rare complication of hepatic involvement. Congestive heart failure is not usually part of the initial presentation. Gastrointestinal disease is equally common and most commonly caused by distal intestinal obstruction syndrome, not by ulcerative colitis. (*Hay et al, 2005, pp. 526–528; Hanley and Welsh, 2003, pp. 92–95*)

40. **(B)** Influenza is transmitted via droplet nuclei. RSV, rhinovirus, and SARS are transmitted via fomites or large particle aerosols. Arbovirus is transmitted by arthropods or ticks and produces a variety of encephalitides including West Nile fever, St. Louis encephalitis, and California encephalitis. (*Tierney et al, 2005, pp. 1324–1339*)

41. **(D)** The most likely diagnosis is pertussis, which is typically preceded by 2 to 3 weeks of cough and coryza without fever: the characteristic "whooping" cough is a high-pitched inspiratory sound. Diphtheria typically presents with sore throat, fever, and malaise and produces a psuedomembrane, most often in the pharynx. H flu type B causes a severe febrile illness that present with meningitis, epiglottitis, septic arthritis, and cellulitis. Legionella causes abrupt onset with fever, chills, and headache, which progress rapidly to pneumonia. In children, pulmonary tuberculosis, when symptomatic, commonly presents with airway obstruction with secondary bacterial pneumonia. (*Hay et al, 2005, pp. 1211–1212, 1227–1238*)

42. **(B)** Erythromycin for 7 to 14 days is the treatment of choice because it promptly terminates respiratory tract carriage of *Bordetella pertussis*. In the later paroxysmal stage it will not effect clinical symptoms. Treatment with clarithromycin and azithromycin may work as well. Household contacts should also be treated. The other drugs listed would not be appropriate for the treatment of pertussis. (*Hay et al, 2005, pp. 1229–1231*)

43. **(C)** A decreased FEV_1 is typically found in patients with CWP. Chest x-ray with eggshell calcifications is found in a small percentage of patients with silicosis. A CT scan showing a ground-glass abnormality may be found in nonspecific interstial pneumonia. A positive antinuclear antibody may be found in silicosis but is nonspecific. A positive rheumatoid factor may be found in rheumatoid arthritis with pulmonary involvement. (*Hanley and Welsh, 2003, pp. 112, 122, 328–329*)

44. **(B)** The initial treatment of choice for IPF is high-dose steroids and immunomodulator

therapy (cyclophosphamide or azothioprine) for at least 3 months. Lung transplantation is considered only if medical therapy fails. Colchine, methotrexate, and broad-spectrum antibiotics are not used in the treatment of IPF. Initial treatment does not generally require hospitalization or intubation. (*Hanley and Welsh, 2003, pp. 110–111*)

45. **(C)** This is Stage 1B. Stage 0 is T is (carcinoma in situ). Stage 1A is T1 N0 M0. Stage 11A is T1 N1 M0 and Stage 11B is T2 N1 M0 or T3 N0 M0. (*Goldman and Ausiello, 2004, p. 1206*)

46. **(D)** Methylxanthines in the form of caffeine citrate (20 mg/kg as loading dose and 5 to 10 mg/kg/d) is the drug of choice. The other treatments offered play no role in treating apnea in the preterm infant. (*Hay et al, 2005, pp. 35–36*)

47. **(D)** Cystic fibrosis is the most common cause of severe lung disease in young adults. It is more common in Whites and is the most common fatal hereditary disorder of whites in the United States. It is an autosomal recessive disorder affecting 1 in 3200 whites. Extrapulmonary manifestations may include disease of the pancreas, distal intestinal obstruction, hepatic disease, nutritional deficiencies, and infertility. It does not affect the thyroid. The median survival is now 31 years of age. (*Tierney et al, 2005, pp. 241–243*)

48. **(A)** In most cases of hyaline membrane disease symptoms will peak within 3 days, after which there is a gradual improvement. Meconium aspiration causes a chest x-ray characterized by patchy infiltrates and coarse streaking, with flattening of the diaphragms. In an infant with ventral septal defect (VSD), the chest x-ray would be normal or show cardiomegaly depending on the size of the VSD. Tetrology of Fallot does not usually cause symptoms at birth. (*Behrman et al, 2004, pp. 575–584, 1508–1509, 1518–1519, 1524–1525*)

49. **(C)** Epidemiologic and clinical data are most helpful. Influenza is otherwise indistinguishable from any number of acute respire illnesses. Leukocytosis may be present but does not assist in making the diagnosis. Chest x-ray findings are nonspecific and may reveal atelectasis and/or an infiltrate in about 10% of children. Lack of vaccination may contribute to the diagnosis but would not by itself be diagnostic. Pneumonia is a common complication of influenza but is not diagnostic. (*Behrman et al, 2004, pp. 1072–1075*)

50. **(A)** Epidemics peak in January—March but may occur as early as in December or as late as in June. The incubation period is 4 days and in urban settings almost all children have been exposed to respiratory syncytial virus by age 2. The virus is transmitted when large infected droplets, either airborne or on hands, are inoculated in the nose or conjunctiva. (*Behrman et al, 2004, pp. 1076–1079*)

51. **(C)** Pregnant women in the second and third trimester are among the groups targeted for influenza vaccine. The vaccine should not be given to children under 6 months old. The live virus vaccine should not be given to children under 5 years. Two doses of vaccine are recommended for children under 9 years who are vaccinated for the first time. (*Hay et al, 2005, pp. 274–275*)

52. **(B)** Amantadine or rimantedine are recommended for treatment of influenza A. Influenza B may be treated with inhaled zanamivir, or oral oseltamivir. Acyclovir, famciclovir, lamivudine, and vidarabine are all antiviral agents used to treat other viral illnesses but are not recommended to treat influenza. (*Goldman and Ausiello, 2004, pp. 1961–1962, 1977–1978, 2188*)

53. **(A)** The pattern described best fits asbestosis. CWP and silicosis cause a nodular pattern with upper lobe to be predominant. Talcosis shows a round and/or irregular pattern on chest x-ray. (*Goldman and Ausiello, 2004, pp. 532–536*)

54. **(A)** Catarrhal: the first stage of illness. The second stage—paroxysmal—is marked by the onset of coughing. The third and final stage is the convalescent stage where the number, severity, and duration of coughing episodes

diminish. There is no formal prodromal phase in pertussis. (*Behrman et al, 2004, pp. 908–912*)

55. **(C)** The description best fits pleuritic chest pain. Chest wall pain is sharp and can be localized and reproducible by palpation. Visceral pain is poorly localized and usually described as aching or heaviness. Ischemic pain and neurologic pain can be very variable in presentation. Neither would fit the description above. (*Tintinalli et al, 2004, sect. 7, ch. 49*)

56. **(A)** Air bronchogram on chest x-ray is found in 80% of patients with noncardiogenic acute respiratory distress syndrome. There may also be peripheral distribution of infiltrates. Kerley B lines and flattened diaphragms are not part of the picture. The heart is usually normal size. (*Goldman and Ausiello, 2004, pp. 594–595*)

57. **(A)** Aphonia, the inability to vocalize is a sign of a complete obstruction as is an inability to cough. Signs and symptoms of a partial obstruction include cough, stridor, and drooling. (*Hay et al, 2005, p. 518*)

58. **(A)** Horner's syndrome (ipsilateral ptosis, miosis, and anhidrosis) is due to involvement of the inferior cervical ganglion and the paravertebral sympathetic chain. Pericarditis, pneumonitis, and systemic acidosis are not components of Horner's syndrome. (*Tierney et al, 2005, p. 264*)

59. **(C)** Sarcoidosis is a systemic disease of unknown etiology which is generally characterized by granulomatous inflammation of the lung. Incidence is high among North American blacks, especially women. Symptoms may include malaise, fatigue, and dyspnea but can also include others. Erythema nodosum is not an uncommon finding. Bronchogenic carcinoma may also present with bilateral hilar adenopathy and a biopsy would also confirm such a diagnosis. Mesothelioma and tuberculosis do not present with these signs or symptoms. (*Papdakis and McPhee, 2005, pp. 854, 984*)

60. **(B)** The findings mentioned are highly suggestive of a benign lesion and evaluation of old radiographs is warranted. A CT should be ordered if it is determined that there is an increase in size. Rapid progression (doubling times less than 30 days) suggests infection; long-term stability (doubling time over 465 days) suggests benignity. (*Tierney et al, 2005, p. 262*)

61. **(D)**. The treatment of choice for *Pneumocystic jiroveci* is trimethoprim-sulfamethoxazole. It is a pneumonia-causing fungus found in mammals and humans worldwide. Patients with HIV and other immunosuppressive disorders are at high risk for developing this infection. Amoxicillin/clavulanate azithromycin and doxycycline are not appropriate for the treatment of *P. jiroveci*. (*Papdakis and McPhee, 2005, p. 754*)

62. **(B)** Ipratropium bromide is considered first-line therapy for patients with chronic obstructive pulmonary disease as it is longer acting and without sympathomimetic side effects. Corticosteroids are generally not recommended as chronic obstructive pulmonary disease is not responsive. Terbutaline and theophylline are other treatments recommended only if the patient is not responsive to ipratropium. (*Papdakis and McPhee, 2005, p. 233*)

63. **(D)** Management of croup is based on the child's level of comfort at rest. If stridor at rest is present, nebulized racemic epinephrine (2.25% solution diluted 1:5 or 1:8 with water and given 4 mL nebulized over 15 minutes) is the recommended treatment. If rebound stridor occurs within 2 hours, a single dose of 0.6 to 1.0 mg/kg of IM dexamethasone is the recommended treatment. (*Biros, 2002, p. 346*)

64. **(C)** Spontaneous pneumothorax may occur in any age group but is most common in males 20 to 40 years of age. Smokers are at greatest risk. (*Goldman and Ausiello, 2004, p. 573*)

65. **(C)** Isoniazid is the appropriate treatment for a recently converted immunocompromised patient. Triple drug treatments would be inappropriate as would no treatment with or without chest x-ray. (*Tierney et al, 2005, p. 260*)

REFERENCES

Ayala C, Spellberg B. *Boards and Wards: A Review for USMLE Steps 2&3*, 2nd ed. Malden, MA: Blackwell; 2003.

Behrman RE, Kliegman RM, Jenson HB. *Nelson Textbook of Pediatrics*, 17th ed. Philadelphia, PA: Saunders; 2004.

Bickley LS, Hoekelman RA. *Bates' Guide to Physical Examination and History Taking*. 8th ed. Philadelphia, PA: Lippincott Williams & Wilkins; 2003.

Biros MH et al. (eds). *Handbook of Urgent Care Medicine*, 2nd ed. Philadelphia, PA: Hanley and Belfus, Inc; 2002.

Goldman L, Bennett JC. *Cecil, Textbook of Medicine*, 22nd ed. Philadelphia, PA: Saunders; 2004.

Goroll AH, Mulley AG. *Primary Care Medicine*. Philadelphia, PA: Lippincott; 2006.

Hanley M, Welsh C. *Current Diagnosis and Treatment in Pulmonary Medicine*. New York: McGraw Hill; 2003.

Hay WW et al (eds). *Current Pediatric Diagnosis and Treatment*, 17th ed. New York: McGraw Hill; 2005.

Papdakis MA, McPhee SJ. *Current Consult: Medicine*. New York: McGraw Hill; 2005.

Tierney LM et al. *Current Medicine Diagnosis and Treatment*. New York: McGraw Hill; 2005.

Tintinalli JE et al. *Emergency Medicine: A Comprehensive Study Guide*, 6th ed. New York: McGraw Hill; 2004.

Way LW, Doherty GM. *Current Surgical Diagnosis and Treatment*. New York: McGraw Hill; 2003.

CHAPTER 12

Rheumatology
Questions

Cathy A Gillespie, DHSc, PA-C

DIRECTIONS (Questions 1 through 25): Each of the numbered items or incomplete statements in this section is followed by answers or by completions of the statement. Select the ONE lettered answer or completion that is BEST in each case.

Questions 1 through 25

1. A 59-year-old female with a known history of rheumatoid arthritis presents with relatively severe complaints of pain, notable boney deformity of the hands with extraarticular findings of cutaneous nodules, scleritis, and pleurisy. On physical exam the patient is found to have splenomegaly. What laboratory evaluation is needed to further evaluate this patient?

   (A) CBC
   (B) erythrocyte sedimentation rate
   (C) C-reactive protein
   (D) antinuclear antibodies
   (E) uric acid

2. Tumor necrosis factor inhibitors are most often considered for use in cases of rheumatoid arthritis that do not respond to conventional therapy. Which of the following side effects must the patient be informed of?

   (A) the potential of exacerbation of congestive heart failure
   (B) increased risk of developing multiple sclerosis
   (C) increased risk of developing opportunistic infections
   (D) should not be used in combination with methotrexate
   (E) injection site at increased risk of abscess formation

3. A 53-year-old obese male presents with a third attack of gout in 1 years time. Following the treatment of this acute attack, further lab testing is performed and the patient is found to have an elevated serum uric acid level, a 24-hour uric acid secretion of 950 mg. Which of the following medications would be most appropriate to initiate for prevention of further gouty attacks?

   (A) colchicine
   (B) probenecid
   (C) prednisone
   (D) allopurinol
   (E) indomethacin

4. A 48-year-old female presents with a chief complaint of gradually progressing difficulty in climbing stairs over the past 3 months. On physical exam there is notable proximal muscle weakness of the upper and lower extremities. The remainder of the exam is unremarkable. On laboratory evaluation a serum creatinine phosphokinase is elevated and a muscle biopsy reveals lymphoid inflammatory infiltrates. What is the appropriate initial treatment of choice in this patient?

(A) prednisone

(B) methotrexate

(C) azathioprine

(D) hydrochloroquine

(E) cyclophosphamide

5. Which of the following treatment options for the prevention of osteoporosis can be used in place of estrogen in postmenopausal women? This medication does not have any effect on the endometrium, coronary plaques, or association with cancer. The use of this medication can produce a reduction in LDL and breast cancer.

(A) raloxifene

(B) alendronate

(C) calcitonin

(D) vitamin D

(E) progestin

6. A 65-year-old male presents with complaints of acute onset of pain and swelling of the right great toe. He denies recent alcohol ingestion or trauma to the area. On physical exam, the patient is afebrile and the first metatarsophalangeal joint is erythematous, swollen, and warm to the touch. Laboratory evaluation reveals a WBC count of 12,000 and a normal differential. Serum uric acid level is 5 mg/dL. Synovial fluid analysis reveals the presence of rhomboid-shaped crystals. What is the most likely diagnosis for this patient?

(A) acute gout

(B) pseudogout

(C) psoriatic arthritis

(D) infectious arthritis

(E) rheumatoid arthritis

7. A 22-year-old male presents with an insidious onset of low back pain over the last 6 months. He describes the pain as dull and has difficulty localizing the pain. The pain often radiates to his thighs. The pain is worse in the morning and associated with stiffening that lessens throughout the day. The patient notes that there is no history of trauma. The initial laboratory evaluation shows an elevated erythrocyte sedimentation rate, positive HLA-B27, and a negative rheumatoid factor. Plain films of the lumbar spine reveal bilateral blurring of the sacroiliac joints. What is the most likely diagnosis with this presentation?

(A) lumbar disc disease

(B) rheumatoid arthritis

(C) ankylosing spondylitis

(D) polymyalgia rheumatica

(E) systemic lupus

8. A 12-year-old female presents with complaints of intermittent pain and stiffness involving her hands. This pain has been progressively worsening over the past 3 years. She relates that for the past 2 months she has been increasingly tired and has experienced swelling and stiffness of her hands, which appears worse in the morning and is relieved as the day goes on. On physical exam she has a low-grade fever. There are multiple symmetrical joint swelling of the proximal interphalangeal and metacarpophalangeal joints with associated warmth, tenderness, and effusion. Initial laboratory findings include a CBC that reveals mild anemia, an elevate erythrocyte sedimentation rate, a positive rheumatoid factor, and a negative antinuclear antibody (ANA) test. X-rays of the hands and wrists show soft tissue swelling and periarticular osteopenia. With this patient presentation what is the most likely diagnosis?

(A) reactive arthritis

(B) infectious arthritis

(C) pauciarticular juvenile rheumatoid arthritis

(D) systemic onset juvenile rheumatoid arthritis

(E) polyarticular onset juvenile rheumatoid arthritis

9. Which of the following is a cause of noninflammatory monarthritis?

   (A) gout

   (B) pseudogout

   (C) osteochondroma

   (D) psoriatic arthritis

   (E) systemic lupus erythematosus

10. A 50-year-old female with known recent diagnosis of rheumatoid arthritis has begun treatment with celecoxib. She has been on this medication for 1 year and notes that her pain continues. Early signs of joint involvement are present in the patient's hands. What medication is the best choice in addition to the celecoxib?

    (A) methotrexate

    (B) tumor necrosis factor inhibitor

    (C) antimalarial

    (D) minocycline

    (E) aspirin

11. Which of the following clinical manifestations does fibromyalgia most commonly present with?

    (A) subcutaneous inflammatory lesions

    (B) abrupt onset of proximal muscle weakness

    (C) insidious onset of symmetrical joint involvement

    (D) widespread musculoskeletal pain and tender points

    (E) symmetrical weakness initially in the legs and progressing caudally

12. These systemic disorders that are HLA-B27 related, including ankylosing spondylitis, reactive arthritis, psoriasis, and Behçet's syndrome are more likely to be associated with this finding?

    (A) vasculitis

    (B) hyperuricemia

    (C) uveitis

    (D) thoracic involvement

    (E) dysentery

13. Skin thickening that begins as swelling of the fingers and hands associated with telangiectasia and Raynaud's phenomenon is most likely seen with which of the following?

    (A) sarcoidosis

    (B) scleroderma

    (C) dermatomyositis

    (D) eosinophilic fasciitis

    (E) eosinophilic-myalgia syndrome

14. Patients with rheumatoid arthritis may require cervical fusion as treatment of chronic instability. Which of the following is the most common complication that may require stabilization with fusion?

    (A) myelodysplasia

    (B) subaxial instability

    (C) cervical spondylosis

    (D) atlantoaxial instability

    (E) superior migration C3 odontoid process

15. A 58-year-old postmenopausal female presents for a routine annual exam. She is concerned about osteoporosis and is currently taking no medications. In counseling the patient about calcium intake along with appropriate vitamin D amounts, what amount of calcium is most appropriate for this patient?

    (A) 700 mg

    (B) 1000 mg

    (C) 1200 mg

    (D) 1500 mg

    (E) 2000 mg

16. A patient with polymyalgia rheumatica has initially responded well to treatment with oral corticosteroids. What is the length of time corticosteroid therapy is required for in most patients?

    (A) 72 hours

    (B) 7 to 10 days

    (C) 6 months

    (D) 12 months

    (E) 24 months

17. Reactive arthritis most commonly presents with a tetrad of urethritis, conjunctivitis, mucotaneous lesions, and oligoarthritis. Which of the following joints are more likely to be involved with this condition?

    (A) small joints of the hands
    (B) small joints of the feet
    (C) upper extremities
    (D) sacroiliac joints
    (E) large weight-bearing joints

18. A 62-year-old male presents with pain and stiffness in his shoulders and hips lasting for several weeks with no history of trauma. In association with these symptoms the patient also has complaints of headache, neck pain, and jaw claudication. It is imperative to diagnose this patient promptly in order to prevent which of the following complication?

    (A) anemia
    (B) cerebral aneurysms
    (C) ischemic optic neuropathy
    (D) mononeuritis multiplex
    (E) respiratory tract complications

19. A 52-year-old male presents with complaint of bilateral knee pain of 2 years duration. The patient states the right knee is more problematic than the left. He states the pain worsens with activity and seems to be progressing. Which of the following diagnostic test is most specific to the diagnosis of this patient?

    (A) erythrocyte sedimentation rate
    (B) C-reactive protein
    (C) serum uric acid
    (D) examination of joint fluid
    (E) x-ray of the knees

20. The diagnosis of systemic lupus erythematosus (SLE) is supported by a positive initial antibody screen. However, this test is not specific. Which of the following test is most specific in the diagnostic evaluation of SLE?

    (A) gliadin antibodies
    (B) anti-dsDNA antibody
    (C) anticentromere antibody
    (D) antiribosomal P antibody
    (E) antinuclear antibodies

21. Which of the following is the most common joint pathology characteristic of rheumatoid arthritis?

    (A) cartilage and bone degenerative changes
    (B) osteophyte proliferation
    (C) spontaneous hemarthrosis
    (D) eburnation of subchondral bone
    (E) inflammation of the synovium and joint capsule

22. Related infections that have been identified as triggers of reactive arthritis include sexually transmitted diseases and which of the following?

    (A) ear infections
    (B) eye infections
    (C) enteric infections
    (D) musculoskeletal infections
    (E) central nervous system infections

23. Patients diagnosed with Sjögren's syndrome should be counseled to avoid which of the following class of medications:

    (A) antihistamines
    (B) decongestants
    (C) corticosteroids
    (D) fluoroquinolones
    (E) penicillins

24. A 6-year-old female is diagnosed with juvenile rheumatoid arthritis. She has a positive antinuclear antibody (ANA) and a negative rheumatoid factor (RF). With this presentation the American Academy of Pediatrics recommends that the patient be referred to which of the following specialist for evaluation:

(A) ophthalmologist for a screening eye examination

(B) otolaryngologist for a screening hearing examination

(C) dermatologist for evaluation of skin expression of the disease

(D) endocrinologist for evaluation of potential growth restriction

(E) gastroenterologist for evaluation of potential peptic ulcer disease

25. A 65-year-old female presents with severe mid back pain of 2 weeks duration. She has no history of trauma. Radiographic evaluation of the patient reveals compression fractures of T11 and T12. The patient is found to have normal findings on complete blood count, erythrocyte sedimentation rate, serum protein, serum calcium, phosphate, and parathyroid hormone level. In addition to dual energy x-ray absorptiometry (DEXA), which of the following laboratory evaluation is most helpful in evaluating this patient for secondary causes of this presentation?

(A) 25-hydroxyvitamin D

(B) rheumatoid factor

(C) serum magnesium

(D) bone biopsy

(E) antinuclear antibodies

Answers and Explanations

1. **(A)** This patient presentation of known rheumatoid arthritis with severe deformities, extraarticular findings, and splenomegaly is most likely Felty syndrome. Felty syndrome is characterized by the triad of deforming rheumatoid arthritis, splenomegaly, and neutropenia. The appropriate lab test to order would be a CBC to evaluate for neutropenia. Ordering an erythrocyte sedimentation rate and C-reactive Protein is not necessarily helpful in diagnosing Felty syndrome; in an acute inflammatory flare both would most likely be elevated. Antinuclear antibodies could be present in 20% to 40% of patients and are not diagnostic of Felty syndrome. Uric acid testing is not relevant to this patient presentation. (*Robbins, 2001, p. 92; Tierney et al, 2005, pp. 480–448*)

2. **(C)** Patients being treated for rheumatoid arthritis with a tumor necrosis factor (TNF) inhibitor are potentially at risk of developing an opportunistic infection. TNF inhibitors have been associated with an increased risk in tuberculosis. It is advised that TNF inhibitors should be discontinued if a patient develops a fever and/or a clinically significant infection, due to this increased risk of infection. Patients with congestive heart failure are not known to react untowardly to TNF inhibitors. Patients who use a TNF inhibitor do not have an increased risk of developing multiple sclerosis, but may in fact have a multiple sclerosis-like reaction to the drug. The use of methotrexate in combination with a TNF inhibitor is suggested, as there is known enhancement of the patients clinical response. Lastly, there is not an increased association of abscess formation at the injection site, but rather patients may have a mild local reaction at the site. (*Tierney et al, 2005, p. 805*)

3. **(D)** Medications used to prevent gout exacerbations include allopurinol and uricosuric drugs, such as probenecid. Allopurinol inhibits the production of uric acid and is indicated for patients who overproduce uric acid, and uricosuric drugs are used in patients who undersecrete uric acid. Criterion to classify a patient as an overproducer is a 24-hour uric acid excretion test. The result of 800 mg or greater indicates that the patient is an overproducer. In this patient scenario there is an overproduction of uric acid, making the case for the use of allopurinol. If this patient's 24-hour uric acid excretion was less than 800 mg, the use of a uricosuric drug would then be appropriate. Prednisone, colchicine, and indomethacin are alternative treatments for acute attacks of gout and not used for preventive measures. (*Tierney et al, 2005, pp. 786–788; Katzung, 2001, pp. 617–619*)

4. **(A)** The most likely diagnosis in this patient presentation is polymyositis. This is supported by the finding of a gradual progressive proximal muscle weakness and elevation of creatinine phosphokinase. The finding of lymphoid inflammatory infiltrates on muscle biopsy confirms the diagnosis. Treatment of choice in this condition is the use of a corticos-

teroid, prednisone. Patients who do not respond to this treatment may benefit from the use of methotrexate or azathioprine. The use of cyclophosphamide, an immunosuppressive agent, is more effective for the treatment of patients with dermatomyositis. Hydroxychloroquine has no apparent effect on the treatment of myositis. (*Tierney et al, 2005, pp. 813–814*)

5. **(A)** There are several treatment options available in the prevention and treatment of osteoporosis; choosing the appropriate regimen should be based upon patient needs. Raloxifene is a selective estrogen receptor modulator, which is best used in the postmenopausal female patient for which estrogen is not an option. Raloxifene increases bone density approximately 1% over a 2-year period and reduces the risk of vertebral fractures up to 40%; however, there appears to be no effect on nonvertebral fractures. It has no effect on the endometrium, coronary plaques, or association with cancer. In fact there is a documented 76% reduction in breast cancer among women taking raloxifene. Alendronate is a bisphosphonate that works by inhibiting osteoclast-induced bone resorption and does reduce the risk of both vertebral and nonvertebral fractures. However, alendronate does not have any effect on LDL or cancer as raloxifene does. Calcitonin does increase bone density 2% to 3% over a 5-year period and reduce the potential of vertebral fractures. Calcitonin does not have the effects noted with LDL and breast cancer reduction. Vitamin D supplementation is a useful mineral in the prevention of osteoporosis along with progestin; both do not have the effects noted with raloxifene. (*Tierney et al, 2005, pp. 1122–1123*)

6. **(B)** Pseudogout presents similarly to acute gout and is best diagnosed by the finding of the rhomboid-shaped crystals of calcium pyrophosphate in joint aspirates. Joints commonly involved in pseudogout are the knees and wrists, and other joints such as the metacarpophalangeals, hips, shoulders, ankles, and elbows. The diagnosis of pseudogout is further supported by the finding of a normal serum uric acid level. Acute gout would more likely be associated with an ele-

vated serum uric acid level. Infectious arthritis is ruled out with the findings of an afebrile patient and WBC count of 12,000. In acute infectious arthritis the WBCs would be expected to be elevated in the range of 50,000 to 200,000. Psoriatic arthritis commonly presents with asymmetrical oligoarticular involvement of two to four joints and in a higher percentage of patients there is known presence of the dermatological expression of psoriasis. Rheumatoid arthritis usually presents with symmetrical polyarticular involvement of three or more joints. (*Tierney et al, 2005, p. 788*)

7. **(C)** Ankylosing spondylosis is the most likely diagnosis in this patient presentation. This disorder is a chronic inflammatory disorder of the joints of the axial skeleton and commonly presents in the late teens or twenties. Males have a more likely incidence than females. The common presentation is pain in the lower back with radiation to the thighs and associated limitation of movement that may lessen during the day. Common laboratory findings are an elevated erythrocyte sedimentation rate and positive HLA-B27. The HLA-B27 is not a specific test for ankylosing spondylitis; a small percentage of the population have positive findings of this antigen. The earliest radiographic findings occur in the sacroiliac joints, with the detection of erosion and blurring of the joint space. Lumbar disc disease is usually seen in the 35 to 45 age group and more likely to be associated with trauma. Rheumatoid arthritis does have the potential to affect this age group, but would more likely be associated with smaller joints of the hands, along with a positive rheumatoid factor. Polymyalgia rheumatica more commonly affects patients over the age of 50 and is associated with fatigue, malaise, chronic pain, and stiffness of the proximal muscles, shoulders, neck, and pelvic girdle. Systemic lupus commonly affects women of childbearing years and presents with exacerbations and remissions of arthritis, rash, fatigue, and the potential for organ system involvement. (*Tierney et al, 2005, pp. 824–825*)

8. **(E)** With this patient presentation the most likely diagnosis is polyarticular onset juvenile

rheumatoid arthritis (JRA). This form of JRA is seen in approximately 40% of JRA patients. It is characterized by a female-to-male ratio of 3:1 and symmetrical involvement of five or more joints. Joints involved are more commonly the small joints of the hands and/or feet. Two subsets of the disease exist that are distinguished by the presence or absence of rheumatoid factor. A positive rheumatoid factor is most commonly seen in girls with later disease onset (at least 8 years old). An antinuclear antibody test (ANA) may be positive in 40% to 50% of patients, but is more likely to be positive with the pauciarticular form. In the early stage of the disease, the x-ray may be normal or show soft tissue swelling and periarticular osteopenia. In addition to the positive ANA found in 75% to 85% of pauciarticular JRA patients, the arthritis must be present in four or less joints. Early onset disease is commonly seen in girls aged 1 to 5 years and has a positive ANA; 30% to 50% of patients will also have eye involvement. Late onset disease is more common in males, with involvement of the large joints. Systemic onset JRA is seen in about 10% of children with JRA. It is characterized by daily intermittent fever. It is characterized by daily intermittent fever spikes and a transient, nonpruritic, pail pink, blanching macular or maculopapular rash found on the trunk. A positive rheumatoid factor is rare in this form of JRA. Reactive arthritis is usually associated with a recent viral or bacterial infection. Infectious arthritis more commonly presents as monarticular and is usually acute in onset. (*Hay et al, 2005, pp. 846–848*)

9. **(C)** Noninflammatory causes of monarthritis include benign tumors, such as osteochondromas, osteoarthritis, trauma, and osteonecrosis. Inflammatory causes include crystal-induced arthritis (gout and pseudogout), psoriatic arthritis, systemic lupus erythematosus, rheumatoid arthritis, and reactive arthritis. (*Tierney et al, 2005, pp. 834–835*)

10. **(A)** The treatment of rheumatoid arthritis is aimed at reduction of pain, preservation of function, and prevention of deformity. Most patients are initially begun on a nonsteroidal anti-inflammatory drug (NSAID) for analgesia and anti-inflammatory control. These drugs do not typically alter progression or prevent erosion of the joint. Consequently, in addition to NSAID therapy, disease-modifying antirheumatological drugs (DMARD) should be started as soon as the diagnosis is confirmed. The most common DMARD used as treatment of choice in rheumatoid arthritis is methotrexate. Antimalarials are usually reserved for mild disease and only 25% to 50% of patients will respond to this treatment and then it may take 3 to 6 months. Tumor necrosis factor (TNF) inhibitor is usually reserved for patients who have failed methotrexate. The use of TNF inhibitor comes along with the potential for serious side-effect profile of increasing the patient's susceptibility to infectious disease and opportunistic infections. Minocycline is used less commonly in mild cases and results only in modest response. Aspirin use would be less likely with this patient due to the history of gastroesophageal reflux. (*Tierney et al, 2005, pp. 801–807*)

11. **(D)** Fibromyalgia syndrome presents with widespread musculoskeletal pain and tender points, referred to as trigger points. Trigger points may be found anywhere on the body, but are most common in the neck, shoulders, hands, low back, and knees. Subcutaneous inflammatory lesions denote erythema nodosum. These lesions are associated with several systemic disorders, such as pregnancy, sarcoidosis, tuberculosis, and streptococcal infections. An abrupt onset of proximal muscle weakness is characteristic of polymyalgia rheumatica. Insidious onset of symmetrical joint involvement most commonly is associated with rheumatoid arthritis. Symmetrical weakness initially in the legs that progresses caudally is characteristic of Guillain–Barré syndrome. (*Tierney et al, 2005, pp. 794–795*)

12. **(C)** Uveitis is an associated finding in patients with Behçet's disease, ankylosing spondylitis, reactive arthritis, psoriasis. These disorders can cause a nongranulomatous anterior uveitis that usually presents unilaterally with pain, redness, photophobia, and visual loss. Uveitis associated with Behçet's disease can be aggressive and result in blindness. Vasculitis is seen with Behçet's disease. Hyperuricemia

may be found with psoriasis. Thoracic involvement is often found in ankylosing spondylitis. Reactive arthritis is more likely to be associated with dysentery. (*Tierney et al, 2005, pp. 160–161*)

13. **(B)** Scleroderma is characterized by diffuse thickening of the skin, associated with areas of telangiectasia and pigmentation changes. Most patients with scleroderma also have an associated polyarthralgia and Raynaud's phenomena. Sarcoidosis more commonly presents with pulmonary symptoms and erythema nodosum. Dermatomyositis presents with scaly patches over the dorsum of the hands (Gottron's sign) and lilac discoloration of the eyelids (heliotrope rash). Eosinophilic fasciitis is a rare disorder associated with skin changes similar to scleroderma; however, there is no association with Raynaud's phenomena. Eosinophilia-myalgia syndrome is associated with chronic ingestion of tryptophan, which is an amino acid previously found in over-the-counter preparations for insomnia and premenstrual syndrome now banned by the food and drug administrators. Cutaneous findings in eosinophilia-myalgia syndrome present with a range of expression from hives to swelling of the extremities. (*Tierney et al, 2005, pp. 811–813*)

14. **(D)** Cervical fusion is frequently needed in patients with rheumatoid arthritis secondary to atlantoaxial instability due to C2 instability. This instability is due to erosion of the ligaments that hold the odontoid in place. This finding is important to establish in rheumatoid arthritis patients prior to surgery that requires intubation or manipulation of the neck. Manipulation of this area of C2 instability can result in quadriparesis or death. Myelodysplasia refers to neural tube defects that can cause complex spinal deformities of the lumbosacral spine. Subaxial instability is the second most common abnormality and may cause subluxation of two or more cervical vertebrae below the level of C2. Cervical spondylosis refers to a form of degenerative joint and disc disease that affects the cervical spine, leading to compression of the associated nerve roots. Superior migration of C3 is a less

common form of cervical spine abnormality. (*Greene, 2001, pp. 73–74*)

15. **(D)** The recommended calcium intake for postmenopausal women not on estrogen replacement therapy is 1500 mg. Outside of menopause the recommended adult dose is 1000 mg. For postmenopausal women on estrogen replacement therapy the dose recommendation is 1000 mg. The average adult has a daily dietary intake of 700 mg of calcium daily, which falls below the standard recommendation. Calcium is found in dairy products, green leafy vegetables, and fish with bones. There is no current recommendation for 2000 mg of calcium intake. (*Tierney et al, 2005, p. 1236*)

16. **(D)** Patients with polymyalgia rheumatica are commonly treated for 1 years time. Six months is too short with most cases. Most patients respond to treatment within 72 hours; if they do not, an alternate diagnosis may be necessary. Tapering doses of prednisone should be monitored closely in all cases; 50% or more of patients may experience exacerbations of the disease while on tapering doses. (*Tierney et al, 2005, pp. 819–820*)

17. **(E)** The most common joints involved in reactive arthritis are the large weight-bearing joints of the knees and ankles. The sacroiliac joints are involved in 20% of patients with reactive arthritis. The small joints of the hands and feet and the upper extremities are not the more likely joints involved in reactive arthritis. (*Tierney et al, 2005, pp. 826–827*)

18. **(C)** The most urgent need for diagnosis of a patient with symptoms of polymyalgia rheumatica (PMR) and giant cell arteritis is to prevent blindness caused by ischemic optic neuropathy as a result of occlusive arteritis of the ophthalmic artery. Early diagnosis is imperative as the neurological damage to the optic nerve is not reversible. Most patients with this diagnosis will have a normochromic, normocytic anemia, but this does not create urgency in treatment. Mononeuritis multiplex commonly presents with painful paralysis of a shoulder and respiratory tract complications

are more nonclassic findings with the presentation of PMR. Cerebral aneurysms are not common findings with PMR; large vessels such as the subclavian and aorta may be involved in giant cell arteritis in 15% of patients. (*Tierney et al, 2005, pp. 819–820*)

19. **(E)** The most likely diagnosis with this patient presentation is osteoarthritis. Typically osteoarthritis presents with an insidious onset of articular stiffness that develops into pain with motion and further aggravation with activity. Pain is then relieved by rest. The most helpful diagnostic test in osteoarthritis is radiographic imaging of the affected joint. Findings common to osteoarthritis are joint space narrowing, sharpened articular margins, osteophyte formation, and lipping of the marginal bones and thickening of the dense subchondral bone. Erythrocyte sedimentation rate and C-reactive protein are commonly negative, as the inflammatory changes are typically minimal. Serum uric acid elevations are more commonly used in diagnosing gout. Examination of the joint fluid is not usually indicated in the early diagnosis of osteoarthritis. (*Tierney et al, 2005, pp. 781–783*)

20. **(B)** Autoantibody production is the primary immunological abnormality seen in patients with systemic lupus erythematosus (SLE); the antinuclear antibody (ANA) is most characteristic of SLE and seen in 95% of patients with SLE, but is not specific for the diagnosis of SLE. A positive ANA can be found in patients with lupoid hepatitis, scleroderma, rheumatoid arthritis, Sjögren's disease, dermatomyositis, and polyarteritis. ANA testing should be employed as the initial screening test in a patient suspected of having SLE. A negative total ANA test is strong evidence against the diagnosis of SLE, where a positive test is not confirmatory of the diagnosis. The most specific antibody tests for SLE are antibodies to double-stranded DNA (anti-dsDNA) and anti-Smith (anti-SM). Although these tests are more specific for SLE, they are less sensitive than ANA. Anti-dsDNA is positive in 60% of patients with SLE and anti-Sm is positive in 30%. Anti-dsDNA is more likely to reflect disease activity. Gliadin antibody assay is utilized to assess patients with suspected celiac disease. Anticentromere antibody is associated with CREST syndrome in scleroderma. Antibodies to ribonucleoprotein are present in patients with a mixture of overlapping rheumatological symptoms known as mixed connective tissue disease. (*Tierney et al, 2005, pp. 809–810*)

21. **(E)** Rheumatoid arthritis is characterized by chronic inflammation of the synovium and joint capsule. This usually progresses to a fibrous ankylosis and less often bony ankylosis. Cartilage degeneration, osteophyte formation, and eburnation of subchondral bone are pathological changes associated with osteoarthritis. Spontaneous hemarthrosis is associated with hemophilia A. (*Tierney et al, 2005, pp. 801–803*)

22. **(C)** Reactive arthritis, previously known as Reiter's syndrome, typically presents with the clinical triad of urethritis, conjunctivitis, and arthritis. The majority of the cases of reactive arthritis are associated with either a sexually transmitted disease (STD) or enteric infection. Common STD etiological triggers are *Chlamydia trachomatis* or *Ureaplasma urealyticum* and enterically *Shigella, Salmonella, Yersinia,* or *Campylobacter* are associated organisms with reactive arthritis. Common ear, eye, musculoskeletal, and central nervous system infections are usually not associated with reactive arthritis. (*Tierney et al, 2005, pp. 826–827*)

23. **(B)** Sjögren's syndrome is an autoimmune disorder that commonly presents with dryness of the eyes, mouth, and other areas of the body covered by mucous membrane. It is frequently associated with rheumatoid arthritis and predominately a disease of women. Due to the chronic dysfunction of the exocrine glands and chronicity of dryness of the eyes and mouth, patients should be counseled to avoid atropinic drugs and decongestants. The use of these medications can further exacerbate their symptoms. Antihistamines, corticosteroids, fluoroquinolones, and penicillins are not directly associated with encouraging exocrine dysfunction. (*Tierney et al, 2005, p. 815*)

24. **(A)** The systemic manifestations of juvenile rheumatoid arthritis (JRA) include fever, erythematous rashes, nodules, leukocytosis, and less commonly iridocyclitis, pleuritis, pericarditis, anemia, fatigue, and growth failure. The American Academy of Pediatrics currently recommends routine eye examinations for patients diagnosed with JRA. Children with JRA and a positive antinuclear antibody screen are at increased risk of having ocular involvement. Eye inflammation develops gradually and is often asymptomatic, routine eye examination, most specifically examination with slit lamp is important in the evaluation of a patient with JRA. This type of examination can detect asymptomatic uveitis, which can lead to visual impairment or blindness. Patients with JRA are not at increased risk of hearing impairment; thus a referral to the otolaryngologist is unnecessary. JRA patients who have a systemic presentation do have a characteristic rash, but a dermatology consult is usually not warranted. Growth restriction may occur with any form of JRA, more commonly may be found in systemic onset and polyarticular onset JRA. There is no current method to predict which patients will have growth restriction and a routine referral is not often indicated. Even though the use of nonsteroidal antiinflammatory drugs are the first line of treatment in JRA, the actual incidence of gastrointestinal ulceration is less common in children than adults. Referral to a gastroenterologist is not indicated. (*Hay et al, 2005, pp. 846–848*)

25. **(A)** This patient has typical findings associated with osteoporosis. Most patients with osteoporosis are asymptomatic until fractures present. Fractures occur spontaneously and are associated with back pain of varied degrees. Serum calcium, phosphate, and parathyroid hormone levels are often normal. Vitamin D deficiency state is common in osteoporosis and important to evaluate for. Rheumatoid factor and antinuclear antibodies would not be of importance with this patient presentation. Serum magnesium is more associated with evaluating for parathyroid or thyroid disorder and has no value with osteoporosis. Bone biopsy is not indicated with this patient; this would be reserved for evaluating for osteomalacia. (*Tierney et al, 2005, pp. 1120–1123; Green, 2001, pp. 57–61*)

REFERENCES

Greene, W (ed). *Essentials of Musculoskeletal Care*, 2nd ed. Rosemont, IL: American Academy of Orthopaedic Surgeons; 2001.

Hay WW, Levin MJ, Sondheimer JM, Deterding RR (eds). *Current Pediatric Diagnosis and Treatment*, 17th ed. New York: McGraw-Hill; 2005.

Katzung, BG (ed). *Basic and Clinical Pharmacology*, 8th ed. New York: McGraw-Hill; 2001.

Robbins L, (ed). *Clinical Care in the Rheumatic Diseases*, 2nd ed. Atlanta, GA: Association of Rheumatology Health Professionals; 2001.

Tierney LM, McPhee, SJ, Papadakis, MA (eds). *2005 Current Medical Diagnosis and Treatment*, 44th ed. New York: McGraw-Hill; 2005.

Obstetrics and Gynecology

Questions

Constance M. Goldgar, MS, PA-C, and Paula B. Phelps, MHE, PA-C

DIRECTIONS (Questions 1 through 80): Each of the numbered items or incomplete statements in this section is followed by answers or by completions of the statement. Select the ONE lettered answer or completion that is BEST in each case.

Questions 1 through 80

1. A 17-year old complains of severe dysmenorrhea since her first menses at age 13. The dysmenorrhea is often accompanied by nausea and vomiting the first 2 days of her menstrual period; analgesics or heating pads do not relieve the pain. She is sexually active and does not want to get pregnant. Her pelvic exam is normal. Which of the following medications is MOST appropriate for this patient?

   (A) narcotic analgesics
   (B) prostaglandin inhibitors
   (C) oxytocin
   (D) oral contraceptives
   (E) luteal progesterone

2. A 25-year-old nullipara consults you because she suddenly stopped menstruating. On questioning her further you find she recently has lost 19 pounds after starting long distance running. The MOST appropriate step in her evaluation is measurement of

   (A) serum TSH concentration
   (B) serum prolactin concentration
   (C) human hCG concentration
   (D) serum estradiol-17b concentration
   (E) serum testosterone concentration

3. Which of the following two causes of nontraumatic vaginal bleeding are seen MOST frequently in the adolescent and reproductive- aged female?

   (A) pregnancy and coagulopathy
   (B) thyroid dysfunction and anovulation
   (C) exogenous hormone use and polyps
   (D) anovulation and pregnancy

4. A 25-year-old nulliparous white female has a chief complaint of heavy and frequent menstrual bleeding for the past year. She has never been sexually active; is moderately overweight; and has hirsutism and acne. She denies vaginal dryness, mood swings, or hot flashes. She also denies hot or cold intolerance, diarrhea, or heart palpitations. Which part of this history suggests polycystic ovarian syndrome?

   (A) her age and parity
   (B) sexual activity
   (C) weight, skin, and hair changes
   (D) moods and temperature

5. Which of the following should NOT be considered in the first line of investigation of an infertile couple?

   (A) semen analysis
   (B) urinary luteinizing hormone
   (C) pelvic and transvaginal ultrasound
   (D) endometrial biopsy
   (E) progesterone test

6. A 39-year-old woman, G3P3, complains of severe, progressive secondary dysmenorrhea and menorrhagia. Pelvic exam demonstrates a tender, diffusely enlarged uterus with no adnexal tenderness. Endometrial biopsy findings are normal. What is the next diagnostic exam needed?

(A) magnetic resonance imaging (MRI)
(B) transvaginal and abdominal ultrasound
(C) hysterosalpingography
(D) laparoscopy
(E) CT scan of the pelvis

7. What is the MOST salient element of the history that suggests the presence of endometrial cancer?

(A) age greater than 70 years
(B) postmenopausal bleeding
(C) obesity
(D) combination progestin and estrogen hormone therapy

8. A 36-year-old G2P2 comes to your office complaining of heavy menstrual bleeding for the past year. The patient is bleeding through a super tampon and a heavy pad every hour of the first three days of her cycle. Her cycle lasts 5 days and cycle length has decreased to having a period every 20 days. She complains of fatigue. Her physical exam and lab workup are normal (negative beta hCG, LH, FSH, prolactin, clotting times, liver function, and renal function tests), except for the CBC and further labs indicating she has iron deficiency anemia. The patient's weight is 298 pounds. In addition to iron supplementation, which of the following is the BEST INITIAL therapy for this patient?

(A) hysterectomy
(B) oral contraceptives
(C) D & C
(D) long-term conjugated estrogen therapy
(E) daily dosing of aspirin

9. A 26-year-old patient is complaining of depression and anxiety just prior to her menses. The symptoms have been going on for over 1 year, but are now starting to interfere with her relationships and her productivity at work. One week prior to menses each month she experiences a depressed mood, a feeling of being on edge, increased irritability, difficulty sleeping, a feeling of being overwhelmed, and is easily fatigued. You have her chart the symptoms daily in a log and return to your office in two cycles. The log is consistent with the history. Her physical exam and general lab profile showed no abnormalities. Which of the following is the MOST effective treatment choice for this disorder?

(A) aprazolam
(B) spironolactone
(C) progestin-only oral contraceptive
(D) fluoxetine
(E) ibuprofen

10. The combination of dysmenorrhea, deep dyspareunia, low back pain, and chronic pelvic pain are symptoms that BEST fit with which of the following conditions?

(A) adenomyosis
(B) ovarian cancer
(C) endometriosis
(D) interstitial cystitis

11. A 25-year-old nulliparous woman complains of dysmenorrhea that has gotten progressively worse over the past 2 years. Her pain is described as a constant, aching pain. It begins 2 to 7 days prior to onset of bleeding and does not subside until the menstrual flow decreases. In addition, she complains of pain on intercourse (dyspareunia). She has never been pregnant and uses condoms and foam for contraception. You make the presumptive diagnosis of endometriosis. Which of the following is the BEST way to confirm the diagnosis definitively?

(A) MRI
(B) pelvic ultrasound
(C) trial of prostaglandin synthetase
(D) laparoscopy
(E) hysteroscopy

12. A 47-year-old G3P1 woman comes into the office complaining of heavy, painful, and irregular menstrual bleeding that has been going on for the past 6 months to a year. She has not been sexually active for the past year. On physical exam, her uterus is estimated to be the size of uterus at 12 weeks' gestation. Pelvic ultrasound confirms the presence of a leiomyoma. Her hematocrit is 29%, mean corpuscular volume (MCV) is 68 fL, and serum ferritin is 10 g/L. What should be the first line therapy?

   (A) myomectomy of leiomyoma
   (B) hysterectomy
   (C) ablation therapy
   (D) oral contraceptive therapy in standard doses
   (E) depot methodroxyprogesterone acetate 150 mg IM every 28 days

13. A woman has undergone a suction curettage for a hydatidiform mole and was diagnosed with benign gestational trophoblastic neoplasia (GTN). Following this INITIAL treatment, which choice of monitoring should be done for patients in order to prevent the development of choriocarcinoma?

   (A) monitor serum radioimmunoassay beta hCG once per week until 3 to 4 normal values are obtained, then monthly for a year
   (B) follow-up every 2 weeks with a urinary pregnancy test
   (C) administer prophylactic chemotherapy
   (D) monitor serum hCG levels after 6 months and again at 1 year
   (E) monitor serum hCG levels monthly accompanied by chest x-ray to rule out metastases

14. A 49-year-old G2P2 patient has a known history of uterine myomata that are approximately 16-week size. Within the past year, her periods have become progressively heavier and longer. A dilation and curettage performed 6 months earlier showed no pathology and failed to decrease the bleeding. Her hematocrit is 34%. The patient is not orthostatic and does not complain of dizziness. Which of the following would be the BEST next step?

   (A) abdominal myomectomy
   (B) laparoscopic-assisted myomectomy
   (C) leuprolide acetate (Lupron Depot)
   (D) transfusion with two units of packed cells
   (E) total abdominal hysterectomy

15. A 20-year-old nulliparous woman presents to the emergency department complaining of pelvic pain and fever and chills. Her symptoms have been going on for 3 days. She has had no new sexual partners, but does not routinely use condoms with her current partner because they "have been dating for 1 year." Clinically, her cervix is erythematous, friable, and there is a mucopurulent discharge. The cervical motion tenderness is significant. Her pregnancy test is negative and there are no adnexal masses. What is the MOST likely pathogen causing her symptoms?

   (A) *Neisseria gonorrhoeae*
   (B) *Chlamydia trachomatis*
   (C) *Haemophilus influenzae*
   (D) *Escherichia coli*
   (E) *Gardnerella vaginalis*

16. A 20-year-old nulligravida comes to your office complaining of pelvic pain and irregular menstrual bleeding. She denies sexual activity, and her beta hCG urine test is negative. She has never been on oral contraceptives. On pelvic exam, you find unilateral tenderness on the left side, and a palpable cystic mass approximately 4 to 5 cm. The MOST likely diagnosis is

   (A) ectopic pregnancy
   (B) functional ovarian cyst
   (C) choriocarcinoma
   (D) sarcoma
   (E) molar pregnancy

17. A 25-year-old G1P1 presents with two days of right-sided pelvic pain and a history of menstrual irregularities for 2 months. She denies fever, chills, or nausea. She has a negative pregnancy test. Her pelvic exam reveals an approximately 5-cm mobile adnexal mass. Which element of the history or physical exam is MOST specific for the diagnosis of ovarian cysts and not for the diagnoses of appendicitis, viral gastroenteritis, endometriotic cysts, carcinoma, or tubo-ovarian abscess?

   (A) right-sided pelvic pain
   (B) denial of fever, chills, or nausea
   (C) menstrual irregularities
   (D) adnexal mass

18. A very firm ovarian mass estimated at 8 cm is found in a 33-year-old female at her annual exam. Which of the following interventions should be considered first?

   (A) combination chemotherapy
   (B) radiation therapy
   (C) surgical consult
   (D) exploratory laparoscopy

19. In women with a *BRCA1* gene mutation, which of the following types of cancer are they MOST at increased risk for?

   (A) cervical cancer
   (B) ovarian cancer
   (C) endometrial cancer
   (D) vaginal cancer

20. You perform a Pap Smear for a 40-year-old patient has not had a Pap smear since the birth of her last baby (15 years ago). Today's Pap smear result indicates squamous cell carcinoma. The reason she sought medical care was for postcoital bleeding. At the time of the Pap smear there was a friable lesion present. At this point, the MOST appropriate step in this patient's management is

   (A) repeat Pap smear in 4 to 6 months
   (B) biopsy visualized lesion and refer patient for gynecologic consult
   (C) colposcopy with endocervical curettage and directed biopsy
   (D) Loop Electrosurgical Excision Procedure (LEEP) or cervical conization
   (E) radical hysterectomy and radiation therapy

21. On physical exam of a 24-year-old nulligravida, an erythematous cervix with a yellow discharge is visualized. The patient has had one new partner in the past 60 days. She uses oral contraceptives for birth control and rarely uses condoms. She has not noticed any pruritis, discharge, or vaginal pain. The wet prep reveals no hyphae or clue cells. Which of the following etiologic organisms BEST fits the clinical information given?

   (A) *Staphylococcus aureus*
   (B) *Chlamydia trachomatis*
   (C) *Gardnerella vaginalis*
   (D) *Candida albicans*
   (E) human papillomavirus (HPV)

22. Cervical cysts are noted while performing a Papanicolaou test. The MOST likely diagnosis is

   (A) Bartholin's cysts
   (B) Nabothian cysts
   (C) cervicitis
   (D) HPV
   (E) cervical carcinoma

23. A 25-year-old G1P1 presents to your clinic for her annual exam. She has no history of abnormal Pap smears, but the results from today's test show squamous intraepithelial lesions (SIL), low grade. Which of the following is the BEST option for what should be done next?

   (A) recheck Pap in 1 year
   (B) repeat Pap smear in 4 to 6 months, using traditional method
   (C) repeat Pap smear in 4 to 6 months, using liquid-based cytology
   (D) HPV testing
   (E) colposcopy

24. A 58-year-old female who is 8-years post-menopausal complains of urinary urgency, frequency, and occasional incontinence. On pelvic exam, her vaginal mucosa appears shiny, pale pink with white patches, and bleeds slightly to touch. Her urinalysis and urine cultures are negative. Which of the following is the BEST treatment for this patient?

   (A) antibiotic by mouth
   (B) testosterone cream to be applied to affected areas
   (C) vaginal suppositories containing sulfa antibiotics
   (D) estrogen-containing vaginal cream or vaginal ring
   (E) surgical procedure

25. It is well established that HPV is very strongly correlated to cervical cancer. HPV testing is becoming more and more common after the finding of an abnormal Pap smear. Not all HPV subtypes cause cancer. Which of the following subtypes is associated with the worst prognosis?

   (A) 16
   (B) 18
   (C) 31
   (D) 33
   (E) 35

26. A 26-year-old mother who is nursing presents to clinic complaining of right breast tenderness and fever. Upon physical exam, she has a 2-cm fluctuant mass at the site of erythema and tenderness. The patient had been seen 4 days ago and was placed on oxacillin, which she has been taking. At this point the BEST treatment is

   (A) changing antibiotic to vancomycin and discontinuing nursing
   (B) surgical drainage and continuation of nursing
   (C) discontinuation of nursing and hot soaks
   (D) incision and drainage, hot soaks, antibiotics, and breast emptying
   (E) hot packs and manual emptying of breasts

27. A 48-year-old woman comes in for her annual physical exam and biannual screening mammogram. Her family history is negative for breast cancer. Her breast physical exam reveals no palpable masses; however, a screening and then diagnostic mammogram demonstrates several coarse calcifications that are suspicious for breast cancer. Which of the following statements is MOST accurate?

   (A) fine needle aspiration would be the BEST diagnostic method for this finding
   (B) since there is no palpable mass on physical exam, the patient may be observed with additional mammography in 3 months
   (C) an image-guided, local excisional biopsy provides the MOST definitive diagnosis
   (D) a reasonable option for this patient is a core tissue biopsy done with stereotaxis
   (E) ultrasound imaging is the diagnostic method of choice for ductal carcinoma in situ (DCIS)

28. A 30-year-old woman who is 6-months post-partum (G2P2) presents to clinic because of a sense of "heaviness and pressure" low in her pelvis. Onset was 2 days ago after a 3-mile run. She was pushing a stroller uphill as she ran. She has dribbling of urine when she coughs or exercises, but denies any other problems with urination. She takes no medications and uses an Intrauterine device (IUD) for contraception. She is lactating. On physical exam it is noted that when the patient is asked to strain, there is a bulging in the upper one third of her vagina, just posterior to her urethra. There is no protrusion noted when the patient is not straining, and with straining the bulge comes to about 0.5 cm, just inside of the introitus. Also noted is a lack of pelvic muscle tone and vaginal dryness. At this point what is the MOST likely diagnosis?

   (A) urethrocele
   (B) enterocele
   (C) cystocele
   (D) rectocele
   (E) uterine prolapse

29. For the patient in question 28, what would be the MOST appropriate therapy?

(A) systemic estrogen therapy

(B) anticholinergics

(C) Kegel exercises

(D) surgery

(E) pessary

30. A 19-year-old female presents to the clinic with complaints of vaginal discharge that started 3 weeks ago. Intercourse is uncomfortable and she is experiencing postcoital bleeding. Her periods have been normal with her last period ending yesterday. She and her new partner use spermicidal foam, but no condoms. Pelvic exam shows mucopurulent discharge from the cervix, left adnexal fullness, and mild cervical motion tenderness. Her pregnancy test is negative. Given the above information, the MOST likely diagnosis is

(A) urinary tract infection

(B) *Trichomonas* vaginitis

(C) intrauterine pregnancy

(D) pelvic inflammatory disease (PID)

(E) cervical dysplasia

31. Which of the following is the MOST common symptom of a cystocele?

(A) difficulty defecating

(B) straining to urinate

(C) low back pain

(D) dribbling urine when coughing

32. Preterm labor occurs more frequently in twin gestations. Which of the following antenatal complications does NOT occur with greater frequency in a twin gestation?

(A) fetal anomalies

(B) preeclampsia

(C) intrauterine growth retardation

(D) gestational diabetes

(E) maternal anemia

33. At 8 weeks' gestation, a 24-year-old primipara was seen a week prior complaining of vaginal bleeding and lower abdominal cramping. Her beta-hCG level was 1,000 mIU/mL at that time. Today, she has no abdominal pain or evidence of tissue passed per vagina. Transvaginal ultrasound (TVUS) shows no adnexal masses as well as no clear pregnancy. Her repeat beta-hCG level is 1,100 mIU/mL. What can be concluded from this information?

(A) the patient has a pregnancy that is non-viable but its location is unknown

(B) she has had a spontaneous abortion and needs a D & C

(C) the hCG level needs to be repeated in 48 hours for more information on viability

(D) this is definitely an ectopic pregnancy

(E) this is a molar pregnancy

34. A 24-year-old Hispanic female (G3P2) presents for routine prenatal care at 20 weeks' gestation. Her urine is positive for glucosuria (2+). This finding would likely indicate

(A) gestational diabetes

(B) need to follow-up with a 3-hour glucose tolerance test

(C) need for a 50-g, 1-hour glucose challenge test

(D) need for instituting dietary control

(E) normal increase in renal threshold for glucose

35. A 39-year-old female G2P2 (SAb 1, living 1) presents to the ED with lower abdominal pain, vaginal bleeding, and a 6-week history of amenorrhea. Her history is significant for oral contraceptive use in the past and a spontaneous miscarriage. In addition, she has had an episode of PID. On presentation she was orthostatic and a culdocentesis performed in the ED was positive for blood. Exploratory laparotomy revealed an ectopic pregnancy. What risk factor did this patient have that has the highest association with developing an ectopic pregnancy?

(A) history of spontaneous abortion

(B) history of oral contraceptive use

(C) advanced maternal age

(D) history of PID

36. A 55-year-old G4P4 presents to your clinic complaining of a vulvar mass. She says she does not know how long it has been there but her husband noticed it two nights ago. She denies any pain, itching, or discharge. She had a complete hysterectomy 10 years ago for fibroid tumors and has been on hormone replacement ever since then. Her history is otherwise unremarkable. On physical exam, the mass appears to be approximately 1 cm and hard. It is located on the right lower labia majora at approximately 4 o'clock. Of the following neoplasms, which is the MOST likely diagnosis?

(A) carcinoma of Bartholin's gland

(B) carcinoma in situ of the vagina

(C) sarcoma botryoides

(D) invasive vaginal cancer

(E) Paget's disease

37. A 35-year-old primipara at 42 weeks' gestation is in the labor and delivery suite for a nonstress test. She has had an uneventful pregnancy but has not felt the fetus moving much in the past 24 hours. A subsequent external fetal monitor tracing demonstrates a repetitive late heart rate deceleration. The first step in managing this patient is

(A) evaluation of maternal hypotension

(B) evaluation of fetal acid–base status

(C) administration of a tocolytic agent

(D) repositioning the patient

(E) checking maternal oxygen saturation

38. A 30-year-old woman who is nursing presents to clinic complaining of breast tenderness. Physical exam reveals a warm, erythematous tender area with induration. The next step in management would be to

(A) prescribe a penicillinase-resistant penicillin, e.g., dicloxacillin

(B) prescribe topical mupirocin and continue breastfeeding

(C) discontinue nursing, empty breasts, and apply hot soaks to affected breast

(D) observe for fever and rest while continuing breastfeeding without medication

(E) breast drainage should be cultured to determine causative organism

39. Fibroadenoma of the breast is a common benign neoplasm. Which of the following clinical descriptions is MOST consistent with the diagnosis of fibroadenoma?

(A) 25-year-old patient with a nontender, round, freely movable breast mass approximately 1 cm in diameter

(B) 55-year-old patient with a 6-cm fixed, hard, breast mass and palpable lymph nodes on the same side

(C) 30-year-old patient with a unilateral, bloody nipple discharge

(D) 40-year-old patient with tender, bilateral breast masses that seem to fluctuate in size monthly

(E) 60-year-old with an erythematous rash on her right breast and nipple

40. A 30-year-old woman presents with bilateral breast pain and nodularity. The tenderness and size of the nodules increase premenstrually. She has no family history of breast cancer. On physical exam, multiple tender "rope-like" nodules are palpated. There is no dominant mass and the lymph nodes are not palpable. After reassuring the patient regarding cancer, you recommend which of the following for INITIAL management

(A) 200-mg danazol daily during luteal phase of menses

(B) decreasing use of caffeine and tobacco

(C) galactography to determine if lesions are focal

(D) fine-needle aspiration to determine atypia

(E) ultrasound for definitive diagnosis

41. A 32-year-old woman (G2P1) with gestational diabetes is delivering at 41 weeks' gestation. The fetus appears to be about 4,100 g. The woman has experienced 5 hours of stage 1 labor, and currently in her second hour of stage 2 labor. The head is delivering but the shoulders are not. Which of the following descriptions include the BEST option for delivering this infant

(A) flexing of the mother's thighs, pitocin augmentation, and suprapubic pressure

(B) flexing of the mother's thighs, suprapubic pressure, and cutting an episiotomy

(C) elevation of the mother's legs, suprapubic pressure, and oxygen for the mother

(D) no elevation of the mother's legs, pitocin, and fundal pressure

(E) no elevation of the mother's legs, suprapubic pressure, and cutting an episiotomy

42. A 32-year-old woman (G1P1) at 35 weeks' gestation presents with a complaint of intermittent bleeding over the past week; however, she has had no evident pain or cramping. Upon physical exam, fetal heart rate is normal. These clinical characteristics are MOST consistent with

(A) placetal abruption

(B) premature labor with bloody mucous discharge

(C) placenta previa

(D) vasa previa

(E) premature rupture of membranes

43. At 33 weeks, a 28-year-old patient (G1P1) calls the office with a complaint of a fluid gush from her vagina. She is not having contractions or evidence of bleeding. You advise her to go to labor and delivery to be examined. Which of the following procedures should be performed first?

(A) induction of labor

(B) nitrazine testing

(C) ultrasound to estimate amniotic fluid volume

(D) digital cervical exam to determine if patient is in labor

(E) administration of antibiotics to prevent infection

44. At 16 weeks' gestation, a 19-year-old G1P0 Asian patient presents with a complaint of vaginal bleeding. She also has been experiencing severe nausea and vomiting. Her quantitative beta hCG is much higher than expected for 16 weeks' gestation, and her fundal height is approximately at 18- to 20-week size. Although she denies a past history of hypertension, her blood pressure is 140/90 mm Hg. No fetal heart sounds can be heard on doptone, and there is no sign of a fetus on ultrasound. What would be her MOST likely diagnosis?

(A) threatened abortion

(B) incomplete abortion

(C) hydatidiform mole

(D) fetal demise at 16 weeks

(E) twin gestation

45. A 66-year-old woman who has had a hysterectomy presents with the complaints of chronic constipation and pelvic fullness. She says that at times it feels as if her insides are falling out. Vaginal prolapse is found on physical exam. On the basis of her history, which of the following types of pelvic relaxation would MOST likely account for her prolapse?

(A) urethrocele

(B) enterocele

(C) cystocele

(D) rectocele

(E) uterine prolapse

46. A 24-year-old G2P1 woman presents during the second trimester complaining of constipation and difficulty passing her bowel movements. Her last delivery was uncomplicated. On physical exam of her introitus and vagina, you notice a bulging of the pelvic floor when she bears down. Your assessment is that the common problem constipation during pregnancy is being made worse because of the presence of a(n)

(A) incompetent cervix
(B) prolapse uterus
(C) cystocele
(D) rectocele
(E) vaginal mass

47. Which of the following BEST describes the clinical characteristics of abruptio placenta?

(A) variable amount of blood loss, no pain, and normal fetal heart rate, no significant maternal history
(B) scant blood loss, soft and nontender uterus, grand multiparity
(C) moderate amount of blood loss, uterine hypertonus, history of maternal hypertension
(D) bloody mucous plug, regular contractions
(E) variable amount of blood loss, abdominal pain, history of caesarian delivery

48. A 20-year-old sexually active woman complains of a profuse, whitish-gray vaginal discharge with a fishy odor that becomes stronger after intercourse and during menses. She denies any irritation and states that her sexual partner has no symptoms. Microscopic evaluation of the discharge reveals granular-appearing epithelial cells ("clue cells"). Which of the following is the BEST therapy?

(A) metronidazole
(B) ciprofloxicin
(C) miconazole cream
(D) fluconazole
(E) doxycycline

49. In a pregnant woman with the diagnosis of vaginal candidiasis, which of the following treatments would be preferred?

(A) metronidazole
(B) ciprofloxicin
(C) miconazole cream
(D) fluconazole
(E) doxycycline

50. Metrodidazole 2 g daily for 3 to 5 days is the treatment regimen for which of the following vaginal infections?

(A) bacterial vaginosis (BV)
(B) candidiasis
(C) trichomoniasis
(D) *Staphylococcus*

51. A lactating woman, diagnosed with mastitis is treated appropriately with dicloxacillin 250 mg q.i.d. She continues her antibiotic therapy and also continues to breastfeed, but her infection does not resolve and after 48 hours is getting worse. At this point what is the appropriate course of action?

(A) increase the dose of doxacillin to 500 mg q.i.d.
(B) discontinue the breastfeeding
(C) refer to a lactation specialist
(D) refer for surgical consult
(E) apply hot compresses

52. Which of the following laboratory tests is essential to good routine prenatal care for the multipara with a normal past history?

(A) plasma blood glucose 1 hour after a 50-g oral glucose load
(B) trichomonas vaginalis screening
(C) x-ray pelvimetry
(D) protein-bound iodine
(E) erythrocyte sedimentation rate (ESR)

53. A 25-year-old G1P0 presents to labor and delivery with increasingly severe and frequent contractions over the previous 5 hours and spontaneous rupture of membranes 1 hour ago. Cervical exam shows dilation to 4 cm. The stage of labor for this patient would be assessed as

(A) second stage
(B) first stage, active phase
(C) first stage, latent phase
(D) cannot be assessed without effacement data
(E) third stage

54. A reactive nonstress test is generally defined as

(A) no change in the fetal heart rate with fetal movements over a 30-minute period
(B) two decelerations with fetal movements over a 40-minute period
(C) one acceleration with fetal movements over a 1-hour period
(D) five decelerations with fetal movements over a 20-minute period
(E) two accelerations with fetal movements over a 20-minute period

55. A 28-year-old primigravid woman at 42 weeks' gestation delivers a 4,000-g (8 lb 13 oz) newborn. Labor stages are as follows: first stage, 17 hours; second stage, 4 hours; third stage, 35 minutes. After a midline episiotomy was performed, the baby was delivered with low forceps. The placenta appeared to be intact. Ten minutes after delivery, she experiences vaginal bleeding estimated to be 500 mL over a 5-minute period. Upon exam, her uterus feels soft and boggy. Which of the following is the MOST likely cause of the hemorrhage?

(A) retained placental tissue
(B) uterine atony
(C) genital tract laceration
(D) disseminated intravascular coagulation
(E) uterine inversion

56. A 22-year-old woman (G1P0) presents at 38 weeks' gestation complaining of dizziness, headache, and fatigue. Pertinent findings include BP of 148/90, 1+ bilateral ankle edema, normal electrolyte levels, normal deep tendon reflexes, and 1+ albuminuria. The MOST appropriate treatment at this time is

(A) immediate delivery
(B) administration of a mild diuretic once daily and prenatal visits every 2 to 5 days
(C) bed rest and prenatal visits every 2 to 5 days
(D) hospitalization with administration of magnesium sulfate via intravenous (IV) pump, 1 to 2 mg/h
(E) hospitalization with constant fetal monitoring

57. A previously unsensitized Rh-negative woman in her second pregnancy is seen in her 26th week. She complains of edema in her legs and some tingling in her left hand. What is the next step in managing this patient?

(A) analysis of the husband's blood type
(B) intramuscular Rho (antiD) immune globulin
(C) ultrasonic evaluation of amniotic fluid volume
(D) Rh antibody titer
(E) amniocentesis

58. For a woman at 34 weeks' gestation who is experiencing preterm labor but has not had rupture of membranes, which of the following drugs is NOT indicated in managing her premature labor?

(A) ritodrine
(B) betamethasone
(C) nifedipine
(D) terbutaline
(E) magnesium sulfate

59. A patient had her last menstrual period on October 10, 2005. Her estimated date of delivery will be on

    (A) July 17, 2006
    (B) July 4, 2006
    (C) August 10, 2006
    (D) June 30, 2006
    (E) July 10, 2006

60. A woman at 22 weeks' gestation presents for her regular check-up. Her hemoglobin level is 10.8 g/dL. Which of the following statements regarding this patient's hemoglobin level is TRUE?

    (A) this patient has iron deficiency anemia
    (B) the reason for this hemoglobin level in this trimester is physiologic: due to the expansion of red cell volume relative to the red blood cell mass
    (C) this patient should receive ferrous sulfate, 300 mg, not more often than twice daily
    (D) screening for anemia should take place later in pregnancy when hemoglobin levels reach their nadir.
    (E) a complete evaluation of the anemia, including serum ferritin, needs to be done.

61. There is a good evidence that screening women at risk for chlamydial infection reduces the incidence of PID. The U.S. Preventive Services Task Force strongly recommends which of the following statements with regard to routine screening for *Chlamydia trachomatis*?

    (A) sexually active women with risk factors should be screened annually
    (B) sexually active women age 30 or younger should be screened
    (C) all pregnant women should be screened at first and third trimesters
    (D) asymptomatic men should be routinely screened for chlamydial infection as it reduces the incidence of new infections in women
    (E) age is the MOST important risk factor in determining whether to screen

62. A thin, white 53-year-old woman who had her last menstrual period 2 years ago presents to your office complaining of hot flashes, vaginal dryness, and sleep loss from night sweats. She inquires about the benefits and risks of hormone replacement therapy (HRT) (combination estrogen–progesterone therapy), especially after hearing so much confusing information from the news media. When you counsel the patient regarding the risks and benefits of a shorter course (< 5 years) of HRT, you tell her that which of the following is a documented risk of HRT?

    (A) increased risk of endometrial cancer
    (B) increased risk of breast cancer
    (C) decreased bone mineral density
    (D) increased risk of thromboembolism
    (E) increased risk of colon cancer

63. A 30-year-old G1P0 woman whose last menses were 8 weeks ago presents with heavy vaginal bleeding and LLQ pain. She had noted passage of something that "looked like liver" the previous day. Pelvic exam reveals 2-cm cervical dilatation. Which of the following is the MOST likely diagnosis?

    (A) incomplete abortion
    (B) complete abortion
    (C) threatened abortion
    (D) incompetent cervix
    (E) missed abortion

64. A 44-year-old G2P2 woman who had two normal pregnancies (13 and 11 years ago) presents with the complaint of amenorrhea for 8 months. She has remarried and would like to become pregnant again. A pregnancy test is negative. Her physical exam is normal. Which of the following tests is next indicated in the evaluation of this patient's amenorrhea?

    (A) endometrial biopsy
    (B) luteinizing hormone (LH), follicle-stimulating hormone (FSH), and estradiol levels
    (C) ovarian antibody assay
    (D) testosterone and Dehydroepiandrosterone (DHEAS) levels
    (E) hysterosalpingogram

65. A 27-year-old G1P0 woman has received regular prenatal care throughout her pregnancy. She presents to the ED at 34 weeks with facial edema, severe headache, and epigastric pain. On physical exam, she has a blood pressure of 160/110 mm Hg, elevated liver function tests, and a platelet count of 60,000/uL. The baby is noted to be alive. Urinalysis indicates 4+ proteinuria. Which therapeutic measure should be taken next in managing this patient?

(A) oral antihypertensive therapy

(B) intravenous immunoglobulin therapy

(C) magnesium sulfate therapy and induction of labor

(D) platelet transfusion

(E) a colloid solution for plasma volume expansion

66. A 28-year-old primagravida presents for routine prenatal care at 32 weeks' gestation. Her pregnancy has been uneventful and she has been receiving regular prenatal care. At her visit today, the fundal height measurement is 36 cm. Of the possibilities below, which would NOT account for the increased fundal height?

(A) fetal macrosomia

(B) multiple gestation

(C) oligohydramnios

(D) fetal position

(E) fibroid uterus

67. A 39-year-old G1P0 at 39 weeks' gestational age is seen for a routine OB visit and has a blood pressure reading of 150/100 mm Hg. During her pregnancy thus far, baseline blood pressures have been 100-120/60-70. She is sent to labor and delivery. She denies any headache, visual changes, nausea, vomiting, or abdominal pain. The cervix is 50% effaced and 2- to 3-cm dilated. A repeat BP shows 160/90. Her hematocrit is 34.0, platelets are 160,000, SGOT is 22, SGPT is 15, and urinalysis is negative for protein. Which of the following is the MOST likely diagnosis?

(A) pregnancy-induced hypertension (gestational hypertension)

(B) chronic hypertension

(C) preeclampsia

(D) eclampsia

(E) HELLP (H-hemolytic anemia EL-elevated liver enzymes LP-low platelet count) syndrome

68. Which of the following statements regarding management of labor in a low-risk pregnancy is TRUE?

(A) food and oral fluids are acceptable if labor is progressing normally

(B) electronic fetal monitoring (EFM) improves perinatal outcomes

(C) walking during labor decreases duration of labor

(D) bed rest is associated with shorter duration of labor, less need for analgesia

(E) perineal shaving decreases maternal febrile morbidity

69. Which of the following statements about hot flashes is FALSE

(A) they usually resolve spontaneously within 2 to 3 years

(B) duration is typically less than 1 minute

(C) when HRT is initiated as a treatment for vasomotor symptoms, hot flashes usually resolve within 1 week

(D) can begin several years before actual menopause

(E) usually are the first physical manifestation of ovarian failure

70. Treating preterm labor with beta-adrenergic agonists has been shown to decrease the rate of which one of the following?

(A) delivery within 48 hours of treatment

(B) low birth weight infants

(C) preterm delivery

(D) perinatal deaths

(E) perinatal infection

71. The MOST common cause of spontaneous abortion in the first 12 weeks of pregnancy is

    (A) the presence of maternal lupus anticoagulant
    (B) chromosomal anomalies
    (C) an incompetent cervix
    (D) maternal drug abuse
    (E) inadequate progesterone

72. In the surgical repair of procidentia, or marked uterine prolapse, which of the following structures MOST likely needs to be repaired in a 45-year-old G4P4?

    (A) transverse and uterosacral ligaments
    (B) sacral nerve
    (C) detrusor muscles
    (D) pelvic floor muscle

73. Which of the following represents the primary effect of oral contraceptives?

    (A) changes in tubal mobility and ovum transport
    (B) sperm penetration
    (C) disruption of implantation
    (D) suppression of FSH and LH
    (E) change in fertile mucus

74. A healthy 20-year-old female is using a low-dose triphasic contraceptive pill for birth control. She experiences break-through bleeding during the third week of each cycle for the past few months. Her pregnancy test is negative. The physical exam is normal. There is no infection or thyroid problem. The patient desires to stay on oral contraceptives. What is the BEST way to manage her therapy?

    (A) continue current oral contraceptive pill (OCP), but add extra estrogen during the third week for a couple of weeks
    (B) prescribe a progestin-only pill
    (C) change to a pill with a higher progestin component
    (D) switch to a pill with a higher estrogenic component
    (E) reassure her and have her return in 1 month

75. Which of the following is the recommended time frame for emergency contraception's greatest effectiveness in preventing pregnancies?

    (A) 0 to 20 hours
    (B) 21 to 40 hours
    (C) 40 to 60 hours
    (D) 60 to 80 hours
    (E) less than 72 hours

76. In a pregnant woman with an incompetent cervix, which of the following is the BEST way to avoid a miscarriage or a premature birth?

    (A) pessary
    (B) bed rest
    (C) cerclage
    (D) magnesium sulfate
    (E) terbutaline

77. Which of the following lists of patient problems BEST typifies the classical presentation of endometriosis?

    (A) dysmenorrhea, deep thrust dyspareunia, infertility, abnormal bleeding, pelvic pain, and headache
    (B) dysmenorrhea, headache, insomnia, infertility, abnormal bleeding, and pelvic pain
    (C) infertility, abnormal bleeding, polycystic ovarian syndrome, insomnia, pelvic pain
    (D) dysmenorrhea, deep thrust dyspareunia, infertility, abnormal bleeding, and pelvic pain

78. When microscopically examining a lesion taken from a fallopian tube, what does the presence of endometrial glands, stroma, and hemosiderin-laden macrophages indicate?

    (A) chronic pelvic inflammatory disease
    (B) cervical cancer
    (C) polycystic ovarian syndrome
    (D) endometriosis

79. A 32-year-old nulliparous, married woman is seeking contraceptive advice. She is a nonsmoker, and has a history of one ectopic pregnancy 5 years ago. She wishes to consider childbearing in the future. Her history includes mild, well-controlled hypertension, and frequent urinary tract infections. Which one of the following contraceptive options would be contraindicated?

(A) condoms and spermicide
(B) intrauterine device
(C) low-dose combined oral contraceptive
(D) diaphragm
(E) progesterone-only oral contraceptive

80. Which one of the following is TRUE regarding emergency estrogen/progesterone postcoital contraception?

(A) it delays the onset of the next menstrual period
(B) it can be used up to 96 hours after intercourse
(C) it is indicated when a condom breaks
(D) it is indicated for patients who have missed a dose of their regular oral contraceptive
(E) it is necessary to have a positive pregnancy test before prescribing emergency contraception

Answers and Explanations

1. **(D)** Conservative measures for treating dysmenorrhea include heating pads, mild analgesics, and outdoor exercise. Evidence suggests that primary dysmenorrhea is due to prostaglandin F2alpha (PGF2alpha), a potent myometrial stimulant and vasoconstrictor, in the secretory endometrium. Prostaglandin synthase inhibitors such as naproxen, ibuprofen, indomethacin, and mefenamic acid can be very effective. However, for patients with dysmenorrhea who are sexually active, oral contraceptives will provide needed protection from unwanted pregnancy and generally alleviate the dysmenorrhea. The OCPs minimize endometrial prostaglandin production during the concurrent administration of estrogen and progestin. (*Alzubaidi et al, 2004*)

2. **(C)** Although exercise-induced secondary amenorrhea may seem apparent in this case, the most common cause of secondary amenorrhea in reproductive age is still pregnancy. Therefore, an hCG test is indicated as a first step in the evaluation of this patient. Sudden weight loss and increased physical activity can cause secondary amenorrhea, as can hypothyroidism and hyperprolactinemia. If ordering serum estradiol concentrations, an FSH level should also be ordered. Alone, serum estradiol levels are less useful than FSH in deciphering cause of amenorrhea. Decreased estradiol occurs with either hypothalamic-pituitary axis failure or ovarian failure. Decreased FSH indicates hypothalamic-pituitary axis failure whereas elevated FSH indicates ovarian failure. Ordering serum testosterone levels should only be considered if the patient has symptoms of androgen excess. (*Nelson, 2005a*)

3. **(D)** Anovulatory bleeding is seen in 10% to 15% of all gynecologic patients and is the most common cause of abnormal vaginal bleeding in adolescents. In perimenarchal adolescents, it is caused by an immature hypothalamic–pituitary–ovarian axis. The top five causes of vaginal bleeding in the adolescent are listed by frequency: anovulation, pregnancy, exogenous hormone use, and coagulopathy. The top six causes of vaginal bleeding in the reproductive-aged women listed by frequency are pregnancy, anovulation, exogenous hormone use, uterine leiomyomas, cervical and endometrial polyps, and thyroid dysfunction. The top four causes of vaginal bleeding in perimenopausal women listed by frequency are anovulation, uterine leiomyomas, cervical and endometrial polyps, and thyroid dysfunction. The top four causes of vaginal bleeding in postmenopausal women listed by frequency are endometrial lesions, exogenous hormone use, atrophic vaginitis, and other tumors. (*Tintinalli, 2004, pp. 647–653*)

4. **(C)** Polycystic ovarian syndrome is suggested by her being moderately overweight, and having hirsutism and acne. As has been claimed in many clinical medicine lectures over the years, 80% to 90% of the diagnosis

comes from the history. The essential parts of the history when investigating the causes of dysfunctional uterine bleeding are age of menarche, menstrual history, date of the first day of the last normal menstrual period, contraceptive use, signs and symptoms of coagulopathy (nosebleeds, petechiae, and ecchymoses), endocrine symptoms, menopause symptoms, weight changes, and stress. *(Tintinalli, 2004, pp. 647–653)*

5. **(D)** In approaching the diagnostic work-up for infertility, with a thorough physical exam and history of both partners, the clinician should establish the following points: (1) Does the woman ovulate? (if not, why not?) (2) Is the semen quality normal? (3) Is there tubal or uterine abnormality? In the initial evaluation of the female partner, noninvasive procedures, such as the measurement of LH and mid-luteal phase progesterone to determine ovulatory function and TVUS to rule out the possibility of fibroids or polycystic ovaries, are first line investigations. Pelvic ultrasound should also be part of the routine gynecologic evaluation because it allows a more precise evaluation of the position of the uterus within the pelvis and provides more information about its size and irregularities. For the male partner, semen analysis is also noninvasive and helpful, though not diagnostic. Endometrial biopsy is no longer recommended for the diagnosis of luteal phase deficiency as it cannot reliably distinguish a fertile window. *(Alper, 2005a; Taylor, 2003, pp. 494–495; Frey and Patel, 2004, pp. 1440–1441; Garcia et al, 2005)*

6. **(B)** The most common causes of secondary dysmenorrhea in this age group are endometriosis, adenomyosis, and the presence of an intrauterine device. For this patient, it would be important also to rule out myomas, polyps, tumors, and leiomyomas. Given the most common causes, endometriosis and adenomyosis, noninvasive studies with transvaginal and abdominal ultrasound would be a reasonable (and economical) first choice. The imaging diagnosis of adenomyosis is usually made by using TVUS or, more expensively, by MRI. Abdominal ultrasound alone can be highly sensitive for detecting masses,

but often lacks specificity for the diagnosis of adenomyosis or endometriosis. Ultrasound, however, is not as specific as MRI in the evaluation of endometriosis. Hysterosalpingography is more invasive and is used to exclude endometrial polyps, leiomyomas, and congenital abnormalities of the uterus. The inability to resolve subtle differences in soft-tissue attenuation limits the usefulness of computerized tomography (CT). Laparoscopy is often needed as a last resort to make the diagnosis of endometriosis where surgical correction can occur simultaneously. *(Reuter, 2004; Daly, 2004)*

7. **(B)** In the United States, there are approximately 36,100 cases of endometrial cancer diagnosed each year and about 6,500 patients die from the disease. For type I endometrial cancers, excessive estrogenic stimuli is a risk factor. Therefore, women who are taking postmenopausal unopposed estrogen replacement or tamoxifen, and women who are 50 pounds above their ideal body weight are at risk for endometrial hyperplasia and endometrial cancer. Type II endometrial cancers tend to occur in older, thinner women without exogenous estrogen exposure. More than 90% of patients with endometrial cancer present with postmenopausal bleeding, thus making it the hallmark history component. *(Goldman and Ausiello, 2004, pp. 1238–1239)*

8. **(B)** Treatment for premenopausal abnormal uterine bleeding is varied. Once infection, fibroid tumors, pregnancy, neoplasm, and iatrogenic causes (e.g., medication related) are ruled out, a woman may be treated hormonally to control bleeding. In this patient, the most likely cause of the bleeding is anovulatory cycles caused by estrogen excess due to her obesity; additionally, the iron deficiency anemia also can cause menometrorrhagia. In patients with irregular cycles, secondary to chronic anovulation, or oligo-ovulation, OCPs help to prevent the risks associated with prolonged unopposed estrogen stimulation of the endometrium. Treatment with cyclic progestins for 5 to 12 days per month is preferred when OCP use is contraindicated, such as in smokers over age 35 and women at risk for thromboembolism. *(Albers et al, 2004, p. 1924)*

9. **(D)** Although approximately 75% of menstruating women experience one or more of the cluster of physical, emotional, or behavioral symptoms associated with the luteal phase of the menstrual cycle (PMS), only 2.5% to 5% of those women have symptoms so severe that they meet the DMS-IV diagnosis of premenstrual dysphoric disorder (PMDD). A recent study of 260 women 18 to 45 years old with PMDD randomized to fluoxetine 20 mg vs. placebo PO qd starting 14 days before expected menses and ending on first day of menses for 3 cycles showed significant reduction in total symptom scores compared with placebo, improved mood-related symptoms, and improved physical symptoms. A dose of 10 mg showed significantly improved mood-related symptoms, but not total or physical symptoms scores. *(Cohen et al, 2002, pp. 439–440)*

10. **(C)** The combination of dysmenorrhea, deep dyspareunia, low back pain, and chronic pelvic pain are most suggestive of endometriosis. The other conditions could all present with a pelvic pain component, but would have a different combination of other symptoms. Adenomyosis is commonly associated with menorrhagia (40% to 50% of patients) and dysmenorrhea (25% to 30% of patients). Ovarian cancer would present with nonspecific findings such as ascites, abdominal discomfort, vague gastrointestinal symptoms, pelvic or abdominal mass, and pain. Interstitial cystitis typically presents with urinary frequency and urgency, as well as suprapubic, perineal, vulvar, or vaginal pain before, during, or after urination. *(Lemcke et al, 2004, pp. 199, 474–477, 494, 532–535)*

11. **(D)** Diagnostic laparoscopy is the only definitive way to diagnosis endometriosis. Ultrasound and MRI may be helpful in the diagnostic workup, but laparoscopy is the most certain method of diagnosing endometriosis. *(Beckmann et al, 2006, p. 368; Tierney et al, 2005, pp. 716–717)*

12. **(E)** This patient has a leiomyoma of the uterus (or fibroid tumors), which is the most common benign neoplasm, but she is also significantly anemic. The labs suggest iron deficiency anemia. It is important to control her bleeding and treat her anemia prior to surgery. The heavy bleeding that typically accompanies fibroid tumors can be minimized by using intermittent progestin supplementation (depot methodroxy-progesterone acetate 150 mg IM every 28 days) and/or prostaglandin synthetase inhibitors. In general, the size of the mass can be decreased, and the bleeding can be lessened, but the only curative treatment is a myomectomy or hysterectomy. *(Tierney et al, 2005, pp. 713–714)*

13. **(A)** GTN consists of benign GTN, most often a hydatidiform mole, and malignant GTN, which includes nonmetastatic and metastatic GTN. Approximately, 5% to 20% of women who have a hydatidiform mole will go on to develop some form of malignant GTN, one of which is choriocarcinoma. To best detect these patients, after molar evacuation, serum radioimmunoassay beta-hCG levels should be monitored weekly until they have been undetectable for three consecutive weeks, followed by monthly monitoring until they have been undetectable for 1 year. Urine pregnancy tests are inadequate, and a sensitive radio-immunoassay is mandatory. Prophylactic chemotherapy is controversial due to significant drug toxicity and possible lack of efficacy; it is usually reserved for highest risk cases or for patients who are unable to return for regular follow-up. Routine chest x-ray at every visit is not warranted unless hCG values rise. *(Moore LE and Ware D, 2005; Hernandez, 2005; Berkowitz and Goldstein, 1996)*

14. **(C)** Leiomyomata are benign growths of the myometrium and the majority of patients do not require surgical or medical treatments. Only if myomas cause significant pressure on the uterus, bladder, or bowel, or if the uterine bleeding causes anemia or a significant alteration in lifestyle or hygiene, medical or surgical therapy is needed. Medical treatment to reduce the size of the tumors may be all the therapy that is necessary. Their growth is stimulated by estrogen; therefore, a 2- to 3-month course of leuprolide acetate (Lupron Depot), a Gn-RH analog, would be the best choice. Gn-RH analogs produce a sustained and continuous release of Gn-RH on the pituitary that

eventually results in a decrease in the release of pituitary gonadotrophins and subsequent decreased production of estrogen from the ovaries. Because the risk of surgical complications increases with the size of the myoma, it is best to reduce the size of the tumor preoperatively and also to treat anemia preoperatively. *(Tierney et al, 2005, pp. 713–714)*

15. **(B)** The patient's diagnosis is PID. For her age group, the most likely pathogens are the sexually transmitted ones, *C. trachomatis* and *N. gonorrhoeae*. Of these two STDs, *C. trachomatis* is more prevalent. Because the causes are often polymicrobial, treatment should be broad based and for a long duration. As long as the patient is medically stable and can tolerate oral medication, she can be treated as an outpatient. One recommended outpatient treatment is ceftriaxone 250 mg, intramuscularly; and doxycycline 100 mg twice daily for 14 days; with or without metronidazole 500 mg twice daily for 14 days. *(Tierney et al, 2005, pp. 718–719; Lemcke et al, 2004, pp. 317–318; http://www.cdc.gov/STD/treatment/TOC2002TG.htm).*

16. **(B)** A functional ovarian cyst is a much more likely diagnosis than any of the others listed. A follicular cyst develops when an ovarian follicle fails to rupture. The granulosa cells lining the cyst continue to enlarge and fluid continues to accumulate. Symptoms associated with a functional ovarian cyst include mild to moderate unilateral pain, and alteration in the menstrual cycle. On occasion, rupture of the follicular cyst causes acute pelvic pain and may need laparoscopic surgery for complete evaluation. In most cases, pain control for 4 to 5 days is what is indicated and consideration of contraception to suppress future ovarian cysts formation. *(Lemcke et al, 2004, pp. 474, 538; Tierney et al, 2005, pp. 720–721).*

17. **(C)** Menstrual irregularities are most specific for the functional ovarian cysts. Right-sided pain could be associated with many items on the differential for abdominal pain. The presence of fever and chills would be more likely seen in appendicitis infections. The negative

pregnancy test makes ectopic pregnancy much less likely. *(Tierney et al, 2005, pp. 720–721, 595)*

18. **(C)** The size and firmness of the ovarian mass suggest endometrioid carcinoma, a tumor in which the potential for malignancy is 100%. Referral to a gynecologic oncologist should be considered first whenever an ovarian malignancy is suspected. Standard of care is complete surgical staging, excision of all visible masses, and abdominal hysterectomy and bilateral salpingo-oophorectomy followed by chemotherapy. Radiation oncology could also be considered. *(Tierney et al, 2005, p. 722)*

19. **(B)** *BRCA1* and *BRCA2* gene mutations are known genetic markers for breast and ovarian cancers. In the 1990s, genetic linkage research was done on families who had strong histories of breast and ovarian cancers. They identified 3 mutations in the two genes *BRCA1* and *BRCA2*. When a woman inherits the *BRCA1*, her lifetime risk of ovarian cancer is 45%, and it is 25% when she has the *BRCA2* gene. *(Tierney et al, 2005, p.719; Lemcke et al, 2004, p. 322)*

20. **(B)** There is no generalized clinical picture of cervical carcinoma, but there are two symptoms often associated with it. They are postcoital bleeding and abnormal uterine bleeding. The average age at diagnosis is 50. Lesions on the cervix that should be considered for immediate biopsy include new exophytic, friable, or bleeding lesions. In this patient, the lesion should have been biopsied at initial exam and this would have helped to make the diagnosis. When lesions are visualized and the biopsy confirms carcinoma, no colposcopic assessment is needed. This patient should definitely not wait 4 to 6 months for a repeat Pap smear. The gynecologic oncologist should stage the cancer and decide on appropriate therapy. *(Beckmann et al, 2006, pp. 268–272, 277)*

21. **(B)** Chlamydia should be suspected when there is eversion of the cervix and a mucopurulent cervicitis. Because of this patient's use of hormonal birth control, her cervix would

likely appear to have erosion, but she has a mucopurulent cervicitis. BV typically presents with a white discharge, amine (or "fishy") odor, and possible itching. Candidiasis often presents with a history of pruritis and a thick white discharge. On wet prep, BV is diagnosed by the presence of clue cells and a positive KOH "whiff test" (amine odor) and vaginal candidiasis is diagnosed by the presence of yeast hyphae. *(Beckmann et al, 2006, pp. 265–267; Tierney et al, 2005, pp. 1391–1392)*

22. **(B)** Nabothian follicles, or epithelial inclusion cysts, present a characteristic appearance: They contain a dense, yellow, mucoid material. A Bartholin's duct cyst is the most common cystic growth in the vulva. When infected, it would be visualized as a fluctuant swelling of the inferior portion of the labia minorae, presenting with periodic pain and dyspareunia. Cervicitis will present with a mucopurulent drainage from the cervical os; occasionally with columnar evasion in chronic cases. Cervical polyps are benign, pedunculated growths of various sizes that extend from the ectocervix or endocervical canal. Cervical carcinoma would appear either grossly on the surface (exophytic) or may not be visible on speculum exam (endophytic) with only the occasional physical exam finding of a firm, expanded cervix. *(Cunningham et al, 2001, pp. 40; Tierney et al, 2005, pp. 709–712)*

23. **(E)** There are several management options, depending on the clinical correlation and whether or not the low squamous intraepithelial lesions (LSIL) finding was accompanied by further information from the pathologist, but most pathologists will recommend that colposcopy should be done next. The 2001 Consensus Guidelines for the Management of Women with Cervical Cytological Abnormalities and the 2001 Guidelines for Management of Women with Cervical Intraepithelial Neoplasia (www.asccp.org) also recommend that colposcopy be done following LSIL on Pap smears. Viewing the cervix and its transformation zone with 10-20X magnification of colposcopy allows for visual assessment. Two solutions are used to further enhance visualization and determination of normal from abnormal tissue. When a dilute solution of acetic acid is applied to the cervix, abnormal areas will look white. After painting the cervix with Lugol's solution (a strong iodine solution), the normal squamous epithelial will take on the stain while the abnormal tissue will not. All abnormal appearing tissue is biopsied. *(Tierney et al, 2005, 710–711)*

24. **(D)** The patient's symptoms describe postmenopausal atrophic changes affecting the vagina, bladder, and urethra. In women with more severe changes, vaginal irritation, dyspareunia, and fragility may become problems. Atrophy is diagnosed by the presence of a thin, clear, or bloody discharge, a vaginal pH of 5 to 7, loss of vaginal rugae, and the finding of parabasal epithelial cells on microscopic exam of a wet-mount preparation. These symptoms are all due to estrogen depletion. Treatment with topical estrogen preparations (cream, tablet, or ring) appears equally effective. Complete relief of symptoms usually occurs within weeks; in the interim, patients may obtain relief through use of vaginal lubricants and moisturizers (e.g., Astroglide, Replens). Minimal doses (e.g., 10 to 25 µg/24 h) should be used and are usually sufficient. Serum studies have shown that when it comes to absorbing estrogen, the vaginal epithelium acts just like the skin and the gut mucosa; therefore, larger doses of vaginal estrogen will result in systemic estrogen levels similar to oral or transdermal administration and will carry an equal risk, benefit, and side-effect profile (uterine bleeding, breast pain, perineal pain). Rarely, endometrial hyperplasia can be a side effect of vaginal estrogen treatment. *(Suckling et al, 2003; Alper, 2005b)*

25. **(B)** Greater than 90% of cervical cancers are associated with HPV. There are many different strains of HPV, some of them causing cervical cancer and some of them not. The strain with the worst prognosis is HPV 18. *(Tierney et al, 2005, p. 1594)*

26. **(D)** A true abscess will require surgical drainage and therapy with antibiotics, rest, warm soaks, and complete emptying of the

breasts every 2 hours. The abscess drainage should be cultured and sensitivities determined. There have been no formal studies of treatment of lactation mastitis associated abscesses. However, incision and draining is recommended along with parenteral antibiotics administered with added coverage for anaerobic bacteria. As soon as the pain of the wound permits, breastfeeding or pumping should be resumed in order to drain the affected breast. Needle aspiration of the abscess, repeated every other day until pus no longer accumulates, has been suggested, as an alternative to open drainage. *(Barbosa-Cesnik et al, 2003, p. 1612)*

27. **(C)** For mammographic abnormalities that are nonpalpable and that require biopsy, image-guided tissue sampling is necessary. Tissue for diagnosis can be obtained by open surgical biopsy with needle localization. The sensitivity of needle-localized excisional biopsy is 99% for nonpalpable lesions. Although it has less morbidity, core-needle biopsy for small foci of highly suspicious microcalcifications with no associated mass is less beneficial because sampling errors are more common and local excision provides definitive treatment. With nonpalpable lesions, core needle or excisional biopsy is preferred over fine needle aspiration biopsy (FNAB) because the sample provides adequate tissue for histologic diagnosis and is more accurate. Ultrasonography is helpful if the radiologist thinks that the lesion has the appearance of a cyst (not this case), but DCIS cannot be diagnosed until tissue samples and pathology are done. *(Kerlikowske et al, 2003, pp. 276–277)*

28. **(C)** Pelvic pressure and stress incontinence in a multiparous woman are common symptoms of pelvic relaxation. The bulging in the anterior portion of the vagina, which was seen on physical exam, confirms the diagnosis of a cystocele. The structures that support the pelvic organs can be weakened by birth trauma, chronic elevation of intra-abdominal pressure (as seen in chronic cough and obesity), intrinsic weaknesses, or atrophic changes from estrogen loss. In the case outlined in the question, the following factors

contributed to her cystocele: birth trauma, decreased estrogen because of lactation, and increased intra-abdominal pressure from pushing a stroller up hill while running. *(Berek, 2002, pp. 685–693; Tierney et al, 2005, pp. 717)*

29. **(C)** The patient may benefit from all of the options to some degree, but the most conservative approach would be to start with Kegel exercises. By strengthening the pelvic floor muscles, this problem may become much less bothersome and once natural estrogen levels are restored after the cessation of breastfeeding, the problem may completely be resolved. Systemic estrogens are contraindicated in breastfeeding because they decrease breast milk production. A pessary may be considered after failure of Kegel exercises. Pessaries could be especially helpful if the patient's symptoms significantly interfere with her lifestyle. Surgery should be reserved for a patient whose symptoms do not improve with conservative therapy or who have significant prolapse. *(Berek, 2002, pp. 685–693; Tierney et al, 2005, pp. 717)*

30. **(D)** PID is a polymicrobial infection of the upper genital tract (cervix, uterus, adnexa). Diagnostic criteria minimally include uterine/adnexal tenderness or cervical motion tenderness, but additional criteria that increase the specificity of the diagnosis are fever (>38.3 °C or > 101° F), abnormal cervical or vaginal mucopurulent discharge, presence of white blood cells (WBCs) on saline microscopy of vaginal secretions, elevated erythrocyte sedimentation rate (ESR), and elevated C-reactive protein (CRP), and laboratory documentation of cervical infection with *Neisseria gonorrhoeae* or *Chlamydia trachomatis*. Unless the patient has acute PID or is unresponsive to therapy, treatment is done on an outpatient basis with oral antibiotics that are effective against *N. gonorrhoeae* and *C. trachomatis*. *(Alper, 2005c)*

31. **(D)** The most common symptom of general pelvic relaxation in general is a feeling of pressure or as if something is protruding from the vagina. With a rectocele, patients may

have difficulty defecating. Straining to urinate may be a symptom of a cystocele, but the most common symptom of a cystocele is stress incontinence, which is often described by patients as dribbling when they cough, sneeze, or jump. Pelvic relaxation may be improved with Kegel exercises, although once the exercises are discontinued the symptoms often return. Pessaries can also be used to prevent stress incontinence. Ultimately, a surgical referral may be needed to correct the problem. *(Beckmann et al, 2006, pp. 289–298)*

32. **(D)** Twin pregnancies have a similar risk of gestational diabetes compared to singleton pregnancies, based on comparison of 89 twin pregnancies with 178 matched singleton pregnancies. Multiple gestations include various complications for the mother and fetus. For the mother, twin pregnancies are associated with higher risk of pregnancy-induced hypertension, anemia, hyperemesis, abruption, placenta previa, postpartum hemorrhage, and increased risk of operative delivery. For the fetus, twin pregnancy increases risk of intrauterine death, spontaneous abortion, congenital anomalies, cerebral palsy, and intrauterine growth retardation. *(Alper, 2005d; Buhling et al, 2003)*

33. **(A)** Since there is a plateau in the hCG level after 1 week (48 hours is usually sufficient), the pregnancy is nonviable. The hCG level need not be repeated at this point. TVUS appears to demonstrate no visualized products of conception. It should be noted, however, that in women with a clinically incomplete abortion, only 50% had retained products of conception. The sensitivity and specificity of cervical status for detecting retained products of conception is approximately 65% and 56%, respectively, whereas the overall sensitivity and specificity of transvaginal sonography in determining products of conception is approximately 100% and 80%, respectively. An ectopic pregnancy cannot be ruled in or out yet. When hCG < 1,200 IU/L and an ectopic pregnancy is not seen, progesterone level needs to be determined. TVUS will show a live embryo (cardiac activity) in the adnexa in only 10% cases (and usually when the hCG is 15 to 20,000 IU/L). If the hCG < 1,200 IU/L, progesterone > 5

ng/mL, and clinical findings are suggestive of ectopic pregnancy, this constellation of findings are highly suggestive of ectopic pregnancy. The low hCG levels and lack of findings on ultrasound (e.g., "snowstorm" appearance) would help rule out a molar pregnancy. *(Yip et al, 2003, pp. 39–41; Wong et al, 2002, p. 430)*

34. **(C)** Although glycosuria is more common during pregnancy because of the lowering of the renal threshold for glucose excretion, this patient may be at an increased risk for gestational diabetes (GDM) due to her ethnicity. Normal screening for GDM occurs at 24 weeks' gestation. Since glycosuria has been detected, screening with a 50-g, 1-hour glucose challenge test would be indicated at this time. Patients do not have to fast for this test. To be considered normal, serum or plasma glucose values should be less than 130 mg/dL (7.2 mmol/L) or less than 140 mg/dL (7.8 mmol/L). Using a value of 130 mg/dL or higher will increase the sensitivity of the test from 80% to 90% and decrease its specificity, compared with using the 140 mg/dL cutoff. An abnormal 1-hour screening test should be followed by a 100-g, 3-hour venous serum or plasma glucose tolerance test. Normal blood sugars at 0, 1, 2, and 3 hours, respectively, are:

- fasting blood sugar 105 mg/dL or less
- 1-hour blood sugar 190 mg/dL or less
- 2-hour blood sugar 165 mg/dL or less
- 3-hour blood sugar 145 or less

A diagnosis of GDM is made if two or more samples are increased or any >200 mg/dL. The patient should be advised regarding dietary control regardless. *(Alper, 2005e; Turok et al, 2003, pp. 1767–1768; Pennison and Egerman, 2001; Thomas et al, 2005)*

35. **(D)** In the general population, PID is the most common risk factor for ectopic pregnancy. Abortion has not been shown to increase the risk of ectopic pregnancy. Birth control pills change the cervical mucosa and make it less permeable to the gonorrhea bacteria. Women on the pill are, therefore, somewhat protected against the development of PID. Advanced maternal age does not place a patient at

increased risk. *(Alper, 2005f; Tenore, 2000, pp. 1086–1088; Shawkat, 2005)*

36. **(A)** Carcinoma of Bartholin's gland is rare (2% to 7% of vulvar cancer), but anytime a new asymptomatic mass in the area of Bartholin's gland is discovered in a postmenopausal woman, it should be investigated aggressively. It is most commonly diagnosed in the fifth decade after the presentation of an asymptomatic vulvar mass. An asymptomatic Bartholin's duct cyst in a young woman typically does not require treatment. *(Berek, 2002, pp. 1340–1341; Tierney et al, 2005, p. 736)*

37. **(D)** Fetal heart rates by EFM are described by rate and pattern of variability. Baseline is defined as 120 to 160 bpm. Late decelerations are a symmetrical fall in FHR beginning at or after the peak of the uterine contraction and returning to baseline only after the contraction has ended. They indicate possible uteroplacental insufficiency and imply some degree of fetal hypoxia. Remedial techniques are empirically designed to overcome uteroplacental insufficiency or to decrease cord compromise and improve placental and fetal oxygenation. Changing maternal position to right/left side lying recumbent or knee–chest position is a reasonable and quick first step. Late fetal heart rate (FHR) decelerations, however, are an ominous sign and should be evaluated quickly and seriously. Persistent non-reassuring tracings indicate the need for emergent delivery. Other remedial techniques include the following: IV infusion, mask oxygen, stopping oxytocics, subcutaneous terbutaline, and amnioinfusion. *(ICSI Guideline, 2004)*

38. **(A)** Mastitis is an inflammation of the breast that is common in breastfeeding women. In order to make a diagnosis of mastitis, there must be an area of hardness, pain, redness, and swelling in the breast. It can be caused by engorgement, a blocked milk duct, or a cracked nipple that allows bacteria to enter. The most common pathogen in infective mastitis is penicillin-resistant *S. aureus*. Less common pathogens are streptococcus or *Escherichia coli*. The preferred antibiotics are usually peni-

cillinase resistant penicillins such as dicloxacillin, with patients usually responding within 24 to 26 hours. In addition to antibiotic treatment, regular emptying of the breast by breastfeeding and/or pumping is necessary to prevent more bacteria from collecting in the breast. There is no evidence of risk to the healthy, term infant of continuing breastfeeding. Symptomatic treatment such as application of heat (e.g., a shower or a hot pack) to the breast prior to feeding may help the milk flow. *(Barbosa-Cesnik et al, 2003, p. 1611)*

39. **(A)** Fibroadenomas are the second most common type of benign breast disease. The most common type is fibrocystic breast changes. A firm, nontender, rubbery, freely movable nodule, 1 to 4 cm, in a young woman is a classic description. Fibroadenoma, unlike fibrocystic changes, do not change with the menstrual cycle. Fine needle aspiration would be acceptable in the diagnostic work-up of a possible fibroadenoma, with confirmation by histology. A physical exam that contains features worrisome for breast cancer includes any mass that is fixed, nipple retraction or bloody nipple discharge, accompanied by lymphadenopathy. An erythematous or eczematous-appearing rash on the breast or nipples brings Paget disease of the breast to mind; ductal carcinoma of the nipple needs to be diagnosed by biopsy and usually requires mastectomy. *(Toy et al, 2003, pp. 220–221)*

40. **(B)** Fibrocystic breast changes are the most common type of benign breast mass. Clinically they are often described as "rope-like," meaning they have the characteristics on palpation of feeling like a coiled rope. There is often diffuse nodularity although solitary cysts may range in size. Also, the size of an individual cyst may fluctuate throughout the menstrual cycle. Pain is the most common presenting symptom of fibrocystic breast change. Often, women will respond to dietary changes, such as decreased caffeine and/or tobacco. Danazol as well as bromocriptine, tamoxifen, and GnRH agonists are usually reserved for women with the most severe symptoms. *(Santen and Mansel, 2005, pp. 275–284)*

41. **(B)** Shoulder dystocia is a complication associated with macrosomia. Although there is no evidence that any one maneuver is superior to another in releasing an impacted shoulder or reducing the chance of injury, American College of Obstetricians and Gynecologists (ACOG) guidelines recommend performance of the McRoberts maneuver (B) as a reasonable initial approach. Fundal pressure (D) should never be attempted. *(ACOG Guideline, 2002)*

42. **(C)** Placenta previa can be distinguished from abruptio placenta by many factors. Placenta previa is characterized by a variable amount of blood loss, no abdominal discomfort, normal FHR, and no significant maternal history associated with the problem. Abruptio placenta, on the other hand, is associated with severe pain, abnormal FHR, usually continuous bleeding, and associated with a history in the mother such as cocaine use, abdominal trauma, maternal hypertension, multiple gestations, and polyhydramnios. In this case, one will need to rule out early labor (accompanying contractions, bloody mucus discharge), coagulopathy, hemorrhoids, vasa previa, cervical or vaginal lesion, or trauma. Vasa previa also occurs late in pregnancy, with vaginal bleeding occurring concomitantly with rupture of membranes. Vasa previa occurs when umbilical cord blood vessels transverse the membranes and cross the cervical os below the fetus. Fetal distress will also accompany vasa previa as the blood loss will be fetal; it requires immediate delivery and is accompanied by over 50% fetal mortality due to fetal exsanguination. *(Moses, 2005a/b; Chamberlain and Steer, 1999, pp. 1342–1345)*

43. **(B)** The accurate diagnosis of spontaneous rupture of membranes is important in order to ascertain whether the patient has begun labor or if the patient has premature rupture of membranes (this patient is 33 weeks). To evaluate for spontaneous rupture of membranes, a sterile speculum exam is performed with the patient in the dorsal lithotomy position. Evidence of rupture of membranes would be clear when blood-tinged fluid in the posterior fornix of the vagina, or pooling, and escape of clear fluid from the cervical os occurs when the patient coughs. Nitrazine testing can distinguish amniotic fluid from urine or vaginal secretion samples from speculum exam. If the pH is 7.1 to 7.3, it will show positive on nitrazine paper (dark blue). False positives can occur, however, with cervical mucus, blood, or semen in the sample. Until rupture of membranes has been ascertained, this patient should not be induced due to risk of prematurity in the fetus. Ultrasound determination of amniotic fluid volume is an important means of evaluating premature and preterm rupture of membranes, but it is not a means of diagnosing rupture of membranes. Digital cervical exam should not be performed as this would increase the risk of ascending infection. When examining the cervix, it might be useful to take a vaginal swab for culture in order to determine appropriate antibiotic if signs of infection develop later. *(Steer and Flint, 1999, p. 1060)*

44. **(C)** Hydatidiform mole is one component of gestational trophoblastic neoplasm (GTN). Moles occur in a gestation in which there is a proliferation of trophoblastic tissue. It can be a complete mole, in which there is no sign of a fetus, or a partial mole, in which the fetus may be viable, or there are findings consistent with a nonviable fetus. Young pregnant women (<20) and older (>40) reproductive ages have increased incidence as do patients with Asian, Latino, or Filipino ethnicity. The most common symptom of hydatidiform mole is several episodes of vaginal bleeding. A size-to-dates discrepancy also is common. Severe nausea and vomiting may occur as well. When signs and symptoms of preeclampsia present earlier than 24 weeks' gestation, molar pregnancy should be high on the differential. The trophoblast is responsible for production of human chorionic gonadotropin (hCG); therefore, the levels of beta hCG in the serum are greater than expected for the weeks of gestation. Ultrasound demonstrates a characteristic "snowstorm" appearance, and is the best means of diagnosing a mole. An incomplete abortion usually occurs prior to 12 to 14 weeks and often characterized by a decreasing

beta-hCG level. A fetal demise at 16 weeks would also have decreasing beta-hCG levels and would not be associated with hypertension. In twin gestation, there would be a higher level of beta hCG and a larger fundal height, but at 16 weeks, fetal heart tones should be heard. (*Alper, 2005g*)

45. **(B)** Enteroceles are common after an abdominal or vaginal hysterectomy and are most likely the result of a weakened support for the pouch of Douglas. An enterocele is a true hernia of the peritoneal cavity. It may be noticed as a separate bulge above the rectocele, and if it is large enough it may prolapse through the vagina. The specific diagnosis of enterocele may be made by transilluminating the bulge and seeing small bowel shadows within the sac. An enterocele contains small bowel and sometimes omentum. (*Stenchever et al, 2001, p. 576*)

46. **(D)** A rectocele is demonstrated on physical exam by asking the patient to strain while the clinician observes the vaginal area. A rectocele will appear as a bulging of the vaginal floor, as opposed to a cystocele, which would appear as a downward bulging of the anterior vagina. Constipation, which is a common problem during pregnancy, is further complicated by a rectocele. Treatment of the constipation is needed, as well as suggesting to the patient she might have to assist with the passage of stool by pressing down on the posterior vagina with her fingers. (*Stenchever et al, 2001, p. 574*)

47. **(C)** Abruptio placentae (i.e., placental abruption) refers to separation of the normally located placenta after the 20th week of gestation and prior to birth. Patients usually present with the following symptoms:

vaginal bleeding, 80%
abdominal or back pain and uterine tenderness, 70%
fetal distress, 60%
abnormal uterine contractions (e.g., hypertonic, high frequency), 35%
idiopathic premature labor, 25%
fetal death, 15%

Maternal and fetal death may occur because of hemorrhage and coagulopathy. The fetal perinatal mortality rate is approximately 15%. Likely risk factors for abruptio placentae are maternal hypertension, abdominal trauma, smoking, cocaine use, and advanced maternal age among others. (*Gaufberg, 2005*)

48. **(A)** The most likely diagnosis of this vaginitis is bacterial vaginosis (BV) and the treatment is metronidazole 500 mg twice daily for 7 days. Other treatments include vaginal preparations of metronidazole and also vaginal preparations of clindamycin. The other treatments would be inappropriate for the treatment of BV. Ciprofloxacin is a treatment for a urinary tract infection. Miconazole cream and fluconazole are treatments for yeast vaginitis. Doxycycline is the treatment for *Chlamydia trachomatis*. (*Tierney et al, 2005, pp. 707–709, 1391*)

49. **(C)** The only acceptable treatment option presented is miconazole cream or any vaginal preparation of an imidazole compound because they are poorly absorbed vaginally. Fluconazole is a category C and therefore should not be used. Metronidazole is a category B, but effectively treats BV, yeast candidiasis. Ciprofloxacin is a category C, but it is ineffective in the treatment of yeast infections. Doxycycline is the treatment for *Chlamydia trachomatis* and is a category C. It can cause permanent discoloration of the tooth enamel and therefore Doxycycline should not be used during the last half of pregnancy, during lactation, and during infancy through age 8 years. (*Lacy et al, 2005, pp. 332–336, 493–495, 630, 996–998; Lemcke et al, 2004, pp. 515–517*)

50. **(C)** The high-dose regimen of metronidazole is for the treatment of Trichomoniasis. *Trichomonas vaginalis* causes this common sexually transmitted disease. The clinical characteristics include a profuse yellow frothy, malodorous, pruritic discharge. Sometimes a strawberry cervix (subepithelial redness) is seen. The pH is between 4.5 and 6. The treatment for BV is also metronidazole, but 500 mg twice daily. Candidiasis would be treated with a imidazole. *Staphylococcus* infection could be treated

by many different antibiotics other than metronidazole. (*Scott et al, 2003, pp. 585–589*)

51. **(D)** The woman was treated appropriately with the doxacillin and it is best if she continues to breastfeed during the mastitis in order that she does not become engorged. Hot compresses may help, but what might be happening now is an abscess that may need surgical drainage. So it is best that she be referred to someone who can perform that procedure. (*Scott et al, 2003, p. 899*)

52. **(A)** Initial screening for gestational diabetes is accomplished by performing a 50-g, 1-hour glucose challenge test at 24 to 28 weeks of gestation. Chest x-ray (and all non-essential radiography) would be contraindicated as part of any antepartum screening. X-ray pelvimetry would not be indicated in a multipara who has previous successful vaginal deliveries. Screening for trichomoniasis is not recommended as it has not been shown to prevent preterm delivery, and treatment of trichomoniasis during pregnancy may be associated with increased low birth weight, preterm birth rate, and 2-year infant mortality rate. Protein-bound iodine and ESR would not be considered a routine test for any normal pregnancy, but may be indicated in specific cases. (*Alper, 2005h*)

53. **(B)** The first stage of labor is divided into two stages: latent and active. The latent stage refers to cervical effacement and early dilation. The active phase occurs when dilation has reached 3 to 4 cm or greater. The second stage of labor begins when cervical dilation is complete and ends with delivery of the infant. The third stage of labor begins after the infant is delivered and ends with placenta expulsion. The percentage of effacement varies with first and subsequent births, and does not necessarily correlate with the stage of labor. By the time the woman is in the first stage active labor (4 cm), 100% effacement has occurred. (*Alper, 2005i*)

54. **(E)** A reactive stress test (normal) is defined as two or more fetal heart rate increases in 20 minutes. The accelerations increase by 15 beats for 15 seconds and are related to fetal movement. A nonreactive stress test (abnormal) requires monitoring for two 20-minute periods where neither period yields adequate accelerations. (*Sweha, 2005*)

55. **(B)** Uterine atony is responsible for ~70% of postpartum hemorrhage (PPH). Muscular contraction of the uterus corpus, rather than coagulation, prevents excessive bleeding from the placental implantation site. Several factors may predispose to uterine atony including conditions that enlarge the uterus (e.g., multiple gestations, multiparity, microsomy, hydramnios), abnormal labor (e.g., precipitous or prolonged delivery, general anesthesia, prolonged labor, use of forceps), and conditions that interfere with uterine contraction (e.g., uterine leiomyomas, magnesium sulfate use). Vaginal and cervical lacerations are less common than uterine atony, but are serious and require prompt surgical attention. Retained placenta, secondary to lack of complete separation from the uterus, and abnormally adherent placenta, such as placenta accreta, are less common causes of postpartum hemorrhage. Although coagulation studies should be part of the work-up, in the immediate postpartum period, disorders of the coagulation system and platelets do not usually result in excessive bleeding. Fibrin deposition over the placental site and clots within supplying vessels play a significant role in the hours and days following delivery, and abnormalities in these areas can lead to late PPH or exacerbate bleeding from other causes, most notably, trauma. Uterine inversion is a rare condition. As a way of remembering the causes of PPH, several sources have suggested using the "4 Ts" as a mnemonic: tone, tissue, trauma, and thrombosis. (*Alper, 2005j; Smith and Brennan, 2004*)

56. **(A)** In this case, the elevated BP, ankle edema, and 1+ albuminuria are indicative of moderate preeclampsia. In addition, complaints of headache and dizziness would indicate a CNS component. Therapy for mild to moderate preeclampsia consists of bed rest and close monitoring, which increases central blood flow to the kidneys, heart, brain, and placenta

and may improve the condition. However, at 38 weeks' gestation, a diagnosis of moderate and certainly severe preeclampsia would likely be managed by induction of labor and delivery, once precise knowledge of the age and maturity of the fetus has been established. *(Sibai et al, 2005, pp. 794–795)*

57. **(D)** An Rh-negative woman must be tested for the presence of antibodies at the beginning of the third trimester so that the rare Rh sensitization of that pregnancy can be detected. She is given Rho (antiD) immune globulin if she is still sensitized, and amniocentesis to determine amniotic bilirubin levels if Rh antibodies are detected at 26 weeks. Cases of Rh sensitization may require intrauterine blood transfusion to prevent erythroblastosis fetalis. *(Kumar and Regan, 2005, p. 1257)*

58. **(E)** Magnesium sulfate is not recommended for preterm labor; evidence suggests no efficacy for preventing or delaying preterm birth, and a Cochrane systematic review (updated 2002) of 23 randomized trials with >2,000 women indicated a possible increase in infant mortality. The use of tocolytics is still controversial, since tocolytic agents do not work effectively for longer than about 48 hours, probably because of tachyphylaxis. Their major use is to postpone delivery and bide time for either maternal transfer or administration of corticosteroids to promote surfactant release (reducing neonatal respiratory distress syndrome by up to 50%). This effect is only significant at gestations up to 34 weeks; after 34 weeks it is usual to allow preterm labor to progress. Significant prolongation of pregnancy has been found for betamimetics (ritodrine, terbutaline). Ritodrine is FDA approved for tocolysis, and is only available in IV form. The betamimetics have many adverse effects including chest pain, dyspnea, tachycardia, palpitation, tremor, headaches, hypokalemia, hyperglycemia, and nausea/vomiting. Terbutaline, though not FDA approved for tocolysis, is widely used and cheaper than ritodrine, and can be delivered IV, subcutaneously, or orally. Nifedipine (calcium channel blocker) may be preferable to betamimetics. When compared to other tocolytic

agents (mainly betamimetics), calcium channel blockers significantly reduced rates of women giving birth within 7 days, if given before 34 weeks' gestation. Nifedipine's adverse effects include neonatal respiratory distress syndrome, necrotizing enterocolitis, intraventricular hemorrhage, and neonatal jaundice. Betamethasone may be given for preterm labor between 26 to 34 weeks' gestation. Steroids given to women expected to deliver preterm reduces mortality, respiratory distress syndrome, and intraventricular hemorrhage in preterm infants. *(Alper, 2005k; Steer and Flint, 1999, pp. 1060–1061)*

59. **(A)** The estimated date of confinement (EDC) or due date is calculated after obtaining a thorough menstrual history. The date of the last onset of normal menses is crucial and a light bleeding episode should not be mistaken for a normal period. A "normal" pregnancy lasts 40 ± 2 weeks. Calculated from the first day of the last normal menses, one adds 7 days to the first day of the last normal menstrual flow and subtracts 3 months. *(Trupin, 2004)*

60. **(B)** In healthy pregnant women who are not deficient in iron or folate, a modest fall in hemoglobin levels at this point of gestation is usually due to the relative greater expansion of plasma volume compared with the increase in hemoglobin mass and red blood cell volume that accompanies normal pregnancy. In the first trimester and at term, the hemoglobin level for most healthy women is ≥11 g/dL. During the second trimester, women experience a nadir in their hemoglobin levels where anemia is defined as less than 10.5 g/dL. *(Leveno et al, 2003, pp. 39–40)*

61. **(E)** Women and adolescents through age 20 years are at highest risk for chlamydial infection, but most reported data indicate that infection is prevalent among women aged 20 to 25. Therefore, age is the most important risk marker. Other patient characteristics associated with a higher prevalence of infection include being unmarried, from African American race, having a prior history of sexually transmitted disease, having new or multiple sex

partners, having had cervical ectopy, and using barrier contraceptives inconsistently. The optimal interval for screening is open to clinical judgment. For example, in women with a previous negative screening test, timing for rescreening should take into account changes in sexual partners. For those at low risk for infection (e.g., in a mutually monogamous relationship with no history of chlamydial infection), it may not be necessary to screen frequently. For previously infected patients, rescreening at 6 to 12 months may be appropriate because of high rates of reinfection. Screening in pregnancy should be done for all women less than age 25. The timing for the screening, however, is also uncertain. Screening early in pregnancy provides a chance to improve pregnancy outcomes associated with chlamydial infection (e.g., low birth weight and premature delivery). Screening in the third trimester could be more effective in preventing transmission to the infant during birth. Until the advent of urine-based screening tests, routine screening of men was rarely performed. Until urine-based screening became available, screening was rarely done in males. Trials are currently underway to assess the effectiveness of screening asymptomatic men for the purpose of reducing infection among women. *(Berg AO, pp. 90–94; U.S. Preventive Services Task Force, 2001)*

62. **(D)** HRT has been shown to cause a small increase in risk of thromboembolism from a baseline risk of 1 in 10,000 women per year to 3 in 10,000 women per year. If there is a past or family history of blood clot, appropriate investigations must be carried out and fully discussed. Estrogen-only therapy given to women with an intact uterus increases the risk of endometrial hyperplasia (thickening of the lining of the uterus) and eventually endometrial cancer. Daily estrogen combined with progestogen given for 10 to 14 days per month (sequential HRT) reduces this risk but does not eliminate it. Sequential HRT given for more than 5 years will increase the risk of endometrial cancer by a small amount but no increased risk appears to apply to estrogen combined with daily progestogen (continuous combined or period-free HRT). Current consensus is that HRT taken

for less than 5 years does not significantly increase the risk of breast cancer; however, studies have shown that after 5 years of use, there is a small increased risk. The largest randomized trial with HRT (Women's Health Initiative (WHI) with 16,608 patients) showed reduction in hip fractures, vertebral fractures, and osteoporotic fractures. However, since fracture-risk reduction may require use of HRT for at least 5 years and its effectiveness appears to diminish rapidly after cessation of treatment, the risks of long-term use likely outweigh the benefits. Estrogen use has been associated with a lower risk of colon cancer, although mechanisms remain unclear. After 6.8 years of follow-up, the Heart and Estrogen/progestin Replacement Study (HERS) study showed a nonsignificant protective effect of estrogen (RR 0.81, 95% CI 0.46–1.45), whereas the WHI trial demonstrated a nominally significant protective effect in healthy postmenopausal women after 3 years of HRT use. *(Hulley et al, 2002, pp. 58–66; Writing Group for the Women's Health Initiative Investigators, 2002, pp. 321–333; Hulley et al, 1998, pp. 611–612)*

63. **(A)** In the classification of spontaneous abortions, an incomplete abortion is characterized by the passage of tissue and an open cervical os. A complete abortion would have a similar history of passing tissue; however, pain or cramping would have subsided and the cervix would be closed. In a threatened abortion, there will be bleeding, but no passage of tissue, and the cervical os would be closed. A missed abortion is defined by no symptoms and a closed os. With an incompetent cervix, women present with painless cervical dilatation. The treatment of an incomplete abortion is dilatation and curettage. Serum-hCG levels are useful to follow after spontaneous abortion; hCG levels should halve every 48 to 72 hours and a plateau could indicate residual retained tissue. *(Toy et al, 2003, pp. 96–98)*

64. **(B)** This patient has secondary amenorrhea. The most common reason for amenorrhea in a woman of reproductive age is pregnancy, which has been ruled out. In the differential diagnosis for her secondary amenorrhea, possibilities include (among others) endometritis,

hypothyroidism, and ovarian insufficiency (or failure). For a patient of this age, ovarian failure is more likely. Studies for establishing the diagnosis of ovarian insufficiency are as follows: (1) serum FSH level, (2) serum LH, and (3) serum estradiol. Persistently elevated gonadotropin levels (especially when accompanied by low serum estradiol levels) are diagnostic of ovarian failure. Ovarian antibody assay is a test with low sensitivity and specificity for determining the diagnosis of autoimmune ovarian failure. Serum testosterone and DHEAS levels should be ordered only if the patient shows symptoms of androgen excess (acne, hirsutism, male-pattern balding, clitoromegaly) or hypertension. The hysterosalpingogram is part of an infertility workup that may demonstrate Asherman syndrome, but is more invasive and not indicated until ovarian failure has been excluded. *(Nelson et al, 2005a; Nelson et al, 2005b; Bakalov and Nelson, 2005)*

65. **(C)** Because pregnancy-induced hypertension (including preeclampsia and eclampsia) has been associated with raised rates of maternal morbidity and mortality and with many increased risks to the fetus, patients with moderate to severe eclampsia should be delivered if the disease develops after 34 weeks' gestation. Magnesium sulfate is the treatment of choice for eclampsia as it reduces the risk of eclampsia and probably maternal death. Oral hypertensive drug therapy, though decreasing the risk of severe hypertension, has not been associated with decreased risk in the infant or mother. There is insufficient evidence for any effects of plasma volume expansion. Intravascular volume expansion carries a serious risk of volume overload, which could lead to pulmonary or cerebral edema. Also, large volume expansion often requires invasive monitoring of intravascular pressure, which includes procedures with risks of their own. Patients with a platelet count greater than $40,000/mm^3$ are unlikely to bleed and do not require transfusion unless the platelet count drops to $<20,000/mm^3$. Patients who undergo cesarean section should be transfused if their platelet count is less than $50,000/mm^3$. *(Alper, 2005k; Sibai et al, 2005, pp. 793–794; Padden, 1999, p. 837; Duley et al, 2003,)*

66. **(C)** Oligohydramnios, diminished amniotic fluid volume, may be associated with intrauterine growth retardation, and would result in a fundal height lower than expected. The fundal height directly correlates with gestational age in weeks from 16 to 38 weeks' gestation—e.g., at 32 weeks it should measure 32 cm. This measurement, however, is subject to measurement problems. In general, a fundal height that is >3 cm larger than the gestational age of the pregnancy in the third trimester requires further testing to determine the cause. *(Jazayeri and Contreras, 2005; Baxter and Sehdev, 2005)*

67. **(A)** Pregnancy-induced hypertension is defined as blood pressure of >140/90 mm Hg on at least two separate occasions that are 6 hours or more apart. It is considered when maternal blood pressure reaches 140/90 or greater for the first time during pregnancy, and proteinuria is not present. Preeclampsia is defined by a blood pressure increase to 140/90 post 20 weeks' gestation with proteinuria. Eclampsia is defined by the development of seizures in a woman with preeclampsia. Chronic hypertension is defined as that occurring prior to the pregnancy or before 20 weeks' gestation (blood pressure of 140/90 or greater). The diagnosis of HELLP syndrome requires the presence of hemolysis based on exam of the peripheral smear, elevated indirect bilirubin levels, or low serum haptoglobin levels in association with significant elevation in liver enzymes and a platelet count below $100,000/mm^3$ after ruling out other causes of hemolysis and thrombocytopenia. *(Alper, 2005k)*

68. **(A)** Eating and drinking during early labor in a low-risk pregnancy has not been associated with dystocia or adverse outcomes. Electronic fetal monitoring in low-risk women may increase the rate of obstetric interventions with no apparent benefit. Bed rest is not recommended as it has been shown to be associated with longer duration of labor, greater need for analgesia, and greater incidence of fetal heart abnormalities. Walking during labor has not been found to have an effect on duration of labor nor affect maternal or fetal outcomes.

There is insufficient evidence to recommend perineal shaving for women on admission for labor, demonstrating no differences in maternal febrile morbidity. (*Alper, 2005l*)

69. **(A)** Hot flashes occur in 70% to 90% of menopausal women. The flashes may begin perimenopausally when relative estrogen deficiency occurs together with cycle irregularity secondary to anovulation, but more often they begin during or after the menopause. Hot flashes usually begin as a sudden sensation of heat centered on the face and upper chest that rapidly becomes generalized and lasts between 2 and 4 minutes. It can be associated with profuse perspiration and occasional palpitations, and is often followed by chills and shivering. More than 80% of women who have hot flashes will continue to have them for more than 1 year. Untreated hot flashes usually stop spontaneously in 2 to 3 years. Estrogen therapy will usually cause resolution of the hot flashes within 3 to 6 weeks. (*Alper, 2005m*)

70. **(A)** In women with premature labor, beta-adrenergic agonists have been clearly shown to reduce the incidence of delivery within 24 and 48 hours of administration. These tocolytic agents have not been shown to consistently reduce the rates of preterm delivery, low birth weight, severe respiratory distress, or perinatal death. A statistically nonsignificant trend toward reduced perinatal mortality has been suggested in women given beta-adrenergic agonists earlier in pregnancy for preterm labor before 28 weeks' gestation. It appears that more effective use of the 24 to 48 hours gained by tocolysis with beta-adrenergic agonists holds promise for reducing perinatal morbidity and mortality, perhaps through more liberal use of predelivery glucocorticoid therapy. (*Alper, 2005n*)

71. **(B)** The most common cause of spontaneous abortion in the first 12 weeks of pregnancy is chromosomal anomalies (accounting for about half of abortions). Cytogenetic evaluations of specimens of sporadic abortions have revealed an overall incidence of chromosomal abnormalities between 50% to 70%. Maternal lupus anticoagulant, incompetent cervix, maternal tobacco abuse, and inadequate progesterone during the luteal phase can also be associated with early abortion. Maternal disease is more likely to be responsible in second trimester miscarriage. (*Leveno et al, 2003, p. 48; Alper, 2005*)

72. **(A)** Childbirth can injure the pelvic floor muscles resulting in a prolapsed uterus. The transverse and uterosacral ligaments are particularly affected. The degree of protrusion of the uterus in relationship to the introitus determines the classification. Slight prolapse is when the uterus descends toward the introitus, but is still in the vagina. Moderate prolapse is when the uterus and cervix descend to the introitus, and marked prolapse, or procidentia, is when the uterus and cervix descend past the introitus and the vagina is inverted. When the prolapse interferes with daily life or quality of life, a surgical repair is indicated. (*Tierney et al, 2005, p.717*)

73. **(D)** Suppression of FSH and LH is the primary effect of oral contraceptives. They may also cause changes in tubal mobility and ovum transport, sperm penetration of the egg, disruption of implantation of a fertilized egg, and change in cervical mucus to make it harder for sperm to swim toward the egg. (*Lemcke et al, 2004, p. 550*)

74. **(C)** During the initial 3 months of oral contraceptive use, break-through bleeding is a common side effect and can be best managed by encouraging the patient to continue. After initiating therapy, when break-through bleeding occurs during the third week of the cycle it is due to a lack of progestin and is best managed by changing to a pill with a higher progestin component. (*Beckmann et al, 2006, pp. 246–247*)

75. **(E)** Emergency contraception is most effective when taken within 72 hours of unprotected intercourse. When taken within the recommended time frame, emergency contraception is 75% effective in preventing pregnancies. It is not an abortive and therefore will not cause an already established pregnancy to be terminated. The Yuzpe method is the most common method. It utilizes four tablets of oral contraceptives containing 0.05-mg ethinyl

estradiol and 0.5-mg DL-norgestrel (Ovral). Two tablets are taken at once and then two more tablets 12 hours later. An alternate regimen is the progestin-only emergency contraceptive (Plan B). *(Beckmann et al, 2006, p. 257)*

76. **(C)** Although all the methods listed (bed rest, devices, and pharmacologic agents and surgery) work to some degree to treat an incompetent cervix, the generally accepted treatment is surgical. A cervical cerclage is a suture or bands that are placed surgically on the cervix to keep it closed prior to delivery. The sutures are removed after fetal maturity has been achieved (about 37 weeks). Labor and delivery occurs rapidly after the removal of the cerclage. The terbutaline and magnesium sulfate are pharmacologic agents used for the medical management of preterm labor with a competent cervix. *(Scott et al, 2003, pp. 83–85)*

77. **(D)** There is great variability in the symptoms with which endometriosis will present. Some women may even be asymptomatic, but endometrial lesions may be found during laparoscopy for other gynecologic reasons. The classic symptoms of endometriosis are dysmenorrhea, deep thrust dyspareunia, infertility, abnormal bleeding, and pelvic pain. Thorough history taking greatly helps in the diagnosis, but the definitive diagnosis is made when the lesions are visualized during laparoscopic surgery or by tissue biopsy. *(Beckmann et al, 2006, pp. 310–307)*

78. **(D)** When the presence of endometrial glands, stroma, and hemosiderin-laden macrophages is noted microscopically on a tissue sample taken from the pelvic cavity, outside of the uterus, the diagnosis of endometriosis can be made. *(Beckmann et al, 2006, pp. 301)*

79. **(B)** A prior tubal pregnancy contraindicates IUD use. Condoms and spermicides are free of hormonal side effects and, if used in combination, are reasonably effective. This patient's hypertension is mild and controlled and unlikely to be negatively affected by either low dose or progesterone-only oral contraceptives. Although there can be an association between urinary tract infections and diaphragm

use in susceptible women, this would not be an absolute contraindication to diaphragm use. *(Lemcke et al, 2004, pp. 549–559)*

80. **(C)** Emergency estrogen/progesterone postcoital contraception (EC) is indicated when a condom breaks, and can be used up to 72 hours after intercourse. It is less effective when given 72 to 120 hours (3 to 5 days) after unprotected intercourse. It is not indicated for a woman who has missed an oral contraceptive pill. A pregnancy test is not useful since emergency contraception prevents a pregnancy rather than aborting an existing pregnancy. If administered before ovulation, EC may inhibit follicular development and maturation, resulting in anovulation and deficient luteal function. Treatment following ovulation may affect the endometrium, thus inhibiting implantation. Menses and fertility, however, will return with the next cycle. *(Samra and Wood, 2004)*

References

Albers JR, Hull SK, Wesley RM. Medical management of anovulatory dysfunctional uterine bleeding. *Am Fam Physician*. 2004; 69:1924.

Alper BS (via DynaMed Systematic Literature Surveillance). Infertility. DynaMed [database online]. 2005a; 9(3). Available at: http://www.DynamicMedical.com. Accessed July 23, 2005.

Alper BS (via DynaMed Systematic Literature Surveillance). Atrophic vaginitis. DynaMed [database online]. 2005b; 9(3). Available at: http://www.DynamicMedical.com. Accessed July 25, 2005.

Alper BS. Pelvic inflammatory disease (PID). Sontheimer D (Reviewer). DynaMed [database online]. 2005c; 9(3). Available at: http://www.DynamicMedical.com. Accessed July 28, 2005.

Alper BS (via DynaMed Systematic Literature Surveillance). Multiple gestations. DynaMed [databse online]. 2005d; 9(3). Available at: http://www.DynamicMedical.com. Accessed July 23, 2005.

Alper BS (via DynaMed Systematic Literature Surveillance). Gestational diabetes. DynaMed [database online]. 2005e; 9(3). Available at: http://www.DynamicMedical.com. Accessed July 28, 2005.

Alper BS. Ectopic pregnancy. Zelnick CJ (Reviewer). DynaMed [database online]. 2005f; 9(3). Available at: http://www.DynamicMedical.com. Accessed July 23, 2005.

Alper BS (via DynaMed Systematic Literature Surveillance). Hydatidiform mole. DynaMed [database online]. 2005g; 9(3). Available at: http://www.DynamicMedical.com. Accessed July 27, 2005.

Alper BS (via DynaMed Systematic Literature Surveillance). Hydatidiform mole. DynaMed [database online]. 2005h; 9(3). Available at: http://www.DynamicMedical.com. Accessed July 23, 2005.

Alper BS Postpartum hemorrhage. Rose D (Reviewer). DynaMed [database online]. 2005i; 9(3). Available at: http://www.DynamicMedical.com

Alper BS (via DynaMed Systematic Literature Surveillance). Premature rupture of membranes (PROM). DynaMed [database online]. 2005j; 9(3). Available at: http://www.DynamicMedical.com

Alper BS (via DynaMed Systematic Literature Surveillance). Pregnancy-induced hypertension (PIH). DynaMed [database online]. 2005k; 9(3). Available at: http://www.DynamicMedical.com. Accessed July 23, 2005.

Alper BS (via DynaMed Systematic Literature Surveillance). Overview of labor and delivery. DynaMed [database online]. 2005l; 9(3). Available at: http://www.DynamicMedical.com. Accessed October 12, 2005.

Alper BS (via DynaMed Systematic Literature Surveillance). Menopause. DynaMed [database online]. 2005m; 9(3). Available at: http://www.DynamicMedical.com. Accessed October 17, 2005.

Alper BS (via DynaMed Systematic Literature Surveillance). Preterm labor. DynaMed [database online]. 2005n; 9(3). Available at: http://www.DynamicMedical.com. Accessed October 13, 2005.

Alper BS. Miscarriage. Prine L (Reviewer). DynaMed [database online]. 2005; 9(3). Available at: http://www.DynamicMedical.com. Accessed October 11, 2005.

Alzubaidi N, Calis KA, Nelson LM. Dysmenorrhea. eMedicine [online]. 2004. Available at: http://www.emedicine.com/med/topic606.htm. Accessed August 12, 2005.

American College of Obstetricians and Gynecologists (ACOG). Shoulder dystocia. Washington, DC 2002; (ACOG practice bulletin; no. 40).Available at: http://www.guideline.gov/summary/summary.aspx?view_id=1&doc_id=3988. Accessed July 23, 2005.

Bakalov V, Nelson LM. Ovarian failure. eMedicine [online]. 2005. Available at: http://www.emedicine.com/med/topic1700.htm#section~workup. Accessed July 29, 2005.

Barbosa-Cesnik C, Schwartz K, Foxman B. Lactation mastitis. *JAMA*. April 2003; 289(13):1612.

Baxter JK, Sehdev HM. Oligohydramnios. eMedicine [online]. 2005. Available at: http://www.emedicine.com/radio/topic898.htm. Accessed March 22, 2006.

Beckmann CR, Ling FW, Smith RP, Barzansky BM, Herbert WN, Laube DW (eds), *Obstetrics and Gynecology*, 5th ed. Philadelphia, PA: Lippincott Williams & Wilkins; 2006.

Berg AO, Allan JD, Frame PS, Homer CJ, Lieu TA, Mulrow CD, Orleans CT, Peipert JF, Pender NJ, Sox HC Jr, Teusch SM, Westhoff C, Woolf SH; US Preventive Services Task Force. Related Articles, Links No abstract Screening for chlamydia infection: recommendations and rationale. U.S. Preventive Services Task Force. *Am J Nurs*. 2002 Oct; 102(10):87–92; discussion 93

Berek, JS (ed), *Novak's Gynecology*, 13th ed., Philadelphia, PA: Lippincott Williams & Wilkins; 2002.

Berkowitz RS, Goldstein DP. Chorionic tumors. *N Engl J Med*. 1996; 335(23):1743–1744.

Buhling KJ, Henrich W, Starr E, et al. Risk for gestational diabetes and hypertension for women with twin pregnancy compared to singleton pregnancy. *Arch Gynecol Obstet*. November 2003; 269(1):34–35.

Chamberlain G, Steer P. ABCs of labour care: Obstetric emergencies. *BMJ*. 1999; 318:1342.

Cohen LS, Miner C, Brown EW, et al. Premenstrual daily fluoxetine for premenstrual dysphoric disorder: A placebo-controlled, clinical trial using computerized diaries. *Obstet Gynecol*. September 2002; 100(3):439–440.

Crowther CA, Hiller JE, Doyle LW. Magnesium sulphate for preventing preterm birth in threatened preterm labour. The Cochrane Database of Systematic Reviews 2002 (4). Art. no.: CD001060.

Cunningham FG, Gant NF, Leveno KJ, Gilstrap LC III, Hauth JC, Wenstrom KD (eds), *Williams Obstetrics*, 21st ed. New York: McGraw Hill; 2001.

Daly S. Endometrioma/Endometriosis. eMedicine [online]. 2004. Available at: http://www.emedicine.com/radio/topic250.htm. Accessed July 29, 2005.

Duley L, Gülmezoglu AM, Henderson-Smart DJ. Magnesium sulphate and other anticonvulsants for women with preeclampsia. The Cochrane Database of Systematic Reviews 2003 (2). Art. no.: CD000025.

Frey KA and Patel KS. Initial evaluation and management of infertility by the primary care physician. *Mayo Clin Proc.* 2004; 79(11):1439–43.

Garcia JE, Nelson LM, Wallach EE. Infertility. eMedicine [online]. 2005. Available at: http://www.emedicine.com/med/topic3535.htm. Accessed July 29, 2005.

Gaufberg SV. Abruptio placentae. eMedicine [online]. 2005. Available at: http://www.emedicine.com/EMERG/topic12.htm. Accessed July 29, 2005.

Goldman L, Ausiello D (eds), *Goldman: Cecil Textbook of Medicine,* 22nd ed. Philadelphia, PA: Saunders; 2004.

Hernandez E. Gestational trophoblastic neoplasia. [online]. 2005. Available at: http://www.emedicine.com/med/topic866.htm. Accessed March 25, 2006.

Hulley S, Furberg C, Barrett-Connor E, Cauley J, Grady D, Haskell W, et al. Noncardiovascular disease outcomes during 6.8 years of hormone therapy. HERS II. *JAMA.* 2002; 288:61–62.

Hulley S, Grady D, Bush T, et al. Randomised trial of estrogen plus progestin for secondary prevention of coronary heart disease in postmenopausal women. *JAMA.* 1998; 280:611–612.

Institute for Clinical Systems Improvement (ICSI) *Intrapartum fetal heart rate management.* Bloomington (MN): ICSI; 2004. (45 references). Available at: http://www.guideline.gov/summary/summary.aspx?view_id=1&doc_id=5992#s24. Accessed August 5, 2005.

Jazayeri A, Contreras D. Macrosomia. eMedicine [online]. 2005. Available at: http://www.emedicine.com/med/topic606.htm. Accessed March 22, 2006.

Kerlikowske K, Smith-Bindman R, Ljung BM, Grady D. Evaluation of abnormal mammography results and palpable breast abnormalities. *Ann Intern Med.* 2003; 139:277–278.

Kumar S, Regan F. Management of pregnancies with RhD alloimmunisation. *BMJ.* 2005; 330:1257.

Lacy CF, Armstrong LL, Goldman MP, Lance LL (eds), *Lexi-Comp's Drug Information Handbook,* 13th ed. Hudson, OH: Lexi-Comp; 2005.

Lemcke DP, Marshall LA, Pattison J, and Crowley DS (eds), *Current Care of Women: Diagnosis and Treatment.* New York: Lange Medical/McGraw-Hill; 2004, pp. 199, 474–477, 494, 532–535.

Leveno KL et al. *Williams Manual of Obstetrics,* 21st ed. New York: McGraw Hill; 2003, pp. 39–40.

Moore LE, Ware D. Hydatidiform mole. eMedicine [online]. 2005. Available at: http://www.emedicine.com/med/topic1047.htm. Accessed March 25, 2006.

Moses S. Vasa previa. Family Practice Notebook [online]. 2005a. Available at: http://www.fpnotebook.com/OB15.htm. Accessed July 29, 2005.

Moses S. Non-stress test. Family Practice Notebook [online]. 2005b. Available at: http://www.fpnotebook.com/OB49.htm. Accessed July 29, 2005.

Nelson LM, Bakalov V, Pastor C. Amenorrhea. eMedicine [online]. 2005a. Available at: http://www.emedicine.com/med/topic117.htm. Accessed July 29, 2005.

Nelson LM, Bakalov V, Pastor C. Ovarian insufficiency. eMedicine [online]. 2005b. Available at: http://www.emedicine.com/med/topic3374.htm#section~workup. Accessed July 29, 2005.

Padden M. HELLP syndrome: Recognition and perinatal management. *Am Fam Physician.* 1999;60:837.

Pennison EH, Egerman RS. Perinatal outcomes in gestational diabetes: A comparison of criteria for diagnosis. *Am J Obstet Gynecol.* May 2001;184(6):1120.

Reuter KL. Adenomyosis (Uterus). eMedicine [online]. 2004. Available at: http://www.emedicine.com/radio/topic737.htm. Accessed July 29, 2005.

Samra OM, Wood E. Contraception. eMedicine [online]. 2004. Available at: http://www.emedicine.com/med/topic3211.htm. Accessed March 22, 2006.

Santen RJ, Mansel R. Benign breast disorders. *N Engl J Med.* July 2005; 353(3):277–278.

Scott JR, Gibbs RS, Karlan BY, Haney AF (eds), *Danforth's Obstetrics and Gynecology,* 9th ed. Philadelphia, PA: Lippincott Williams & Wilkins; 2003.

Shawkat E. Risk factors for ectopic pregnancy. BestBets [online]. 2005. Available at: http://www.bestbets.org/cgi-bin/bets.pl?record=00921. Accessed July 29, 2005.

Sibai B, Dekker G, Kupferminc M. Preeclampsia. *Lancet* 2005; 365:794–795.

Smith JR, Brennan BG. Postpartum hemorrhage. eMedicine [online]. 2004. Available at: http://www.emedicine.com/med/topic3568.htm. Accessed July 29, 2005.

Steer P, Flint C. ABCs of labour care: Preterm labour and premature rupture of membranes. *BMJ*. 1999; 318:1060–1061.

Stenchever MA, Droegemueller W, Herbst HA, Mishell DR (eds), *Stenchever: Comprehensive Gynecology*, 4th ed. St. Louis, MO: Mosby; 2001.

Suckling J, Lethaby A, Kennedy R. Local oestrogen for vaginal atrophy in postmenopausal women. The Cochrane Database of Systematic Reviews 2003 (4). Art. no.: CD001500.

Sweha A, Hacker TW, Nuovo J. Interpretation of the electronic fetal heart rate during labor. American Family Physician [online]. 2005. Available at: www.aafp.org/afp/990501ap/2487.html. Accessed July 29, 2005.

Taylor A. ABCs of subfertility: Making a diagnosis. *BMJ* [online]. 2003; 327. Available at: http://bmj.bmjjournals.com/. Accessed July 27, 2005.

Tenore JL. Ectopic pregnancy. *Am Fam Physician*. 2000; 61:1080–1088.

Thomas R, Moore TR, Warshak C. Diabetes mellitus and pregnancy. eMedicine.[online]. 2005. Available at: http://www.emedicine.com/med/topic3249.htm. Accessed July 29, 2005.

Tierney LM, Jr., McPhee SJ, Papadakis MA (eds), *Current Medical Diagnosis & Treatment 2005*, 44th ed. New York: McGraw-Hill; 2005.

Tintinalli JE, Kelen JD, Stapczynski JS (eds), *Emergency Medicine, A comprehensive Study Guide*, 6th ed. New York: McGraw-Hill; 2004.

Toy EC, Baker III B, Ross PJ, Gilstrap III LC. *Case Files: Obstetrics Gynecology*. New York: McGraw-Hill (Lange Medical Books); 2003, p. 220–221.

Trupin SR. Common pregnancy complaints and questions. eMedicine [online]. 2004. Available at: http://www.emedicine.com/med/topic3238.htm. Accessed July 29, 2005.

Turok DK, Ratcliffe SD, Baxley EG. Management of gestational diabetes mellitus. *Am Fam Physician*. 2003; 68:1767–1772, 1767–1768.

U.S. Preventive Services Task Force. Screening for chlamydial infection—including ocular prophylaxis in newborns. *Guide to Clinical Preventive Services*, 2nd ed. Baltimore, MD: Williams & Wilkins; 1996. (Updated in 2001)

Wong SF, Lam MH, Ho LC. Transvaginal sonography in the detection of retained products of conception after first-trimester spontaneous abortion. *J Clin Ultrasound*. September 2002; 30(7):430.

Writing Group for the Women's Health Initiative Investigators. Risk and benefits of estrogen plus progestin in healthy postmenopausal women. Principal results from the Women's Health Initiative randomized controlled trial. *JAMA*. 2002; 288:321–333.

Yip SK, Sahota D, Cheung LP, Lam P, Haines CJ, Chung TK. Accuracy of clinical diagnostic methods of threatened abortion. *Gynecol Obstet Invest*. 2003; 56:39–41.

SECTION III
Pediatrics

Questions

Rachel A. Carlson, MSBS, PA-C

DIRECTIONS (Questions 1 through 65): Each of the numbered items or incomplete statements in this section is followed by answers or by completions of the statement. Select the ONE lettered answer or completion that is BEST in each case.

Questions 1 through 65

1. Which of the following sets gives the three MOST common bacterial pathogens for acute otitis media in an 18-month-old child?

   (A) *Streptococcus pneumoniae, Staphylococcus aureus, Haemophilus influenzae*

   (B) *Streptococcus pneumoniae, Moraxella catarrhalis, Haemophilus influenzae*

   (C) *Streptococcus pneumoniae, Moraxella catarrhalis, Mycoplasma pneumonia*

   (D) *Streptococcus pyogenes, Haemophilus influenzae, Pseudomonas aeruginosa*

2. A 9-month-old Caucasian male is being evaluated at the pediatrician's office. He is slightly irritable and extremely pale. His physical exam is otherwise unremarkable. Dietary history reveals a "picky eater," but he eagerly takes six 8-ounce bottles of regular cow's milk per day. The following laboratory tests were obtained:

   Hemoglobin 4.3 mg/dL (normal: 10.5 to 14.0)
   Hematocrit 13.1% (normal: 33 to 42)
   Mean corpuscular volume (MCV) 65 fL (normal: 74 to 91)

   Which of the following is the MOST likely diagnosis?

   (A) acquired aplastic anemia

   (B) beta thalassemia major

   (C) iron deficiency anemia

   (D) megaloblastic anemia

3. A 5-year-old child presents to the office with complaints of a sore throat and fever for 2 days. She is diagnosed with acute pharyngitis. Which of the following is the MOST common organism for her infection etiology?

   (A) adenovirus

   (B) group A beta-hemolytic streptococcus

   (C) group C streptococcus

   (D) *Streptococcus pneumoniae*

4. All of the following are cardinal signs of pediatric congestive heart failure EXCEPT

   (A) bradycardia

   (B) cardiomegaly

   (C) hepatomegaly

   (D) tachypnea

5. A 14-year-old girl presents to the office for a third visit over the past month complaining of fatigue and pain in her pelvic bones. Her previous evaluation included the following laboratory tests:

Heterophile antibody test: negative
Hematocrit: 34%

Since her last visit to the office, she has lost 4 pounds. Her mother reports she has a poor appetite. On physical exam, she is pale with several large ecchymotic areas on her legs and inguinal lymphadenopathy. Which of the following is the MOST likely diagnosis?

(A) anorexia nervosa
(B) acute lymphoblastic leukemia
(C) Crohn's disease
(D) infectious mononucleosis/Epstein–Barr virus

6. A 4-month-old infant presents with lethargy, fever, marked irritability, a bulging fontanelle, and positive Kernig's and Brudzinski's signs. A lumbar puncture reveals elevated lymphocytes, normal protein concentration, and normal glucose concentration. Which of the following is the MOST likely diagnosis?

(A) bacterial meningitis
(B) infectious mononucleosis
(C) tuberculous meningitis
(D) viral meningitis

7. Three weeks ago, an 8-year-old female was diagnosed with strep pharyngitis based upon a positive throat culture for group A beta-hemolytic streptococcus. Today, she returns to the clinic with evidence of polyarthritis. The differential diagnosis includes rheumatic fever. What additional finding would allow you to make the diagnosis of rheumatic fever based upon the modified Jones criteria?

(A) acute pharyngitis
(B) arthralgia
(C) carditis
(D) erythema multiforme

8. Idiopathic thrombocytopenia purpura is the most common thrombocytopenia of childhood. Which of the following laboratory tests should be ordered to substantiate this diagnosis?

(A) antinuclear antibody test
(B) bleeding time
(C) differential count
(D) platelet count

9. A patient is seen at the clinic for her health maintenance checkup. She claims to have started her first menstrual period last week. On physical exam, her breast development shows the areola and papilla, forming a secondary mound. Her genital exam reveals an abundance of coarse, curly pubic hair covering the labia and mons pubis. According to Tanner's stages of sexual maturation, at what stage would you assess her sexual maturity?

(A) Tanner stage II
(B) Tanner stage III
(C) Tanner stage IV
(D) Tanner stage V

10. During the first year of life, what would be the expected average growth for an infant who weighs 7 pounds at birth?

(A) 6 pounds at 2 weeks, 12 pounds at 5 months, 18 pounds at 12 months
(B) 6 pounds at 3 weeks, 21 pounds at 4 months, 30 pounds at 12 months
(C) 7 pounds at 2 weeks, 14 pounds at 4 months, 21 pounds at 12 months
(D) 7 pounds at 2 weeks, 21 pounds at 6 months, 30 pounds at 12 months

11. A 3-year-old child presents to the emergency department with bruises on his body. His mother claims that her son sustained these bruises when he tumbled down the stairs 8 days ago. Which of the following colors would you expect the bruises to be if this occurred as stated?

(A) brown
(B) purple
(C) red
(D) yellow

12. An 8-month-old infant presents with a 5-day history of a runny nose in late January. Then over the past 3 days she has developed a temperature of 101.2°F and vomiting (three times in 24 hours). This morning she developed watery, nonbloody, nonmucous diarrhea. Which of the following is the MOST likely causative organism for her illness?

    (A) *Clostridium difficile*
    (B) *Giardia lamblia*
    (C) adenovirus
    (D) rotavirus

13. With normal growth and development, the angular alignment of children's legs progresses through a series of developmental stages. Which of the following children have angular development in the lower extremities considered to be PATHOLOGIC?

    (A) 12-month-old male with genu varum
    (B) 36-month-old female with genu valgum
    (C) 36-month-old female with genu varum
    (D) 60-month-old male with genu valgum

14. Which of the following is the first sign of puberty in a normal male?

    (A) appearance of axillary hair
    (B) appearance of pubic hair
    (C) deepening of the voice
    (D) enlargement of the testes

15. A previously healthy, active 18-month-old child presents with unilateral nasal obstruction and foul-smelling discharge. The child's physical exam is otherwise unremarkable. Which of the following is the MOST likely diagnosis?

    (A) choanal atresia, unilateral
    (B) deviated nasal septum
    (C) nasal foreign body
    (D) nasal polyp

16. A 9-year-old child, who was diagnosed with a viral upper respiratory infection 2 weeks ago, returns to the clinic with a complaint of a 2-day history of drooping of one side of her mouth. She is afebrile with a blood pressure of 110/60 mm Hg. Her physical exam reveals an inability to completely close her left eye, inability to wrinkle her forehead, and drooping of her mouth on the left side. Her smile is asymmetric. The remainder of her exam is otherwise normal. Which of the following is the MOST likely diagnosis?

    (A) Bell's palsy
    (B) botulism
    (C) brain stem glioma
    (D) Guillain–Barré syndrome

17. A 5-year-old child presents to the office for a school physical exam. His past medical history is unremarkable, including normal growth and development. His physical exam is normal except for a grade II/VI high-pitched, vibratory, systolic ejection murmur heard best at the left lower sternal border with radiation to the apex. When the child is in a supine position, the murmur is louder. Which of the following murmurs is the MOST likely diagnosis?

    (A) physiologic peripheral pulmonic stenosis murmur
    (B) pulmonary ejection murmur
    (C) Still's murmur
    (D) venous hum

18. Which of the following sleeping positions for a healthy infant should be recommended to parents during anticipatory guidance in order to reduce the risk for sudden infant death syndrome?

    (A) prone position
    (B) seated position
    (C) side position
    (D) supine position

19. A previously healthy 12-month-old infant has been coughing and experiencing fever on and off for 2 months. He was diagnosed and treated for pneumonia approximately 3 months ago. On physical exam, he is in no acute respiratory distress, however is tachypnic with bibasilar rales and scattered rhonchi. Which of the following is the MOST likely diagnosis?

(A) bronchiectasis

(B) chronic bronchitis

(C) croup

(D) bronchopulmonary dysplasia

20. In reference to Question 19, which of the following is the MOST likely pathogen responsible for the infant's condition?

(A) *Corynebacterium diphtheriae*

(B) *Streptococcus pneumoniae*

(C) parainfluenza virus

(D) rhinovirus

21. At 12 hours of age, a physical exam is performed on a neonate with intrauterine growth retardation. He is noted to have microcephaly, jaundice, and hepatosplenomegaly. Which of the following is the MOST likely congenital viral infection in this neonate?

(A) cytomegalovirus

(B) herpes simplex virus

(C) rubella

(D) syphilis

22. A previously healthy, 5-month-old infant is admitted to the hospital due to lethargy progressing to semiconsciousness. The physical exam reveals a depressed mental status and bilateral retinal hemorrhages. Which of the following is the MOST likely diagnosis?

(A) child abuse

(B) retinitis pigmentosa

(C) Reye's syndrome

(D) viral encephalitis

23. A 2-year-old child presents to the emergency department via ambulance due to a seizure lasting approximately 2 minutes with jerking and somnolence. En route in the ambulance her vital signs are temperature 39°C rectal; pulse 120/min; respiration 32/min; blood pressure 110/64 mm Hg. Upon further questioning, her mother claimed she had a runny nose yesterday. On physical exam she is sleepy, but arousable with negative Kernig's and Brudzinski's signs. Which of the following seizures is the MOST likely diagnosis?

(A) absence seizure

(B) complex partial seizure

(C) febrile seizure

(D) simple partial seizure

24. A 6-month-old uncircumcised male presents with a 2-day history of a fever (39.6°C rectal today), vomiting, and poor feeding. Urinalysis of a catheterized specimen reveals 50 to 100 white blood cells/high-power field and moderate bacteria. Two days later, the urine culture results are available. Which of the following is the MOST common pathogen responsible for this infant's first urinary tract infection?

(A) *Enterococcus*

(B) *Escherichia coli*

(C) *Klebsiella*

(D) *Staphylococcus saprophyticus*

25. A 6-month-old infant presents to the emergency department with a 2-day history of vomiting and diarrhea. Upon physical exam she appears to be intermittently irritable and restless with minimal tearing when crying. Her capillary refill is 3 to 4 seconds. She has decreased skin turgor, sunken eyes, and a depressed anterior fontanel. Based on these clinical manifestations, what is the magnitude of her dehydration?

(A) less than 3%

(B) approaching 3% to 5% (mild)

(C) approaching 6% to 10% (moderate)

(D) approaching 11% to 15% (severe)

26. A previously well, 15-month-old male is brought to the emergency department in the middle of the night with increased irritability and severe paroxysmal colicky abdominal pain followed by vomiting. On physical exam, a tubular mass is palpated in the abdomen. The rectal exam reveals bloody mucus. Which of the following is the MOST likely diagnosis?

    (A) appendicitis
    (B) infectious enteritis
    (C) intussusception
    (D) pyloric stenosis

27. Which of the following daily maintenance fluid requirements is the closest approximation for an 18-kg child who is refusing to eat?

    (A) 900 mL
    (B) 1200 mL
    (C) 1400 mL
    (D) 1800 mL

28. A 4-year-old child has been hospitalized for suspected meningococcal meningitis. Cerebrospinal cultures are positive for *Neisseria meningitidis*, which confirms this diagnosis. Family members and close contacts need to be treated with prophylactic medication. Which of the following medications should be administered?

    (A) penicillin
    (B) rifabutin
    (C) rifampin
    (D) rimantadine

29. At a 2-month-old well-child checkup, a female infant is noted to have the following physical findings: widely open anterior and posterior fontanels, large protruding tongue, coarse facial features, low-set hair line, and an umbilical hernia. In the newborn period, there was a prolongation of physiologic icterus. The results of the newborn screening test are abnormal. Which of the following is the MOST likely diagnosis?

    (A) congenital adrenal hyperplasia
    (B) congenital hypothyroidism
    (C) Crigler–Najjar syndrome
    (D) galactosemia

30. A 48-hour-old healthy infant is noted to have a superficial swelling over the right parietotemporal region that does not extend across the suture line. Which of the following conditions is it MOST likely to be?

    (A) subperiosteal hemorrhage
    (B) cephalohematoma
    (C) craniotabes
    (D) subgaleal hemorrhage

31. A 2-year-old child is brought to the emergency department by his mother with sudden onset of choking, gagging, coughing, and wheezing. Vital signs are temperature 37°C; pulse 120/min; and respiration 28/min. The physical exam reveals decreased breath sounds over the right lower lobe with inspiratory rhonchi and localized expiratory wheezing. The chest x-ray reveals normal inspiratory views but expiratory views show localized hyperinflation with mediastinal shift to the left. Which of the following is the MOST likely diagnosis?

    (A) asthma
    (B) epiglottitis
    (C) foreign body aspiration
    (D) pulmonary embolism

32. A 16-year-old girl is brought to the emergency department by ambulance after reportedly ingesting "a bottle of aspirin." Vital signs are temperature 37.8°C oral; pulse 94/min; respiration 30/min; blood pressure 100/68 mm Hg. What would you expect the blood gases to show that would confirm she had swallowed the aspirin?

    (A) metabolic acidosis with respiratory acidosis
    (B) metabolic acidosis with respiratory alkalosis
    (C) metabolic alkalosis with respiratory acidosis
    (D) metabolic alkalosis with respiratory alkalosis

33. A 16-year-old high school male presents to the emergency department 4 hours after sustaining an abrasion to his knee after a fall while roller blading on the school playground. His school immunization record reveals that his last diphtheria, tetanus, and pertussis (DPT) booster was at 4 years of age. In this situation, which of the following is the MOST appropriate plan?

(A) administer tetanus toxoid

(B) administer adult tetanus and diphtheria toxoid (Td)

(C) administer diphtheria and tetanus toxoid, and cellular pertussis (Tdap) vaccine

(D) administer tetanus immune globulin

34. All of the following primitive reflexes should be elicited in the physical exam of a normal 4-week-old infant EXCEPT

(A) asymmetric tonic neck

(B) moro's

(C) palmar grasp

(D) parachute

35. A 3-day-old infant has bilateral copious, yellow-green eye discharge and conjunctival inflammation. A Gram stain of this discharge reveals Gram-negative intracellular diplococci. Which of the following antibiotics is the drug of choice for this infection?

(A) ceftriaxone

(B) cephalexin

(C) erythromycin

(D) gentamicin

36. A 10-year-old boy, the son of a migrant worker, presents to the emergency department complaining of a painful, swollen area along his right jaw and neck. On physical exam, he is febrile and has diffuse tenderness over the right parotid gland. His laboratory tests include an elevated serum amylase. In this patient, which of the following is a complication of his disease?

(A) hepatitis

(B) nerve deafness

(C) pneumonitis

(D) testicular torsion

37. Which of the following physical exam findings in a newborn infant should cause the clinician to suspect a genetic disorder?

(A) Café au lait spots

(B) subconjunctival hemorrhages

(C) miliaria

(D) vernix caseosa

38. The newborn exam at 1 minute shows a heart rate of 120 bpm, strong cry, some flexion in the upper extremities, sneezing with nasal catheter suction, and bluish hands and feet; but the remainder of the body is pink. What is the Apgar score?

(A) 7

(B) 8

(C) 9

(D) 10

39. Which of the following is the most common congenital heart malformation?

(A) atrial septal defect

(B) tetralogy of Fallot

(C) ventricular septal defect

(D) transposition of the great vessels

40. A 5-year-old male presents to the office for his kindergarten physical exam. Assuming that the patient's immunizations have been up to date, which of the following are the immunizations that the patient will receive at the end of today's visit?

(A) hepatitis B, inactivated poliovirus (IPV), diphtheria, tetanus, acellular pertussis (DTaP), measles, mumps, rubella (MMR), varicella

(B) IPV, DTaP, MMR, pneumococcal (PCV)

(C) IPV, DTaP, MMR, *Haemophilus influenzae* type b (Hib)

(D) DTaP, IPV, MMR

41. Which of the following is an absolute contraindication to breast-feeding?

    (A) tuberculosis of the mother
    (B) methadone treatment (20 mg/d)
    (C) maternal smoking
    (D) infant with cystic fibrosis

42. A 4-month-old infant presents to the office for her "well-check." The parents state that they have no concerns and think she is doing well. She is being breast-fed every 4 to 6 hours and has four wet diapers a day and two dirty diapers a day. Her birth weight was 7 pounds 7 ounces (50th percentile); she missed her 2-month appointment and at today's visit her weight is 11 pounds 5 ounces (5th percentile). The clinician however is very concerned and diagnoses the infant with which of the following?

    (A) dwarfism
    (B) failure to thrive
    (C) lactose intolerance
    (D) Beckwith–Wiedemann syndrome

43. During influenza season a 15-year-old presents to the emergency department unresponsive. The parents state that when they tried to wake him up in the morning he would not get up and was barely breathing. They deny any drug or alcohol use and state that he just had some cold symptoms the previous few days. A spinal tap shows decreased glucose, increased pressure, and increased proteins, but there were no cells found. The rest of the blood work shows elevated liver enzymes, but normal serum bilirubin and alkaline phosphatase. A liver biopsy demonstrates microvesicular steatosis without glycogen and large mitochondria. Which of the following is the best treatment for this patient?

    (A) high-dose steroids
    (B) broad-spectrum antibiotics until the cultures come back
    (C) supportive treatment, including maintenance fluids and hyperventilation
    (D) liver transplant

44. A 5-year-old female presents for her kindergarten physical exam and her mother mentions that she thinks she looks a bit yellow to her. The clinician notes diffuse jaundice, icterus, and Kayser–Fleischer rings. Which of the following is the treatment of choice for this patient?

    (A) alpha-interferon therapy
    (B) D-penicillamine therapy
    (C) methylprednisolone
    (D) protease inhibitor therapy

45. A 24-month-old infant presents for his routine physical exam. The parents state that he has been following all of his developmental milestones. On exam the clinician hears a grade II/VI murmur along the left sternal border, which radiates into the left axilla and the left side of the back. The child also has decreased femoral pulses bilaterally. The clinician orders a chest x-ray. Which of the following is the expected finding on x-ray based on the presentation?

    (A) notching or scalloping of the ribs
    (B) boot shaped heart—right ventricular hypertrophy
    (C) "egg on string"—narrowed mediastinum
    (D) absence of the main pulmonary artery

46. An 8-year-old female presents to the emergency room with her parents. They state she has been coughing all night the past few nights, to the point she sounds like she is choking. On exam, the clinician notes mild retractions at rest and more with the lung examination with diffuse stridor. Pulse oximetry is 92% on room air and the child is afebrile. Which of the following is the recommended treatment for this patient?

    (A) supportive care only—mist therapy
    (B) IV antibiotics, with Gram-negative coverage
    (C) intramuscular dexamethasone
    (D) nebulized racemic epinephrine and oral dexamethasone

47. A neonate presents with meconium ileus and it is successfully unobstructed. The infant returns at her 4-month appointment with signs of failure to thrive. Which of the following is the most likely diagnosis for this patient?

(A) cystic fibrosis
(B) Wilson's disease
(C) intussusception
(D) volvulus

48. Which of the following is NOT a cyanotic heart lesion?

(A) transposition of the great arteries
(B) atrioventricular septal defect
(C) hypoplastic left heart syndrome
(D) tricuspid atresia

49. A 2-week-old infant male presents for a routine checkup. The mother complains that he nurses every hour, but vomits (nonbilious) after every time he eats. He has only had three bowel movements since he has been home. On exam the infant has not gained any weight since leaving the hospital and the clinician notes gastric peristaltic waves. Which of the following is the treatment of choice for this patient?

(A) pyloromyotomy
(B) metoclopramide
(C) laparotomy
(D) omeprazole

50. A 6-month-old infant presents for her checkup. He father mentions that they started solid foods after her 4-month check and that she has had foul-smelling diarrhea off and on for the first month of solids and now it is everytime she eats and it looks greasy. They have tried different formulas, different cereals without improvement. What is the diagnostic test of choice for the most likely disorder?

(A) sweat chloride test
(B) RAST (radioallergosorbent assay test)
(C) gastrin level
(D) intestinal biopsy

51. A 9-year-old child presents to the urgent care center with her mother. The child is complaining of dark colored urine. The mother mentions that the child was complaining of sore throat and cold symptoms a few weeks ago. The urine shows gross hematuria without nitrites or leukocytes. Which of the following is the best test to help the clinician confirm the diagnosis?

(A) monospot
(B) antistreptolysin O titer
(C) immunoglobulin electrophoresis
(D) renal biopsy

52. Upon performing a newborn exam, the clinician notes a widened pulse pressure, paradoxical splitting of S_2, and a "machine" like murmur heard best at the second intercostal space, left sternal border, and inferior to the clavicle. Which of the following is the most likely diagnosis?

(A) tetralogy of Fallot
(B) ventricular septal defect
(C) atrial septal defect
(D) patent ductus arteriosus

53. Which of the following is the most common cause of sudden death in an adolescent athlete?

(A) mitral valve prolapse
(B) surgically corrected aortic stenosis
(C) hypertrophic cardiomyopathy
(D) rheumatic heart disease

54. A 7-year-old male presents to the emergency room with complaints of severe dyspnea, dysphagia, drooling, muffled voice, and fever. The pulse oximetry is 91% on room air; lung exam shows stridor and inspiratory retractions. Which of the following is the expected chest x-ray finding for the suspected diagnosis?

(A) thumb sign
(B) Scottie dog sign
(C) steeple sign
(D) figure 3 sign

55. Which of the following is the most common lethal genetic disorder in the United States?

    (A) trisomy 13
    (B) trisomy 21
    (C) cystic fibrosis
    (D) neurofibromatosis

56. Which of the following is the initial treatment step in an adolescent who presents to the emergency room with status epilepticus?

    (A) IV glucose
    (B) stabilize airway
    (C) arterial blood gas
    (D) IV diazepam therapy

57. A 12-year-old male presents to the urgent care center complaining of burning pain in his lower extremities with weakness. On exam, the clinician notes symmetric weakness with severely decreased active range of motion of the lower extremities, additionally decrease position and vibratory sensation in the distal portions bilaterally. Upon further questioning, the patient does admit to being diagnosed with mononucleosis 2 weeks ago. Which of the following is the most likely diagnosis?

    (A) poliomyelitis
    (B) botulism
    (C) Tick–bite paralysis
    (D) Guillain–Barré syndrome

58. Which thoracic curvature is an indication for treatment with bracing in an adolescent with scoliosis?

    (A) less than 20°
    (B) 20° to 40°
    (C) 40° to 60°
    (D) 40° with lumbar curvature of 30°

59. A 6-year-old female presents with complaints of hip pain so severe that she has not been able to walk to the school bus. Exam shows severe tenderness at the left hip with markedly decreased active and passive range of motion of the left hip. Radiologic exam demonstrates joint effusion with widening. Which of the following is the most likely diagnosis?

    (A) osteochondritis dissecans
    (B) slipped capital femoral epiphysis
    (C) septic hip arthritis
    (D) Legg–Calvé–Perthes disease

60. A 16-year-old male presents to the office with thumb pain. He just returned from a skiing trip. On exam the practitioner notes markedly decreased passive range of motion of the wrist with the ulnar collateral ligament. What is the most likely diagnosis?

    (A) mallet finger
    (B) gamekeeper's thumb
    (C) boxer's fracture
    (D) nondisplaced scaphoid fracture

61. A 3-year-old child is brought in by her parents to the urgent care center stating that the child will not bend her arm. They are obviously worried and distraught. The clinician notices the elbow is held in strict pronation and there is tenderness over the radial head. X-ray examination shows no findings. Which of the following is the treatment of choice for this disorder?

    (A) place elbow in full supination and move from full flexion to extension
    (B) immobilization of the elbow in a splint for 2 weeks
    (C) referral to the orthopedic surgeon for suspected radial head fracture
    (D) call child protective services for suspected battery

62. A 7-year-old child is brought in to the office by her mother who states that the child is still wetting the bed at night. She is worried that there is something wrong with the child. Upon examination there is no abnormality. Urinalysis is negative. Which of the following is the treatment of choice for this disorder?

(A) bed-wetting alarm

(B) desmopressin acetate (DDAVP)

(C) imipramine

(D) amitriptyline

63. A 13-year-old male presents with fever and blood in his urine. Examination shows an asymptomatic mass in the left lower quadrant. Urinalysis shows hematuria and small leukocytes. Which of the following is the most likely diagnosis?

(A) renal cell carcinoma

(B) intussusception

(C) volvulus

(D) nephroblastoma

64. A mother brings in her 20-month-old infant girl to the office because she noticed pubic hair growing. On exam the clinician notices that the clitoris is enlarged; the rest is unremarkable. Which of the following is an expected lab finding on this patient?

(A) increased aldosterone

(B) increased estrogen

(C) increased androstenedione

(D) increased luteinizing hormone

65. A 5-year-old presents for her kindergarten checkup. The clinician notes that over the past couple years, her height decreased from the 50th percentile to the 5th percentile. On exam, the clinician also notes truncal adiposity. All of her lab tests are normal. Which of the following is the most likely diagnosis?

(A) growth-hormone deficiency

(B) Cushing's disease

(C) congenital hypothyroidism

(D) congenital adrenal hyperplasia

DIRECTIONS (Questions 66 through 72): Each group of items in this section consists of lettered headings followed by a set of numbered words or phrases. For each numbered word or phrase, select the ONE lettered heading that is most closely associated with it. Each lettered heading may be selected once, more than once, or not at all.

Questions 66 through 72

Select the ONE lettered *pattern of inheritance* to correlate with the numbered *disease*.

(A) autosomal dominant

(B) autosomal recessive

(C) X-linked dominant

(D) X-linked recessive

66. vitamin D-resistant rickets

67. achondroplasia

68. Duchenne's muscular dystrophy

69. Hunter's syndrome

70. neurofibromatosis

71. hemophilia A

72. sickle cell anemia

DIRECTIONS (Questions 73 through 100): Each of the numbered items or incomplete statements in this section is followed by answers or by completions of the statement. Select the ONE lettered answer or completion that is BEST in each case.

Questions 73 through 100

73. You are seeing a 7-year-old Caucasian female in your office for her complaint of "an itchy head." The girl's mother, who is with her, states that this has been bothering her daughter for about a week and she has noticed a lot of "dandruff" in the girl's hair that will not come out. She also tells you that several of her daughter's friends are having the same problem. Based on the most likely diagnosis, what is the best treatment for this patient?

(A) permethrin 1% shampoo

(B) ketoconazole cream

(C) tar-based shampoo

(D) silver sulfadiazine 1% cream

74. A young mother brings her 4-year-old son to your clinic for evaluation of a rash on his umbilicus and hands that she has been treating with an over-the-counter ointment for about a week, without success. She says that she has noticed that he scratches the rash periodically, and it seems to bother him the most at night. She also says that she noticed this same rash on the hands on one of the other boys at his daycare center. On exam there are excoriated papules and nodules on his hand and umbilicus. What is the most likely diagnosis?

(A) herpes simplex

(B) scabies

(C) pediculoses

(D) tinea corporis

75. A new mother brings her 3-month-old daughter to your clinic for a rash on the infant's head. On exam, you notice the skin affected by the rash is thickened, yellowish-white in color, scaly, and looks waxy. Additionally, it only involves the scalp and bilateral postauricular areas. What is the most likely diagnosis?

(A) contact dermatitis

(B) lichen planus

(C) pityriasis rosea

(D) seborrheic dermatitis

76. You have been seeing an 8-year-old male in your office for brown, nonpruritic, annular lesions on the back of his hands, feet, and extensor surface of the elbows and knees that have been present for several months. At today's visit you notice the lesions are essentially unchanged since you last saw him about a month ago. What is the best treatment for this suspected disorder?

(A) excision and biopsy

(B) no treatment

(C) topical steroids

(D) wet to dry dressings

77. Which of the following is the recommended treatment of a 2 to 5-cm, single, nonpainful, common wart on the hand of a 7-year-old?

(A) 40% salicylic acid plaster

(B) burning laser surgery

(C) electrocautery

(D) liquid nitrogen

78. In treating uncomplicated, comedonal acne (open and closed comedones) in adolescents, which of the following treatments is best?

(A) topical antibiotics

(B) topical keratolytics

(C) oral retinoids

(D) systemic antibiotics

79. The most common fracture of newborns is a fracture of the

(A) clavicle

(B) humerus

(C) radius

(D) ulna

80. A 13-year-old male presents to the clinic for a complaint of right knee pain that he first noticed about a year ago. It started out as just some mild discomfort in the area just below the kneecap, but has been getting progressively worse and now it hurts anytime he uses his leg, even when walking. He does not remember any injury to his knee. When you examine his knee you notice swelling and exquisite tenderness over the tibial tubercle. X-rays are normal. What is the most likely diagnosis?

(A) chondromalacia patellae

(B) Osgood–Schlatter disease

(C) patellar subluxation

(D) patellofemoral overuse syndrome

81. The eggs of this parasite are detected by microscopic examination of clear adhesive tape that has been pressed to the child's anus in the morning, prior to bathing. What parasite is most likely to be identified by this test method?

(A) *Ancylostoma duodenale* (hookworm)
(B) *Ascaris lumbricoides* (ascarias)
(C) enterobiasis (pinworm)
(D) trichuriasis (whipworm)

82. A 13-year-old male presents with complaints of pain in both knees, and his right ankle. The pain is worse in the morning. He denies any injuries, but does notice he tires more easily when playing baseball. He says this has been going on for about the last 8 weeks. His father admits to having chronic low back pain but otherwise the family medical history is non-contributory. Based on this history which of the following is the most likely diagnosis?

(A) juvenile rheumatoid arthritis
(B) Lyme arthritis
(C) psoriatic arthritis
(D) enteropathic arthritis

83. An 8-year-old female presents with complaints of 3-day duration of a red itchy right eye with a lot of yellowish-green color discharge. She denies any injury. Her visual acuity is normal but she does have moderate tearing and mild photophobia. What is the most likely diagnosis?

(A) allergic conjunctivitis
(B) bacterial conjunctivitis
(C) viral conjunctivitis
(D) Reiter's syndrome

84. While seeing a 12-week-old female for her well-child checkup, you notice she has tearing from her left eye with a small reddened area that is swollen and she cries when you touch it. The swollen area is just below the medial inferior eyelid. There is also constant tearing from this same eye. Her mother says it just started about 2 days ago and is getting worse. What is the most likely cause of this problem?

(A) blepharitis
(B) conjunctivitis
(C) dacryocystitis
(D) anterior uveitis

85. The majority of cases of halitosis in young children can be traced to which of the following causes?

(A) dental caries
(B) nasal foreign body
(C) poor dietary habits
(D) upper respiratory infection

86. Of the following, which is the most frequent cause of epistaxis in children?

(A) bleeding disorders
(B) choanal atresia
(C) digital trauma
(D) foreign bodies

87. You are seeing a 5-year-old male in your clinic for evaluation of a firm, painful lump that is slightly reddened and approximately 3 cm in diameter, in his right axilla. His mother tells you the lump has been there for a couple of days. The boy does not look acutely ill. The mother informs you they got a new kitten and puppy about a month ago but otherwise nothing else is new at home. Which of the following is the most likely etiology for his rash?

(A) *Bartonella henselae*
(B) parvovirus
(C) Hodgkin's disease
(D) Osgood–Schlatter disease

88. When considering infections caused by nematodes, which of the following is most consistent with iron deficiency anemia, abdominal discomfort, weight loss, and the presence of ova in the feces?

(A) ascariasis
(B) hookworm
(C) pinworms
(D) whipworm

89. Erythema migrans, the characteristic rash of Lyme disease, occurs in what percent of patients with this disease?

    (A) 20% to 40%
    (B) 40% to 60%
    (C) 60% to 80%
    (D) 80% to 100%

90. A 2-week-old male is being seen in your clinic for a profuse mucoid discharge from both eyes, with some associated tearing. On exam, you notice both eyes are hyperemic and the eyelids are red and swollen. Which of the following is the most likely cause of this patient's ophthalmia neonatorium (conjunctivitis in the newborn)?

    (A) allergic
    (B) gonococcal
    (C) chlamydial
    (D) viral

91. Of the following, which neurological problem is *not* associated with Lyme disease?

    (A) aseptic meningitis
    (B) Bell's palsy
    (C) polyradiculitis
    (D) seizures

92. A young mother brings her 3-week-old daughter for care of a rash in her mouth. The mother indicates the baby was doing fine until 2 days ago when she noticed white spots in the infant's mouth. On exam they do not come off with a tongue blade. She is bottle-feeding the infant without any problem. Which of the following is the most likely diagnosis of this problem?

    (A) leukoplakia
    (B) hand–foot–mouth disease
    (C) herpangina
    (D) oral candidiasis

93. You are seeing a 14-year-old male in your office for evaluation of the following behavior problems that according to his mother have been present for about a year, and in the past few months have been getting worse. She complains that her son has been having problems in school, is not behaving, and is getting into fights. He seems to only want to talk about science fiction movies and occasionally seems to be talking to people who aren't really there. Sometimes, he seems really depressed and at other times, "full of energy and happy." Based on this mother's observations, which of the following is the most likely diagnosis?

    (A) attention deficit hyperactivity disorder (ADHD)
    (B) bipolar disorder
    (C) conduct disorder
    (D) depression

94. A 9-year-old male presents in August with complaints of a red rash on the palms of his hands, soles of his feet, and a little on his legs. His mother states that this rash started about 2 days ago, and just before it appeared her son had been complaining of a severe headache and that he was aching all over. She said he also felt "hot to the touch" during that time, as well. He mentions he was camping in Arkansas about 10 days ago with his dad, but did not eat anything abnormal. Based on this history, what is the most likely diagnosis?

    (A) endemic typhus
    (B) human ehrlichiosis
    (C) Q fever
    (D) rocky mountain spotted fever

95. In young children, which of the following is the most common cause of lower respiratory tract infections?

    (A) adenovirus
    (B) human parvovirus
    (C) parainfluenza virus
    (D) respiratory syncytial virus

96. A 3-year-old male presents to the clinic for a cough that his mother says occurs only after he has been running. She says she first noticed this about 6 months ago, after he had had one of his usual winter colds, and his cough persisted for about a week. Based upon this history, what is the most likely diagnosis?

    (A) airway foreign body
    (B) asthma
    (C) cystic fibrosis
    (D) laryngomalacia

97. You are seeing a 12-month-old male for his mother's concerns that he does not seem to play with other children as his brother and sister did at this age. She indicates she has noticed that he does not seem to respond when she or other children call him by name, he is indifferent to other children or adults when they are present, and he does not seem to know any, "just grunts." Based upon this history, your most likely diagnosis for this problem is which of the following?

    (A) attention deficit hyperactivity disorder (ADHD)
    (B) autism
    (C) fragile X syndrome
    (D) schizophrenia

98. When evaluating a newborn, the inability to pass a small catheter through the nasal cavity is most indicative of which of the following conditions?

    (A) choanal atresia
    (B) meconium ileus
    (C) nasal infection
    (D) nasal polyps

99. Anorexia nervosa is an eating disorder commonly affecting teenage girls. Which of the following best represents the percentage of the teenage girls affected?

    (A) 1% to 5%
    (B) 5% to 10%
    (C) 10% to 15%
    (D) 15% to 20%

100. The most common childhood nutritional disorder, in the United States, is which of the following?

    (A) binge eating disorder
    (B) folate deficiency
    (C) obesity
    (D) rickets

Answers and Explanations

1. **(B)** Acute otitis media (AOM) is primarily a disease of early childhood. The bacterial pathogens differ in the various ages of pediatric patients with AOM. In an 18-month-old child, the three most common bacterial pathogens are *Streptococcus pneumoniae*, *Haemophilus influenzae*, and *Moraxella catarrhalis*. Other less common bacterial pathogens include *Streptococcus pyogenes*, *Staphylococcus aureus*, anaerobic organisms, and Gram-negative enteric organisms (such as *Pseudomonas aeruginosa*). In early infancy (less than 6 weeks of age), AOM is also caused by group B streptococcus and *S. aureus*. *Chlamydia trachomatis* and *Mycoplasma pneumoniae* are uncommon pathogens for AOM. *P. aeruginosa* is often the causative organism for chronic suppurative otitis media. (*Behrman and Kliegman, 2002, pp. 388–389; Hay et al, 2005, pp. 472–483*)

2. **(C)** Iron deficiency anemia is the most common cause of anemia in the United States in term infants between 6 months and 3 years of age. Both breast milk and regular cow's milk are low in iron and in a form not easily absorbed. During periods of rapid weight gain in infancy and adolescence there is an increase in the need for total body iron. Without supplementation of iron-rich foods or vitamins during the period of rapid weight gain, the patient becomes deficient. Characteristic laboratory values for iron deficiency anemia include low mean corpuscular volume (MCV), low mean corpuscular hemoglobin (MCH), low mean corpuscular hemoglobin concentration (MCHC), low hemoglobin (Hgb), elevated red blood cell distribution width (RDW), and a blood smear with hypochromic, microcytic cells. Acquired aplastic anemia is usually a normocytic anemia with a normal MCV and RDW. Megaloblastic anemia is caused by a nutritional deficiency (such as vitamin B_{12} or folate), cancer chemotherapy, or rare metabolic disorders resulting in an elevated MCV and MCH. Beta-thalassemia major is the most common cause of transfusion-dependent anemia. It is more common among infants of Mediterranean, Middle Eastern, or Asian descent who are normal at birth but develop severe anemia in the first year of life. Laboratory findings include severe hypochromic, microcytic anemia with marked anisocytosis and poikilocytosis and an elevated serum bilirubin level. Lead poisoning, or plumbism, is a normocytic, slightly hypochromic anemia. The MCV is low with a characteristically elevated blood lead level. (*Hay et al, 2005, pp. 857, 862–864, 869–871*)

3. **(A)** In children who present with symptoms of sore throat and fever, over 90% of these cases are due to a viral infection. Adenovirus is one of the most common etiologic viral agents. The four remaining choices are bacterial pathogens of which group A beta-hemolytic streptococcus is the most common followed by the less common pathogens (group C streptococcus, *Arcanobacterium haemolyticus*, and *Streptococcus pneumoniae*). (*Hay et al, 2005, pp. 495–497, 1136; Behrman and Kliegman, 2002, pp. 390–391*)

4. **(A)** In left-sided congestive heart failure, the signs of tachycardia, tachypnea, intercostal retractions, rales, and rhonchi are found. Hepatosplenomegaly is a sign of right-sided congestive heart failure. Bradycardia is not associated with either left- or right-sided congestive heart failure in the pediatric patient. (*Behrman and Kliegman, 2002, pp. 557–558*)

5. **(B)** Leukemia is the most common form of childhood cancer. Acute lymphoblastic leukemia is the most common form of leukemia, accounting for approximately 4/100,000 children under 15 years. The clinical presentation is variable, ranging from severe with a life-threatening infection to asymptomatic at a routine well-child visit. Often there is a 3- to 4-week history of an illness prior to the diagnosis, with signs and symptoms including malaise, anorexia, intermittent fever, bone tenderness, pallor, petechiae, purpura, and abdominal pain. Findings noted on the physical exam include pallor, petechiae, purpura, retinal hemorrhages, lymphadenopathy (either localized or generalized to cervical, axillary, or inguinal areas), bone and joint tenderness (especially in the pelvis, lower vertebral bodies, and femur), hepatosplenomegaly, and nephromegaly. Initially, the most useful test is a complete blood count with differential, revealing multiple cytopenias and leukemic blasts. The bone marrow examination is diagnostic, revealing a homogeneous infiltration of leukemic blasts replacing normal marrow. Patients with chronic Epstein–Barr virus infections present with sore throat, fever, posterior cervical lymphadenopathy, and malaise associated with atypical lymphocytosis and a positive heterophile antibody test. Clinical findings of anorexia nervosa include bradycardia, reduced peripheral circulation, and interruption of pubertal development. Significant weight loss with secondary amenorrhea is an important diagnostic clue. Crohn's disease is an idiopathic, chronic inflammatory bowel disease of childhood involving any region of the alimentary tract from the mouth to the anus. Symptoms include crampy, abdominal pain, diarrhea (possibly bloody), weight loss, fever, malaise, fatigue, and growth retardation. (*Hay et al, 2005, pp. 166–168, 654–656, 911–915, 1156–1157; Behrman and Kliegman, 2002, pp. 657–659*)

6. **(D)** In most cases of acute viral meningitis, the cellular response is predominately mononuclear cells upon examination of the cerebral spinal fluid (CSF). In bacterial meningitis, the differential classically shows a predominance of polymorphonuclear cells. Glucose is an important indicator of severe brain involvement. It is equally important in the differential diagnosis of bacterial meningitis and a more chronic infection such as tuberculosis. The CSF protein level in viral meningitis usually ranges from 50 to 150 mg/dL. In bacterial meningitis, the CSF protein level increases, with a range between 100 and 500 mg/dL. It is very uncommon for infectious mononucleosis to advance to the point of central nervous system symptoms. (*Behrman and Kliegman, 2002, pp. 382–386; Hay et al, 2005, pp. 787–790*)

7. **(C)** The diagnosis of rheumatic fever is based on clinical rounds using the modified Jones criteria. Two major manifestations or one major and two minor manifestations in addition to supporting evidence of a preceding streptococcal infection are needed to make the diagnosis of rheumatic fever. The major manifestations are polyarthritis, carditis, erythema marginatum, subcutaneous nodules, and Sydenham chorea. The minor manifestations are fever, arthralgia, previous rheumatic fever or rheumatic heart disease, an elevated sedimentation rate or C-reactive protein, and a prolonged P–R interval. The supporting evidence of a preceding streptococcal infection includes elevated titers of antistreptolysin O or other streptococcal antibodies and positive throat culture for group A beta-hemolytic streptococcus. (*Behrman and Kliegman, 2002, p. 591; Hay et al, 2005, pp. 599–601*)

8. **(D)** In idiopathic thrombocytopenia purpura (ITP), the platelet count is reduced to less than 20,000/mm (some authors say less than 50,000/mm). Clot retraction, bleeding time, and the tourniquet test depend on platelet function and are abnormal in ITP. The white blood cell count is normal and anemia usually is not present. Although the differential smear

may show decreased platelets, the working diagnosis is made by a platelet count and confirmed by bone marrow examination revealing normal granulocytic and erythrocytic series. In adolescents, systemic lupus erythematosus is a consideration in the differential diagnosis of thrombocytopenia purpura. This would make the antinuclear antibody test appropriate for ruling out that disease, but would not substantiate the diagnosis of ITP. (*Behrman and Kliegman, 2002, p. 637; Hay et al, 2005, pp. 887–888*)

9. **(C)** Tanner's stages of sexual maturation categorize the progression of pubertal development in girls according to pubic hair and breast development. Menarche usually occurs 18 to 24 months following the onset of breast development. In female breast development, Tanner stage I is an absence of breast development; stage II is a small, raised breast bud. Stage III shows further enlargement/elevation of breast and alveolar tissue; stage IV is the areola and papilla forming a secondary mound on breast contour; and stage V is the mature breast with alveolar area as part of the breast contour. For the stages of pubic hair development, stage I is prepubertal, an absence of hair; stage II shows sparse, fine, hair, primarily on the border of labia; stage III is pigmented and curly and increases in quantity on the mons pubis; stage IV is increased quantity of coarser texture with labia and mons pubis well covered; and stage V is mature adult distribution with spreading to medial thighs. (*Hay et al, 2005, p. 112; Gunn and Nechyba, 2002, pp. 102–103*)

10. **(C)** During the first year of life, the average, normal expected increase in weight of a full-term infant is to regain the birth weight by 2 weeks of age, double the birth weight by 4 months of age, and triple the birth weight by 1 year of age. (*Hay et al, 2005, pp. 66–70*)

11. **(D)** When evaluating children with physical injuries, the major difficulty is distinguishing between intentional and unintentional injuries. Inconsistencies between the stated story and the injury are suspect. Discoloration caused by healing bruises tends to follow a distinctive pattern. On the first day, there is swelling without discoloration. From day 1 through day 5, the bruise is purple in color. For days 5 through 7, the bruise is green. Then, from day 7 through day 10, the bruise is yellow, followed by a brownish color from day 10 to day 14. (*Gunn and Nechyba, 2002, pp. 81, 94–96*)

12. **(D)** Rotavirus is one of the most important causes of acute gastroenteritis in infants and young children primarily 6 to 24 months of age. In the United States, there are 65,000 to 70,000 hospitalizations and 200 deaths per annum. Peak incidences occur in the fall and winter. Most initial infections are characterized by diarrhea (watery, nonbloody, nonmucous), fever, and vomiting. Nasal congestion and coryza often precede the gastrointestinal symptoms. *Clostridium difficile* produces a toxin that causes a self-limited diarrhea in which symptoms characteristically begin following the administration of antibiotics that reduce normal bowel flora. *Giardia lamblia*, a flagellated protozoa, characteristically causes a mild diarrhea, with or without a low-grade fever, anorexia, flatulence, and abdominal cramps. It is not associated with vomiting nor upper respiratory symptoms. Shigella gastroenteritis in young children classically presents acutely with a high fever or seizures along with vomiting followed by bloody, mucoid, diarrheal stools. (*Jenson and Baltimore, 1995, pp. 1075–1077, 1092–1095, 1114–1115; Hay et al, 2005, pp. 641–643*)

13. **(C)** The normal variation in the angular alignment of the lower extremities changes with age. Physiologic bow legs (genu varum) and knock knees (genu valgum) occur in a sequence that follows a normal developmental pattern. Although bowing of the lower legs may be appreciated at birth, the relative bowing of the legs is most prominent during the second year of life. During the third and fourth years of life, physiologic knock knees develop. There is resolution of the knock knees between 5 and 7 years of age when normal adult alignment occurs. However, some normal adults may have a slight appearance of the knock knees. If there is development

out of this sequence, such as persistent bowing beyond 2 years of age, bowing that is increasing rather than decreasing, or unilateral bowing, then an evaluation is indicated to determine the pathologic cause. (*Hay et al, 2005, p. 816; Behrman and Kliegman, 2002, pp. 832–834*)

14. **(D)** The first sign of pubertal development in boys is the enlargement of testicular size and occurs at the mean age of 11.6 years. Genital stages accelerate before pubic hair development, which occurs, on average, at 13.4 years of age. The deepening of the voice and the development of chest and axillary hair usually occurs in midpuberty or 2 years after the growth of pubic hair. (*Hay et al, 2005, p. 111; Gunn and Nechyba, 2002, pp. 104–105*)

15. **(C)** Foreign bodies of the nose are common in children and often are unsuspected until the child presents with a persistent unilateral, foul-smelling, purulent rhinorrhea. Choanal atresia is the most common congenital anomaly of the nose and may be either unilateral or bilateral. With unilateral choanal atresia, newborns may be asymptomatic until the first respiratory infection, when they present with nasal obstruction and difficulty breathing. Infants with bilateral choanal atresia often present at birth with difficulty in mouth breathing, leading to cyanosis. A nasal polyp causes nasal obstruction, leading to hyponasal speech and mouth breathing with profuse mucoid or mucopurulent rhinorrhea. On physical exam of the nasal passage, a glistening gray, grape-like mass may be noted. Mild septal deviations are usually asymptomatic. Clinically, the deformity is apparent and there may be edema. (*Hay et al, 2005, pp. 492–494*)

16. **(A)** Bell's palsy is the acquired peripheral facial weakness (cranial nerve VII) of sudden onset and unknown etiology. It often follows a viral illness with notable improvement within 2 weeks and near complete recovery within 2 months. Prednisone therapy may promote recovery of facial strength. Guillain–Barré syndrome (acute idiopathic polyneuritis) generally presents with symmetrical weakness of the lower extremities, which may ascend rapidly to the arms, trunk, and face.

Nonspecific respiratory or gastrointestinal symptoms may occur 5 to 14 days preceding the infection. Physical exam will yield symmetric flaccid weakness, which is usually proximal in distribution. Rarely, there is cranial nerve (III–VI, IX–XI) involvement. Botulism is most often caused by the ingestion of food containing the *Clostridium botulinum* toxin or rarely from an infected wound. Children will present with blurred or double vision, ptosis, or choking. Physical findings include a weak, swallow paralysis of accommodation and eye movements. In this case, there was not a history of food ingestion or wound infection to support this diagnosis. Children with a brain stem tumor may present with facial and extraocular muscle palsies, hemiparesis, gait disturbances, and hydrocephalus (25%). Changes in personality such as lethargy, irritability, and aggressive behavior are particularly common findings. Speech and swallowing difficulties are not unusual. Later in the illness, patients will develop vomiting and headaches. (*Behrman and Kliegman, 2002, pp. 399–400, 772, 812; Hay et al, 2005, pp. 792–793, 802*)

17. **(C)** Still's murmur is the most common innocent murmur of early childhood and is usually appreciated in children from 3 to 6 years of age. It is a grade I–III/VI early systolic ejection murmur of musical or vibratory quality heard best between the apex and the left lower sternal border. It is loudest when the patient is in a supine position. The murmur may diminish or disappear with inspiration, during the Valsalva maneuver, or when the patient is standing or seated. A physiologic peripheral pulmonic stenosis murmur is a soft, short, high-pitched, grade I–II/VI systolic ejection murmur. Typically, it is auscultated with equal intensity at the left upper sternal border, along the back, and in both axillae. It is usually found in newborns and generally disappears by 3 to 6 months of age. A pulmonary ejection murmur is the most common innocent murmur of later childhood and is usually seen in children 8 to 14 years of age. It is a soft, early to midsystolic ejection, grade I–III/ VI murmur heard best along the left upper sternal border. It is louder when the

patient is supine or with increased cardiac output. It diminishes with standing or during the Valsalva maneuver. A venous hum is a continuous musical, grade I–II/VI murmur heard at the right or left superior infraclavicular area. The murmur is obliterated when the patient is in a supine position, with head rotation, and with compression of the jugular vein. It is usually auscultated in children from 3 to 6 years of age. (*Hay et al, 2005, pp. 560–561; Behrman and Kliegman, 2002, p. 560*)

18. **(D)** Sudden infant death syndrome (SIDS) is defined as the sudden, unexplained death of an apparently healthy infant that is unexpected and not adequately explained by a comprehensive medical history, a postmortem physical, and investigation of the death scene. SIDS is the second leading cause of death in infants between 1 month and 1 year of age, second only to congenital anomalies. The exact etiology of SIDS is unclear. Prevention of SIDS has become a focus of public health measures. In 1994, The American Academy of Pediatrics initiated a campaign called "Back to Sleep," which recommended placing infants in the supine position for sleep. Following the institution of this campaign in the United States, the annual death rate decreased from 1.3 per 1000 to 0.7 per 1000. (*Behrman and Kliegman, 2002, p. 546; Hay et al, 2005, pp. 554–555*)

19. **(A)** Bronchiectasis, meaning "dilation of the bronchi," results from destruction of the airway and poor drainage often associated with cystic fibrosis, foreign body aspiration or an infection. It is uncommon in the general population. The presentation may vary from a chronic productive cough to recurrent pneumonia with or without hemoptysis. Persistent rhonchi, rales, and decreased breath sounds are noted over the affected atelectatic area. Croup is an inflammatory disease of the larynx most frequently affecting young children during the fall and early winter months. Typically, there is an upper respiratory tract prodrome followed by stridor and a "barky cough" in the absence of drooling. Subglottic narrowing with a normal epiglottis is diagnostic on a lateral neck x-ray. The most com-

mon pathogen is parainfluenza virus. Bronchopulmonary dysplasia is most commonly seen in infants in the neonatal intensive care unit. It is a chronic condition seen in patients whose clinical course included hyaline membrane disease. These infants typically need oxygen for a few months as they grow and some need permanent tracheostomy and ventilation for up to 2 years. Chronic bronchitis falls into the chronic obstructive pulmonary disease category typically seen in older adults and does not typically present with acute symptoms. (*Hay et al, 2005, pp. 513–514, 519–526*)

20. **(B)** Bronchiectasis has numerous etiologies. Most commonly cultures reveal normal oral flora from the lower respiratory tract: *Streptococcus pneumoniae, Staphylococcus aureus, Haemophilus. influenzae, Pseudomonas aeruginosa.* Parainfluenza viruses typically are responsible for croup. *Corynebacterium diphtheriae* is the causative organism for diphtheria. Rhinovirus is the most common pathogen isolated with acute viral rhinitis or the common cold. (*Hay et al, 2005, pp. 519–526*)

21. **(A)** Cytomegalovirus (CMV) is one of the congenital neonatal TORCH infections (*t*oxoplasmosis, *o*ther [syphilis, varicella-zoster, and parvovirus in this list], *r*ubella, *c*ytomegalovirus, and *h*erpes simplex/*h*epatitis/ HIV). CMV is the most common congenital infection. The disease-specific manifestations for CMV include microcephaly with periventricular calcifications, neonatal jaundice with direct hyperbilirubinemia, and hepatosplenomegaly. Other associated manifestations include intrauterine growth retardation, thrombocytopenia, and purpura. Disease-specific manifestations for herpes simplex virus include skin/eye/mouth vesicles, encephalitis, respiratory distress, and sepsis. Disease-specific manifestations of rubella include congenital heart lesions (patent ductus arteriosus, pulmonary artery stenosis, aortic stenosis, ventricular defects), thrombocytopenic purpura characterized by purple macular lesions ("blueberry muffin" appearance), cataracts, retinopathy, and sensorineural deafness. Disease-specific manifestations of

syphilis include mucocutaneous lesions (snuffles), periostitis, osteochondritis, and hemolytic anemia. Often these babies are stillborn. Syphilis is caused by a spirochete, *Treponema pallidum*, not a virus. (*Hay et al, 2005, 1146–1149,1152–1156, 1165–1166; Behrman and Kliegman, 2002, pp. 438–446*)

22. **(A)** Approximately 40% of children who have been physically abused showed evidence of ocular trauma. Retinal hemorrhages are the most frequent ocular finding that result from violent shaking. This form of child abuse is termed shaken baby syndrome. The finding of retinal hemorrhages in an infant without an appropriate medical condition (e.g., clotting disorder, leukemia) should raise concerns about nonaccidental trauma. Some of the most common presenting complaints of infants with shaken baby syndrome are lethargy, coma, seizures, vomiting, and respiratory distress. Retinal hemorrhages are not associated with retinitis pigmentosa, retinoblastoma, Reye's syndrome, or viral encephalitis. With Reye's syndrome, an antecedent viral illness is followed by vomiting and progressive lethargy. On exam, there is usually fever, tachypnea, lethargy, and stupor. Laboratory hallmarks include elevated serum hepatocellular enzyme assays and elevated serum ammonia. Retinitis pigmentosa is a progressive retinal degeneration and is characterized by pigmentary changes, optic atrophy, and progressive impairment of visual function. The presenting clinical manifestation is usually an impairment of dark adaptation or night vision. Clinical manifestations of viral encephalitis vary in severity depending upon the etiologic organism (e.g., cytomegalovirus, mumps, echovirus). Some children will have mild symptoms lapsing into a coma leading to death, whereas others are febrile, with convulsions and hallucinations followed by full recovery. (*Hay et al, 2005, pp. 221–225, 460, 685–686, 1160*)

23. **(C)** A febrile seizure is a brief (less than 15 minutes), generalized, symmetric, tonic-clonic seizure associated with a febrile illness (temperature greater than 38.8°C) without any central nervous system infection or neu-

rologic cause. An absence (petit mal) seizure is a brief (2 to 25 seconds) loss of consciousness that can occur multiple times per day. There is no loss of tone, and frequently the only observable behaviors are staring or minor movements such as lip smacking and semipurposeful movements of the hands. There is no postictal period. Complex partial seizures (psychomotor) have varied symptoms including alterations in consciousness, unresponsiveness, and repetitive complex motor activities that are purposeless. Often, at the beginning of the attack, there is a psychoillusory phenomenon such as hallucinations, visual distortions, visceral sensations, or feelings of intense emotions. Simple partial seizures include focal motor, adversive, and somatosensory seizures. Manifestations of these seizures are varied including hallucinatory, psychoillusory or complex emotional phenomena. Children will interact normally with their environment, with the exception of those limitations imposed by the seizure. Following the seizure (minutes to hours), there may be transient paralysis of the affected body part. (*Hay et al, 2005, pp. 743–759; Behrman and Kliegman, 2002, pp. 793–800*)

24. **(B)** Urinary tract infections (UTIs) are one of the most common infections in children. Clinical features of a UTI vary depending upon the age and sex of the child. In newborns, the most common symptom is failure to thrive associated with poor feeding, diarrhea, and vomiting. In infants, the symptoms may be relatively nonspecific, such as poor feeding, failure to gain weight, vomiting, fever, strong-smelling urine, and irritability. As children grow older, the initial signs and symptoms become more specific to the urinary tract. In early infancy, males are two times more likely than girls to have a UTI. Also, uncircumcised males are 10 times more likely to be affected than circumcised males. *Escherichia coli* is the most common pathogen for the first UTI (80%) and of recurrent infections (75%). Other organisms that cause infections include *Pseudomonas aeurginosa, Proteus, Enterobacter, Klebsiella,* and *Enterococcus.* An infection with *Staphylococcus saprophyticus,* a coagulase-negative staphylococcus, is primarily seen in

adolescents with a UTI. (*Hay et al, 2005, pp. 729–731; Behrman and Kliegman, 2002, pp. 707–709*)

25. **(C)** Dehydration is a common pathophysiologic alteration in fluid and electrolyte balance in children. Children are at an increased risk for dehydration because of their decreased oral intake, especially when ill, and their higher ratio of surface area to body weight, promoting significant evaporative losses. Important clinical features to estimate the degree of dehydration include postural blood pressure, changes in heart rate, capillary refill time, skin turgor and color, lack of tears, lack of external jugular venous filling when supine, sunken fontanel (if present), and altered mental status. This infant was estimated to have moderate dehydration (6% to 10% decrease in body weight) with decreased skin turgor (minimal tears), slightly longer capillary refill time (3 to 4 seconds), depressed anterior fontanel, and intermittent irritability and restlessness. Severe dehydration (11% to 15% decrease in body weight) manifests as markedly decreased skin turgor with parched or mottled mucous membranes, absence of tears, tachycardia, capillary refill greater than 4 seconds, hypotension, circulatory collapse, and anuria. Mild dehydration (3% to 5% decrease in body weight) manifests as normal to slightly decreased skin turgor; dry mucous membranes; decreased tearing; mild oliguria; and normal pulse, blood pressure, and perfusion. (*Hay et al, 2005, pp. 1323–1325*)

26. **(C)** Intussusception is the most common cause of intestinal obstruction between 3 months and 6 years of age. It is twice as common in males than females. It is caused by intestinal invagination, usually around the ileocecal valve. The classic presentation is intermittent severe colicky abdominal pain with legs drawn up, followed by periods of comfort or falling asleep. Vomiting usually occurs in the early phase, which later becomes bilious. A passage of blood and mucus in the stool ("currant jelly stools") occurs in 60% of the cases. Palpation of the abdomen usually reveals a sausage-shaped mass in the right upper quadrant. The classic presentation of

pyloric stenosis is in first-born males, 3 to 6 weeks of age, presenting with nonbilious projectile vomiting leading to dehydration with hypochloremia, hypokalemia, and metabolic alkalosis. A firm, movable, 2-cm olive-shaped mass ("olive") is palpable superior and to the right of the umbilicus in the midepigastrum. Additionally, peristaltic waves may be visible on the physical exam. The classic presentation of appendicitis presents with a period of anorexia followed by steady periumbilical pain shifting to right lower quadrant pain; nausea and vomiting is followed by a low-grade fever. Diarrhea (nonbloody and mucous), if it occurs, is infrequent. Peritoneal signs are present. The incidence increases with age and peaks during adolescence. Infective enteritis usually begins with emesis followed by crampy abdominal pain of hyperperistalsis. This sequence of symptoms with emesis preceding pain is an important factor in distinguishing it from intussusception. Masses are not palpated with infective enteritis. (*Behrman and Kliegman, 2002, pp. 492, 499; Hay et al, 2005, 628–629, 636–638, 641–643*)

27. **(C)** Dehydration is a common pathophysiologic alteration in fluid balance in children. The body has a maintenance fluid requirement to replace daily normal losses that occur through the skin, kidney, intestines, and respiratory tract. The following formula can be used to calculate the usual amount of fluid a healthy child requires by mouth to maintain hydration:

100 mL/kg for the first 10 kg body weight

50 mL/kg for the next 10 kg body weight

20 mL/kg for the weights above 20 kg

For this question, an 18-kg child would require:

100 mL/kg × 10 kg =	1000 mL for the first	10 kg
50 mL/kg × 8 kg =	400 mL for the next	8 kg
Total =	1400 mL	18 kg

(*Hay et al, 2005, pp. 1322–1323, Gunn and Nechyba, 2002, pp. 234–235*)

28. **(C)** Meningococcal meningitis is caused by *Neisseria meningitidis*, a Gram-negative diplo-

coccus. Household, school, or child-care contacts exposed to the respiratory secretions of the patient are at a high risk for developing the infection and should receive chemoprophylaxis with rifampin. Alternative chemoprophylactic medications include ciprofloxacin and ceftriaxone. Aqueous penicillin G is the drug of choice for treatment of meningococcal meningitis, but it is not a chemoprophylactic medication because it does not eradicate nasopharyngeal carrier state. Rifabutin is an alternative prophylactic agent for infections with nontuberculous mycobacteria. Rimantadine is a chemoprophylactic agent for influenza A in children and adults. (*Gunn and Nechyba, 2002, p. 837; Hay et al, 2005, pp. 1201–1203*)

29. **(B)** Congenital hypothyroidism is one of the most common disorders tested for in newborn screening tests, revealing an elevated TSH (thyroid stimulating hormone) and a decreased T_4 (thyroxine). Symptoms suggestive of congenital hypothyroidism in the neonate include hypotonia, coarse facial features, hirsute forehead, large fontanels (anterior and posterior), widely open sutures, umbilical hernia, protruding/large tongue, hoarse cry, distended abdomen, and prolonged jaundice. Signs of congenital hypothyroidism include lethargy or hypoactivity, poor feeding, constipation, mottling, and hypothermia. Congenital adrenal hyperplasia (CAH) is not universally screened for in the newborn screening test, as it is included in only 14 of the 50 states. In females with CAH, there may be virilization with abnormalities of the external genitalia varying from mild enlargement of the clitoris to complete fusion of the labioscrotal folds. Signs of adrenal insufficiency (salt loss) may present in the first few days of life. Crigler–Najjar syndrome is not one of the disorders tested for in the standard newborn screening tests. It is an inherited disease producing congenital nonobstructive, nonhemolytic, unconjugated severe hyperbilirubinermia. The physical findings in this infant do not correlate with Crigler–Najjar syndrome. Galactosemia is tested for in the newborn screening test in nearly all 50 states. The infant may have symptoms of cataracts, he-

patomegaly, and prolonged jaundice. Often these neonates have *Escherichia coli* sepsis, leading to death in the first 2 weeks of life if not treated promptly. (*Hay et al, 2005, pp. 14, 973–976, 998–1000, 1020*)

30. **(B)** A cephalohematoma is a firm, tense external swelling of the cranium that does *not* extend across suture lines because it is limited to the surface of one cranial bone. It occurs most often in the parietal area. This subperiosteal hemorrhage usually is not present at birth, but develops within the first 24 hours of life. Craniotabes is a condition caused by the osteoporosis of the outer table of the involved membraneous bone, generally over the temporoparietal or parietooccipital areas, creating a "ping-pong ball" sensation when gentle pressure is applied. A subgaleal hemorrhage is a firm, fluctuant external swelling of the cranium that does extend across suture lines and increases in size after birth. (*Behrman and Kliegman, 2002, pp. 201–202, 210; Hay et al, 2005, p. 22*)

31. **(C)** Foreign body aspiration into the respiratory tract is associated with an acute choking or coughing episode with expiratory wheezing (indicative of a lower airway obstruction) in children 6 months to 4 years of age. Often, there is a history of the child playing with small toys that are commonly aspirated. Asymmetrical physical findings of decreased breath sounds and localized wheezing are present with foreign body aspiration. A positive forced expiratory chest x-ray shows a mediastinal shift away from the affected side. Radiolucent foreign bodies such as plastic toys may not appear on an x-ray, but there will be evidence of this mediastinal shift. Asthma is generally characterized by wheezing, but it is not unilateral nor is it of sudden onset. A chest x-ray reveals bilateral hyperinflation with flattening of the diaphragm. Epiglottitis is a life-threatening upper airway obstructive condition that presents with a sudden onset of fever, dysphagia, drooling, and inspiratory retractions with stridor. A lateral neck x-ray reveals an enlarged, indistinct epiglottis ("thumb sign"); however, the chest x-ray is normal. Pulmonary embolism, rare in

children, presents clinically with acute dyspnea, tachypnea, and tachycardia. There may be mild hypoxemia, rales, and focal wheezing. Chest x-rays may be normal, or there may be a peripheral infiltrate, small pleural effusion, or elevated hemidiaphragm. (*Hay et al, 2005, pp. 514–515, 518–519, 546, 1080–1085; Behrman and Kliegman, 2002, p. 551*)

32. **(B)** An acute salicylate overdose (greater than 150 mg/kg) will produce symptoms of salicylate intoxication. Chronic salicylate intoxication occurs with ingestion of greater than 100 mg/kg/day for at least 2 days. Salicylates affect most organ systems, leading to various metabolic abnormalities. Because salicylates are a gastric irritant, symptoms of vomiting and diarrhea occur soon after the overdose, which may contribute to the development of dehydration. Salicylates stimulate the respiratory center leading to hyperventilation and hyperpnea resulting in respiratory alkalosis and compensatory alkaluria. A characteristic feature of salicylate intoxication is the coexistence of a respiratory alkalosis with a widened anion gap metabolic acidosis. (*Behrman and Kliegman, 2002, pp. 104–107; Hay et al, 2005, pp. 1327–1329*)

33. **(C)** Generalized tetanus (lockjaw) is a neurologic disease caused by *Clostridium tetani*. Although any open wound is a potential source for contamination with *C. tetani*, those with dirt, soil, feces, or saliva are at increased risk. Tetanus-prone wounds contain devitalized tissue, especially those caused by punctures, frostbite, crush injury, or burns. Recommendations for tetanus prophylaxis in a child with a laceration or abrasion depend upon the number of previous vaccinations, occurrence of last booster, type of wound (clean or tetanus-prone), and age of child. In this case, the patient is older than 7 years and had all of his previous immunizations; however, his most recent booster was greater than 10 years ago. Thus, he should receive an adult type diphtheria and tetanus toxoid with acellular pertussis. In most cases, when tetanus toxoid is required for wound prophylaxis in a child older than 7 years, the Td instead of tetanus toxoid alone is recommended so that diphtheria immunity is maintained. If tetanus immunization is not up to date at the time of wound treatment, then the immunization series should be completed according to the primary immunization schedule. If a child is younger than 7 years, then the diphtheria, tetanus, acellular pertussis (DTaP) booster is indicated, unless there is a contraindication for pertussis, in which case the diphtheria and tetanus (DT) booster should be administered. Tetanus immune globulin (TIG) is recommended for treatment of tetanus. Under special circumstances a patient infected with the human immunodeficiency virus (HIV) with a tetanus-prone wound should also receive TIG in addition to the prophylactic vaccine. (*Hay et al, 2005, pp. 1208–1210; Centers for Disease Control, 2006*)

34. **(D)** Normally, primitive reflexes are present at birth and should not persist beyond 6 months of age. Some primitive reflexes include asymmetric tonic neck, moro, palmar grasp, and rooting. The absence or persistence beyond a certain time indicates a dysfunction of the central nervous system. The parachute reflex is a postural response that normally appears around 7 months of age to coincide with volitional movement. It occurs when an infant is held prone by the waist over a surface and lowered with the head downward and extends the arms and legs as a form of protection. (*Hay et al, 2005, p. 7; Behrman and Kliegman, 2002, p. 770*)

35. **(A)** Gonococcal ophthalmia neonatorum presents as a unilateral or bilateral serosanguineous discharge and then within 24 hours the discharge becomes mucopurulent, followed by conjunctival injection and edema of the eyelids. The usual incubation period for *Neiserria gonorrhea* is 2 to 5 days; however, the infection may be present at birth or delayed greater than 5 days if there has been instillation of silver nitrate prophylaxis. A presumptive diagnosis is made by the demonstration of Gram-negative intracellular diplococci on Gram stain. Definitive diagnosis is made by culture. Following a positive Gram stain and pending culture results, treatment should be promptly initiated with ceftriaxone (50 mg/kg/24 hours IV or IM for one dose not to

exceed 125 mg). An alternate drug is cefotaxime (100 mg/kg/24 hours IV or IM every 12 hours for 7 days or 100 mg/kg as a single dose). Although erythromycin drops (0.5%) are used prophylactically for *N. gonorrhea*, this is not an effective treatment. Neonatal conjunctivitis caused by *Chlamydia trachomatis* is treated with a 2-week course of oral erythromycin. Staphylococcal neonatal conjunctivitis is treated with parenteral methicillin. *Pseudomonas aeruginosa* neonatal conjunctivitis is treated with an aminoglycoside and gentamicin ophthalmic ointment. (*Hay et al, 2005, p. 58; Behrman and Kliegman, 2002, p. 204*)

36. **(B)** The most likely diagnosis in this patient is mumps. It is endemic in most unvaccinated populations. The onset is characterized by pain and swelling in one or both parotid glands. The pain can be exacerbated by tasting sour liquids such as lemon juice. An elevated serum amylase level is common and coincides with the parotid swelling. Unilateral, rarely bilateral, nerve deafness is a complication of mumps that may be transient or permanent. Other complications include meningoencephalomyelitis, orchitis, epididymitis, pancreatitis, arthritis, and rarely thyroiditis and myocarditis. (*Behrman and Kliegman, 2002, p. 453; Hay et al, 2005, pp. 1167–1169*)

37. **(A)** Café au lait spots are brown macules which may be found on any part of the body. The presentation of six or more spots greater than 1.5 cm is a sign of neurofibromatosis, a genetic disorder which results in neurofibromas that can develop in any organ/tissue system. Miliaria are blocked sweat gland ducts that are commonly found on the face, scalp or intertriginous areas. Vernix caseosa is a normal finding in newborns and is a whitish, greasy layering on the body—it decreases as an infant comes to full term. Subconjunctival hemorrhages are a common finding in infants secondary to birth trauma.(*Hay et al, 2005, pp. 5–6, 415*)

38. **(B)** The Apgar score assesses the newborn at 1-minute and 5-minute intervals to determine the need for resuscitative care. The infant is evaluated by heart rate, respiratory effort, muscle tone, response to catheter in nostril, and color, and each is rated on a scale of 0, 1, or 2 for a total score of 10. The heart rate is scaled 0–2 for absent, <100 bpm (slow) and >100 bpm; respiratory effort of absent, slow/irregular and good/crying. Muscle tone scale (0–2) consists of limp, some flexion, and active motion; response to catheter stimulation (0–2) is scaled no response, grimace and cough/sneeze. Finally, color is scored 0–2 for blue/pale, body pink with blue extremities and completely pink. (*Hay et al, 2005, p. 4*)

39. **(C)** Ventricular septal defect, a hole between the two ventricles and can be cyanotic or acyanotic based on the size of the defect, accounts for 30% of cases of congenital heart disease. Atrial septal defect occurs in approximately 10% of congenital heart disease cases. Transposition of great vessels is an embryonic malformation resulting in the aorta arising from the right ventricle and the pulmonary artery arising from the left ventricle. It is responsible for about 10% of all congenital malformations. Tetralogy of Fallot, consisting of a ventricular septal defect, overriding aorta, pulmonic/subpulmonic stenosis, and right ventricular hypertrophy, accounts for 10% of congenital heart disease. (*Hay et al, 2005, pp. 772–794*)

40. **(D)** The immunization schedule is developed biannually by the Centers for Disease Control and Prevention. Assuming that the child has had the appropriate immunizations at their regularly scheduled exams, the recommended immunizations at the 4- to 6-year-old range are the DTaP (diptheria, tetanus, acellular pertussis), IPV (inactivated polio), and the MMR (measles, mumps, and rubella). The hepatitis series should have been completed by 6 months of age, the Hib should be completed by 12 to 15 months. Varicella is given from 12 to 18 months and the PCV (pneumococcal) should be finished by 12 to 15 months. (*Centers for Disease Control and Prevention, 2006b*)

41. **(A)** There are only two known absolute contraindications to breast-feeding: tuberculosis

of the mother and galactosemia of the infant. The highly contagious nature of tuberculosis makes the risk greater than the benefit and infants with galactosemia are unable to digest any lactose due to an enzyme deficiency. Infants of mothers in a methadone program may be breast-fed as long as the mother's dose is less than 40 mg. While nicotine is transmitted in breast milk and is therefore strongly discouraged, it is not an absolute contraindication. As long as a breast-fed infant with cystic fibrosis is maintaining normal growth with supplemented pancreatic enzymes, breast-feeding is encouraged. (*Hay et al, 2005, pp. 288, 299–301*)

42. **(B)** Failure to thrive is diagnosed in infants under 6 months with a decrease in growth velocity that results in a decrease in two major percentile lines on the growth chart. In the case of this patient, she was initially in the 50th percentile and crossed the 25th and 10th percentile and fell into the 5th percentile. Failure to thrive is also known as growth deficiency and may also be diagnosed if the child under 6 months has not grown for two consecutive months or if a child over 6 months has not grown for 3 consecutive months. Growth hormone deficiency/dwarfism may present with decreased growth velocity later in childhood; the drop in percentiles is grossly below the 5th percentile mark. Lactose intolerance presents with varying gastrointestinal symptoms without the marked decrease in weight. Beckwith–Widemann syndrome consists of macrosomia, macroglossia, and omphalocele and they are at increased risk for malignancies, hypoglycemia, and dysmorphism (usually of the ears). (*Hay et al, 2005, pp. 247, 288, 964–968, 1069*)

43. **(C)** This patient has presented with classical findings of Reye's syndrome—upper respiratory infection followed by unresponsiveness. Reye's syndrome is usually preceded by an upper respiratory tract illness which progresses into vomiting, strange behavior, stupor, and coma. Liver function tests (LFTs) will be markedly elevated (without jaundice); however, the serum bilirubin and alkaline phosphatase are normal. Unresponsive patients who have a spinal tap will show no cells in the CSF and glucose may be low with increased CSF pressure. If arterial blood gases are ordered, they will show a mild respiratory alkalosis and metabolic acidosis. A liver biopsy will show little inflammatory changes with diffuse microvesicular steatosis and absent glycogen from the hepatocytes. The mitochondria of the hepatocytes are large and polymorphic with decreased matriceal density. Treatment for patients with Reye's syndrome is largely supportive—specifically decreasing cerebral edema. There is no place for antibiotics or steroids. The liver will fully recover if the cerebral edema is decreased. (*Hay et al, 2005, pp. 685–686*)

44. **(B)** Wilson's disease is a result in a genetic mutation on chromosome 13 which causes decreased bile excretion of copper and results in accumulation of copper by the liver, specifically the ceruloplasmin. The build-up of copper causes damage to the liver, basal ganglia, and other tissues. Physical exam shows jaundice, hepatosplenomegaly, Kayser–Fleischer rings (a brown band at the junction of the iris and cornea under slit-lamp), and neurologic manifestations later in the disease process. Laboratory tests show marked decrease in ceruloplasmin of the liver, anemia, hemoloysis, and severely elevated bilirubin with decrease alkaline phosphatase. Urinalysis shows severe elevation in copper excretion, glycosuria, and aminoaciduria. Liver biopsy is conclusive with evidence of copper greater than 250 µg/g of dry tissue. Treatment requires copper chelation with D-penicillamine or trientine hydrochloride. Liver transplant may be required with noncompliance and in acute fulminant disease. Copper chelation is continued for life with the addition of zinc (decrease copper absorption) and vitamin B_6 (decrease optic neuritis). Genetic screening of siblings and future children should be strongly encouraged. Alpha-interferon therapy is mainly used to treat hepatitis patients. There is no place for steroids in therapy and protease inhibitors are antiviral medications that are typically used in HIV patients. (*Hay et al, 2005, pp. 683–685*)

45. **(A)** The patient's presentation is consistent with findings of coarctation of the aorta. The pathognomonic finding in coarction is decreased or absent femoral pulses. However, the majority of children show no signs of coarctation in infancy and develop signs and symptoms as children, most notably unequal pulses and blood pressure between arms and legs (arms lower than legs). Additionally, a grade II/VI ejection murmur is heard at the aortic area and left sternal border that radiates into the left axilla and left back. Chest x-ray shows a normal sized heart, the aorta is prominent, indents at the level of the coarctation, and the poststenotic segment is dilated resulting in the "figure 3" sign. Scalloping or notching of the ribs is due to enlargement of the intercostal arteries. Echocardiography is used to directly visualize the coarctation and estimate the obstruction. Asymptomatic infants and children are encouraged to have corrective surgery prior to age 5, after which they are at increased risk for myocardial dysfunction and hypertension and require exercise testing prior to participation in aerobic activities. The boot shaped heart is seen in patients with tetralogy of Fallot secondary to right ventricular hypertropy; the narrowed mediastinum finding with "egg on a string" is typically seen in patients with transposition of the great vessels. (*Hay et al, 2005, pp. 582– 594*)

46. **(D)** Viral croup usually presents with cough that may sound like dog barking or a seal. The patients are usually afebrile and also present with stridor either at rest, in severe cases, or when agitated, in mild cases. Additionally, the patient may be cyanotic and have retractions and acute shortness of breath. Radiologic exam of the neck shows subglottic narrowing with a normal epiglottis, "steeple sign." However, x-rays are usually not indicated in patients with the common presenting symptoms. Treatment for viral croup is mainly symptomatic especially in mild cases consisting of oral hydration and mist therapy. Severe cases (stridor at rest) call for oxygen for patients who have desaturated, nebulized racemic epinephrine, and glucocorticoids. Dexamethosone as an intramuscular injection or oral one time dose is effective in alleviating symptoms, decreasing the need for intubation and decreasing hospital stays. Inhaled budesonide is also effective in decreasing hospital stays and improving symptoms, but dexamethosone is more cost-effective. Patients who are unable to be stabilized need airway maintenance either by intubation with endotracheal tube or by tracheostomy if intubation fails. Since it is a self-limiting disorder, unless there is a secondary infection most children recover in a few days. (*Hay et al, 2005, pp. 513–514*)

47. **(A)** Cystic fibrosis (CF) is a major cause of gastrointestinal and pulmonary morbidity in children due to mutations in the CF genes. The mutations lead to a deficiency in cystic fibrosis transmembrane conductance regulator protein that controls movement of salt and water into and out of epithelial cells and results in production of abnormally thick mucus. About 15% of patients with CF present with meconium ileus at birth. This is typically treated with enema for disimpaction and rarely surgery. Approximately half of infants with CF will present with failure to thrive which is diagnosed by lack of growth for two consecutive months in patients under 6 months of age. They may also present with respiratory compromise. However, not all patients present in childhood. Diagnosis of CF is confirmed by a sweat chloride level above 60 meq/L or with genetic testing. Treatment for patients with CF is mainly symptomatic therapy for obstructions of the digestive and respiratory tract. Additionally there is pancreatic enzyme supplementation to aid in digestion and vitamin and calorie supplementation for deficiencies in the diet. Gene therapy is now being looked at for future treatment. Intussusception (telescoping of the small intestine) typically presents in an infant with paroxysmal abdominal pain, vomiting, and diarrhea that may progress into bloody stools. Volvulus is normally the result of intestinal malrotation that causes occlusion of the superior mesenteric artery and eventual bowel necrosis. Infants typically present within 3 weeks of life with bile-stained vomiting and bowel obstruction. Wilson's disease is defect in the

ability to excrete copper in the bile that results in liver accumulation of copper. (*Hay et al, 2005, pp. 526–528, 631, 637–638*)

48. **(B)** Cyanotic heart lesions are a result of a right-to-left shunt. These include tetralogy of Fallot, pulmonary atresia with and without ventricular septal defect, tricuspid atresia, hypoplastic left heart syndrome, and transposition of the great arteries. The right-to-left shunt results in deoxygenated blood reaching the left venticle, aorta, and systemic arteries. The decreased oxygen in the blood results in decreased oxygen to the tissue and subsequently causes cyanosis. Atrial septal defect, ventricular septal defect, atrioventricular septal defect, and patent ductus arteriosus most commonly present with a left-to-right shunt. (*Hay et al, 2005, pp. 571–599*)

49. **(A)** This infant is presenting with signs and symptoms of pyloric stenosis. Infants typically have vomiting (projectile at times) after every feeding and it normally starts between 2 and 4 weeks of age. The infant nurses fervently and is hungry. Additionally, there may be dehydration, constipation, weight loss, and apathy. Abdomen may be distended with gastric peristaltic waves. Occasionally an olive-sized mass can be felt in the right upper quandrant with deep palpation after the child has vomited. Vomitus is typically nonbilious. Diagnosis is confirmed by an upper gastrointestinal series with delayed gastric emptying, enlarged pyloric muscle, and characteristic semilunar impressions on the gastric antrum. Additionally, an ultrasound is needed to verify the hypertrophic muscle. The treatment of choice for these patients is pyloromyotomy which can be done laparoscopically. These patients make full recoveries and have an excellent prognosis. (*Hay et al, 2005, p. 628*)

50. **(D)** Celiac disease or gluten enteropathy typically initially presents with diarrhea episodes in the first 6 to 12 months of life—when whole grains are first fed. Therefore, in strictly breast-fed babies, symptoms may not be noticed until solid foods are begun. The diarrhea is usually intermittent at first and then typically progresses into pale, greasy, foul-smelling, frothy stools. Additional symptoms may be constipation, vomiting, and abdominal pain, which may lead the clinician to think intestinal obstruction. Other findings may be failure to thrive, anemia, and vitamin deficiencies. Stool sample demonstrates excessive fecal fat excretion. Blood tests show hypoproteinemia and impaired carbohydrate absorption. Intestinal biopsy is the diagnostic test of choice for celiac disease. Results show shortened celiac mucosa, absent villi, lengthened crypts of Lieberkuhn, plasma cell infilation of the lamina propria, and intraepithelial lymphocytes. Treatment consists of dietary restriction of gluten—wheat, rye, and barley. Steroids are given on an as-needed basis. Sweat chloride testing is utilized in patients suspected of cystic fibrosis. Gastrin level is taken in patients suspected of Zollinger–Ellison syndrome and RAST (radioallergosorbent assay test) is used in patients to determine different environmental-type allergens. (*Hay et al, 2005, pp. 646–647*)

51. **(B)** The most likely diagnosis for this patient is post-streptococcal glomerulonephritis. The diagnosis is supported by a documented culture of group A beta-hemolytic streptococcus infection. If a culture is not available like the patient in this scenario, the clinician can order an anti-streptolysin O titer. Antistreptolysin is an enzyme released by group A streptococcus and is elevated for up to 1 month after strep infection. Glomerulonephritis presents with gross hematuria with or without edema. Hyptertension, proteinuria, ascites, and headache may also be present. Treatment with antibiotics is useful if infection is still present, and symptomatic treatment for renal failure with hemodialysis, if necessary. Symptoms typically resolve within a few weeks. The monospot is used to diagnose infectious mononucleosis. Renal biopsy could be performed on extreme cases of glomerulonephritis but is not typically necessary. Immunoglobulin electrophoresis would be utilized in patients suspected of having immunoglobulinopathies or IgA-mediated glomerulonephritis. (*Hay et al, 2005, p. 713*)

52. **(D)** Patent ductus arteriosus (PDA) is an isolated abnormality that occurs in infants. The

ductus arteriosus is a normal fetal vessel that joins the aorta and the pulmonary artery and spontaneously closes after 3 to 5 days. Lack of closure results in the audible murmur that is "machine-like" and maximal at the second intercostal space (ICS) at the left sternal border (LSB) and inferior to the clavicle. It is typically a pansystolic murmur with bounding pulses and a widened pulse pressure. There is also a paradoxical splitting of S1 and S2. Echocardiography confirms the PDA, the direction and degree of shunting, and the presence of lesions for which the PDA is needed to keep. If there are no other cardiac malformations requiring the PDA, then if the PDA is large, surgery should be completed before 1 year of age. Symptomatic PDAs that are relatively small may be closed with indomethacin in preterm infants. The mumur heard in atrial septal defect (ASD) usually is an ejection type, systolic murmur heard best at the LSB, 2nd ICS with a wide, fixed S_2 and normal pulses. Ventricular septal defect (VSD) presents with a harsh, pansystolic murmur heard best at the 3rd and 4th ICS. With increasing size of the VSD, heaves, thrills, and lifts are present along with radiation throughout the chest. Tetralogy of Fallot presents with a rough ejection, systolic murmur heard best at the LSB and the 3rd ICS with radiation to the back. (*Hay et al, 2005, pp. 572–574, 577–579, 588–590*)

53. **(C)** Hypertrophic cardiomyopathy in adolescence is typically due to familial hypertrophic cardiomyopathy with an incidence of 1:500. Many patients are asymptomatic until a sporting event which may cause symptoms, specifically sudden cardiac death. Examination may demonstrate a palpable or audible S_4, an LV (left ventricular) heave, systolic ejection murmur (may need to stimulate cardiac activity), and/or a left precordial bulge. Echocardiography is the gold standard for diagnosis but family history should be assessed. Stress testing is indicated to assess for ischemia and arrhythmias. Strenuous activities are prohibited for these patients. The other cardiomyopathies (dilated and restrictive) are next but are not as common. Congenital structural abnormalities of the coronary arteries are the next most common cause. Valvular

disorders, including surgically repaired aortic stenosis, are typically not causes of sudden death, but these patients should be screened for symptoms, and stress tested as necessary. (*Hay et al, 2005, pp. 604–605, 622*)

54. **(A)** This patient presentation describes epiglottitis. Although there is a decreased incidence of epiglottitis secondary to the introduction of the vaccine for *Haemophilus influenzae* type b (Hib), patients still present with suddent onset of fever, dysphagia, muffled voice, drooling, cyanosis, inspiratory retractions, and soft stridor. The patients are usually sitting in a tripod position to aid their breathing. Recognition of the classic symptoms needs to be immediate to stabilize the patient's airway, as these patients will decompensate into respiratory failure quickly. In the event that there is time, a lateral neck x-ray will show the "thumb sign," which is an enlarged, indistinguished epiglottis. Treatment for the patient requires intubation for airway stabilization, blood cultures and throat/epiglottis cultures, and antibiotic coverage for *H. influenzae*. The steeple sign is seen in patients with croup and is due to a subglottic narrowing. The "figure 3" sign is seen in patients with coarctation of the aorta. The "Scottie dog" sign is seen in oblique lumbar films and is a normal finding representing the pars interarticularis. Its absence signifies spondylolysis. (*Hay et al, 2005, pp. 514–515; Erkonen, 2000, p. 317f; Gunn and Nechyba, 2002, p. 536t*)

55. **(C)** With an incidence of 1:3000 to 1:4000 Caucasians, cystic fibrosis is the most common lethal genetic disorder in the United States. While trisomy 21 (Down syndrome) is one of the most common genetic disorders with 1:500 newborns, it is typically not a fatal disease. It is characterized with mental retardation and physical malformations. Trisomy 13 is a fatal trisomy, with most deaths occurring in early infancy or by the age of 2, but its incidence is approximately 1:12,000 live births. Neurofibromatosis, a genetic disorder of typical autosomal dominant inheritance, occurs in approximately 1:3000 live births. Most affected children have the skin lesions (café au

lait macules or neurofibromas) and other minor problems. (*Hay et al, 2005, pp. 526–528, 1061, 1064–1065*)

56. **(B)** Status epilepticus is a medical emergency and is defined as seizure activity that lasts a minimum of 30 minutes. This results in hypoxia, acidosis, cerebral edema, and structural damage. Additionally, fever, respiratory depression, hypotension, and death may occur. There are both convulsive and nonconvulsive types of status epilepticus. Due to its emergency status and potential complications, the clinician needs to initiate the ABCs (airway, breathing, circulation). Therefore the first line of treatment is to establish and maintain an airway, oxygen is next, and then circulation, which encompasses pulse, blood pressure, and IV access. Once the IV is established the orders should be for glucose-containing fluids and IV drug therapy with diazepam, lorazepam, or midazolam; and phenytoin and phenobarbital. Arterial blood gases should be ordered and any abnormalities should be corrected appropriately. Finally, the clinician should determine the underlying cause: trauma, structural disorder, infection, lactic acidosis, toxins, and uremia. Maintenance drug therapy is necessary until the underlying cause is determined and rectified. (*Hay et al, 2005, pp. 744–750*)

57. **(D)** Guillain–Barré syndrome is most likely due to a delayed hypersensitivity with T-cell–mediated antibodies to mycoplasma and viral infections (CMV, EBV, hepatitis B, *campylobacter jejuni*). The patients may mention a nonspecific respiratory or gastrointestinal infection 1 to 2 weeks prior to symptoms. Complaints may be paresthesias, weakness in bilateral lower extremities with occasional ascension into the arms, trunk, and face, and rarely ataxia and ophthalmoplegia in the Miller–Fisher variant. Exam findings demonstrate symmetric flaccid weakness, with impariment of position, vibration, and touch in the distal portions of the extremeties. If a spinal tap is performed, it may show few polymorphonuclear neutrophils with high protein and normal glucose. EMG is positive for decreased nerve conduction. Laboratory tests may show high titers of suspected infec-

tions or active infection of hepatitis/bacterial pathogens. Gullain-Barre is normally a self-limiting disorder within a few weeks, unless there are issues with respiratory depression. Poliomyelitis is secondary to polioviruses and presents with fever, paralysis, meningeal signs, and asymmetrical weakness. Botulism secondary to infection with *Clostridium botulinum* in older children presents with blurred vision, diplopia, ptosis, choking, and weakness. In infants, botulism presents as constipation, poor suck and cry, apnea, lethargy, and choking. Tick-bite paralysis presents with rapid onsent with ascending flaccid paralysis reaching upper extremities in a couple of days of onset and patients often present with paresthesia and pain. Finding of a tick is usually confirmatory for these patients. (*Hay et al, 2005, pp. 792–793t*)

58. **(B)** Scoliosis is defined by lateral curvature of the spine with rotation of vertebrae and is typically located in the thoracic or lumbar spine in the right or left directions. Idiopathic scoliosis most commonly presents as a right thoracic curve in females from 8 to 10 years of age. Scoliosis is typically asymptomatic unless curvatures are so severe that there is pulmonary dysfunction or there is an underlying disorder (bone or spinal tumor) that is causing the scoliosis. X-rays need to be taken of the entire spine to help determine the degree of curvature. Treatment modalities are based on the degree of curvature: 20° or less does not normally require treatment; 20° to 40° (is an indication for bracing in an immature child; and 40° and greater is resistant to bracing and requires surgical fixation with spinal fusion, which is best done at special centers. (*Hay et al, 2005, pp. 814–815*)

59. **(D)** Legg–Calvé–Perthes disease is also known as avascular necrosis of the proximal femur. It typically occcurs in children between 4 and 8 years old and persistent hip pain is the main symptom, and on exam the clinician notices a limp and/or limitation of motion of the affected hip. Radiologic exam demonstrates the necrosis with effusion and joint space widening with a negative aspirate. Treatment involves surgical hip replacement. Slipped capital femoral epiphysis (SCFE) is

due to the displacement of the proximal femoral epiphysis owing to disruption of the growth plate. The head is normally displaced medially and posteriorly relative to the femoral neck. It typically occurs in adolescence, specifically obese males, and can also be associated with hypothyroidism. SCFE usually occurs after direct trauma to the hip or a fall. Patients complain of vague symptoms at first that progress into pain of the hip or of the knee. On exam there is decreased internal rotation of the hip and can be confirmed by lateral x-ray of the hip. Septic hip arthritis is not common in children and will have a positive aspirate. Osteochondritis dissecans typically presents in the knee, elbow, and talus and is characterized by a wedge-shaped necrosis of bone. (*Hay et al, 2005, pp. 815–816, 824–825*)

60. **(B)** Gamekeeper's thumb is a result in damage to the ulnar collateral ligament during forced abduction of the metacarpalphalangeal joint, an injury that is most commonly seen in skiers. An avulsed fragment may or may not been seen on radiologic exam. If it is smaller than 2 mm, there is no fragment, a thumb spica cast can be used as seen in patients with no fragment. If the fragment is larger than 2 mm, surgery is required. Mallet finger is an avulsion of the extensor tendon and occurs in ball-handling sports. Boxer's fracture is a distal neck fracture of the 5th metacarpal. Scaphoid fractures are due to hyperextension of the wrist injuries and present with pain in the anatomic snuffpox and swelling. (*Hay et al, 2005, p. 840*)

61. **(A)** Nursemaid's elbow is the subluxation of the radial head due to a child or infant being lifted or pulled by the hand. The patient will present with the elbow pronated and painful and he or she will not bend the elbow. During the radiologic exam, the dislocation is usually reduced by placing the elbow in full supination and moving it slowly from flexion to extension. This typically provides immediate relief of pain and a sling may be given for comfort for a couple of days. Otherwise x-rays are normal. Child protective services should be considered if this is a recurrent problem or if there are other associated signs

and symptoms of battery. There is no need for orthopedic referral unless reduction is not commonly done in your setting. Immobilization of the elbow is not recommended as the patient then may have to recover from frozen shoulder. (*Hay et al, 2005, p. 819*)

62. **(A)** This patient is presenting with signs and symptoms of primary nocturnal enuresis, which is the wetting only at night during sleep without any sustained period of dryness. It is mainly considered a parasomnia occurring in deep-sleep. The incidence of enuresis is higher in boys, is typically related to a developmental delay, and most children become continent by adolescence. Patients need to be tested for structural abnormalities and infections, in addition to neurologic diseases, diabetes mellitus and insipidus, and seizure disorders. Treatment includes limiting liquids at bedtime and routine bathroom training during the day. If these are unsuccessful, the next option is a bed-wetting alarm. This device is attached to the child's undergarment and vibrates wthen the child is wet to arouse the child to be aware of their need to urinate. If the alarm is unsuccessful, then the next step is medication—DDAVP (desmopressin acetate) or imipramine. (*Hay et al, 2005, pp. 207–208*)

63. **(D)** Nephroblastoma also known as Wilms' tumor typically presents with an asymptomatic abdominal mass noticed by the parent or an increasing size of the abdomen. On exam, the mass feels smooth and firm, is well defined, and usually does not cross the midline. Gross hematuria may be present, but rare, and some patients have microscopic hematuria when tested. Wilms' tumor accounts for approximately 5% of cancers in children under 15 years. Wilms' tumor arises from the kidney and the average age at diagnosis is 4 years old. Ultrasound and CT of the abdomen can be used to confirm the presence of an intraabdominal mass. Treatment includes exploratory abdominal surgery for removal and staging with a mixture of chemotherapy. Intussusception (telescoping of the small intestine) typically presents as an infant with paroxysmal abdominal pain,

vomiting, and diarrhea that may progress into bloody stools. Volvulus is normally the result of intestinal malrotation that causes occlusion of the superior mesenteric artery and eventual bowel necrosis. Infants typically present within 3 weeks of life with bile-stained vomiting and bowel obstruction. (*Hay et al, 2005, pp. 930–932*)

64. **(C)** Infant girls presenting with signs of precocious puberty need to be screened for congenital adrenal hyperplasia (CAH). CAH most commonly presents with pseudohermaphroditism in females—urogential sinus, enlarged clitoris, or other signs of virilization. In males there tends to be isosexual precocity in older males and salt-losing crisis in infant males. Both children show increased linear growth and skeletal maturation. The most common type of CAH is a deficiency in the enzyme 21-hydroxylase and laboratory tests demonstrate increased urinary and plasma androgens (DHEA, androstenedione). There may be elevated progesterone, but typically there is no effect on estrogen. There is also decreased aldosterone and elevated urinary ketosteroids. There is also no effect on the levels of leutenizing hormone or follicle-stimulating hormone. Treatment usually involves glucocorticoids, mineracorticoids, and reconstructive surgery if needed. (*Hay et al, 2005, pp. 998–1000*)

65. **(A)** Growth hormone (GH) deficiency is defined as a decreased growth velocity, delay in skeletal maturation, absence of other explanations for poor growth (lack of intake), and laboratory tests demonstrating decreased GH secretion. Etiology of GH deficiency can be congenital, genetic, acquired, or idiopathic, which is the most common. Infants usually have a normal birth weight and may have a slightly decreased length. Additionally, most infants present with other endocrine deficiencies like hypoglycemia, hypothyroidism, and/or adrenal insufficiency. Children may present with truncal adiposity because growth hormone promotes lipolysis. Serum GH or intrinsic growth factor levels may or may not be decreased. In patients who do not have a demonstrated decrease in these hor-

mones, a trial period with GH is indicated. These patients and positive GH-deficient patients receive a once-daily subcutaneous injection of recombinant human GH. Congential hypothyroidism typically presents with short stature (typically noted after the 4-month newborn visit), delayed epiphyseal development, delayed closure of fontanelles, and retarded dental eruption in addition to other signs of hypothyroidism. Cushing's disease typically presents with truncal adiposity with thin extremities, muscle wasting, decreased growth rate, and moon facies. Lab results show elevated adrenocorticosteroids both in urine and serum, hypokalemia, eosinopenia, and lymphocytopenia. Typically in patients under 12 years of age, Cushing's disease is secondary to administration of ACTH or glucocorticoids. Congential adrenal hyperplasia typically presents with pseudohermaphroditism in females or salt-losing crisis in males with or without isosexual precocity. There is an increased linear growth and advanced skeletal maturation. (*Hay et al, 2005, pp. 964–969, 973–975, 998–1001*)

66. **(C); 67. (A); 68. (D); 69. (D); 70. (A); 71. (D); 72. (B)** Disorders caused by an abnormality in a single gene, except for new mutations, are either autosomal or X-linked. The disorders that follow an autosomal dominant inheritance are neurofibromatosis and achondroplasia. The disorders that follow an autosomal recessive inheritance are sickle cell anemia and cystic fibrosis. The disorder that follows an X-linked dominant inheritance is vitamin D-resistant rickets. The disorders that follow an X-linked recessive inheritance are Duchenne's muscular dystrophy, Hunter's syndrome, and hemophilia A. (*Hay et al, 2005, pp. 727–728, 871–873, 1034t, 1064–1067*)

73. **(A)** The most likely diagnosis is pediculosis. This parasitic infestation is most commonly seen in the young school-aged child, and more often in female and Caucasian children. The pediculosis louse lives in the hair and on the scalp and intermittently "bites" into the skin to feed. Discrete urticarial papules or erosions may arise at the bite site. By visualizing the live louse on the scalp, or in the hair, one

can easily make the diagnosis. However, the louse may be difficult to see, as it is only 1 to 3 mm in size. Otherwise, nits, or the casings of the eggs laid by the louse, can often be seen on the proximal portion of the hair shaft. The nit adheres to the hair shaft and is often difficult to remove. Brown nits are representative of current infestations and white nits past infestations. Treatment of head lice can be difficult due to the increasing resistance to some of the current treatment options. First-line treatment includes permethrin (1%) and permethrin-based products. Secondary treatment options for resistant infestations may include Malathion (0.5%). Regardless of treatment, viable ova should be removed by combing the patient's wetted hair with a finely toothed comb until all are removed. Ketoconazole cream and tar-based shampoos are utilized in fungal and seborrheic dermatitis infections. Silver sulfadiazine cream is a topical antibiotic. (*Behrman and Kliegman, 2002, p. 882; Gunn and Nechyba, 2002, p. 843*)

74. **(B)** Scabies, *Sarcoptes scabiei*, is the most common arthropod infestation of children, and it is highly contagious. However, its presentation varies widely and is dependent on the child's age, duration of the infestation, and immune status. Most often, the presenting complaint is severe intermittent itching. The linear papule or burrow commonly associated with scabies is often difficult to identify. Instead, most children will present with eczematous eruptions of red, excoriated papules and nodules. Usually, the distribution of the papules are the most diagnostic finding, and may include the web spaces of the fingers and toes, axillae, umbilicus, groin, penis, and the instep of the feet. Usually, in older children and adults, the face and scalp are spared. The treatment for scabies is a 12-hour application of permethrin 5% lotion. In addition, the parents and all caregivers should be treated at the same time. Clothing and bedding should be washed and dried (heat kills scabies). The family should also be educated in the treatment and prevention of future infestations. Moreover, they should be advised that the itching associated with scabies could persist for 7 to 14 days after successful treatment. Pediculosis is an infestation of louse

in the hair. Tinea corporis is a fungal infection of the torso or "ring worm" and presents with annual scaly plaques with central clearing and pustules. Herpes simplex typically presents with grouped vesicles on erythematous base and is painful. It typically is located in the lips, eyes, cheeks, or hands of children. (*Behrman and Kliegman, 2002, pp. 868–869, 882*)

75. **(D)** Seborrheic dermatitis is common in all age groups. In infants, this inflammatory skin disease is often manifested as thickened, yellowish-white, scaly, waxy appearing skin of the scalp and commonly involves the postauricular areas and the forehead. The more common name is "cradle cap." Cradle cap is a self-limiting disease of infants and resolves by the child's first birthday. In all ages, the scalp scale can be treated by shampooing with zinc pyrithione (Head and Shoulders), selenium sulfide 1% to 2.5%, salicylic acid (Tsal), or ketoconazole (Nizoral). The primary lesion in lichen planus presents on the flexor surfaces and is characterized by pruritic papules that are polygonal and flat-topped. Pityriasis rosea typically presents with the "herald patch" that is a solitary pink, round patch with some central clearing typically found on the torso. The rest of the eruption is described as papulovesicular and develops a Christmas tree pattern. Contact dermatitis usually presents with red patches and plaques with scales and localized to the area exposed to the irritant. (*Behrman and Kliegman, 2002, pp. 875–877*)

76. **(B)** This presentation is typical for granuloma annulare, which is a benign skin disorder, and treatment is not warranted. It is most commonly seen in children aged 6 to 10. The red to brown lesions are annular or circinate. These asymptomatic lesions are often confused with tinea corporis. The lesions will disappear on their own over a couple of years. (*Behrman and Kliegman, 2002, p. 878*)

77. **(D)** Liquid nitrogen is the treatment of choice for a single isolated wart. Forty percent salicylic acid in a plaster application is the most effective treatment of large and painful warts. Electrosurgery, burning laser surgery and other destructive treatments should be

avoided because of the potential for scarring and subsequent problems often associated with scars, as well as the possible recurrence of the wart after destructive treatment. (*Hay et al, 2005, pp. 423–424; Behrman and Kliegman, 2002, p. 881*)

78. **(B)** Topical keratolytic agents applied to the skin either as a single, once a day agent or in combination regime (retinoic acid cream, azelaic acid, and adpalene) once a day in the evening and benzoyl peroxide gel in the morning will control approximately 80% to 85% of cases of adolescent acne. When treating inflammatory acnes, papular or pustular, a daily topical antibiotic such as tetracycline, minocycline, or erythromycin can be used in addition to a daily keratolytic. The oral retinoid, 13-cis-retinoic acid (isotretinoid), accutane is reserved for treating nodulocystic acne (severe cystic acne). This medication is not effective for the milder forms of acne such as comedonal. Isotretinoin is teratogenic in women of childbearing age and has other side effects. Because of this, isotretinoin is not recommended unless strict adherence to FDA guidelines can be ensured. (*Hay et al, 2005, pp. 417–420; Behrman and Kliegman, 2002, pp. 284–285*)

79. **(A)** Clavicular factures are the most common fractures in infants and children. In newborns, this fracture is usually unilateral and often occurs after a difficult delivery. Many times no treatment is required or a figure-of-eight bandage can be used. For infants and children, a sling can be used. The bump that can be seen after fracture consolidation will usually resolve in a few months to a year. The next most common fractures are of the extremities, humerus being the most common and then the femur, but still much less common than the clavicle. (*Hay et al, 2005, p. 820; Behrman and Kliegman, 2002, p. 202*)

80. **(B)** Osgood–Schlatter disease is caused by microfractures of the patellar ligament where it inserts into the tibial tubercle. This condition usually occurs in the preteen and adolescent years, and is more common in males than females. The history of injury can be vague

and the patient may not remember a specific injury that precipitated the pain. Often the pain progresses to the point of interference of even routine physical activities. X-rays may or may not show any abnormalities. Upon x-ray, Type I disease appears normal, but Type II will reveal fragmentation of the tibial tubercle. Often, after healing there will be enlargement of the tibial tubercle. Generally, treatment consists of rest, limitation of activities, and isometric exercises. Chondromalacia patellae can only be diagnosed under an arthroscopic exam, not based on clinical features. Patellofemoral overuse syndrome presents with medial knee pain and subpatellar pain. Additional signs are swelling and crepitus in the knee and it is more common in females than males. It is diagnosed by increased Q-angles (anterior superior iliac spine through center of patella to tibial tubercle). Subluxation of the patella or dislocation is more common in adolescent girls and the patient presents with acute knee pain. The knee is in flexion with a mass lateral to the knee and with absence of the bony prominence of the patella (flat). X-ray confirms the dislocation. (*Hay et al, 2005, pp. 819, 841–842; Behrman and Kliegman, 2002, pp. 836–837*)

81. **(C)** Enterobiasis or pinworms is a worldwide infection that affects people of all ages and socioeconomic levels. It especially affects children. The classic manifestation of this problem is nocturnal anal pruritis and sleeplessness. The sleeplessness may be secondary to the migration of female worms to the perianal area to lay eggs, during which the tape may pick up the larvae. Transmission of the worms occurs when children ingest the eggs that are present on their hands (from scratching), in the bed clothes, or in house dust. After hatching in the stomach, the larvae migrate to the cecum where they mature into adults. The treatment of choice for pinworms is pyrantel pamoate or nebendazole. Albendazole may also be used. For eradication of this parasite, often the entire family must be treated at once. Ascarias is a helminthiasis infection that is ingested and excreted in the stool. Diagnosis is made by stool examination for the characteristic eggs. Hookworms are found in warm,

damp soil and penetrate the skin. From there the infection can spread to the lungs where they ascend into the trachea to be swallowed and live in the intestine. Diagnosis is made by stool examination for the eggs. Whipworm is ingested from the soil and lives in the intestine; detection is also made by egg in the feces. (*Hay et al, 2005, pp. 1267–1268; Behrman and Kliegman, 2002, pp. 466–467*)

82. **(A)** Juvenile rheumatoid arthritis (JRA) presents as three distinct types. The types are based upon clinical manifestations during the first 6 months of the illness. The most common type is pauciarticular as presented by this 13-year-old in the scenario above. Second is polyarticular disease with five or more joints being affected and the third is systemic onset of disease that begins with high spiking fevers that are often associated with a rash that comes and goes with the fever elevations. It is recommended that patients with pauciarticular JRA have an ophthalmologic evaluation and slit lamp exam every 3 months if the antinuclear antibody test (ANA) is positive and every 6 months if the ANA is negative, for 4 years after the JRA is identified to catch iridocyclitis (untreated results in blindness). Lyme arthritis usually presents with a monoarticular rash that typically affects the larger joints, without morning stiffness. Enteropathic arthritis is associated with gastrointestinal symptoms occurring simultaneously as lower extremity arthritis. It encompasses Reiter's syndrome, reactive arthritis (e.g., post-salmonella, shigella), and arthritis associated with celiac disease and inflammatory bowel disease. Psoriatic arthritis is the arthritis accompanying the dermatological disorder of psoriasis. The build-up of epidermal cells over the joints causes inflammation and thickening that results in arthralgia. (*Hay et al, 2005, pp. 846–849; Behrman and Kliegman, 2002, pp. 344–349*)

83. **(B)** Bacterial conjunctivitis is often unilateral and presents with a mucopurulent discharge. Common bacterial causes of this problem include nontypable *Haemophilus, Streptococcus pneumoniae, Moraxella catarrhalis,* and *Staphylococcus aureus.* These infections usually respond to topical antibiotics such as sulfacetamide, erythromycin. Systemic treatment is indicated for conjunctivitis caused by *chlamydia trichomatis, Neisseria gonorrhea,* or *Neisseria meningitides.* Allergic conjunctivitis is usually associated with moderate to severe itching of the eyes and clear mucoid drainage. Viral conjunctivitis is usually associated with minimal itching, profuse tearing, and minimal clear mucoid drainage. While Reiter's syndrome typically presents with a conjunctivitis, it is also concomitantly presents with arthritis and urethritis. (*Hay et al, 2005, pp. 444–447; Behrman and Kliegman, 2002, pp. 429–430*)

84. **(C)** Dacryocystitis, whether acute or chronic, is usually secondary to bacterial infections. It presents as an acutely inflamed swelling and tender area over the lacrimal sac just medial and inferior to the inner canthus of the eye. Because the lacrimal sac is inflamed and blocked there is tearing and usually a purulent discharge from the eye. There may also be an orbital cellulitis. Treatment consists of oral and topical antibiotics, warm compresses, and surgical drainage may be indicated. After the acute episode and for chronic cases, surgical correction of the nasolacrimal obstruction is required. Anterior uveitis typically presents with pain, photophobia, blurred vision, and injection without exudates. Blepharitis is an inflammation of the lid margin that presents with crusty debris along the lashes. Unless there is a concomitant conjunctival infection, there is typically no injection noted. (*Hay et al, 2005, pp. 441–449; Behrman and Kliegman, 2002, pp. 429–430t*)

85. **(B)** While halitosis can be caused by pharyngitis, sinusitis, and poor hygiene, the most common cause of halitosis in children is a nasal foreign body. Seeds and beads are the leading objects inserted into the nose. If not promptly removed, they can cause nasal obstruction, infection, rhinorrhea, bleeding, halitosis, or a foul smell. They are usually easy to remove, but if there is difficulty in removing the foreign body, the child should be referred to an otolaryngologist for definitive care. Tobacco use in adolescents is a common cause of halitosis. Dental disease is the most common

cause of halitosis in adults. (*Hay et al, 2005, pp. 494, 504*)

86. **(C)** Most cases of epistaxis in the anterior portion of the nose are caused by digital trauma (nose picking) or some other mechanical cause such as nose blowing or repeated nose rubbing. Other causes may include incorrect use of steroid nasal sprays. Examination of the anterior nose will usually reveal irritation of the Kiesselbach area. Less than 5% of recurrent nosebleeds are caused by bleeding disorders. Choanal atresia, unilateral, usually appears as a chronic nasal discharge that may be mistaken for chronic sinusitis. Foreign bodies typically present with purulent discharge instead of bleeding. (*Hay et al, 2005, p. 493*)

87. **(A)** Cat scratch disease (CSD) is caused by the Gram-negative bacillus, *Bartonella henselae*. The disease is more common in the fall and winter months and more males than females are affected. Typically (approximately 90%), patients report handling a cat or kitten, and up to 70% will report a scratch by a cat. The most common complication of CSD is encephalitis. About half of the patients with CSD will develop a primary cutaneous papule at the site of inoculation, most often (approximately 50%) on the hands or upper extremities, 3 to 10 days after the exposure. Regional lymphadenopathy will usually develop in about 1 to 7 weeks after the cutaneous lesions, and will affect the nodes draining the site of the scratch or bite. The affected lymph nodes may be inflamed and are usually tender. Occasionally, the involved nodes may suppurate. The lymphadenopathy resolves in about 2 months, but may last as long as 4 to 8 months. Treatment is usually not indicated for this self-resolving disease. However, suppurative lesions may need to be aspirated for pain relief. It has been shown that 5 days of treatment with azithromycin has helped to speed recovery for some patients. Because Hodgkin's disease involves the lymph nodes, it should be considered as a differential diagnosis when evaluating a child for CSD. However, it typically presents as a cervical lymphadenopathy. Fifth disease (erythema infectiosum) is a childhood disease caused by the human parvovirus. This common community acquired disease does not usually require treatment, but respiratory isolation is recommended for 7 days following the onset of symptoms. The initial stage of the disease presents as red cheeks that appear to be "slapped" or "slapped cheeks" with circumoral pallor. Osgood–Schlatter disease is an orthopedic problem in children. It is the result of repetitive microtraumas to the patellar ligament at its point of insertion into the tibial tubercle. Usually, rest and anti-inflammatory medications are helpful in alleviating the pain associated with this condition. (*Behrman and Kliegman, 2002, pp. 437, 836–837; Hay et al, 2005, pp. 923–925, 1240–1241*)

88. **(B)** Hookworm (*Ancylostoma duodenale* and *Nectar ameruanus*) infections, if severe, can cause iron deficiency anemia. Abdominal discomfort, weight loss, and ova in the stool are more commonly associated with these nematodes. Both types of human hookworms are found in tropic and subtropic climates, which include the southeastern United States, primarily the coastal areas. The larva of this parasite is passed in the feces and incubates in warm, damp soil when they hatch into larvae. The larvae penetrate directly into the skin of humans, enter the bloodstream, and migrate to the lungs. From the lungs they move up to the trachea and are swallowed. Once swallowed, they mature in the intestines. The worms attach their mouth to the mucosal lining of the intestine where they suck blood and shed new ova. Mild infections are usually asymptomatic, but severe infestations can cause anemia. Treatment for the infestation is achieved with albendazole. In severe cases of anemia, parenteral iron or transfusion may be indicated. Pinworms are associated only with localized pruritus, specifically the anus. Treatment may help recurrent urinary tract infections in some young girls. Ascariasis is usually asymptomatic; however, in severe cases it may be associated with anorexia, diarrhea, vomiting, weight loss, and abdominal pain. Whipworm is also asymptomatic until the infection is severe, with general gastrointestinal symptoms—pain, diarrhea, and mild

abdominal distention. Eosinophilia may also be present, although slight. (*Hay et al, 2005, pp. 1267–1269; Behrman and Kliegman, 2002, pp. 466–467*)

89. **(C)** Appearing in 60% to 80% of cases, the characteristic rash may not be present in all cases of acute Lyme disease. Following the bite of a deer tick (*Ixodes* species), infected with the spirochete *Borrelia burgdorferi*, an erythematous ring forms around the bite site and spreads outward. The ring may have a raised border and usually a clear center. The ring can attain a diameter of up to 20 cm. Multiple rings may form and rings can form at sites distal to the original bite site. If left untreated, the rash will usually resolve within 3 weeks. Erythema migrans is a minimally tender to nontender, nonscaly rash that persists longer than many of the other erythematous rashes of childhood. (*Hay et al, 2005, pp. 1247–1249*)

90. **(C)** Chlamydial infections are the most common cause of conjunctivitis in newborns in developed countries. Other causes of ophthalmia neonatorium include reactions to silver nitrate prophylaxis, other bacterial infections, such as gonococcal or staphylococcal, or viral organisms, such as adenovirus or echovirus. *Chlamydia trachomatis* causes conjunctivitis and pneumonia in neonates. Treatment for chlamydial conjunctivitis should be with systemic erythromycin to treat the conjunctivitis and as prophylaxis against pneumonia. (*Hay et al, 2005, p. 444; Behrman and Kliegman, 2002, pp. 428–429*)

91. **(D)** Seizures have not been associated with Lyme disease. Neurologic manifestations occur in up to approximately 20% of patients with Lyme disease. Primarily, these are Bell's palsy, lymphocytic, aseptic meningitis, and polyradiculitis. Cranial neuropathies, such as Guillain–Barré' syndrome and ataxias are less common. Additional neurologic manifestations include peripheral neuropathy, pseudotumor cerebri, and encephalitis. If untreated, most neurological symptoms are self-limited, but some will persist or become permanent. (*Hay et al, 2005, pp. 1247–1249; Behrman and Kliegman, 2002, p. 427*)

92. **(D)** Oral candidiasis (thrush) is very common in the first few weeks of infancy. The diagnosis is usually done by visual inspection and does not usually require further laboratory testing. On visual exam, white, creamy plaques are found on the buccal mucosa and occasionally the gingival and lingual mucosa. For this age group, direct topical application of nystatin in oral suspension to the lesions should suffice. If the lesions are resistant to treatment or if they occur in older children, consideration should be given to the possibility of the patient being immunocompromised. All sources of candida, such as toys and bottle nipples, should be sterilized daily. Herpangina and hand–foot–mouth disease are ulcerating lesions of the oral cavity due to viruses and are self-limiting, but can be very painful. Leukoplakia is a precursor lesion to oral cancer, seen most commonly in oral tobacco users. (*Hay et al, 2005, pp. 1277–1280*)

93. **(B)** Bipolar affective disorder is the most likely diagnosis for this patient. Although ADHD, bipolar disorder, and conduct disorder share many similarities in behavior disorders, such as varying degrees of school and behavior problems, defiant attitude, and distractibility, the obsession with ideas (in this case science fiction movies) is not present in ADHD and conduct disorder. The mood swings described here as depression and elation are consistent with bipolar disorder, which is confirmed by the presence of hallucinations. Hallucinations, when considering a differential diagnosis in a behavior disorder, are diagnostic for bipolar disorder. In up to 70% of patients with bipolar disorder, their first symptom of the disorder may be depression. However, hallucinations are not typically a manifestation of depression. (*Hay et al, 2005, pp. 194–195*)

94. **(D)** Rocky mountain spotted fever (RMSF) is the most common rickettsial infection in the United States, especially in the eastern, southeastern, and western states, and it is very common in 5- to 9-year-old children. A known tick exposure may or may not be documented. Most exposures to ticks carrying *Rickettsia sichettsii*, the causative organism of

this disease, occur in the warmer months of April to September when victims are most likely to participate in outdoor activities in wooded areas. The incubation period of RMSF is 3 to 12 days (mean 7) after a tick exposure. The tick must be attached for 6 hours or greater in order to transmit the disease. Clinical presentation includes fever, often >40ºC, myalgias, headache, and less characteristic, red-rose macular or macropapular rash. The rash usually appears within 2 to 6 days, after the fever. The rash is especially prevalent on the palms, soles, and extremities. After several days, the rash, which starts peripherally and spreads centrally, becomes petechial. Conjunctivitis, edema, splenomegaly, meningismus, and confusion may occur. Up to 5% to 7% of patients with RSMF will die, and therefore, delays in treatment should be avoided. Treatment for children is doxycycline, regardless of age and despite the possible side effect of stained teeth. In endemic areas, treatment should be started early and is often based on suspicion alone, and prior to the appearance of the rash. Endemic typhus (murine typhus) is not transmitted by ticks but instead by the fleas from infected rodents. The rash of endemic typhus differs from that of RMSF in that it does *not* involve the palms and soles. Q fever is spread by inhalation instead of ticks. The cause of this rickettsial disease is *Coxiella burrettii* hosted by domestic animals including dogs, cats, cattle, and sheep. Unpasteurized milk from infected animals may also be a source of this infection. One form of human monocytic ehrlichiosis is carried by ticks that have fed on infected hosts that may include deer, wild rodents, and sheep, most commonly in the southeast, north, and south central United States. The presentation is usually a viral syndrome without any rash. Although this is usually a self-limiting disease, deaths do occur in children; therefore treatment should be carried out with the antibiotic of choice, doxycycline, regardless of side effects. (*Hay et al, 2005, pp. 1171–1173; Behrman and Kliegman, 2002, pp. 460–462*)

95. **(D)** In young children, respiratory syncytial virus (RSV) accounts for over 70% of bronchiolitis, approximately 40% of the cases of pneumonia, and about 10% of cases of croup. This seasonal disease occurs in the winter and early spring months of the year. Over 50% of children have been infected with RSV by age 1, and by the age of 2, almost all children have been infected. Reinfection commonly occurs but is mild. Adenovirus infections, though common in early childhood, only account for approximately up to 10% of all respiratory diseases. The peak incidence of adenovirus respiratory infections occurs in the spring, summer, and early winter. Human parvovirus infection is known as erythema infectiosum or Fifth disease and usually affects school aged children. This disease is characterized by the "slapped-cheek" appearing rash on the face that appears about 10 to 17 days following the infection. About 2 days after the appearance of this facial rash, a similar rash appears on the extremities, trunk, neck, and buttocks. The rash often persists for a few days to a few weeks (average of 10 days) and often will recur with exposure to bathing in warm water, exercise, sunlight, and stress. Parainfluenza viruses fall into four categories and are responsible for the majority of cases of croup (65%), laryngitis (50%), and tracheobronchitis (25%). Types 1 to 3 occur as seasonal outbreaks with types 1 and 2 in the fall and type 3 in the spring and summer. Type 4 is an endemic virus. Clinical symptoms of these viruses include laryngeotracheitis (croup), laryngitis, bronchiolitis, and less commonly pneumonia (especially in immunocompromised children). (*Hay et al, 2005, pp. 1138–1140; Behrman and Kliegman, 2002, pp. 454–455*)

96. **(B)** Asthma, in this case exercise-induced, is the most likely cause of this problem. The symptoms commonly associated with acute exacerbations of asthma include wheezing, cough, dyspnea, and chest pain. Some symptoms that might be suggestive of asthma include exercise-induced cough, nighttime cough, cough after cold air exposure, and cough after laughing. Airway foreign bodies, though not common, are an acute problem that may present as sudden cough, choking, and wheezing. Cystic fibrosis (CF) is the most common, lethal, genetic disease affecting the

Caucasian population. Up to 50% of patients with CF are diagnosed in infancy, but others may not be diagnosed until adolescence or adulthood. Chronic or recurrent cough should be an indicator for consideration of CF as a differential diagnosis. Laryngomalacia is the most common cause of stridor in infants. It is the incomplete development of the cartilaginous support of the laryngoglottic structures. This congenital condition is usually self-limiting and occurs most commonly in infants at or just after birth. The inspiratory collapse of the epiglottis or arytenoid cartilages is heard as stridor. (*Hay et al, 2005, pp. 513–518; Behrman and Kliegman, 2002, pp. 531–532*)

97. **(B)** Autism is the most likely diagnosis for this child. Autism often presents before the second year of life as the child's failure to respond to their name, failed speech development, and appearing self-absorbed and withdrawn in the presence of other children or adults are noticed. Often in childhood, autistic children may develop ritualistic behaviors and intense interests that if interrupted may cause tantrums and rages. When speech does begin to develop, it may be nonsensical: reversal of speech patterns, echolation, and other abnormal patterns. Goals of treatment include early intervention to address behavior and communications skills. ADHD is characterized by easy distractibility, inattention, and overactivity. Estimates for the presence of ADHD in school aged children range from 2% to 20%. Fragile X syndrome is the most common cause of functional mental retardation. This syndrome, affecting approximately 1 in 1250 males, is caused by a trinucleotide expansion (CGG repeated sequence) in the Fragile X Mental Retardation I (FMR1) gene. Fragile X syndrome is characterized by a wide range of symptoms, which may include language delay, hyperactivity, autistic behavior, and variable levels of mental retardation. Schizophrenia is usually detected in adolescence, with prepubertal onset occurring rarely. Patients may initially present with somatic or social behavior problems. Schizophrenic children and adolescents often have the same symptoms as adults, such as

hallucinations, bizarre thought processes, and rambling speech. (*Hay et al, 2005, pp. 94–95, 189–190, 198–199, 1070; Behrman and Kliegman, 2002, pp. 53–54, 56, 95, 294*)

98. **(A)** Choanal atresia, whether unilateral or bilateral, is a nasal obstruction that occurs relatively rarely in newborns. If bilateral choanal atresia occurs at birth, it causes a respiratory distress that requires immediate treatment (due to infants being obligate nose breathers) by placing an oral airway and subsequent surgical correction. Unilateral choanal atresia can present as a chronic, single-sided, nasal discharge that may not appear until later in childhood. Meconium ileus, intestinal obstruction secondary to inspissated meconium, occurs in approximately 10% of newborns with cystic fibrosis. Cystic fibrosis affects approximately 1 in 2500 live Caucasian births, and is a leading cause of death in young adults. Nasal infections may occur secondary to a furuncle (infected hair follicle) in the anterior nares or as a nasal septal abscess following spread of a furuncle. Common causes of nasal infections include picking at the nose and pulling out nose hairs. Nasal polyps are uncommon in children under 10, and when they do occur it is usually in older children and adults with allergic rhinitis. (*Hay et al, 2005, pp. 492–493; Behrman and Kliegman, 2002, pp. 328, 531, 535–538*)

99. **(A)** It is estimated that 1% to 5% of teenage girls are affected by anorexia nervosa. There are two types of anorexia nervosa. The first is the nonpurging type when girls restrict their total caloric intake and the second involves binge eating and purging in association with the restrictive dietary habits. Otherwise, intensive exercise regimes may be used as a means to control weight. Anorexia nervosa may also occur in boys but is more prevalent in girls (20:1). The cause of this familial problem is unknown. DSM-IV criteria also include refusal to keep weight at 85% of ideal, intense fear of gaining weight even though underweight, amenorrhea, and disturbance in way one's body is shaped. (*Hay et al, 2005, pp. 173–174; Behrman and Kliegman, 2002, pp. 68–69*)

100. **(C)** Obesity is the number one nutritional disorder in children in the United States. In 1999, 14% of American adolescents were considered obese. Risk factors for obesity include other obese family members and infants born to diabetic mothers. Associated environmental factors include sedentary lifestyle, total caloric intake, television watching, and computer games. All are considered contributory factors in childhood obesity. Binge eating disorder is a relatively new eating disorder category. It is most frequent in overweight or obese individuals. This disorder includes recurrent episodes of binge eating (eating more than most individual would in a 2-hour period) and a sense of lack of control over the impulse to eat, marked distress over the episodes occurs at least 2 days a week, and is not associated with regular compensatory activity such as purging or fasting. Folate deficiency anemia (megaloblastic) can occur in infants within a few weeks after birth. This deficiency may be a result of malabsorption, low dietary intake such as with goat's milk or home prepared formulas that have been sterilized by heating, or formulas based on pasteurized milk. Infants who are breast-fed or given supplemented cows' milk formulas do not have a problem with folate deficiency. In children, vitamin D deficiency results in rickets. Rickets is a result of poor dietary intake of vitamin D and inadequate exposure to direct sunlight. Vitamin D sources include milk, cheese, and baby formula. Vitamin D in humans is produced by activation of its inactive precursors in the skin after exposure to ultraviolet light. (*Hay et al, 2005, pp. 169–170, 305–307, 727–728, 298–299t; Behrman and Kliegman, 2002, pp. 65–69, 81–84*)

REFERENCES

Behrman RE, Kliegman, RM (eds). *Nelson's Essentials of Pediatrics*, 4th ed. Philadelphia: WB Saunders; 2002.

Centers for Disease Control and Prevention (a). Summary of recommendations for tetanus toxoid, reduced diphtheria toxoid and acellular pertussis vaccine (Tdap) and tetanus and diphtheria toxoids (Td) use among adolescents aged 11–18 years; February, 2006. Available at http://www.cdc.gov/mmwr/preview/mmwrhtml/rr55e223a4.htm Retrieved on August 1, 2006.

Centers for Disease Control and Prevention (b). *2006 Childhood & Adolescent Immunization Schedule*; 2006. Available at: http://www.cdc.gov/nip/recs/ child-schedule.htm. Retrieved March 1, 2006.

Erkonen WE. *Radiology 101: The Basics and Fundamentals of Imaging*. Philadelphia: Lippincott Williams & Wilkins; 2000.

Gunn VL, Nechyba C. *The Harrriet Lane Handbook: A Manual for Pediatric House Officers*, 16th ed. St. Louis: Mosby; 2002.

Hay WW, Levin MJ, Sondheimer JM, Deterding RR (eds). *Current Pediatric Diagnosis and Treatment*, 17th ed. New York: McGraw-Hill; 2005.

Jenson HB, Baltimore RS (eds). *Pediatric Infectious Diseases, Principles and Practice*. Stamford, CT: Appleton & Lange; 1995.

Pharmacology

Questions

Raymond Pavlick, PhD

1. Which of the following warrants special consideration when initially prescribing levothyroxine?

   (A) a history of peptic ulcer disease
   (B) a history of stable angina
   (C) obesity
   (D) rheumatoid arthritis
   (E) Parkinson's disease

2. Which of the following medications is capable of causing agranulocytosis?

   (A) insulin
   (B) metformin (Glucophage)
   (C) methimazole (Tapazole)
   (D) prednisone
   (E) desmopressin (DDAVP)

3. Of the following choices, which regimen of combination therapy would be most appropriate for the treatment of stage 2 hypertension (systolic blood pressure (SBP) >160 mm Hg or diastolic blood pressure (DBP) >100 mm Hg) in a 44-year-old white male with a past medical history of myocardial infarction ?

   (A) verapamil and hydrochlorothiazide
   (B) verapamil and metoprolol
   (C) metoprolol and captopril
   (D) doxazosin and hydrochlorothiazide
   (E) captopril and spironolactone

4. A 4-year-old child swallows several tablets of a medication that he found in his parent's bathroom cabinet underneath the sink. Approximately 2 to 3 hours after ingesting the tablets, there were no symptoms other than nausea and vomiting. Thirty hours after ingesting the tablets, elevated aminotransferase levels were detected followed by jaundice, hepatic encephalopathy, renal failure, and death. The tablets most likely were

   (A) diazepam
   (B) aspirin
   (C) oxycodone
   (D) acetaminophen
   (E) phenobarbital

5. Which of the following requires drug-free periods to avoid a tolerance effect when used as prophylaxis for chronic stable angina?

   (A) digoxin
   (B) diltiazem
   (C) metoprolol
   (D) isosorbide dinitrate
   (E) propanolol

6. A patient with chronic-stable angina is being treated with daily doses of metoprolol and sublingual nitroglycerin PRN to control occasional angina attacks. Approximately 45 minutes after taking sildenafil, the patient suffers a severe attack and takes several nitroglycerin tablets within a short time frame, which ultimately leads to his death. Which of the following best explains what occurred?

   (A) the nitroglycerin/sildenafil combination led to a fatal arrhythmia

   (B) the metoprolol/sildenafil interaction triggered acute arterial thromboembolism

   (C) severe hypotension developed from the nitroglycerin/sildenafil interaction

   (D) the metoprolol/sildenafil combination led to a fatal coronary vasospasm

   (E) the metoprolol/sildenafil combination led to severe bronchospasm

7. Which of the following medications is often prescribed in combination with digoxin for managing moderate to severe congestive heart failure, but can also be a cause of digoxin toxicity?

   (A) nitroglycerin

   (B) furosemide (Lasix)

   (C) triamterene (Dyrenium)

   (D) verapamil

   (E) ramipril (Altace)

8. Of the following choices, which regimen is considered first-line therapy for *Helicobacter pylori*-positive individuals with peptic ulcer disease?

   (A) omeprazole (Prilosec) + clarithromycin (Biaxin) + amoxicillin (Amoxil)

   (B) omeprazole (Prilosec) + rantidine (Zantac) + clarithromycin (Biaxin)

   (C) esomeprazole (Nexium) + clarithromycin (Biaxin) + ampicillin (Principen)

   (D) rantidine (Zantac) + amoxicillin (Amoxil) + bismuth subsalicylate

   (E) misoprostol (Cytotec) + clarithromycin (Biaxin) + metronidazole (Flagyl)

9. Following a gunshot wound to the lower abdomen, a 29-year-old male is hospitalized and treated with clindamycin for a potential anaerobic infection. After 3 days of clindamycin therapy while recuperating in the hospital, he develops severe diarrhea, dehydration, and lower abdominal cramping. A stool culture is ordered and later discovered to contain *Clostridium difficile*. After discontinuing the clindamycin, which of the following would be the most appropriate treatment?

   (A) cefaclor (Ceclor)

   (B) doxycycline (Monodox)

   (C) amoxicillin (Amoxil)

   (D) metronidazole (Flagyl)

   (E) cephalexin (Keflex)

10. Which of the following medications is most appropriate for the treatment of an initial case of acute uncomplicated cystitis in a 23-year-old female?

   (A) amoxicillin (Amoxil)

   (B) ciprofloxacin (Cipro)

   (C) doxycycline (Monodox)

   (D) azithromycin (Zithromax)

   (E) gentamicin (Garamycin)

11. All of the following are generally effective at quickly managing an acute asthma attack in the adult patient EXCEPT

   (A) albuterol

   (B) levalbuterol (Xopenex)

   (C) metaproterenol (Alupent)

   (D) salmeterol (Serevent)

   (E) pirbuterol (Maxair)

12. Which of the following type 2 diabetes medications is INCORRECTLY paired with its mechanism of action?

    (A) glyburide (Diaβeta): increases pancreatic secretion of insulin

    (B) metformin (Glucophage), decreases hepatic glucose production

    (C) acarbose (Precose), increases cellular uptake of glucose

    (D) rosiglitazone (Avandia), increases insulin sensitivity of tissues

    (E) repaglinide (Prandin), increases pancreatic secretion of insulin

13. The preferred methods for monitoring warfarin therapy and unfractionated heparin (UFH) therapy is to measure the _____ and _____, respectively

    (A) aPTT (activated partial thromboplastin time); INR (international normalized ratio)

    (B) ACT (activated clotting time); INR

    (C) INR; aPTT

    (D) INR; ACT

    (E) ACT; aPTT

14. A 61-year-old male arrives at the emergency department (ED) suffering an acute myocardial infarction as a result of coronary artery thrombosis. One of the agents administered to the patient is a thrombolytic agent. From the choices below, which drug is a thrombolytic agent?

    (A) abciximab (ReoPro)

    (B) alteplase (tPA)

    (C) warfarin

    (D) heparin

    (E) clopidogrel (Plavix)

15. A patient on a 16 mg daily dose of hydromorphone is being switched to morphine sulfate for pain control. If 7.5 mg of hydromorphone is equianalgesic with 30 mg of morphine sulfate, what dose of morphine sulfate should be prescribed if you account for 25% cross-tolerance?

    (A) 30 mg

    (B) 36 mg

    (C) 48 mg

    (D) 64 mg

    (E) 80 mg

16. It is recommended that baseline liver function tests (LFTs) be ordered before starting therapy with all of the following medications EXCEPT

    (A) pioglitazone (Actos)

    (B) simvistatin (Zocor)

    (C) extended-release niacin (Niaspan)

    (D) gemfibrozil (Lopid)

    (E) clopidogrel (Plavix)

17. One of the most common adverse effects with spasmolytics like carisoprodol (Soma) and cyclobenzaprine (Flexeril) is their tendency to cause

    (A) rash

    (B) drowsiness

    (C) hypertension

    (D) myalgia

    (E) hyperglycemia

18. A 44-year-old male has periodic attacks of gout that are secondary to hyperuricemia. Plasma uric acid levels can be decreased with

    (A) allopurinol (Zyloprim) or prednisone

    (B) allopurinol (Zyloprim) or probenecid (Benemid)

    (C) colchicine or probenecid (Benemid)

    (D) indomethacin (Indocin) or colchicine

    (E) aspirin or prednisone

19. One of the common tendencies associated with antiarrhythmic drugs is their ability to produce "proarrhythmic" effects. What does this mean?

(A) they suppress the arrhythmia that they are being used for without any serious side effects

(B) they selectively block certain ion channels in the heart that are responsible for triggering the arrhythmia

(C) they create a new and often worse arrhythmia in the heart

(D) they increase the resistance of cardiac cells to premature activation by prolonging the refractory period

(E) they decrease conduction velocity through the sinoatrial (SA) and atrioaventricular (AV) nodes

20. Taking aspirin or other nonsteroidal anti-inflammatory drug 30 to 45 minutes prior to taking _____ blunts side effects and may increase patient compliance.

(A) atorvastatin (Lipitor)

(B) warfarin

(C) niacin

(D) insulin

(E) metformin (Glucophage)

21. A 24-year-old male college student presenting to your clinic 1 week ago was diagnosed with depression and subsequently prescribed 10 mg/day of fluoxetine (Prozac). He unexpectedly shows up today and states that he is not experiencing any improvement since starting the medication. What is the best treatment option at this time?

(A) double the dose of fluoxetine to 20 mg/day

(B) maintain the 10 mg/day dose of fluoxetine and comfort the patient that the medication may still take at least one to two more weeks to work

(C) discontinue the fluoxetine and start sertraline (Zoloft)

(D) discontinue the fluoxetine and start amitriptyline

(E) maintain the current dose of fluoxetine and prescribe phenelzine (Nardil) to be used in combination

22. Assuming no contraindications to their use, the antihypertensives of first choice for treating high blood pressure in the type 2 diabetic patient are

(A) angiotensin converting enzyme inhibitors (ACEIs)

(B) Ca^{+2} channel blockers

(C) β-blockers

(D) thiazide diuretics

(E) α-receptor blockers

23. From the choices below, which medication would be the most appropriate for an otherwise healthy 57-year-old male seeking relatively quick relief from urinary obstructive symptoms with slight prostatic enlargement due to benign prostatic hyperplasia (BPH)?

(A) finasteride (Proscar)

(B) doxazosin (Cardura)

(C) testosterone

(D) desmopressin (DDAVP)

(E) atropine

24. Chronic therapy with which drug can potentially lead to abrupt, unpredictable, and transient motor fluctuations (from mobility to immobility) often referred to as the "on–off phenomenon"?

(A) cyclobenzaprine (Flexeril)

(B) diazepam (Valium)

(C) methotrexate (Rheumatrex)

(D) levodopa/carbidopa (Sinemet)

(E) carbamazepine (Tegretol)

25. A 5-year-old boy with no known drug allergies is diagnosed in your clinic with bilateral acute otitis media. Which of the following is the drug of choice?

(A) levofloxacin (Levaquin)

(B) nitrofurantoin (Macrobid)

(C) amoxicillin (Amoxil)

(D) doxycycline (Monodox)

(E) gentamicin (Garamycin)

26. Which of the following drugs is indicated for the treatment of anemia associated with chronic renal failure?

(A) deferoxamine
(B) warfarin
(C) protamine sulfate
(D) Epogen
(E) Argatroban

27. A 60-year-old man with active peptic ulcer disease and a 22-year history of type 2 diabetes mellitus complains of pain in his left lower extremity that started about 3 months ago. He describes the pain as burning, tingling, and "electric-like" that varies in intensity throughout the day, but is most severe at night. He also says that when he wears long pants or socks the pain is agonizing. Since he first noticed the pain 3 months ago, he has tried acetaminophen, naproxen, and hydrocodone, but nothing has provided any significant relief. All of the following medications would be considered an appropriate choice to prescribe at this time EXCEPT

(A) gabapentin (Neurontin)
(B) amitriptyline
(C) cyclobenzaprine (Flexeril)
(D) duloxetine (Cymbalta)
(E) desipramine (Norpramin)

28. Which of the following is considered a stimulant laxative (cathartic)?

(A) senna (Senokot)
(B) polyethylene glycol (PEG)
(C) docusate sodium (Colace)
(D) methylcellulose (Citrucel)
(E) bismuth subsalicylate (Pepto-Bismol)

29. All of the following are capable of producing orthostatic hypotension EXCEPT

(A) hydrochlorothiazide
(B) chlorpromazine (Thorazine)
(C) amitriptyline
(D) diazepam (Valium)
(E) doxazosin (Cardura)

30. RS is a 23-year-old male visiting your clinic today for a preemployment physical. He has a past medical history of asthma that is currently being managed PRN with a multidose inhaler of albuterol. RS tells you he has been using it daily for the last month due to increased shortness of breath and that it does not seem to be working too well. The most appropriate step at this time is to

(A) add ipratropium bromide (Atrovent) for use on a daily basis and continue albuterol PRN
(B) add fluticasone (Flovent) for use on a daily basis and continue albuterol PRN
(C) discontinue the albuterol and prescribe fluticasone for use on a daily basis
(D) add methylpredisone for use on a daily basis and continue albuterol PRN
(E) increase the dose of albuterol and keep using PRN

31. All of the following could be a warning sign of an underlying problem with combined oral contraceptive (COC) use shortly after starting therapy EXCEPT

(A) blurred vision
(B) calf pain
(C) right upper quadrant pain
(D) increased thirst and urination
(E) chest pain

32. Which of the following should be used cautiously in patients with chronic pulmonary disease or elevated intracranial pressure (ICP)?

(A) morphine sulfate
(B) nalaxone
(C) carbamazepine
(D) methylphenidate
(E) verapamil

33. Which of the following is the drug of choice for treating herpes simplex virus (HSV) types 1 and 2?

(A) amantadine (Symmetrel)

(B) acyclovir (Zovirax)

(C) zidovudine (Retrovir)

(D) nystatin (Mycostatin)

(E) zanamivir (Relenza)

34. Oral desmopressin (DDAVP) can be used to manage which two conditions?

(A) primary nocturnal enuresis and neurogenic (central) diabetes insipidus

(B) primary nocturnal enuresis and nephrogenic diabetes insipidus

(C) neurogenic (central) diabetes insipidus and primary adrenal insufficiency

(D) SIADH and primary hyperaldosteronism

(E) primary nocturnal enuresis and primary hyperaldosteronism

35. A 35-year-old male is brought to the ED with unremitting, generalized convulsive status epilepticus. The initial, preferred treatment is intravenous administration of

(A) phenobarbital

(B) valproic acid (Depakote)

(C) phenytoin (Dilantin)

(D) lorazepam (Ativan)

(E) donepezil (Aricept)

36. A 58-year-old male with a history of hyperlipidemia takes 40 mg of lovastatin daily. After he was recently diagnosed with pneumonia and started on antibiotic therapy as an outpatient, he complains of progressive muscle weakness, tenderness, and pain in his lower extremities. Which antibiotic was this patient most likely prescribed?

(A) clarithromycin (Biaxin)

(B) doxycycline (Monodox)

(C) levofloxacin (Levaquin)

(D) amoxicillin + clavulanate (Augmentin)

(E) cefuroxime (Ceftin)

37. Following chronic therapy for its listed indication, all of the following medications are typically tapered prior to discontinuation EXCEPT

(A) tricyclic antidepressants (TCAs) for depression

(B) β-blockers for hypertension

(C) prednisone for systemic lupus erythematosus

(D) selective serotonin reuptake inhibitors (SSRIs) for depression

(E) ezetimibe for hyperlipidemia

38. According to the most recent NCEP/ATP (National Cholesterol Education Program/Adult Treatment Panel) guidelines, the LDL-C threshold for starting pharmacologic therapy in high-risk, hyperlipidemic patients is

(A) ≥200 mg/dL

(B) ≥160 mg/dL

(C) ≥140 mg/dL

(D) ≥130 mg/dL

(E) ≥100 mg/dL

39. From the choices below, which medication would be considered the safest for use in pregnancy?

(A) warfarin

(B) captopril (Capoten)

(C) isotretinoin (Accutane)

(D) esomeprazole (Nexium)

(E) misoprostol (Cytotec)

40. β-blockers are used in all of the following situations EXCEPT

(A) chronic management of glaucoma

(B) prophylaxis of migraine headaches

(C) symptom control in hypothyroidism

(D) prophylaxis of chronic stable angina

(E) control of ventricular arrhythmias or sinus tachycardia

41. Drug X is an antiepileptic medication that is labeled as a "CYP2D6 inducer." CYP2D6 enzymes do not metabolize drug X. Drug Y is an antihypertensive medication that is typically metabolized to inactive products by CYP2D6 enzymes. Assuming drugs X and Y are taken simultaneously by a patient, which of the following statements is TRUE?

(A) the patient will be at greater risk for having a seizure

(B) the patient will be at lesser risk for having a seizure

(C) the patient will likely experience hypertension

(D) the patient will likely experience hypotension

(E) the patient will likely experience hypotension and be at greater risk for having a seizure

42. A 50-year-old male presents to the ED with an episode of paroxysmal supraventricular tachycardia (PSVT). He is hypotensive (BP 108/70), does not feel faint nor is complaining of any chest pain. ECG shows a regular arrhythmia with no P waves, narrow QRS complexes, and an HR of 172 bpm. Successive valsalva maneuvers fail to terminate the PSVT. Which of the following is considered the treatment of choice for this patient at this time?

(A) synchronized direct current cardioversion (DCC)

(B) intravenous amiodarone

(C) intravenous atenolol

(D) intravenous adenosine

(E) intravenous digoxin

43. Which of the following is the primary site of action for wafarin?

(A) kidneys

(B) liver

(C) blood

(D) small intestine

(E) red bone marrow

44. All of the following are TRUE of radioactive iodide EXCEPT

(A) it can be used to help detect metastatic differentiated thyroid cancer

(B) it is indicated for the treatment of Graves' disease

(C) its use is contraindicated in pregnant females

(D) it raises the risk of cancer and leukemia in patients who have used it

(E) a common side effect of its use is thyroiditis, which typically causes sore throat

45. Which of the following exerts its action by inhibiting cell wall synthesis?

(A) amoxicillin (Amoxil)

(B) ciprofloxacin (Cipro)

(C) doxycycline (Monodox)

(D) erythromycin

(E) gentamicin (Garamycin)

46. The use of triptans is contraindicated in patients with a history of

(A) kidney stones

(B) gall bladder disease

(C) cerebrovascular disease

(D) peptic ulcer disease

(E) psychosis

47. Two 0.75-mg tablets of levonorgestrel taken 12 hours apart are effective as

(A) emergency contraception following unprotected intercourse

(B) analgesia for pain associated with endometriosis

(C) a method to increase the chances of becoming pregnant by inducing ovulation

(D) a method for preventing hot flashes in postmenopausal women

(E) a method of protection against HIV transmission

48. Which drug can potentially lead to oropharyngeal candidiasis and which agent can be used to treat this type of infection?

    (A) albuterol; ketoconazole (Nizoral)
    (B) triamcinolone (Azmacort); fluconazole (Diflucan)
    (C) fluticasone (Flovent); amantadine (Symmetrel)
    (D) cromolyn sodium (Intal); levofloxacin (Levaquin)
    (E) flunisolide (Aerobid); metronidazole (Flagyl)

49. A 19-year-old female presents to the clinic with complaints of nausea, diarrhea, flatulence, stomach cramps, and bloating. A stool sample provided while at the clinic has frothy and greasy characteristics, but is free of any visible blood. She explains that she just returned from a 2-week camping trip where she did a great deal of swimming in a couple of lakes. This patient should be started on treatment with

    (A) metronidazole (Flagyl)
    (B) nystatin (Mycostatin)
    (C) sulfamethoxazole/trimethoprim (Septra)
    (D) doxycycline (Monodox)
    (E) erythromycin

50. A 34-year-old woman presents to the clinic with complaints of intermittent flushing and blushing that started 3 to 4 weeks ago. Since then, she has noticed several inflammatory papules on the cheeks, nose, and chin. Upon exam, you notice an overall rosy hue to the face and the absence of any comedones. Which of the following would be the best course of topical therapy at this time?

    (A) mupirocin ointment
    (B) permethrin cream
    (C) tretinoin gel
    (D) hydrocortisone 1% cream
    (E) metronidazole gel

51. DJ is a 55-year-old African American male with a past medical history of

    • moderate persistent asthma for which he takes an inhaled corticosteroid and long-acting β_2-agonist for long-term control, plus a short-acting β_2-agonist for acute exacerbations
    • hypertension for which he takes hydrochlorothiazide

    DJ's asthma appears well controlled, but his blood pressure is elevated at 142/90. He also presents today with new onset atrial fibrillation. If DJ's atrial fibrillation does not spontaneously revert to sinus rhythm and continues to persist, which of the following would be the most appropriate therapy for DJ?

    (A) propanolol
    (B) diltiazem
    (C) captopril (Capoten)
    (D) losartan (Cozaar)
    (E) methyldopa

52. RK is a 52-year-old male who recently underwent surgery for a hip replacement. Upon discharge, he is prescribed oxycodone 7.5 mg + acetaminophen 325 mg (Percocet 7.5/325) and told to take one to two tablets every 6 hours as needed to help manage the pain he is expected to encounter as he recovers at home. Which of the following medications would you also recommend for RK to help minimize potential side effects associated with his pain medication?

    (A) esomeprazole (Nexium) + TUMS
    (B) diphenhydramine
    (C) guaifenesin
    (D) hydrocortisone 1% cream
    (E) senna + docusate (Senokot)

53. A 53-year-old female with a past medical history of rheumatoid arthritis presents to the clinic with a chief complaint of bilateral swelling of the knees, morning stiffness, and chronic fatigue. She states that the stiffness has gotten worse over the last 6 months. She is currently taking naproxyn 500 mg twice per day. All lab reports are normal, with the exception of an elevated ESR. Which of the following agents would be most appropriate to initiate at this time?

   (A) indomethacin (Indocin)
   (B) sulindac (Clinoril)
   (C) sulfasalazine (Azulfidine)
   (D) methotrexate (Rheumatrex)
   (E) acetaminophen

54. Activated charcoal can be an effective gastrointestinal decontamination therapy in overdoses of all of the following EXCEPT

   (A) carbamazepine (Tegretol)
   (B) iron
   (C) oxycodone
   (D) salicylates
   (E) TCAs

55. According to the American Diabetes Association (ADA), the drug therapy goals for a sustained $HbA1_C$ and blood pressure in the type 2 diabetic patient are

   (A) < 8%; <120/80
   (B) < 7%; <120/80
   (C) < 7%; <130/80
   (D) < 6%; <120/80
   (E) < 6%; <130/80

56. All of the following are TRUE in regards to growth hormone therapy EXCEPT

   (A) growth hormone is typically administered subcutaneously or intramuscularly for the management of growth hormone deficiency
   (B) growth hormone has been used in patients suffering from AIDS wasting or cachexia
   (C) the initial use of growth hormone may require the adjustment of oral antidiabetic medications in diabetic patients
   (D) all growth hormone currently available in the United States are derived via recombinant DNA techniques
   (E) the effects of growth hormone are antagonized by cephalosporins

57. Omega-3 fatty acids (fish oils) have recently received a great deal of attention, as the FDA has now approved the first prescription product. What is the main therapeutic effect of omega-3 fatty acids?

   (A) lower blood glucose levels in the diabetic patient
   (B) prevent hot flashes in postmenopausal women
   (C) lower systolic pressure in the hypertensive patient
   (D) lower plasma triglycerides
   (E) reduce the risk of prostate cancer in men

58. A 28-year-old woman in the ED is administered an intravenous paralytic agent prior to endotracheal intubation. The agent produces transient muscle fasciculations, particularly over the thorax and abdomen, prior to paralysis. The agent is most likely

   (A) tubocurarine
   (B) rocuronium (Zemuron)
   (C) carbamazepine (Tegretol)
   (D) succinylcholine
   (E) pyridostigmine (Mestinon)

59. A 22-year-old man with pernicious anemia can be given which of the following to correct any hematologic and neurologic defects of his condition?

(A) vitamin K

(B) folic acid

(C) ferrous (iron) sulfate

(D) vitamin B_{12}

(E) Procrit

60. Common adverse reactions associated with aminoglycosides include

(A) diarrhea and bone marrow depression

(B) ototoxicity and nephrotoxicity

(C) blurred vision and hyperglycemia

(D) headache and hypoglycemia

(E) rash and dyspepsia

61. All of the following are indicated for the treatment of insomnia EXCEPT

(A) zolpidem (Ambien)

(B) zaleplon (Sonata)

(C) triazolam (Halcion)

(D) meclizine (Antivert)

(E) eszopiclone (Lunesta)

62. A patient presents with signs and symptoms of moderate congestive heart failure that includes a modest degree of left ventricular dysfunction, shortness of breath, fatigue, reduced exercise tolerance and ankle edema. Which of the following drug combinations would be the best choice for initial treatment?

(A) digoxin and hydrochlorothiazide (Hydrodiuril)

(B) metoprolol (Toprol) and triamterene (Dyrenium)

(C) metoprolol (Toprol) and enalapril (Vasotec)

(D) enalapril (Vasotec) and furosemide (Lasix)

(E) isosorbide dinitrate and furosemide (Lasix)

63. All of the following are indicated for the treatment of postmenopausal osteoporosis EXCEPT

(A) calcitonin (Miacalcin)

(B) raloxifene (Evista)

(C) alendronate (Fosamax)

(D) ibandronate (Boniva)

(E) topiramate (Topamax)

64. Whether used for smoking cessation (Zyban) or depression (Wellbutrin XL), one of the potential adverse effects of bupropion is

(A) neutropenia

(B) erectile dysfunction

(C) urinary retention

(D) a lowering of seizure threshold

(E) gynecomastia

65. A 25-year-old male is hospitalized with symptoms of delusion, paranoia, rambling statements coupled with disorganized thought, and flattened affect. The companion who brings him to the hospital claims this is the first time she has ever witnessed any of these symptoms and is not aware of any medication he is currently taking. Which of the following is the most appropriate drug for this patient?

(A) sertraline (Zoloft)

(B) topiramate (Topamax)

(C) olanzapine (Zyprexa)

(D) clomipramine (Anafranil)

(E) thioridazine (Mellaril)

66. Grapefruit juice can significantly _____ of some benzodiazepines and statins, thereby _____ their clinical effects.

(A) decrease renal excretion; intensifying

(B) displace plasma protein binding; intensifying

(C) increase oral absorption; intensifying

(D) increase renal excretion; diminishing

(E) stimulate hepatic metabolism; diminishing

67. The JNC7 guidelines recommend which type of medication as first-line therapy for most patients (without compelling indications) suffering from stage 1 hypertension?

(A) calcium channel blockers

(B) β-blockers

(C) thiazide diuretics

(D) ACEIs

(E) α-blockers

68. Hyperkalemia is a contraindication to the use of which of the following medications?

(A) metformin (Glucophage)
(B) cimeditine (Tagamet)
(C) triamterene (Dyrenium)
(D) glipizide (Glucotrol)
(E) verapamil

69. Which of the following drugs block the actions of leukotrienes and can be used for long-term control of mild persistent asthma?

(A) cromolyn sodium (Intal)
(B) omalizumab (Xolair)
(C) zafirlukast (Accolate)
(D) nedocromil sodium (Tilade)
(E) ipratropium bromide (Atrovent)

70. All of the following may result from the use of thiazide diuretics EXCEPT

(A) hypoglycemia
(B) hyperuricemia
(C) hyperlipidemia
(D) hypokalemia
(E) hypercalcemia

71. Which of the following therapeutic regimens is most appropriate for a 17-year-old female diagnosed with gonococcal and chlamydial urethritis?

(A) amoxicillin + clavulanate (Augmentin)
(B) sulfamethoxazole + trimethoprim (Septra)
(C) metronidazole (Flagyl)
(D) ceftriaxone (Rocephin) + azithromycin (Zithromax)
(E) doxycycline (Monodox) + amoxicillin (Amoxil)

72. All of the following are noncontraceptive, beneficial effects of COCs EXCEPT

(A) reduced risk of ovarian cancer
(B) reduced risk of symptomatic pelvic inflammatory disease
(C) decreased frequency of menstrual cramps
(D) reduced risk of liver cancer
(E) reduced risk of functional ovarian cysts

73. Which of the following is a potential adverse effect associated with UFH?

(A) hyperglycemia
(B) hypothyroidism
(C) thrombocytopenia
(D) excessive cough
(E) muscle cramps

74. A 31-week pregnant female is diagnosed with an uncomplicated urinary tract infection (UTI). Which of the following would be most appropriate in this situation?

(A) doxycycline (Monodox)
(B) sulfamethoxazole + trimethoprim (Bactrim)
(C) metronidazole (Flagyl)
(D) nitrofurantoin (Macrodantin)
(E) levofloxacin (Levaquin)

75. It is important to educate nonpregnant females prescribed progestin-only pills (POPs; minipills) to take them within 3 hours of the same time every day because

(A) follicular development is then less likely to happen
(B) ovulation is then less likely to happen
(C) the endometrium is then more likely to be thin and atrophic
(D) the effect on cervical mucus decreases after 22 hours and is gone after 27 hours
(E) amenorrhea is then more likely to happen

76. An antimuscarinic drug produces all of the following effects EXCEPT

(A) mydriasis
(B) bronchodilation
(C) decreased gastric acid secretion
(D) decreased lacrimation
(E) bradycardia

77. Which property accounts for why some β-blockers produce dizziness and drowsiness, whereas other β-blockers are not as likely to cause these problems?

    (A) selectivity for certain β-receptors
    (B) degree of lipophilicity
    (C) degree of intrinsic sympathomimetic activity (ISA)
    (D) serum half-life
    (E) margin of safety

78. Which of the following antineoplastic medications is most likely to cause cardiac toxicity and precipitate heart failure?

    (A) doxorubicin
    (B) cisplatin
    (C) cyclophosphamide
    (D) tamoxifen
    (E) 6-mercaptopurine

79. Which of the following is considered a first-line agent for the long-term treatment of panic disorder?

    (A) propanolol (Inderal)
    (B) buspirone (BuSpar)
    (C) bupropion (Wellbutrin)
    (D) aripiprazole (Abillify)
    (E) fluoxetine (Prozac)

80. All of the following have been shown to be somewhat effective for migraine prophylaxis EXECPT

    (A) valproic acid (Depakote)
    (B) hydrocodone
    (C) propanolol (Inderal)
    (D) amitriptyline
    (E) topiramate (Topamax)

81. Which of the following agents is the treatment of choice to reverse an opioid overdose?

    (A) buprenorphine (Subutex)
    (B) butorphanol
    (C) nalbuphine (Nubain)
    (D) methadone (Dolophine)
    (E) naloxone (Narcan)

82. Which compound can be applied topically and acts as a keratolytic to remove corns, calluses, and common warts?

    (A) acetaminophen
    (B) salicylic acid
    (C) flurbiprofen (Ansaid)
    (D) hydroxychloroquine (Plaquenil)
    (E) colchicine

83. All of the following drugs can cause bradycardia EXCEPT

    (A) verapamil
    (B) diltiazem
    (C) amlodipine (Norvasc)
    (D) propanolol
    (E) metoprolol

84. In addition to insulin and fluid replacement with 0.9% saline, which electrolyte is commonly infused in the type 2 diabetic patient who arrives in the ED in a hyperglycemic, hyperosmolar, nonketotic state?

    (A) bicarbonate
    (B) potassium
    (C) calcium
    (D) magnesium
    (E) sulfate

85. Both rifampicin (Rifampin) and certain antiepileptics (AEDs) such as phenytoin and carbamazepine (Tegretol) have been shown to reduce the effectiveness of

    (A) nicotine replacement therapy
    (B) COCs
    (C) HMG-CoA reductase inhibitors (statins)
    (D) NSAIDs
    (E) proton (acid) pump inhibitors (PPIs)

86. The administration of tissue plasminogen activator (tPA) must occur within what time from the onset of ischemic stroke in order to be potentially effective and safe?

    (A) <1 hour
    (B) <3 hours
    (C) <5 hours
    (D) <8 hours
    (E) <12 hours

87. Drugs such as donepezil (Aricept) and rivastigmine (Exelon) that are used for Alzheimer's disease exert their effect by

    (A) blocking muscarinic receptors
    (B) blocking serotonin receptors
    (C) inhibiting acetylcholinesterase
    (D) binding to muscarinic receptors
    (E) binding to serotonin receptors

88. Which agent is indicated for a 31-year-old female with constipation-predominant irritable bowel syndrome who has not responded to increases in dietary fiber and bulk forming laxatives?

    (A) loperamide (Imodium)
    (B) granisetron (Kytril)
    (C) trimethobenzamide (Tigan)
    (D) sucralfate (Carafate)
    (E) tegaserod (Zelnorm)

89. Which agent is most appropriate for the treatment of seasonal allergies in a 32-year-old male taxi driver?

    (A) diphenhydramine (Benadryl)
    (B) clemastine (Tavist)
    (C) ergotamine tartrate (Cafergot)
    (D) promethazine (Phenergan)
    (E) loratadine (Alavert)

90. Which class of medications now include a boxed warning and expanded warning statements about the increased risk of suicidality in children and adolescents being treated with these drugs?

    (A) benzodiazepines
    (B) typical antipsychotics
    (C) atypical antipsychotics
    (D) opiates
    (E) antidepressants

91. When used chronically in the adult patient, oral corticosteroids can produce all of the following EXCEPT

    (A) sodium and water retention
    (B) hypoglycemia
    (C) osteoporosis
    (D) impaired would healing
    (E) central redistribution of fat

92. Which of the following is the primary emergency treatment for anaphylaxis?

    (A) epinephrine
    (B) antihistamines
    (C) atropine
    (D) aminophylline
    (E) dopamine

93. A 12-year-old boy reaches under his friend's porch to retrieve a baseball and suffers a small puncture wound to his left hand as a result of a bite by the friend's cat. Within a few hours, he becomes febrile and complains of chills. Which drug would be the most appropriate to give this patient?

    (A) amoxicillin + clavulanate (Augmentin)
    (B) erythromycin
    (C) doxycycline (Monodox)
    (D) levofloxacin (Levaquin)
    (E) gentamicin (Garamycin)

94. Which of the following regimens has superior efficacy in treating acute nausea and vomiting associated with high doses of cyclophosphamide?

    (A) metoclopramide (Reglan)
    (B) metoclopramide (Reglan) + dexamethasone (Decadron)
    (C) ondansetron (Zofran) + dexamethasone (Decadron)
    (D) lorazepam (Ativan)
    (E) prochlorperazine (Compazine)

95. A 52-year-old male is brought to the ED by his daughter because she recently notices that he gets extremely tired, has periodic tremors in his hands, and suffers from increasing memory lapses. Initial lab work shows a serum creatinine of 2.2 mg/dL. His past medical history is significant for bipolar disorder, for which he has been taking the same drug for the past 32 months. Which of the following is most likely responsible for the patient's symptoms?

    (A) valproic acid (Depakote)
    (B) lithium carbonate (Lithobid)
    (C) carbamazepine (Tegretol)
    (D) olanzapine (Zyprexa)
    (E) risperidone (Risperdal)

96. Angiotensin receptor blockers (ARBs) are not as likely to produce cough and angioedema compared to ACEIs because they do not

    (A) cause hyperkalemia
    (B) cause hyponatremia
    (C) increase bradykinin levels
    (D) undergo a first pass effect
    (E) cross the blood–brain barrier

97. Which of the following drugs used for the management of obesity increases the fat content of the stool and can potentially cause fecal urgency and incontinence?

    (A) dexfenfluramine (Redux)
    (B) orlistat (Xenical)
    (C) sibutramine (Meridia)
    (D) phentermine (Adipex-P)
    (E) benzphetamine (Didrex)

98. Which of the following medications increases the risk of developing Reye's syndrome in the pediatric patient when used to treat influenza and other viral illnesses?

    (A) acetaminophen
    (B) aspirin
    (C) ibuprofen
    (D) oseltamivir (Tamiflu)
    (E) naproxen

99. All of the following are effective in relieving and preventing ischemic episodes in patients with variant (Prinzmetal's) angina EXCEPT

    (A) verapamil
    (B) diltiazem
    (C) atenolol
    (D) isosorbide dinitrate
    (E) nifedipine

100. A 24-year-old male is on a 2-injection regimen for his type 1 diabetes mellitus that includes NPH and regular insulin taken before breakfast and then again before dinner. One evening, he has an abnormally light dinner and in the middle of the night, he awakens in a cold sweat with his heart pounding. He obtains a glucometer reading and discovers that his blood glucose is 44 mg/dL. He eats some candy and then goes back to sleep. Immediately after awakening the next morning, his blood glucose is 277 mg/dL. What should he do at this time?

    (A) take the usual morning insulin regimen after breakfast instead of before breakfast
    (B) decrease the morning NPH dose and leave the morning regular insulin dose unchanged
    (C) increase the morning NPH dose and leave the morning regular insulin dose unchanged
    (D) leave the morning NPH dose unchanged and increase the morning regular insulin dose
    (E) increase both the morning NPH and regular doses

Answers and Explanations

1. **(B)** Multiple factors influence the initial dose of levothyroxine when used for thyroid replacement therapy, including age, the duration and severity of hypothyroidism, and the presence of certain underlying conditions. Thyroid hormones are known to elevate heart rate and increase cardiac contractility, both of which demand more oxygen utilization by the heart. In hypothyroid patients with a history of stable angina, initial levothyroxine doses are typically smaller and then titrated upward. This regimen prevents a more immediate increase on the heart's workload that could occur with usual doses and minimizes the chances of an exacerbation of angina. *(DiPiro et al, 2005, pp. 1384; Ganong, 2003, pp. 328)*

2. **(C)** Methimazole is an antithyroid agent known as a thionamide or thiourea drug. It decreases the synthesis of thyroid hormone by inhibiting the oxidation of iodide and the coupling of iodotyrosines. Minor adverse reactions include skin rash, nausea, vomiting, and drowsiness. The main risk of thionamides, however, is agranulocytosis, with the incidence varying between 0.5% to 6.0%. Patients who receive methimazole should be closely supervised and cautioned to report immediately any evidence of illness, including sore throat, skin eruptions, fever, headache, or general malaise. In such cases, methimazole should be discontinued and white blood cell and differential counts should be made to determine whether agran-

ulocytosis has developed. Since the onset is sudden, routine monitoring is not required. It is particularly important for the patient to carefully monitor for signs and symptoms during the early stages of methimazole therapy, since methimazole-induced agranulocytosis usually occurs within the first 3 months of therapy. *(DiPiro et al, 2005, pp. 1378)*

3. **(C)** Once a patient suffers a myocardial infarction, regulating blood pressure is imperative for reducing the risk of a recurrent cardiovascular event. Hypertension significantly raises the afterload of the heart. This causes its workload to increase and may also induce myocardial hypertrophy if the hypertension is chronic. Together, these lead to additional oxygen demands, which could precipitate another myocardial infarction, particularly in the heart that is already compromised because of a prior event.

In addition to their antihypertensive properties, ACEIs have been shown to have many other beneficial effects. These include prolonging survival, improving cardiac function, and reducing subsequent cardiac events in patients with a history of myocardial infarction. Similarly, non-ISA (intrinsic sympathomimetic agents) β-blockers have been shown to reduce the risk of recurrent myocardial infarction.

The seventh report of the Joint National Committee on the Prevention, Detection,

Evaluation, and Treatment of High Blood Pressure (JNC-7) recommends a 2-drug combination for stage 2 hypertension and lists postmyocardial infarction as a compelling indication for choosing a non-ISA β-blocker and ACEI over other hypertension therapies. *(Chobania et al, 2003, p. 2568; DiPiro et al, 2005, p. 199)*

4. **(D)** Acetaminophen toxicity may result from a single toxic dose, from repeated ingestion of large doses of acetaminophen (e.g., 7.5 to 10 g daily for 1 to 2 days), or from chronic ingestion of the drug. Dose-dependent, hepatic necrosis is the most serious acute toxic effect associated with overdose and is potentially fatal. Acetaminophen is the second most common cause of liver failure requiring transplantation in the United States. *(Tierney et al, 2006, pp. 1615–1616)*

5. **(D)** According to the American College of Cardiology/American Heart Association practice guidelines for chronic stable angina, β-blockers like metoprolol are generally considered among the initial anti-anginal drugs of choice in the long-term prophylactic management of chronic stable angina. Long-acting nitrates such as isosorbide dinitrate can be used alone or in combination as second-line therapy in patients previously treated with a β-blocker. However, the development of tolerance is a major limiting step in their efficacy when used long-term. The degree of tolerance can be limited by utilizing a regimen that includes a minimum 8- to 10-hour period per day without nitrates no matter the route of delivery (ointment, patch, or tablets). *(DiPiro et al, 2005, p. 273; Gibbons et al, 2002, p. 47; Tierney et al, 2006, p. 348)*

6. **(C)** Sildenafil and other selective phosphodiesterase (PDE) inhibitors (e.g., tadalafil, vardenafil) profoundly potentiate the vasodilatory effects (e.g., a greater than 25 mm Hg decrease in systolic blood pressure) of organic nitrates, and potentially life-threatening hypotension or hemodynamic collapse can result. Nitrates promote the formation of cyclic guanosine monophosphate (cGMP) by stimulating guanylate cyclase, and sildenafil acts to decrease the degradation of cGMP via PDE type 5 by inhibiting this enzyme, resulting in increased accumulation of cGMP and more pronounced smooth muscle relaxation and vasodilation than with either sildenafil or nitrates alone. In this scenario, the profound hypotension led to a significant decrease in coronary blood flow, thereby worsening the patient's ischemia that he was experiencing during his angina attack. Because of the serious risk of concomitant use of organic nitrates and selective PDE inhibitors, such combined use is contraindicated. *(DiPiro et al, 2005, pp. 1522–1525)*

7. **(B)** Digoxin binds to Na^+/K^+ ATPases on the sarcolemmal membranes of cardiac muscle cells and inhibits them from working. This raises intracellular Na^+ levels, which facilitates Na^+/Ca^{+2} exchange. The resulting increase in intracellular Ca^{+2} enhances contractile protein cross-bridge formation and cardiac contractility, resulting in a positive inotropic effect.

    One of the parameters often monitored in the heart-failure patient taking digoxin is serum K^+. Potassium and digoxin inhibit each others binding to the Na^+/K^+ ATPases; therefore, hyperkalemia reduces the actions of digoxin, whereas hypokalemia increases its effect. As a result, hypokalemic patients are more susceptible to the many cardiac manifestations of digoxin toxicity, particularly ventricular arrhythmias. Rhythm disturbances are a major concern in heart failure patients, as they are already at an elevated risk for sudden cardiac death that can be linked to ventricular arrhythmias.

    Furosemide is a K^+-wasting, loop diuretic that is often prescribed with digoxin to provide symptomatic relief due to fluid retention, particularly in patients with moderate to severe congestive heart failure. Hence, loop diuretics should be used cautiously as a result of their potential to cause hypokalemia and subsequently, an elevated risk of cardiac arrhythmias. *(DiPiro et al, 2005, pp. 235–237, 243–244)*

8. **(A)** Triple therapy regimens consisting of a PPI and two antibiotics are considered first-line

therapy for the eradication of *Helicobacter pylori*. PPI-based regimens that combine clarithromycin and amoxicillin, clarithromycin and metronidazole, or amoxicillin and metronidazole have been shown to have the most effective eradication rates. Due to lower eradication rates, it is recommended that histamine receptor antagonists like rantidine not be substituted for a PPI. Misoprostol is used for reducing the risk of nonsteroidal anti-inflammatory agent (NSAIA)-induced gastric ulcer in patients at high risk of developing complications from these ulcers and in patients at high risk of developing gastric ulceration. It has no effect on *H. pylori* eradication. *(DiPiro et al, 2005, pp. 637–640)*

9. **(D)** *Clostridium difficile* is a gram-positive, anaerobic, spore-forming bacillus that is responsible for the development of antibiotic-associated diarrhea and colitis. *C. difficile* colitis results from a disturbance of the normal bacterial flora of the colon, colonization with *C. difficile*, and release of toxins that cause mucosal inflammation and damage. Antibiotic therapy is the key factor that alters the colonic flora. Specific therapy aimed at eradicating *C. difficile* is indicated if symptoms are persistent or severe. The drug of choice is metronidazole, 500 mg orally three times daily. Oral metronidazole and vancomycin are equally effective in treating diarrhea caused by *C. difficile*. Despite the isolation of metronidazole-resistant strains of *C. difficile*, metronidazole is the drug of first choice because of its lower cost. *(DiPiro et al, 2005, p. 1920; Tierney et al, 2006, pp. 618–620)*

10. **(B)** Acute uncomplicated cystitis is predominately caused by *E. coli*. While trimethoprim-sulfamethoxazole has been used to treat uncomplicated cystitis in numerous cases, it is becoming more ineffective due to the emergence of resistant strains of *E. coli*. As a result, fluoroquinolones such as ciprofloxacin are now considered the drugs of choice over all other antibiotics. Three-day courses of fluoroquinolones have been shown to be more effective than single-dose therapies. *(DiPiro et al, 2005, pp. 2086–2088; Tierney et al, 2006, p. 938)*

11. **(D)** Albuterol, metaproterenol, and pirbuterol are all short-acting β_2-agonists that have an onset of action within minutes. They are available as metered dose inhalers (MDLs) and can typically produce maximal bronchodilation within 30 minutes of administration. Levalbuterol is also a short-acting β_2-agonist that is administered via nebulizer. As a group, the short-acting β_2-agonists are the most effective bronchodilators and are considered the treatment of choice for the management of severe acute asthma according to the National Asthma Education and Prevention Program's Guidelines for the Diagnosis and Management of Asthma.

Salmeterol is a long-acting β_2-agonist, as it can take up to 20 minutes for onset and 1 to 4 hours for maximal bronchodilation following inhalation. Hence, salmeterol is not effective for severe acute asthma, but it can be used adjunctively with low to medium doses of inhaled corticosteroids (e.g., flunosilide, fluticasone) for long-term control (preventative) of chronic asthma. *(DiPiro et al, 2005, pp. 518–519, 529; Katzung, 2004, pp. 324–325; Murphy et al, p. 108)*

12. **(C)** Sulfonylureas like glyburide enhance insulin secretion by the pancreas; hence, they are typically known as insulin secretagogues. Their net effect leads to increased responsiveness of β-cells to both glucose and non-glucose secretagogues (such as amino acids), resulting in more insulin being released at all blood glucose concentrations. Repaglinide is considered a non-sulfonylurea insulin secretagogue. It is structurally different than glyburide, but it acts similarly to enhance insulin secretion. Metformin helps control glucose levels by decreasing hepatic glucose production, while rosiglitazone improves glycemic control by making tissues more sensitive to the effects of endogenous insulin. Acarbose is an alpha-glucosidase inhibitor (AGI). Taken orally, AGIs inhibit the upper gastrointestinal enzymes α-glucosidases) that readily convert carbohydrates into monosaccharides in a dose-dependent fashion. Hence, as digestion is slowed, AGIs ultimately decrease the absorption of glucose into the bloodstream. *(Katzung, 2004, pp. 704–711)*

13. **(C)** Because of their unpredictable and varied anticoagulant responses among patients, routine monitoring of warfarin or UFH therapy is essential in achieving desired therapeutic outcomes and minimizing bleeding complications. The aPTT is the most commonly used test to determine the degree of anticoagulation produced by UFH. The therapeutic range of aPTT is often considered to be 1.5 to 2.5 times the mean normal control value.

The INR consists of a ratio of prothrombin times (patient/control) that is normalized, which removes the variability of a patient's own prothrombin time due to differences in laboratory reagents and methods. The recommended target INR is typically based on the therapeutic indication, which for most, is between 2.0 and 3.0. *(DiPiro et al, 2005, pp. 382, 392)*

14. **(B)** Both warfarin and heparin are anticoagulants that are indicated for the prevention of thrombi. They do not actively lyse clots, but are capable of preventing further thrombogenesis. Both abciximab and clopidogrel are considered antiplatelet agents. Abciximab inhibits the activation of glycoprotein IIb/IIIa receptors on platelets, which helps to reduce platelet aggregation. Clopidogrel blocks adenosine diphosphate (ADP) receptors on platelets. The binding of ADP to these receptors is an important cellular mechanism in stimulating platelet aggregation. Alteplase converts plasminogen to plasmin, which then actively dissolves the fibrin threads associated with a thrombus. *(Katzung, 2004, pp. 543–555)*

15. **(C)** Opioid rotation is a common practice of switching a patient from one opioid to another. This typically occurs when patients are not getting sufficient pain relief with one opioid (despite increasing its dose) or are complaining of its side effects. Opioid rotation requires the provider to determine approximate equianalgesic dosing conversions, as different opioids usually have different potencies.

In this particular problem, 6 mg of hydromorphone is equianalgesic with 24 mg of morphine

sulfate. Using this ratio of relative potencies, the first step is to determine how many milligrams of morphine sulfate is equianalgesic with 16 mg of morphine sulfate:

$$\frac{7.5 \text{ mg hydromorphone}}{30 \text{ mg morphine sulfate}} = \frac{16 \text{ mg hydromorphone}}{X \text{ mg morphine sulfate}}$$

Solving for X, the calculation is 64 mg.

Due to wide ranges in individual responses to the various opioids and also because of potential cross-tolerance between opioids, the calculated dose of the new opioid is typically reduced by at least 25% to ensure safety:

$$64 \text{ mg} - 16 \text{ mg} (25\% \text{ of } 64) = 48 \text{ mg}$$

(DiPiro et al, 2005, p. 1096; Obenrader, 2004; Tierney et al, 2006, p. 74)

16. **(E)** Thiazolidinediones ("glitazones") such as pioglitazone; HMG-CoA reductase inhibitors or "statins" such as simvistatin; niacin; and fibric acid derivatives or "fibrates" such as gemfibrozil have all been shown to cause liver enzyme elevation. Each of these drugs comes with the recommendation of having LFTs checked prior to therapy and have suggested threshold values that determine if therapy should be initiated. Although clopidogrel should be used cautiously in hepatically impaired patients, there are no data to suggest that it significantly raises liver enzymes. *(Tierney et al, 2006, pp. 1211, 1250; PRESCRIBER'S LETTER)*

17. **(B)** Spasmolytics like carisoprodol and cyclobenzaprine are indicated as an adjunct to rest and physical therapy for relief of muscle spasm associated with acute, painful musculoskeletal conditions. Some of the more common adverse effects include drowsiness, dizziness, and dry mouth. These effects appear to be related to the drug's antimuscarinic properties. Patients should be advised not to use these drugs with alcohol or other central nervous system (CNS) depressants, as these combinations can cause significant sedation. Operating machinery or driving a motor vehicle should be avoided while taking carisoprodol or cyclobenzaprine. *(Katzung, 2004, pp. 444)*

18. **(B)** Probenecid is considered a uricosuric agent, as it decreases the reabsorption of uric acid in the proximal convoluted tubules of nephrons. Hence, more uric acid is excreted via the urine, which leads to a decrease in plasma levels. Allopurinol inhibits the key enzyme (xanthine oxidase) involved in uric acid synthesis. This also leads to a reduction in the amount of uric acid found in the plasma. Colchicine and indomethacin can be used to alleviate the inflammation associated with acute gouty arthritis, but they do not affect plasma uric acid levels. *(Katzung, 2004, pp. 596–599)*

19. **(C)** Many antiarrhythmic drugs have the potential for causing new arrhythmias or even worsening arrhythmias for which the drug is indicated. This phenomenon is referred to as a "pro-arrhythmic" effect. For example, treatment with the class 1A agent quinidine for supraventricular arrhythmias can precipitate torsade de pointes (a form of ventricular tachycardia) in 4% to 8% of patients using the drug due to its ability to prolong the QT interval.

Long QT interval syndrome (LQTS) can often lead to an abrupt loss of consciousness and death. It is characterized by QT prolongation accompanied by tachycardia. In patients with LQTS that develop torsade de pointes, the symptoms can range from syncope (where the torsade de pointes stops suddenly) to cardiac arrest (when it results in ventricular fibrillation). Hence, torsade de pointes can have a particularly poor prognosis. *(DiPiro et al, 2005, pp. 347–348; Woelfel, 2004)*

20. **(C)** Of all the therapeutic agents currently on the market, niacin has the greatest potential to raise high-density lipoproteins (HDL-C), often by as much as 25% to 35%. The amount of niacin needed to achieve this therapeutic effect is very high compared to the recommended daily allowance (RDA) for niacin (3.0 to 4.5 g/day vs. 20 mg/day). Unfortunately, compliance with niacin therapy is high due to intense (yet harmless) flushing of the skin that is quite similar to hot flashes experienced in many postmenopausal women. Aspirin and other NSAIDs can often blunt this prostaglandin-mediated response to high doses of niacin, as their mechanism of action is to decrease prostaglandin synthesis. *(DiPiro et al, 2005, p. 444; Tierney et al, 2006, pp. 1249–1250)*

21. **(B)** Alleviation of symptoms associated with depression is typically slow in onset following initiation with SSRIs. Fluoxetine, for instance, can take anywhere between 2 to 6 weeks to achieve substantial benefit when used for depression. After just 1 week of therapy, there is little justification to increase the current dose or switch to another SSRI like sertraline. Switching the patient to a TCA like amitriptyline at this point would further delay symptom relief, as TCAs can also take several weeks to produce improvement. Compared to SSRIs, TCAs are also more likely to create unwanted side effects such as weight gain, orthostatic hypotension, and constipation. Combining an SSRI with a monoamine oxidase inhibitor (MAOI) such as phenelzine can cause serotonin syndrome that can be lethal. In order to avoid interaction between SSRIs and MAOIs, it is recommended that at least 4 to 5 weeks pass after discontinuing one and starting the other. *(Tierney et al, 2006, pp. 1070–1073; Katzung, 2004, p. 490)*

22. **(A)** Aggressive treatment of hypertension in diabetic patients is essential in preventing many comorbidities, including nephropathy, myocardial infarction, and stroke. The American Diabetes Association (ADA) currently recommends the use of ACEIs as first-line agents for the treatment of hypertension in diabetic patients. This recommendation is based on a number of studies that have demonstrated a clinically significant decrease in the development and progression of diabetic nephropathy, a so-called "protective renal effect." The majority of diabetics will actually require the use of multiple antihypertensive agents to reach their goal blood pressure, as one medication alone is often ineffective. Whatever combination regimen is selected, it should include an ACEI. *(Tierney et al, 2006, p. 433; ADA Guidelines, 2006)*

23. **(B)** α1-adrenergic antagonists (blockers) such as doxazosin cause relaxation of the internal urethral sphincter and also decrease prostatic smooth muscle tone. As a result, urinary outflow from the bladder is enhanced and the patient is less likely to experience obstructive symptoms such as weak urine flow, straining to initiate urine flow, dribbling after urination, and the constant feeling of a full bladder.

5α-reductase inhibitors such as finasteride and dutasteride (Avodart) decrease the production of intraprostatic dihydrotestosterone (DHT) by inhibiting the enzyme type II 5α-reductase. Within the prostate, this enzyme converts testosterone into DHT, which causes prostatic enlargement and growth. As a result, 5α-reductase inhibitors shrink the prostate, which subsequently can provide relief of obstructive symptoms.

α1-adrenergic antagonists are faster acting in providing symptom relief compared to the 5α-reductase inhibitors, which often take up to 6 months to maximally shrink an enlarged prostate gland. Hence, patients with troublesome symptoms seeking quick relief generally do not prefer 5α-reductase inhibitors.

The use of testosterone would not be indicated as this could raise DHT levels and cause further prostatic enlargement. Desmopressin is a synthetic analog of antidiuretic hormone (ADH) and would cause urinary retention, thus exacerbating symptoms. Atropine is a muscarinic antagonist and would also worsen symptoms. *(DiPiro et al, 2005, pp. 1536–1543)*

24. **(D)** One of the drug therapies used to manage the symptoms of Parkinson's disease is the combination of levodopa (L-DOPA) and carbidopa. Levodopa is the precursor to dopamine, which is the neurotransmitter whose decreased concentrations in the substantia nigra lead to symptoms of tremor, rigidity, bradykinesia, and postural instability. Levodopa is converted into dopamine by dopa decarboxylase, an enzyme found within the nervous tissue and also the peripheral circulation. Levodopa is used instead of dopamine because it can cross the blood–brain barrier. While

levodopa can improve symptoms, it does not halt progression of the disease. Carbidopa inhibits peripheral dopa decarboxylase, which allows more levodopa to cross the blood–brain barrier instead of being converted into dopamine within the circulation. Carbidopa itself does not cross the blood–brain barrier.

A complication that can potentially develop over time with this therapy is the "on–off phenomenon," which is characterized by abrupt, unpredictable, and transient fluctuations in motor symptoms. The patient experiences a good response to therapy during the "on" phase, but then encounters symptoms of their underlying parkinsonism during the "off" period. Dyskinesias can occur in the "on" periods, but overall, mobility is improved. *(Tierney et al, 2006, pp. 1008–1009)*

25. **(C)** First-choice antibiotic treatment for acute otitis media includes a 10-day course of amoxicillin (80 to 90 mg/kg/day in two divided doses) or a combination of erythromycin (50 mg/kg/day) and a sulfonamide (150 mg/kg/day). Reasons for amoxicillin therapy include spectrum of activity including both susceptible and intermediate resistant *S. pneumoniae*, safety, cost, and tolerability. *(O'Mara, 2004; Tierney et al, 2006, p. 185)*

26. **(D)** Epogen is a synthetic form of erythropoietin (EPO), a naturally-occurring hormone synthesized and secreted by the kidneys. EPO works at the red bone marrow to stimulate erythropoiesis or red blood cell production. In patients with chronic renal failure, EPO production is usually impaired, and this EPO deficiency leads to anemia.

Deferoxamine is an iron-chelating compound that can be given systemically in situations of iron overdose. Warfarin and argatroban are both anticoagulants and do not typically affect red cell count. Protamine sulfate is a heparin-chelating compound that can be given in cases of heparin overdose. *(Tierney et al, 2006, p. 910)*

27. **(C)** The patient's diabetic condition, report of his pain characteristics (burning, tingling, and

"electric-like") and allodynia (pain from stimuli that are not normally painful) are suggestive of neuropathic pain. Whereas nociceptive pain is often acute and typically relieved with conventional analgesics (e.g., opioids, acetaminophen, NSAIDs), chronic neuropathic pain syndromes like peripheral diabetic neuropathy are not. The patient has already tried courses of conventional analgesics that have not provided any significant pain relief. TCAs (amitriptyline, desipramine) have been recommended and shown to provide pain relief in diabetic neuropathy, as have antiepileptic drugs like gabapentin that decrease neuronal excitability. The serotonin and norepinephrine reuptake inhibitor duloxetine is indicated for pain associated with diabetic neuropathy. Spasmolytics like cyclobenzaprine are not indicated for diabetic neuropathy, nor have studies confirmed a role as analgesics for neuropathic pain. *(DiPiro et al, 2005, pp. 1091, 1102; Tierney et al, 2006, pp. 1223–1224)*

28. **(A)** Senna is a plant derivative found in preparations such as Senokot and Ex-Lax. While the exact mechanism is unknown, it is believed that cathartics induce peristalsis by directly stimulating the enteric nervous system of the bowel. PEG is an example of an osmotic laxative that leads to water retention in the bowel. It is often used when complete colonic cleansing is required prior to gastrointestinal endoscopic procedures. Docusate is a typical ingredient found in stool softeners, whereas methylcellulose is a plant product used in bulk forming laxatives. Bismuth subsalicylate is not a laxative, but rather an antidiarrheal agent. *(Katzung, 2004, pp. 1046–1047)*

29. **(D)** Orthostatic hypotension is a common adverse reaction associated with many different medications and can lead to injuries caused by falls. Antihypertensive medications such as the thiazide diuretics (e.g., hydrochlorothiazide) and $\alpha1$-adrenergic antagonists (e.g., doxazosin) can produce orthostatic hypotension via dehydration and peripheral vasodilation, respectively. $\alpha1$-adrenergic antagonists are known for producing "first-dose effects" that include syncope, dizziness, and orthostatic hypotension. Some of the TCAs like

amitriptyline exert strong antimuscarinic properties that can also lead to peripheral vasodilation. The phenothiazines (e.g., chlorpromazine) are a group of typical antipsychotics (neuroleptics), some of whose members (known as low potency) also have similar $\alpha1$-adrenergic-blocking actions. Benzodiazepines (e.g., diazepam) are not known to produce orthostatic hypotension. *(DiPiro et al, 2005, pp. 1541–1542; Tierney, et al, 2006, p. 1071; Katzung, 2004, pp. 468–473)*

30. **(B)** The patient is in need of long-term control therapy due to his worsening symptoms. Whenever increased use of a quick-relief medication such as a β_2-agonist (albuterol) occurs, it is usually indicative of needing to add a long-term control agent to the therapeutic regimen or to increase the dose of an already prescribed long-term control medication. Inhaled corticosteroids like fluticasone are considered first-line long-term control medications for patients with persistent asthma. *(Tierney et al, 2006, pp. 230–237)*

31. **(D)** COCs are associated with an increased risk of each of the following: myocardial infarction, thromboembolic disease, cerebrovascular disease, and hypertension. Furthermore, they have also been shown to worsen all of the named conditions, as well as other disorders such as current breast cancer, benign liver adenomas, liver cancer, and active viral hepatitis. A fairly common mnemonic known as "ACHES" can be used to remember potential problems that can occur with COC use.

Abdominal pain can be indicative of a thrombus in the pelvis or liver, a benign liver tumor or gall bladder disease.

Chest pain can be suggestive of a thrombus in the lungs or in coronary arteries leading to angina or myocardial infarction.

Headaches may be suggestive of stroke or hypertension.

Eye problems such as blurred vision, double vision, or loss of vision may indicate stroke or blood clots in the eyes.

Severe leg pain can be indicative of inflammation and venous thrombosis in the lower extremity. *(Tierney et al, 2006, pp. 752–753)*

32. **(A)** Via its interaction with mu (μ) receptors throughout the CNS, morphine and other related opioids not only produce an analgesic effect, but they also can cause respiratory depression, particularly as doses are increased. Typically, morphine will reduce the respiratory rate, which then leads to an increase in the levels of carbon dioxide (CO_2) in the blood and cerebrospinal fluid (CSF). In the patient with underlying pulmonary disease, whose ventilation and gas exchange efficiency may already be compromised, morphine has the potential to raise the CO_2 level further and also limit how much oxygen (O_2) can be breathed into the lungs. Excess CO_2 also has the effect of causing pronounced vasodilation of cerebral blood vessels, which results in an increase in ICP. Elevations in ICP can also reduce ventilation further. *(DiPiro et al, 2005, pp. 1094–1095; Ganong, 2003, p. 599)*

33. **(B)** Acyclovir is the treatment of choice for HSV disease, typically in oral doses of 200 mg five times daily or 400 mg three times daily. In situations where oral acyclovir cannot be absorbed effectively by the GI tract or tolerated by the patient, intravenous acyclovir can be administered at a rate of 15 mg/kg/day). *(DiPiro et al, 2005, p. 2271)*

34. **(A)** Desmopressin is a synthetic analog of ADH. In neurogenic or central diabetes insipidus, there is lack of ADH synthesis and secretion for the hypothalamus and posterior pituitary gland, respectively. Desmopressin can be used as ADH replacement therapy in this situation. Since ADH inhibits diuresis, desmopressin is also indicated for the treatment of primary nocturnal enuresis (bedwetting), particularly in young children. Desmopressin is largely ineffective in nephrogenic diabetes insipidus, since in this condition, the kidneys are insensitive to the effects of ADH. Syndrome of inappropriate ADH secretion (SIADH) is characterized by excess ADH production

despite normal blood volume and plasma osmolality; hence, desmopressin would exacerbate this condition.

Primary hyperaldosteronism is treated surgically (adrenalectomy), with sprinolactone (a K^+-sparing diuretic) and/or antihypertensives depending upon the etiology and symptoms.

Primary adrenal insufficiency is generally treated with glucocorticoids (e.g., hydrocortisone) and/or mineralocorticoids (e.g., fludrocortisone acetate) depending upon the clinical findings. *(Tierney et al, 2006, p. 868, 1109–1110, 1164–1167, 1172–1173)*

35. **(D)** In most patients suffering from generalized convulsive status epilepticus (GCSE), benzodiazepines such as lorazepam and diazepam are effective initial therapies due to their relatively high lipid solubility. As a result, they are able to cross the blood–brain barrier easily, which gives them the potential to stop seizures quickly. Lorazepam's lipid solubility is less compared to diazepam and it also redistributes to fat more slowly. Hence, lorazepam tends to have a longer duration of action (12 to 24 hours) than diazepam (20 to 30 minutes).

Phenytoin is often used as a second-line agent in patients whose seizures do not terminate with benzodiazepines. It can also be used immediately after benzodiazepine administration for seizure control. This is more likely to occur with diazepam whose duration of action is shorter than for lorazepam. Phenytoin has a long half-life (20 to 36 hours) compared to diazepam and can provide long-term seizure control. Phenytoin is not considered a first-line agent because its lipid solubility is less than the benzodiazepines and therefore cannot enter the brain quickly enough to terminate seizure activity. *(DiPiro et al, 2005, pp. 1053–1056; Tierney et al, 2006, p. 986)*

36. **(A)** Macrolides are known to interact with HMG-CoA reductase inhibitors ("statins") by inhibiting CYP3A4 isoenzymes in the

liver. These enzymes metabolize many of the statins, including lovastatin. When macrolides such as clarithromycin are administered, they inhibit these enzymes, resulting in higher levels of statins remaining in the blood for longer periods of time. One of the potential adverse effects of statins, particularly when their blood concentrations elevate, is myositis or myopathy. (*Katzung, 2004, pp. 568–570*)

37. **(E)** Abrupt cessation of TCAs can lead to a withdrawal syndrome that is linked to their strong antimuscarinic properties. A "cholinergic rebound" consisting of dizziness, nausea, diarrhea, insomnia, and restlessness can occur if the dose is not tapered over several days.

Sudden β-blocker withdrawal can produce "adrenergic rebound" effects that include hypertension and cardiac arrhythmias, such as sinus tachycardia. For those patients with particularly high coronary disease risk, additional problems such as unstable angina or myocardial infarction may occur. To minimize these effects, β-blockers are recommended to be tapered over 1 to 2 weeks.

A withdrawal syndrome has also been linked to sudden discontinuation of SSRIs. It is characterized by dysphoric mood, agitation, and flu-like symptoms. To minimize these effects, SSRIs should be tapered gradually over a period of weeks to months before eventually discontinuing the drug.

Chronic therapy with systemic corticosteroids can induce atrophy of the adrenal glands, which significantly depresses the adrenal response to adrenocorticotropic hormone (ACTH). Stopping prednisone suddenly would leave the body without a source or glucocorticoids, as the hypothalamic–pituitary–adrenal axis needs time to reestablish its normal functioning. As a result, an acute adrenal crisis (Addisonian crisis) that is marked by dehydration with severe vomiting and diarrhea, hypotension, shock, and loss of consciousness can develop and potentially lead to a fatality.

Sudden discontinuation of ezetimibe, a drug that blocks cholesterol absorption in the small intestine, is not known for precipitating withdrawal reactions. It is not generally tapered when switching to another drug for hyperlipidemia or discontinuing therapy altogether. (*DiPiro et al, 2005, p. 208, 1242; Tierney et al, 2006, p. 1071; Ganong, 2003, pp. 377–378, 384*)

38. **(E)** In 2004, the NCEP/ATP guidelines were updated with several new recommendations that reflected a more aggressive approach in treating and preventing hyperlipidemic conditions. One of those new recommendations was that the LDL-C threshold for starting pharmacologic therapy in high-risk patients be lowered from 130 mg/dL or higher to 100 mg/dL or higher. The previous recommendation released in 2001 stated that pharmacologic therapy for an LDL-C level between 100 to 129 mg/dL in high-risk individuals was optional. High-risk individuals are defined as those with coronary heart disease (CHD) or a CHD equivalent such as peripheral arterial disease, carotid artery disease, or diabetes mellitus. (*Grundy et al, 2004*)

39. **(D)** Warfarin is contraindicated in all trimesters and is listed as category X by the FDA, as it has been shown to induce fetal bleeding and cause several teratogenic effects including CNS malformations, structural deformities of the nose, and bone dysplasias.

ACEIs (e.g., captopril) should not be used, especially during the second and third trimesters of pregnancy, due to their increased risk of causing fetal hypotension and fetal renal damage, which can be fatal.

Isotretinoin is also listed as category X and a known teratogen causing malformations of the CNS, face, and ears.

Misoprostol is a synthetic prostaglandin analog indicated for reducing the risk of NSAID-induced gastric ulcers in patients at high risk of complications from gastric ulcer. It also has oxytotic properties, meaning that it can induce uterine contractions that may endanger pregnancy. The drug comes with a black box warning stating that administration to women who are pregnant can cause abortion, premature birth, or birth defects.

Esomeprazole is category B and has not been shown to cause birth defects or threaten pregnancy.

(DiPiro et al, 2005, pp. 643, 1430; Katzung, 2004, pp. 178, 999–1000; Tierney et al, 2006, p. 117)

40. **(C)** β-blockers are not indicated for use in hypothyroidism. Instead, they are used frequently (especially propanolol) for symptom control in patients suffering from hyperthyroidism until the condition is resolved with thionamides, radioactive iodine therapy, or thyroid surgery. No matter the etiology of hyperthyroidism, the tremulousness, tachycardia, diaphoresis, and anxiety associated with the condition can all be effectively relieved with β-blockers. *(Tierney et al, 2006, p. 1138)*

41. **(C)** As a CYP2D6 inducer, the antiepileptic medication will stimulate or increase the activity of the enzymes responsible for metabolizing the antihypertensive medication into harmless by-products. As a result, the patient is more susceptible to having his/her blood pressure elevate, since the dose of the antihypertensive drug is being cleared from the body more quickly. *(Katzung, 2004, pp. 53–56)*

42. **(D)** Synchronized DCC is the treatment of choice in patients with severe symptoms such as syncope, anginal pain, and heart failure. This patient only has mild symptoms resulting from his PSVT. In these situations, nonpharmacologic measures that increase vagal activity (e.g., Valsalva maneuver) to the heart can be attempted to help restore a sinus rhythm. Since this failed in our patient, drug therapy is the best option.

Both the American Heart Association and American College of Cardiology recommend adenosine as the drug of first choice in patients with PSVT, as it slows conduction and interrupts the reentry pathways through the AV node. Adenosine is capable of producing hypotension and would need to be used cautiously. However, adenosine has a short duration of action (6 to 10 seconds). Intravenous verapamil is equally efficacious in terminating PSVT and could also be used in this situation. *(Blomström-Lundqvist et al, 2003; DiPiro et al, 2005, pp. 337)*

43. **(B)** Warfarin interferes with the actions of vitamin K in the liver. Within hepatocytes, vitamin K is a cofactor required for the activation of clotting factors II (prothrombin), VII, IX, and X. By disrupting the actions of vitamin K, warfarin indirectly results in a slowed rate of synthesis of these four clotting factors, thereby creating the anticoagulant effect. *(DiPiro et al, 2005, pp. 388–389; Katzung, 2004, p. 550)*

44. **(D)** The main organs that take up iodine are the thyroid gland, which absolutely requires it for thyroid hormone (T_3 and T_4) production and the kidneys, which filter it from the blood and excrete it in the urine. Radioactive iodine (RAI) in the form of ^{131}I is one of the many therapies that can be used in the treatment of Graves' disease. Others include thyroid surgery and thionamides (thiourea drugs). RAI selectively destroys the thyroid follicular cells that concentrate it, thereby decreasing T_3 and T_4 production and lowering T_3 and T_4 levels in the blood. When used therapeutically, a common side effect of RAI is thyroiditis due to edema and leukocyte infiltration. RAI should not be administered to pregnant females, since it crosses the placenta and could be harmful to the developing fetus. Use of ^{123}I or ^{131}I with scanning can help determine if cancerous thyroid cells have spread to extra-thyroidal tissues. The administration of RAI has never been demonstrated to increase the risk of cancer or leukemia. *(DiPiro et al, 2005, p. 1379; Ganong, 2003, p. 321; Katzung, 2004, p. 634; Tierney et al, 2006, pp. 1139–1140)*

45. **(A)** All β-lactam antibiotics, including the penicillins (e.g., amoxicillin) and cephalosporins, prevent bacterial growth by inhibiting cell wall synthesis. Fluoroquinolones (e.g., ciprofloxacin) block bacterial DNA synthesis. Erythromycin,

doxycycline, and gentamicin all inhibit protein synthesis, but via different mechanisms. *(Katzung, 2004, pp. 734, 756, 758, 764, 777)*

46. **(C)** Triptans such as sumitriptan (Imitrex) and eletriptan (Relpax) are serotonin receptor agonists that are taken to help terminate and relieve pain associated with acute migraine attacks. During an attack, vasodilation of intracranial blood vessels occurs, leading to dural plasma extravasation, perivascular inflammation, and subsequent pain. Triptans help minimize these reactions by causing vasoconstriction of intracranial blood vessels. However, in the patient who has underlying cerebrovascular disease, vasoconstriction can further diminish blood flow, creating potentially dangerous hypoxic conditions in the brain. *(DiPiro et al, 2005, pp. 1106, 1114–1115)*

47. **(A)** There are a few products on the market that are FDA-approved specifically for emergency contraception. These include *Plan B* (two 0.75-mg tablets of levonorgestrel taken 12 hours apart) and *Preven* (four tablets, each containing 0.25 mg of levonorgestrel and 50 mcg of ethinyl estradiol, to be taken two at a time 12 hours apart). Several oral contraceptives contain doses of the steroids used in Plan B and Preven and can therefore also be used as emergency contraception. *(Tierney et al, 2006, p. 757)*

48. **(B)** If they coat the mouth and throat, inhaled corticosteroids (e.g., triamcinolone, fluticasone, flunisolide) can alter the local bacteria and fungal population thereby enhancing fungal growth. In cases of oropharyngeal candidiasis (thrush), white spots on the tongue and hard palate can be visualized, and the patient usually has pain on swallowing. In the asthma patient, the utilization of a spacer with a MDI can help minimize the chances of oropharyngeal candidiasis, as can routine gargling and rinsing following each inhaled treatment. Fluconazole is an antifungal agent that is effective in treating oropharyngeal candidiasis. *(DiPiro et al, 2005 pp. 528–529; Katzung, 2004, pp. 328–329; Tierney et al, 2006, pp. 203, 231)*

49. **(A)** The patient is most likely suffering from giardiasis that could have been contracted on her camping trip. While swimming, she may have inadvertently swallowed water contaminated with *Giardia lamblia*, whose incubation period is generally 1 to 3 weeks, after which symptoms develop. An effective treatment is metronidazole 250 mg taken three times daily for 5 to 7 days. *(Tierney et al, 2006, pp. 1478–1480)*

50. **(E)** Metronidazole is the topical treatment of choice for rosacea, which is consistent with the clinical findings in this 34-year-old female patient. Mupirocin ointment is a treatment option for impetigo, while permethrin is indicated for scabies. Tretinoin is effective and indicated for comedonal acne. Topical hydrocortisone has not been shown to be effective for rosacea. *(Tierney et al, 2006, pp. 117–118)*

51. **(B)** In DJ's situation, the choice of initial medication should be guided by his past medical history of asthma and also his recent elevation in blood pressure. Hypertensive patients with new onset atrial fibrillation are typically prescribed either B-blockers or calcium channel blockers. The use of propanolol (a nonselective β-blocker) would be discouraged because it may exacerbate DJ's asthma, plus decrease the efficacy of the β$_2$-agonists he is taking for long-term control and quick relief of exacerbations. Both captopril (ACEI) and losartan (angiotensin receptor blocker; ARB) are ineffective for rate control. In addition, ACEIs and ARBs have been shown to be relatively less effective in treating hypertension in African American patients. Methyldopa is not indicated for atrial fibrillation. Diltiazem offers the most effective treatment for both DJ's hypertension (in combination with the hydrochlorothiazide he is already taking) and atrial fibrillation. *(Tierney et al, 2006, pp. 374–375, 428–437)*

52. **(E)** Constipation is a common adverse effect of opioid therapy. In order to minimize or prevent constipation, the use of stool softeners (docusate) and a stimulant laxative (senna) can be initiated when opioid therapy is begun. The use of TUMS could actually make

things worse for RK, as antacids containing calcium carbonate alone can cause constipation. *(Tierney et al, 2006, pp. 81, 541)*

53. **(D)** In rheumatoid arthritis patients who fail to achieve pain relief with NSAIDs, methotrexate is often the treatment of choice. Methotrexate is the most common disease-modifying antirheumatic drug (DMARD) used in rheumatoid arthritis patients. Since the patient is not responding to naproxyn, switching to another NSAID (e.g., indomethacin, sulindac) is not likely to help the patient's symptoms. Acetaminophen is not an anti-inflammatory agent and would most likely provide less relief than naproxyn. Sulfasalazine is another DMARD, but is considered a second-line agent for rheumatoid arthritis. *(Katzung, 2004, pp. 588; Tierney et al, 2006, pp. 830–832)*

54. **(B)** Iron is one of the few substances that activated charcoal is ineffective against when swallowed in overdose. Whole bowel irrigation with an osmotic laxative containing PEG, such as GoLYTELY, can be effective for iron ingestion when introduced into the stomach via a gastric tube. *(Tierney et al, 2006, pp. 1612, 1619, 1625–1626, 1631, 1634, 1637–1638)*

55. **(C)** Data collected from several studies (e.g., UK Prospective Diabetes Study (UKPDS) and Diabetes Control and Complications Trial (DCCT)) have consistently demonstrated that tight glycemic control leads to decreased rates of diabetic complications, including retinopathy, nephropathy, and neuropathy. This decreased risk of complications was significant when therapeutic regimens lowered the average $HbA1_C$ to 7.0%. On the basis of this evidence, the ADA currently recommends that all diabetic patients have a management plan that achieves normal or near-normal glycemia with an A1C goal of <7%.

Similarly, other data (e.g., from the UKPDS and Hypertension Optimal Treatment trial (HOT)) have shown several benefits of lowering blood pressure <130/80 in the diabetic patient, including a reduction in stroke, nephropathy, and coronary heart disease.

Therefore, a target blood pressure goal of <130/80 is considered reasonable by the ADA if it can be safely achieved. *(ADA Guidelines, 2006)*

56. **(E)** There are no data to suggest that the effects of growth hormone are affected by cephalosporins.

All growth hormone formulations are synthesized by recombinant DNA techniques. In 1985, human pituitary growth hormone was withdrawn from the U.S. market following reports of patients who developed Creutzfeldt–Jakob disease (CJD) after receiving therapy. It is believed that CJD was transmitted via contaminated human pituitary-derived growth hormone.

Because it is a protein, synthetic growth hormone is typically given subcutaneously to avoid metabolism by the stomach.

In addition to its role in treating growth hormone deficiency, growth hormone has also been used recently to minimize and slow the muscle-wasting associated with AIDS, as it can stimulate protein synthesis in skeletal muscle cells.

Physiologically, growth hormone tends to elevate blood glucose levels by stimulating hepatic gluconeogensis and decreasing tissue glucose uptake.

(DiPiro et al, 2005, pp. 1408–1416, 2583)

57. **(D)** Omega-3 fatty acids have been linked to a reduction in plasma triglycerides. The FDA approved Omacor in November 2004 for the management of hypertriglyceridemia, and the drug is expected to reach market in late 2005. *(Scott, 2005; DiPiro et al, 2005, p. 443)*

58. **(D)** Tubocurarine and rocuronium are classified as nondepolarizing neuromuscular blocking drugs, whereas succinylcholine is depolarizing. Nondepolarizing agents competitively block nicotinic receptors on skeletal muscle, which leads to flaccid muscle paralysis.

Depolarizing agents, on the other hand, activate nicotinic receptors on skeletal muscle cells leading to membrane depolarization, initial fasciculations, and intense contractions. Succinylcholine is not metabolized efficiently at neuromuscular junctions; hence, the cells remain depolarized and are unable to repolarize or recover back to a resting state. This failure to repolarize then leads to a flaccid muscle paralysis.

Pyridostigmine in an acetylcholinesterase inhibitor indicated for myasthenia gravis and causes an increase in skeletal muscle activity. *(Katzung, 2004, pp. 104–105, 433–434)*

59. **(D)** Pernicious anemia is a chronic illness caused by impaired absorption of vitamin B_{12} due to a lack of intrinsic factor (IF) production by the gastric mucosa. Replacement therapy with intramuscular injections of vitamin B_{12} is often used to treat this condition. An alternative is Nascobal, a synthetic form of vitamin B_{12} in a nasally administered gel. *(Tierney et al, 2006, pp. 487–488)*

60. **(B)** All aminoglycosides are ototoxic and nephrotoxic. The likelihood of experiencing these toxicities occurs when treatment lasts beyond 5 days, at higher doses, in elderly patients, and those suffering from renal insufficiency. Other agents that produce either of these toxicities should not be used concurrently. *(Katzung, 2004, p. 767)*

61. **(D)** Zolpidem, zaleplon, and triazolam are all indicated for short-term treatment of insomnia, whereas eszopiclone can be used for long-term treatment.

Meclizine is used in the prevention and treatment of nausea, vomiting, and/or vertigo associated with motion sickness. It has also been used in the symptomatic treatment of vertigo associated with diseases affecting the vestibular system (e.g., labyrinthitis, Meniere's disease). *(Tierney et al, 2006, pp. 192–193, 540, 1079–1080)*

62. **(D)** A combination of a loop diuretic and an ACE inhibitor is typically the initial treatment in most symptomatic patients with congestive heart failure. ACE inhibitors have been demonstrated to not only reduce symptoms but also mortality in patients with symptomatic heart failure. Loop diuretics offer the best option to reduce the congestive symptoms in the lungs and fluid retention in the ankles. *(Tierney et al, 2006, pp 390–392)*

63. **(E)** Both alendronate and ibandronate are oral bisphosphanates that have been shown to increase bone mineral density and reduce the risk of osteoporosis-related fractures of the vertebrae, hip, and other sites. Similar reports also exist for calcitonin, but are limited to the vertebrae. The calcitonin that is used clinically is derived from salmon and typically administered intranasally. Oral raloxifene is a selective estrogen receptor modulator (SERM) that increases bone mineral density of the spine and hip, but not to the same extent as the bisphosphonates. *(DiPiro et al, 2005, pp. 1658–1659)*

64. **(D)** One of the potentially serious adverse effects of bupropion is a reduction in seizure threshold. However, seizures remain a relatively uncommon adverse effect of bupropion therapy, particularly when current recommended dosages for depression are not exceeded and underlying predisposing factors are not present. Nonetheless, bupropion is contraindicated in seizure disorder and it should not be used concomitantly with other medications known to lower seizure threshold. Furthermore, it should be discontinued and not restarted in patients who experience a seizure while on treatment. *(DiPiro et al, 2005, pp. 1024, 1137, 1204, 1247)*

65. **(C)** The patient is showing symptoms and signs of schizophrenia for which antipsychotic agents are the treatment of choice. Olanzapine is an atypical antipsychotic (e.g., second generation) that has less risk of causing extrapyramidal side effects (EPS) compared to typical antipsychotics (e.g., first-generation) such as thioridazine. Because of the risk of EPS, typical antipsychotics are not considered first-line treatments. *(DiPiro et al, 2005, pp. 1213–1215; Tierney et al, 2006, pp. 1058–1061)*

66. **(C)** Some of the active ingredients in grapefruit juice inactivate cytochrome P450 enzymes

(CYP3A4 isoenzymes) in both the intestine and liver. The intestinal CYP3A4 enzymes typically metabolize a percentage of oral benzodiazepines (e.g., alprazolam) and statins (e.g., atorvastatin) before they are absorbed into the blood. If these enzymes are inhibited, then more of the drug is absorbed, and its effect is enhanced. *(DiPiro et al, 2005, p. 106; Katzung, 2004, p. 62)*

67. **(C)** The JNC7 guidelines recommend thiazide diuretics (e.g., hydrochlorothiazide, chlorthalidone) as first-line therapy for those patients without compelling indications (heart failure, post myocardial infarction, high coronary disease risk, diabetes mellitus, chronic kidney disease, and recurrent stroke prevention). The recommendation is based on the evidence that has shown them to reduce the risk of morbidity and mortality associated with cardiovascular complications of hypertension compared to other agents. While a compelling indication will often dictate the use of another antihypertensive agent and classify it as first-line, thiazide diuretics can also be beneficial and may be used in combination. *(Chobania et al, 2003)*

68. **(C)** Triamterene is a K^+-sparing diuretic based on its mechanism of action. In the kidneys, it will lead to less K^+ excretion in the urine and hence retention of plasma K^+. In patients with elevated plasma K^+, triamterene can cause further hyperkalemia, which can impact neuromuscular and cardiac function. *(DiPiro et al, 2005, p. 205; Katzung, 2004, pp. 250–252.)*

69. **(C)** Leukotrienes are inflammatory mediators that are generated within the lungs. When they bind to specific receptors, they induce a variety of responses, including bronchospasm and mucus production. Zafirlukast (and also montelukast) are leukotriene receptor antagonists that block these effects in the lungs and improve asthma symptoms. Zafirlukast is considered an alternative therapy for long-term control of asthma, as it has been shown to be less effective than inhaled corticosteroids.

Both cromolyn and nedocromil are mast cell stabilizers and can also be used as an alternative treatment to inhaled corticosteroids. Omalizumab is an anti-IgE antibody, while ipratropium bromide is a muscarinic receptor antagonist. *(DiPiro et al, 2005, pp. 507, 523, 525, 530–531)*

70. **(A)** Hyperglycemia can be an adverse effect of thiazide diuretic use. Hyperuricemia, hyperlipidemia, hypokalemia, and hypercalcemia are all possible side effects. Hence, patients should be assessed for electrolyte imbalances, lipid abnormalities, gout, and diabetes mellitus prior to prescribing thiazide diuretics. *(DiPiro et al, 2005, pp. 204–205)*

71. **(D)** It is estimated that in females with gonorrhea, coexisting chlamydial infection occurs 50% of the time. For gonococcal urethritis, the treatments of choice include ceftriaxone or cefixime (Suprax). In cases of coexistent chlamydial infection, either doxycycline or azithromycin are recommended. *(DiPiro et al, 2005, p. 2100; Tierney et al, 2006, pp. 1432)*

72. **(D)** There are several noncontraceptive benefits associated with oral contraceptive use, but a reduction in the risk of liver cancer is not one of them. Moreover, females with a history of or existing liver cancer should avoid oral contraceptives altogether. Oral contraceptives have been shown to worsen the prognosis of existing liver cancer. *(DiPiro et al, 2005, pp. 1451–1455)*

73. **(C)** Heparin-induced thrombocytopenia (HIT) is a potentially serious complication of UFH therapy, usually occurring within 4 to 10 days after heparin treatment has started. Fortunately, current estimates show that it is infrequent, occurring in approximately 0.3% to 3.0% of patients receiving UFH for more than 4 days. HIT should immediately be suspected in a patient who develops deep vein thrombosis or pulmonary embolism while receiving UFH. *(DiPiro et al, 2005, pp. 406–408)*

74. **(D)** Nitrofurantoin has been shown to be a safe and effective drug during pregnancy for treating UTIs. Tetracyclines, fluoroquinolones, and sulfonamides are not recommended for use in pregnancy because of various risks they pose on the fetus. *(Tierney et al, 2006, pp. 782, 1571)*

75. **(D)** In order for POPs to be maximally effective in preventing a pregnancy in a non-breastfeeding woman, they should be taken within 3 hours of the same time every day. Their main mechanism of action is to induce thickening of the cervical mucus, thereby providing a barrier to sperm transport. Unlike COCs, they do not inhibit ovulation on a consistent basis. *(DiPiro et al, 2005, p. 1455; Tierney et al, 2006, pp. 753–754)*

76. **(E)** Muscarinic receptor antagonists block the peripheral responses produced by the parasympathetic nervous system, which, in turn, leads to the opposite effects. Physiologically, the parasympathetic nervous systems causes miosis, bronchoconstriction, increased gastric acid secretion, increased lacrimation, and bradycardia. Hence, an antimuscarinic drug would be cause of the following choices, but instead produce tachycardia. *(Ganong, 2003, pp. 229–231)*

77. **(B)** β-blockers are capable of crossing the blood–brain barrier, and hence can cause CNS side effects. In general, drugs that are more lipophilic can cross the blood–brain barrier more efficiently compared to drugs that are less lipophilic. Each β-blocker has a different degree of lipophilicity based on its chemical structure. *(DiPiro et al, 2005, pp. 207)*

78. **(A)** Doxorubicin is a common antineoplastic drug used for a variety of cancers, including breast, bladder, ovarian, and endometrial, among many others. Unfortunately, it has a well-established, dose-dependent adverse effect on the heart that is linked to free-radical formation. *(DiPiro et al, 2005, pp. 227, 2303–2305; Katzung, 2004, 913–914)*

79. **(E)** Because of their limited side effects, SSRIs such as fluoxetine are first-line medications for panic disorder. Benzodiazepines, as well as some of the TCAs and MAO inhibitors, have also been used but are considered second-line agents. *(DiPiro et al, 2005, pp. 1296–1297)*

80. **(B)** Whereas opioids may be effective for acute migraine treatment in some patients, they are generally not considered for use as prophylactic therapy. Frequent use of opioids can lead to tolerance and dependence, plus they have also been associated with rebound headache. *(DiPiro et al, 2005, pp. 1111, 1113, 1115–1116)*

81. **(E)** Naloxone is a specific opioid antagonist administered intravenously in cases of opioid overdose. It is a short-acting drug that may require repeated doses if the offending opioid has a long duration of action. *(Tierney et al, 2006, p. 1631)*

82. **(B)** Salicylic acid is a commonly used keratolytic that is typically applied as a lotion or gel (2% to 10% concentration) to corn pads. It is also indicated for the treatment of common warts, but is used in higher concentrations (17%). *(DiPiro et al, 2005, pp. 1773–1774; Tierney et al, 2006, pp. 128–129)*

83. **(C)** Both nonselective (propanolol) and cardioselective (metoprolol) β-blockers cause bradycardia. The same is true of calcium channel blockers that are classified as nondihydropyridines such as the benzothiazepines (verapamil) and diphenylalkylamines (diltiazem). These drugs block calcium channels in both the heart and vascular smooth muscle. Hence, vasodilation (with a subsequent drop in blood pressure) and bradycardia both occur. Dihydropyridines (amlodipine) have a greater effect on calcium channels in vascular smooth muscle compared to those in the heart. As a result, they are more potent vasodilators than the nondihydropyridines, which can lead to reflex tachycardia. *(DiPiro et al, 2005, pp. 208–209)*

84. **(B)** Insulin not only causes cellular uptake of glucose, but also of potassium. Hypokalemia may develop when insulin is infused to correct either a hyperglycemic hyperosmolar state or a diabetic ketoacidosis. Hence, in order to avoid hypokalemia, potassium chloride can be added to the saline solution, as long as the serum potassium is not elevated. *(Tierney et al, 2006, p. 1232)*

85. **(B)** Several medications have been implicated in decreasing the efficacy of oral contraceptives,

including rifampicin and several of the antiepileptics (AEDs). A back-up method of contraception is suggested for females taking rifampicin and COCs concomitantly on a short-term basis. If they are taken for longer periods of time, the patient should consider an alternative method of contraception. Similarly, for those patients taking either phenytoin or carbamazepine for seizure disorder, an alternative method of contraception is highly recommended. *(DiPiro et al, 2005, pp. 1457–1458)*

86. **(B)** Early reperfusion of brain tissue with tPA is critical in reducing disabilities in those patients who ultimately survive ischemic stroke. Several studies involving patients who presented more than 3 hours after the onset of neurological symptoms have failed to demonstrate a distinct benefit. Furthermore, some of these studies have suggested a higher risk of intracerebral hemorrhage when tPA is administered beyond this 3-hour time window. *(DiPiro et al, 2005, pp. 419–420)*

87. **(C)** Acetylcholinesterase inhibitors for Alzheimer's disease were designed around the "cholinergic hypothesis," which stated that the replenishment of acetylcholine could help restore memory and cognitive ability, both of which are lost as the disease progresses. While numerous cholinergic pathways are destroyed during Alzheimer's disease, many others are also lost. Even though these acetylcholinesterase inhibitors are indicated for Alzheimer's disease, they are not curative and do not restore function. *(DiPiro et al, 2005, pp. 1159–1160, 1162–1166)*

88. **(E)** Tegaserod is a serotonin receptor (5-HT$_4$ subtype) agonist. The stimulation of these receptors in the gastrointestinal (GI) tract leads to increases in both GI motility and secretions, both of which help facilitate the passage of stools. It also appears that the tegaserod enables patients to become less sensitive to some of the symptoms of their disease particularly bloating and abdominal discomfort. *(DiPiro et al, 2005, pp. 690–69; Tierney et al, 2006, p. 618)*

89. **(E)** The second generation antihistamines such as loratadine, fexofenadine, and desloratadine are nonsedating when taken at recommended doses. Since the patient is employed as a taxi driver, remaining alert is of prime importance. First-generation antihistamines (e.g., diphenhydramine, clemastine) have a much higher potential for causing sedation and should be avoided in this particular patient. *(DiPiro et al, 2005, pp. 1734–1735; Tierney et al, 2006, p. 789)*

90. **(E)** In October 2004, the FDA instructed manufacturers off all antidepressants to include in their labeling a boxed warning and expanded warning statements about the increased risk of suicidal thinking and behavior in children and adolescents being treated with these drugs. This directive was based on a combined analysis of several studies that concluded the risk of suicidal behavior to be twice as high (4% vs. 2%) in children and adolescents receiving antidepressants versus placebo. *(FDA)*

91. **(B)** Chronic therapy with oral corticosteroids can lead to many of the same symptoms associated with Cushing's syndrome. The natural glucocorticoids synthesized and secreted by the adrenal glands act to raise glucose levels. Hence, oral corticosteroid therapy is likely to produce hyperglycemia, which could lead to a diabetic state. *(DiPiro et al, 2005, pp. 522–523; Katzung, 2004, pp. 645, 650–651)*

92. **(A)** Intramuscular administration of epinephrine is the drug of choice to quickly reverse the considerable vasodilation (and subsequent drop in blood pressure) and bronchoconstriction that often occurs with anaphylaxis. Several adjunctive therapies (e.g., intravenous fluids, antihistamines, corticosteroids) may also be necessary to help maintain blood pressure, reduce inflammation, and prevent bronchospasm. However, epinephrine should be the first drug administered. *(DiPiro et al, 2005, pp. 1608–1609; Tierney et al, 2006, p. 792)*

93. **(A)** *Pasteurella multocida* is the typical cause of an early infection (within 24 hours) due to a cat bite. Penicillins offer the best coverage for *P. multocida*, compared to other antibiotics. *(DiPiro et al, 2005, 1991–1992)*

94. **(C)** Chemotherapy-induced nausea and vomiting (CINV) is a common problem for cancer patients that can lead to decreased compliance. Cyclophosphamide is a chemotherapeutic agent that is highly emetogenic. Antiemetics, known as selective serotonin receptor inhibitors (e.g., ondansetron, granisetron, dolasetron), are the drugs of choice for CINV, and their efficacy is enhanced when used concomitantly with dexamethasone. *(DiPiro et al, 2005, pp. 667–672; Tierney et al, 2006, p. 1682)*

95. **(B)** The patient's symptoms are consistent with long-term lithium therapy, which can cause a variety of neuropsychiatric side effects (e.g., tremor, ataxia, mental confusion, fatigue, poor concentration). Lithium is also known to produce adverse effects on the kidneys that can lead to nephrogenic diabetes insipidus and increased serum creatinine concentrations. *(DiPiro et al, 2005, pp. 1277–1278; Tierney et al, 2006, pp. 1076–1077)*

96. **(C)** Cough and angioedema are believed to be bradykinin-mediated effects. ACEIs not only inhibit angiotensin converting enzyme, but they also block the activity of kininase II, which is the enzyme responsible for degrading bradykinin. Hence, with ACEI use, bradykinin levels rise. ARBs possess an entirely different mechanism of action, as they do not inhibit either kininase II or ACE, but instead are receptor antagonists. *(DiPiro et al, 2005, pp. 205–207; Ganong, 2003, p. 603)*

97. **(B)** Dexfenfluramine was pulled from the market in 1997 after reports linking it with cardiac valve damage and pulmonary hypertension. Sibutramine inhibits the neuronal reuptake of serotonin and norepinephrine, which is thought to be related to appetite suppression. Phentermine and benzphetamine are both sympathomimetics that have also been linked to appetite suppression. Orlistat is the only medication that works in the GI tract, as it blocks the absorption of fat. This leads to increased fat content of the stool, which can cause a variety of side effects, including flatulence, bloating, abdominal pain, fecal urgency, and incontinence. *(DiPiro et al, 2005, pp. 2667–2670; Tierney et al, 2006, p. 1269)*

98. **(B)** The pathogenesis of Reye's syndrome is unknown, but there appears to be a potential association between aspirin use and the development of the disease. Reye's syndrome is marked by hepatic failure and encephalopathy and has a poor prognosis. *(DiPiro et al, 2005, pp. 1946; Tierney et al, 2006, p. 1383)*

99. **(C)** Both nitrates and calcium channel blockers have been shown to be effective in variant angina, which is characterized by coronary artery spasm. β-blockers are not recommended due to their potential to cause coronary artery vasoconstriction, which would exacerbate the condition. *(DiPiro et al, 2005, pp. 284–285; Tierney et al, 2006, p. 347)*

100. **(D)** Regular insulin is a short-acting insulin that starts working 30 to 60 minutes after administration. Increasing the dose by a few units can help quickly restore a normoglycemic state. NPH is an intermediate-acting insulin, which has an onset of action of 2 to 4 hours. Therefore, adjusting the NPH dose at breakfast time will not correct the morning hyperglycemia. If the NPH dose was increased, it could cause him to experience hypoglycemia in the middle of the day once it starts to work. *(DiPiro et al, 2005, pp. 1345–1346)*

REFERENCES

American Diabetes Association: Standards of Medical Care in Diabetes 2006. *Diabetes Care.* January 2006; 29 (Supplement 1; pp. S4–S42).

Blomström-Lundqvist C, Scheinman MM, Aliot EM, Alpert JS, Calkins H, Camm AJ, Campbell WB, Haines DE, Kuck KH, Lerman BB, Miller DD, Shaeffer CW, Stevenson WG, Tomaselli GF. ACC/AHA/ESC guidelines for the management of patients with supraventricular arrhythmias—executive summary: A report of the American College of Cardiology/American Heart Association Task Force on Practice Guidelines, and the European Society of Cardiology Committee for Practice Guidelines (Writing Committee to Develop Guidelines for the Management of Patients With Supraventricular Arrhythmias.). *J Am Coll Cardiol.* 2003; 42:1493–1531.

Chobania AV, Bakris GL, Black HR, Cushman WC, Green LA, Izzo JL, Jr., Jones SW, Materson BJ, Oparil S, Wright JT Jr., Roccella EJ. The Seventh Report of the Joint National Committee on Prevention, Detection, Evaluation, and Treatment of High Blood Pressure: The JNC 7 Report. *JAMA*. 2003; 289:2560–2571.

DiPiro JT, Talbert RL, Yee GC, Matzke GR, Wells BG, Posey LM (eds), *Pharmacotherapy: A Pathophysiologic Approach, 6th ed.* New York: McGraw-Hill; 2005.

Ganong WF. *Review of Medical Physiology*, 21st ed. New York: Lange Medical Books/McGraw-Hill; 2003.

Gibbons RJ, Abrams J, Chatterjee K, Daley J, Deedwania PC, Douglas JS, Ferguson TB Jr., Fihn SD, Fraker TD Jr., Gardin JM, O'Rourke RA, Pasternak RC, Williams SV. ACC/AHA 2002 Guideline Update for the Management of Patients with Chronic Stable Angina: A Report of the American College of Cardiology/American Heart Association Task Force on Practice Guidelines (Committee to Update the 1999 Guidelines for the Management of Patients with Chronic Stable Angina). 2002. Available at: www.acc.org/clinical/guidelines/stable/stable.pdf.

Grundy SM, Cleeman JI, Merz CNB, Brewer HB, Clark LT, Jr., Hunninghake DB, Pasternak RC, Smith SC, Stone NJ, Jr., for the Coordinating Committee of the National Cholesterol Education Program. Implications of recent clinical trials for the National Cholesterol Education Program Adult Treatment Panel III Guidelines. *Circulation*, 2004; 110:227–239.

Katzung BG (ed), *Basic & Clinical Pharmacology*, 9th ed. New York: Lange Medical Books/McGraw-Hill; 2004.

Liver Function Test Scheduling. *Pharmacist's Letter/Prescriber's Letter*, 2005; 21(12):211210.

National Heart, Lung and Blood Institute, National Asthma Education and Prevention Program. *Expert Panel Report 2. Guidelines for the Diagnosis and Management of Asthma. NIH Publication No. 97-4051. Bethesda, MD, US Department of Health and Human Services, 1997.* Available at http://www.nhlbi.nih.gov/guidelines/asthma/asthgdln.pdf.

Obenrader J. Equianalgesic dosing of opioids for pain management. *Pharmacist's Letter/Prescriber's Letter*, 2004; 20 (200915).

O'Mara NB. Guidelines for the treatment of otitis media. *Pharmacist's Letter/Prescriber's Letter*, 2004; 20 (200505).

Scott GN. Omega-3 fatty acids. *Pharmacist's Letter/Prescriber's Letter*, 2005; 21 (210709).

Tierney LM, Jr., McPhee SJ, Papadakis MA (eds), *Current Medical Diagnosis & Treatment 2005*, 44th ed. New York: Lange Medical Books/McGraw-Hill; 2005.

Woelfel JA. Drug-induced long QT interval and sudden cardiac death. *Pharmacist's Letter/Prescriber's Letter*, 2004; 20 (201111).

Psychiatry

Questions

Michelle Heinan, EdD, PAC

DIRECTIONS (Questions 1 through 70): Each of the numbered items or incomplete statements in this section is followed by answers or by completions of the statement. Select the ONE lettered answer or completion that is BEST in each case.

Questions 1 through 70

1. The histrionic personality would be listed in what cluster?

   (A) Cluster A
   (B) Cluster B
   (C) Cluster C
   (D) Cluster D
   (E) Cluster E

2. Which complication can be found in anorexia nervosa and not bulimia?

   (A) salivary gland hypertrophy
   (B) reversible cerebral atrophy
   (C) petechial hemorrhages
   (D) hypokalemia
   (E) osteoporosis

3. What is another name for multiple personalities?

   (A) dissociative amnesia
   (B) dissociative fugue
   (C) depersonalization
   (D) dissociative disorder not otherwise specified
   (E) dissociative identity disorder

4. The diagnostic criteria for anorexia nervosa include

   (A) less than 85% of normal weight for their height
   (B) patient feels lack of control over eating
   (C) use of inappropriate compensatory behaviors
   (D) two binge episodes a week for 3 months
   (E) patient is concerned about weight and shape of their body

5. Which of the following medications interact to decrease lithium levels?

   (A) indomethacin
   (B) potassium sparing diuretics
   (C) theophylline
   (D) valproic acid
   (E) COX-2 inhibitors

6. What disorder may have an abnormal dexamethasone suppression test?

   (A) personality disorder
   (B) anxiety disorder
   (C) dissociative disorder
   (D) adjustment disorder
   (E) mood disorder

7. What personality type may have "slow" activity seen on EEG?

   (A) avoidant personality
   (B) paranoid personality
   (C) histrionic personality
   (D) schizoid personality
   (E) borderline personality

8. A patient presented to your office with multiple somatic complaints. During the mental status exam you notice that the patient loses the thread of conversation and discusses irrelevant topics based on an external stimuli. The patient never gets back to the main point he or she was trying to express. What is this thought process called?

   (A) tangentiality
   (B) circumstantiality
   (C) looseness of association
   (D) word salad
   (E) neologisms

9. Which of the following personality disorders is listed in Cluster C?

   (A) avoidant
   (B) antisocial
   (C) borderline
   (D) schizoid
   (E) paranoid

10. Treatment for a paranoid personality disorder would include

   (A) confirm paranoid beliefs
   (B) challenging paranoid ideas
   (C) confrontation of delusions
   (D) do not empathize with patient
   (E) outline a treatment plan in detail

11. Which of the following lab results would be found in a patient with anorexia nervosa?

   (A) elevated T3
   (B) elevated LH and FSH
   (C) elevated cholesterol
   (D) decreased transaminases
   (E) leukopenia

12. Mr. Smith leaves home and does not return, nor does he go to work. A friend of Mr. Smith's sees him in another state while on vacation. When he approaches Mr. Smith, he does not recognize him and has a total different demeanor. What type of disorder does Mr. Smith have?

   (A) amnesia
   (B) fugue
   (C) schizophrenia
   (D) dissociative identity disorder
   (E) depersonalization

13. What type of disorder develops within 3 months of an identified stressor such as finances, going to school, divorce, or illness in their life. The stressor causes impairment in their job and relationships, but the symptoms resolve within 6 months. What is the most likely diagnosis?

   (A) depression
   (B) bereavement
   (C) posttraumatic stress disorder
   (D) personality disorder
   (E) adjustment disorder

14. *DSM IV* classifies disorders into five axes. What type of information should be provided on Axis IV?

   (A) global assessment
   (B) clinical disorders
   (C) medical conditions
   (D) psychosocial stressors
   (E) personality disorders

15. Which medication should be prescribed for generalized anxiety in a patient who has a history of alcohol dependence?

   (A) lorazepam
   (B) paroxetine
   (C) venlafaxine
   (D) buspirone
   (E) sertraline

16. Personality disorders would be listed on which axis?

    (A) Axis I
    (B) Axis II
    (C) Axis III
    (D) Axis IV
    (E) Axis V

17. Generally, patients who are malingering

    (A) use illness to attain a goal
    (B) are perfectionists
    (C) are workaholics
    (D) have a history that agrees with their physical symptoms
    (E) will demonstrate function only when being observed

18. Which of the following statements is true regarding the avoidant personality disorder?

    (A) symptoms do not improve in time
    (B) symptoms of anxiety do not need to be treated
    (C) can use beta-blockers
    (D) they seek interpersonal contact
    (E) will stay in treatment

19. Which of the following criteria is considered to be a high risk factor for "successful" suicide?

    (A) people who live in climates with limited amount of sun
    (B) lower socioeconomic status
    (C) female
    (D) committed religious beliefs
    (E) divorced

20. A patient that has depressive symptoms on more days than not for greater than 2 years would be diagnosed as

    (A) major depressive disorder
    (B) psychotic
    (C) bipolar
    (D) dysthymic
    (E) situational depression

21. Performing a mental status exam will assist in showing how the patient's brain is currently processing. Upon completion of the exam, the one process that CANNOT be determined is

    (A) thought disorders
    (B) affect
    (C) intelligence quotient
    (D) cognition and memory
    (E) insight and judgment

22. A patient presents to your office claiming that the FBI is trying to poison him. These types of beliefs would be onsidered to be a(n)

    (A) somatic delusion
    (B) delusion of persecution
    (C) illusion
    (D) delusion of grandeur
    (E) hallucination

23. What question does the "C" represent in the alcohol abuse screening tool CAGE?

    (A) Have you ever felt the need to *cut down*?
    (B) Has anyone ever *cautioned* you not to drink?
    (C) Have you been *caught* having an "eye opener" in the morning?
    (D) Has anyone ever *criticized* you about your drinking?
    (E) Do you *care* that you are feeling guilty about drinking?

24. A phobia is an excessive fear of an object or place that leads to or can be preceded by

    (A) panic attack
    (B) depression
    (C) hallucinations
    (D) delusions
    (E) confabulations

25. Comorbidity for this personality disorder includes ADHD, paraphilias, somatization disorder, and pathological gambling. Learning disabilities are also associated. What is the most likely diagnosis?

(A) borderline

(B) antisocial

(C) narcissistic

(D) avoidant

(E) histrionic

26. Which one of the following disorders would NOT be included in the differential diagnosis for dissociative identity disorder?

(A) schizophrenia

(B) complex partial seizures

(C) rapid cycling bipolar disorders

(D) malingering

(E) obsessive compulsive personality disorder

27. The hallmark of a manic episode is

(A) hypersomnolence

(B) psychosis

(C) depression

(D) anxiety

(E) euphoria or irritability

28. Ms. Smith is diagnosed with an anxiety disorder. Based on the history gathered from the patient, you decide to treat her with phenelzine 15 mg one tablet twice a day to start. Which of the following side effects is considered common for this medication?

(A) dizziness

(B) urinary retention

(C) sexual dysfunction

(D) weight gain

(E) blurred vision

29. What type of pharmacological agent would be used as a first-line medication to treat obsessive compulsive disorder?

(A) risperidone

(B) lonazepam

(C) fluoxetine

(D) trazadone

(E) venlafaxine

30. Ms. Jones wakes up from a deep sleep after having a nightmare. The nightmare caused her to reexperience the time she received third degree burns on her arms. The next day at work, she was very jumpy and had difficulty concentrating. What diagnosis would be given to Ms. Jones?

(A) adjustment disorder

(B) posttraumatic stress disorder

(C) personality disorder

(D) anxiety

(E) schizophrenia

31. ECT is effective in several conditions. What condition would NOT be appropriate for treatment with ECT?

(A) severe depression

(B) manic disorders

(C) psychosis during pregnancy

(D) obsessive compulsive disorder

(E) depression unresponsive to medication

32. A patient who is intoxicated presents to the emergency department. On ocular exam, you notice mydriasis. Which one of the following substances could he have been using?

(A) sedatives

(B) ETOH

(C) opiods

(D) cocaine

(E) PCP

33. Which one of the following symptoms is related to delirium tremens?

(A) hypersomnolence

(B) normal temperature

(C) bradycardia

(D) hypotension

(E) perceptual distortions

34. A student is told that he failed a course in school and forgets that he has been given this information. The defense mechanism utilized by this student is

(A) sublimation
(B) reaction formation
(C) displacement
(D) repression
(E) denial

35. Which of the following statements is true regarding vascular dementia?

(A) occurs more frequently in females
(B) those patients with a stroke are at increased risk
(C) chronic onset
(D) the patient has a normal funduscopic exam
(E) the cardiac chambers are normal size

36. Which of the following personality disorders can become less intense with age?

(A) dependent
(B) borderline
(C) antisocial
(D) avoidant
(E) obsessive compulsive

37. Mr. Johnson comes to the clinic today. Based on the history, you suspect he is the victim of domestic violence occurring in the home. Which of the following would not be an indicator for domestic violence?

(A) bruises at different stages of healing
(B) delay in treatment for an injury
(C) eye contact with provider
(D) inconsistent explanation for injuries
(E) repeated office visits for nonspecific complaints

38. A misinterpretation of an external stimulus is

(A) delusions
(B) hallucinations
(C) illusions
(D) neologisms
(E) tactile hallucinations

39. ECT postprocedural hypertension can be treated. Which one of the following pharmacological agents is contraindicated for this treatment?

(A) angiotensin-converting enzyme inhibitors
(B) nicardipine
(C) IV nitroglycerin
(D) clonidine
(E) beta-blockers

40. Which personality disorder is characterized by eccentricities, social isolation, "magical thinking," and suspiciousness?

(A) avoidant
(B) antisocial
(C) borderline
(D) schizoid
(E) schizotypal

41. Which of the following diseases is known for "plaques and tangles"?

(A) Parkinson's disease
(B) vascular dementia
(C) Huntington's chorea
(D) Alzheimer's disease
(E) ALS

42. You are asked to see a patient that was admitted to the hospital. Upon attempts to obtain a history, you notice the patient states words that sound similar, but do not have the same meaning. He also does some rhyming of his words. What type of thought process would this be?

(A) flight of ideas
(B) circumstantiality
(C) looseness of association
(D) word salad
(E) clanging

43. Which one of the following antidepressants has the longest half-life?

(A) amoxapine
(B) clomipramine
(C) fluoxetine
(D) protriptyline
(E) paroxetine

44. A patient presents to the emergency room with alcohol withdrawal syndrome. What is the pharmacological agent of choice to be administered?

   (A) clonidine
   (B) phenobarbital
   (C) neuroleptics
   (D) benzodiazepines
   (E) methadone

45. Which of the following agents does not cause erectile disorders?

   (A) desipramine
   (B) amitriptyline
   (C) digoxin
   (D) trazodone
   (E) HCTZ

46. A 56-year-old man presents to your office stating he has no desire to have sex. He has recently gotten back into dating after being divorced for 10 years and is being pressured by his current girlfriend. The gentleman states he has no desire to be with his girlfriend or any other person. What would be the most likely diagnosis?

   (A) sexual aversion disorder
   (B) hypoactive sexual desire
   (C) hyperactive sexual desire
   (D) erectile disorder
   (E) sexual arousal disorder

47. A 60-year-old woman states that she has difficulty maintaining sexual excitement when being intimate with her husband. She states she is not able to attain enough lubrication to enjoy the sexual encounter. What is the most likely diagnosis?

   (A) hypoactive sexual disorder
   (B) sexual aversion disorder
   (C) hyperactive sexual disorder
   (D) sexual arousal disorder
   (E) vaginismus

48. Women most commonly commit suicide by what method?

   (A) overdose
   (B) jumping
   (C) hanging
   (D) firearms
   (E) slashing wrists

49. Suicide victims have associated stressors depending on their age. The most common stressor of suicide victims over the age of 30 is

   (A) separation
   (B) illness
   (C) rejection
   (D) unemployment
   (E) legal problems

50. A 19-year-old female college student is brought to the emergency room by emergency medical service. The paramedics were called to a frat house when the patient was found passed out on the floor. People at the party stated they had seen her take some pills, but were not sure what they were. After taking the pills, the patient became confused, depressed, and paranoid. She also became chilled, dizzy, and nauseated. Which street drug do you suspect she has taken?

   (A) ketamine (special K)
   (B) PCP
   (C) GHB (gamma hydroxybutyrate)
   (D) MDMA (ecstasy)
   (E) Rohypnol

51. A mother brings her 5-year-old child to the hospital after the child collapses at home. The mother states the child has been having diarrhea for the last 3 days. She has tried to get him to drink fluids. Upon further questioning, the mother states the child has had 12 loose stools a day for the last 3 days. Examination reveals the child to be responsive, but lethargic and dehydrated. The child is admitted to the hospital and mom is very involved in the child's care. While mom is there, the child is improving slightly, but still having multiple loose stools. When the mother had to

leave to go to work, the child responded well to treatment without any further episodes of diarrhea. What is the most likely diagnosis?

- (A) Munchausen syndrome
- (B) schizophrenia
- (C) malingering
- (D) Munchausen by proxy
- (E) factitious disorder

52. Which of the following signs/symptoms is NOT found in toxic psychosis?
- (A) cerebellar signs
- (B) excessive salivation
- (C) increased deep tendon reflexes
- (D) dilated pupils
- (E) muscle twitching

53. QT interval delay may occur in which antipsychotic medication's?
- (A) Risperidone
- (B) Olanzapine
- (C) Ziprasidone
- (D) Quetrapine
- (E) aripiprazole

54. Which of the following statements is INCORRECT related to the treatment of bipolar disorder?
- (A) start lithium and have levels checked frequently
- (B) start psychotherapy
- (C) add an antipsychotic medication
- (D) continue drug therapy for 2 to 4 months
- (E) hospitalize if the patient is in full manic state

55. What type of schizophrenia is characterized by self-injury, harm to others, mutism, or rigidity?
- (A) paranoid
- (B) undifferentiated
- (C) disorganized
- (D) catatonic
- (E) schizophreniform

56. Which disorder is characterized by episodes of hypomania and depression for greater than 2 years?
- (A) dysthmia
- (B) major depressive disorder
- (C) cyclothymia
- (D) bipolar
- (E) mood disorder

57. Which of the following disorders is NOT treated with an SSRI?
- (A) posttraumatic stress disorder
- (B) anorexia
- (C) panic attacks
- (D) general anxiety disorder
- (E) obsessive compulsive disorder

58. A 32-year-old male presents to your office with the complaint of low back pain for 7 months. The patient states he was initially injured on the job while trying to lift a 50-poundbarrel off a truck. He denies any paresthesias or bowel/bladder problems associated with the low back pain. The patient states that he had been given NSAIDs and a muscle relaxer, followed by physical therapy treatments. X-rays that were taken 5 months ago were reported as normal. He was placed on light duty at that time. The patient has seen many practitioners who have "not helped him." Another person who works with this patient was at the clinic and stated the patient has had problems with one of his other coworkers. You consider trying the patient on an antidepressant first and then possibly sending him to a pain clinic if no success. What is the most likely diagnosis?
- (A) somatoform disorder
- (B) hypochondriasis
- (C) drug addiction
- (D) somatoform pain disorder
- (E) schizophreniform

59. Which of the following problems would NOT be considered in a differential diagnosis for schizophrenia-like behavior?

    (A) panic attacks
    (B) autistic disorder
    (C) normal adolescence
    (D) borderline personality disorder
    (E) obsessive compulsive disorder

60. What type of finding would be necessary to determine if a child has shaken baby syndrome versus a viral illness?

    (A) poor feeding
    (B) lethargy
    (C) retinal hemorrhages
    (D) irritability
    (E) vomiting

61. A child who has oppositional defiant disorder is at high risk for developing which disorder?

    (A) mood disorder
    (B) personality disorder
    (C) conduct disorder
    (D) ADHD
    (E) developmental disorder

62. A 24-year-old female comes to your office complaining of anxiety. The patient had witnessed a traumatic event 3 days earlier that made her feel fearful. She has not been able to tell her family about this experience. She now feels like she is numb and in a dazed, dreamlike state with poor concentration, and difficulty sleeping. She experienced a flashback of the event yesterday. What is the most likely diagnosis?

    (A) posttraumatic stress disorder
    (B) dissociative fugue
    (C) psychosis
    (D) acute stress disorder
    (E) depersonalization

63. Sensorium on mental status exam would include

    (A) judgment
    (B) insight
    (C) thought
    (D) concrete thinking
    (E) concentration

64. Which of the following symptoms would be found in amphetamine withdrawal?

    (A) fatigue
    (B) arrhythmias
    (C) confusion
    (D) seizure
    (E) tension

65. Sleepwalking disorders occur during what part of the night?

    (A) first one-third
    (B) second half
    (C) second one-third
    (D) last third
    (E) first half

66. Several complications can occur from shift workers sleep disorder. Which one of the following is NOT a complication of this disorder?

    (A) low morale
    (B) cardiovascular symptoms
    (C) gastrointestinal problems
    (D) decreased alcohol abuse
    (E) increased absenteeism

67. Severely impaired comprehension associated with a nonsensical speech is called

    (A) bradylalia
    (B) aculalia
    (C) dysprosody
    (D) dysarthria
    (E) cluttering

68. Orthostatic hypotension is most frequently found in the use of

    (A) quetiapine
    (B) clozapine
    (C) risperidone
    (D) olanzapine
    (E) ziprasidone

69. A 4-month-old is brought to your office by his mother due to failure to thrive. The child was eating fine until a month ago when he started regurgitating the food. What is the most likely diagnosis?

(A) pica

(B) rumination

(C) general medical condition

(D) oppositional defiant disorder

(E) mental retardation

70. Which one of the following are criteria used to diagnose depression in geriatric patients?

(A) increased concentration

(B) increased energy

(C) decreased guilt

(D) increased interested

(E) suicidal ideation

Answers and Explanations

1. **(B)** Histrionic personality disorder is listed under Cluster B characterized by their emotional behavior. The behavior is very dramatic and erratic. Cluster B also includes the antisocial, narcissistic, and borderline personality disorders. (*Toy and Klamen, 2004, p. 88*)

2. **(E)** Osteoporosis is found in anorexia nervosa due to a lack of calcium intake, decreased estrogen, and increase in cortisol. Bulimia nervosa has multiple medical complications in the cardiovascular, dental, dermatologic, endocrine, gastrointestinal, and neurologic systems. There are also associated dehydration and electrolyte disorders. Salivary gland hypertrophy, reversible cerebral atrophy, petechial hemorrhages, and hypokalemia are all part of the complications. (*Ebert et al., 2000, pp. 424, 428*)

3. **(E)** Dissociative identity disorder is also called multiple personality disorder. There are usually at least two personalities both distinct in their own rights. The dominant personality at the time determines the behavior and attitudes. (*Sadock and Sadock, 2002, p. 680*)

4. **(A)** Diagnostic criteria for anorexia nervosa include a weight loss to 85% of the required body weight. Both anorexia and bulimia patients are concerned about their body image, but bulimics feel a lack of control over eating with episodes of binge eating. (*Labus, 2004, p. 791*)

5. **(D)** Valproic acid decreases lithium levels when taken concurrently. The other medica-tions listed increase lithium levels. (*Tierney et al, 2005, p. 1046*)

6. **(A)** Diagnosis of personality disorder should be made on patient history. However, in some cases an abnormal dexamethasone suppression test can be found in people with personality disorders. (*Labus, 2004, p. 806*)

7. **(E)** EEG changes may be seen in borderline or antisocial personalities. Diagnosis should be made based on history. (*Labus, 2004, p. 807*)

8. **(A)** Tangentiality is a disturbance in thought causing the person to start a train of thought, but never getting to the point. Circumstantiality is seen in someone who eventually gets to the point after a delay in the thought process. Word salad is a mixture of words and phrases that are incoherent. Looseness of association is when the ideas shift between subjects that are totally unrelated to each other. Neologisms are the creation of new words. (*Sadock and Sadock, 2002, p. 283*)

9. **(A)** Avoidant personality disorder is listed under Cluster C characterized by an anxious behavior. Obsessive compulsive and dependent personality disorders are also listed in this cluster. (*Toy and Klamen, 2004, p. 88*)

10. **(E)** Treating paranoid personality disorders can be litigious. It is important to document everything and outline the treatment plan to the patient in detail. The practitioner needs to

avoid challenging ideas of paranoia, be supportive, avoid confronting delusions, let the patient have as much control over treatment as possible, medicate with low-dose neuroleptics, and initiate assertiveness training. (*Moser, 2001*)

11. **(E)** Anorexics may show decreased levels of T3, LH, and FSH. Elevated levels can be found in growth hormone, plasma cortisol, transaminases, and serum cholesterol. Leukopenia may be present. EKG changes reveal a sinus bradycardia and arrhythmias. (*Labus, 2004, p. 794*)

12. **(B)** Dissociative or psychogenic fugue is precipitated by a stressful event that causes the patient to develop amnesia, leave home, and assume another identity. (*Labus, 2004, p. 815*)

13. **(E)** A response to a stressor that disturbs the mood of the patient causes impairment in function. The symptoms occur within 3 months of the stressor and last no longer than 6 months. Anxiety, depression, or combination is associated with adjustment disorders. (*Labus, 2004, p. 779*)

14. **(D)** The *Diagnostic and Statistical Manual* (*DSM*) is a classification system developed by the American Psychiatric Association. Each axis provides different types of information in order to assist providers in improving their treatment of patients and for coding purposes. Axis IV lists the psychosocial and environmental stressors in a person's life. These stressors may be positive or negative related to occupation, housing, education, economic, or support problems. This axis also includes difficulty accessing health-care services. (*Sadock and Sadock, 2002, p. 290*)

15. **(D)** Buspirone is recommended in treating generalized anxiety disorders in a patient who has a history of drug or alcohol dependence because of its nonaddictive nature. (*Labus, 2004, p. 785*)

16. **(B)** Personality disorders and mental retardation are listed on Axis II. (*Sadock and Sadock, 2002, p. 290*)

17. **(A)** Patients who are malingerers do not want to improve until their goal is met. Goals may be financial, occupational, or legal. These patients will act differently when they think they are not being observed. (*Ebert et al, 2000, p. 384*)

18. **(C)** Avoidant personality disorders will avoid some medical treatments and interpersonal contact because they fear embarrassment or are not willing to take risks. Symptoms will resolve in time. Any anxiety or depression associated with avoidant personality disorders should be treated. (*Moser, 2001*)

19. **(C)** Risk factors for successful suicide include being male, prior suicide attempts, depression, unemployment, being single, divorced, or widowed, alcoholism, or older than 45 years. (*Feibusch et al, 2002, p. 382*) Older than 45 year of age for men and over 55 years of age for women are risk factors. (*Sadock and Sadock, 2002, p. 914*)

20. **(D)** Dysthymic disorder is characterized as depressive symptoms lasting more than 2 years. Men and women are equally as likely to get dysthymia. The patient should have two associated symptoms of depression such as lack of concentration, hopelessness, low self-esteem, changes in appetite, and changes in sleep patterns. (*Feibusch et al, 2002, pp. 384–385*)

21. **(C)** The mental status exam is able to evaluate appearance, affect, mood, speech, activity, and behavior, thought processes, cognition, fund of knowledge, judgment, content of thought, and insight. You can obtain a basic knowledge of the level of intelligence based on information provided by the patients and their behavior. Intelligence quotient is measured through IQ tests. (*Tierney et al, 2005, p. 1008; Lange, p. 99*)

22. **(B)** Patients who have delusions of persecution often feel that people are taking pictures and tape recording them. Patients often believe that external agencies or relatives are attempting to harm them. (*Ebert et al, 2000, p. 108*)

23. **(A)** The screening test of alcohol abuse is called CAGE. The four questions to ask for the screening test are "Have you ever felt the need to cut down on drinking?" "Have you ever felt annoyed by criticism of your drinking?" "Have you ever felt guilty about your drinking?" and "Have you ever taken a morning eye opener?" If a patient responds yes to two of the questions, it is considered to be positive for abuse. (*Tierney et al, 2005, p. 18*)

24. **(A)** Patients who have a phobia realize it is an irrational fear and try to avoid whatever they have the fear of. In attempts to avoid the "problem," patients can develop anxiety or panic attacks. (*Sadock and Sadock, 2002, p. 609; Ebert et al., 2000, p. 109*)

25. **(B)** Antisocial personality disorder is associated with ADHD, pathological gambling, somatization disorder, paraphilias, and learning disabilities. The patient may also meet the criteria for other personality disorders. (*Moser, 2001*)

26. **(E)** Schizophrenia would be a possible differential diagnosis for multiple personality dissociative identity disorder because of the delusions found in schizophrenics. Schizophrenics believe they have separate identities. Rapid cycling bipolar disorders are similar, but the dissociative identity disorder has distinctive personalities. Malingerers look for secondary gains and that becomes obvious. Partial complex seizures are also included in the differential. (*Sadock and Sadock, 2002, p. 684*)

27. **(E)** The hallmark of mania is euphoria or irritability. Early in the illness, euphoria is predominant. Later on, euphoria switches to irritability. (*Sadock and Sadock, 2002, p. 553*)

28. **(A)** Phenelzine has common side effects of dizziness, nausea, nervousness, myoclonus, hypertensive reactions, drowsiness, and dry mouth. (*Ebert et al, 2000, p. 333; Sadock and Sadock, 2002, p. 981*).

29. **(C)** Fluvoxamine, paroxetine, and sertraline are all approved for the treatment of obsessive compulsive disorder. Use of an SSRI in combination with behavioral therapy is recommended. (*Sadock and Sadock, 2002, p. 622*)

30. **(B)** Posttraumatic stress disorder is a type of anxiety disorder characterized by reexperiencing a traumatic event. Patients have difficulty concentrating, insomnia, illusions, nightmares about the event, and startle reactions. Treatment needs to begin as soon as possible, though sometimes the symptoms do not occur until quite a while after the initial traumatic event. (*Tierney et al, 2005, p. 1011*)

31. **(D)** ECT is used for treating severe depression or when patients do not respond to medication for depression, manic disorder, chronic schizophrenia, and psychoses during pregnancy, but not obsessive compulsive disorder. To achieve a quick response to relieve depressive symptoms, ECT can also be used. (*Tierney et al, 2005, p. 1043; Tess and Smetana, 2005*)

32. **(D)** Patients intoxicated with cocaine present with mydriasis. In opiod intoxication, the pupils are constricted. (*Ebert et al, 2000, p. 246*)

33. **(E)** Fever, tremor, tachycardia, perceptual distortions, diaphoresis, perceptual distortions consisting of visual or tactile hallucinations, hypertension, as well as changes in the psychomotor activity levels are all symptoms of delirium tremens. (*Sadock and Sadock, 2002, p. 405*)

34. **(E)** The person denies reality from an external source so that it never existed or happened. Denial is a defense mechanism that can be benign or pathological. (*Sadock and Sadock, 2002, p. 207*)

35. **(B)** Vascular dementia is an abrupt onset in comparison to Alzheimer's, which is slower in onset. Vascular dementia can be prevented by reduction of risk factors such as hypertension and diabetes. The disease typically occurs in males. Carotid bruits, cardiac chamber enlargement, and abnormalities on funduscopic exam may be found. (*Gabbard, 2001; Sadock and Sadock, 2002, p. 333*)

36. **(B)** Borderline personality disorder has been found to become less intense after the age of

35. However, this is not the case for all borderline personality disorders. People with this disorder tend to undermine themselves just before reaching a goal. (*Moser, 2001*)

37. **(C)** Signs and symptoms of domestic violence can include delay in treatment of an injury or denying the seriousness of the injury, joint pains, bruises, or broken bones that are at various stages of healing; repeated office visits for nonspecific complaints; or inconsistent explanations for injuries. There is lack of eye contact with the provider. Patients will turn their eyes downward due to fear of making eye contact. (*Kirk et al, 2003, p. 193; American College of Physicians, 2005*)

38. **(C)** Illusions are associated with external stimuli whereas hallucinations are not. Delusions are beliefs that are false based on wrong inference by the patient about what is happening in reality. (*Sadock and Sadock, 2002, p. 285*)

39. **(A)** Persistent or severe tachycardia with hypertension may occur postprocedurally. Short-acting beta-blockers can all be used to treat ECT postprocedure hypertension. (*Tess and Smetana, 2005*)

40. **(E)** Schizotypal personality disorder is male dominated and may be genetically related to schizophrenia. Patients who are schizotypal are eccentric in their behavior. They have "magical thinking," cognitive/perceptual distortions, and peculiar behavior. (*Moser, 2001*)

41. **(D)** Neurofibrillary tangles are found in Alzheimer's disease. The tangles occur in the hippocampus, cortex, locus ceruleus, and substantia nigra. Plaques, commonly referred to as senile or amyloid plaques, are also found in Alzheimer's disease. (*Tierney et al, 2005, pp. 331–332*)

42. **(E)** Clanging is a disturbance in thought in which the person selects words that are similar by sound, but do not mean the same. Sometimes the person will rhyme the words. Flight of ideas is rapid transitioning between subjects, but tend to be connected.

Looseness of association is when a person changes subjects, but there is no connection between the subjects. Circumstantiality is where the person has a point and eventually gets to that point, but with delay in the thought process. Word salad is a mixture of words that have no sense. (*Sadock and Sadock, 2002, p. 283*)

43. **(D)** Protriptyline has the longest half-life at 126 hours. Clomipramine has 54 to 77 hours, and fluoxetine 24 to 72 hours. (*Lange, p. 302*)

44. **(D)** Benzodiazepines are the first line of treatment for alcohol withdrawal. Dosage should start out high and titrate downward as the patient improves. Carbamazepine has also been found to be beneficial in the treatment of alcohol withdrawal in place of the benzodiazepines. (*Sadock and Sadock, 2002, p. 404; Lange, p. 253*)

45. **(D)** Trazodone does not impair erection or ejaculation. Desipramine and amitriptyline impair both erection and ejaculation. Digoxin and HCTZ only impair erection. (*Sadock and Sadock, 2002, p. 708*)

46. **(B)** Hypoactive sexual disorder can occur in both men and women and is a loss of desire for sexual activity. The clinician must take into consideration the patient's life stressors, medical condition, age, and desire for sexual activity prior to this event. (*Sadock and Sadock, 2002, p. 702*)

47. **(D)** Both males and females can have sexual arousal disorder. It is manifested in females by lack of adequate lubrication maintained or attained during sexual excitement. The male counterpart would be erectile dysfunction. (*Sadock and Sadock, 2002, p. 703*)

48. **(A)** Women frequently select overdose for committing suicide. The trend is now changing where women are using firearms instead. Men typically use firearms or hanging. Women attempt suicide more frequently than men, whereas men are more successful at completed suicides. (*Moser, 2001*)

49. **(B)** Stressors associated with suicide over the age of 30 typically are related to illness. Stressors for those under the age of 30 usually are related to unemployment, legal problems, separation, and rejection. (*Sadock and Sadock, 2002, p. 915*)

50. **(D)** Club drugs consist of MDMA, Rohypnol, GHB, and ketamine. MDMA is ecstasy and has both hallucinogenic and stimulant properties. People who ingest the drug while in areas that are confined can develop severe hyperthermia, dehydration, possible fibrillation, brain damage, and death. Rohypnol is the "date rape" drug. GHB has anabolic, euphoric, and sedative properties. This drug is called "liquid ecstasy." Ketamine has also been used as a date rape drug. It can be mixed into drinks, injected, or snorted. Another name for ketamine is special K. (*Kirk et al, 2003, pp. 162–163*)

51. **(D)** Munchausen by proxy is when a parent, usually the mother, exaggerates, induces, or creates an illness in their child. The parent remains very involved in the child's care. The problem seems to originate when the parent is around and disappears if the parent is away from the child for a period of time. (*Tierney et al, 2005, p. 1018; Kirk et al, 2003, p. 252*)

52. **(E)** Phencyclidine may cause a reaction that is difficult to differentiate from psychosis. Toxic psychosis is characterized by cerebellar signs, dilated pupils, excessive salivation, and increased deep tendon reflexes. (*Tierney et al, 2005, p. 1028*)

53. **(C)** Ziprasidone has been found to induce a QT interval delay in some patients. It is important to screen patients for cardiac risk factors. (*Tierney et al, 2005, p. 1030*)

54. **(D)** Treatment of bipolar disorder would include starting lithium, and continuing this medication for 4 to 6 months, checking lithium levels frequently, beginning psychotherapy, adding an antipsychotic medication, and hospitalizing the patient if he or she is in the full manic state. (*Labus, 2004, p. 802*)

55. **(D)** Catatonic schizophrenia is characterized by self-injury or violence to others, mutism, posturing, and other motor symptoms such as rigidity. (*Labus, 2004, p. 812*)

56. **(C)** Cyclothymia is characterized by symptoms of depression and hypomania for at least 2 years. Symptoms are milder than a regular depressive or manic episode. Occasionally patients will have regular depressive or manic symptoms at which time they need to be reclassified as bipolar. (*Tierney et al, 2005, p. 1036*)

57. **(B)** SSRIs have been effective in the treatment of PTSD, panic attacks, obsessive compulsive disorder, generalized anxiety disorder, and bulimia. (*Tierney et al, 2005, p. 1038*)

58. **(D)** Somatoform pain disorder is a focus on pain for greater than 6 months. The subjective findings outweighs the objective findings. Pain in the neck, pelvic, or low back areas are frequent sites, as well as headaches. The disorder may be precipitated by an injury. The patient will have a history of seeing multiple providers and possibly many medical and surgical treatments. The patient is unresponsive to treatment. Stressors can aggravate or precipitate the pain. There may be an expectation of secondary gains. Age of onset is around 30s and 40s. Treatment consists of placing the patient on an antidepressant and sending the patient to a pain clinic. (*Labus, 2004, pp. 815–824*)

59. **(A)** Panic attacks would not be included in the differential diagnosis for schizophrenia-like behavior. Autistic disorder, malingering, normal adolescence, obsessive compulsive disorder, personality disorders such as paranoid, schizotypal, borderline, or schizoid, and factitious disorders would be considered as part of the differential diagnosis. (*Labus, 2004, p. 813*)

60. **(C)** It is sometimes difficult to tell if shaken baby syndrome has occurred or a child is having a viral illness unless identifiable signs of fractures, bruises, retinal hemorrhages, or subdural hemorrhage can be found. (*Kirk et al, 2003, pp. 210–211*)

61. **(C)** Oppositional defiant disorder is a less intense form of conduct disorder. Children who continue with the chronic behavior are at risk of developing conduct disorder. This disorder is most often seen in boys, with problems being worse at school. The behavior can occur at home and with peers. (*Auth and Kerstein, 2005, p. 93*)

62. **(D)** Acute stress disorder is characterized by experiencing or witnessing a traumatic event where the person felt threatened by death or injury or the people they witnessed. The person feels fearful and helpless. Symptoms usually occur within a month of the event, last 2 days, and resolve in a month. The person feels numb, has lack of awareness of surroundings, and sees everything in a dreamlike state. Sometimes they develop amnesia. Flashbacks or recurrent images can occur with acute stress disorder. Difficulty sleeping, poor concentration, anhedonia, irritability and despair are associated with this disorder. If not treated at the early stages, the patient is at risk of developing PTSD. (*Auth and Kerstein, 2005, p. 110*)

63. **(E)** Sensorium includes alertness, orientation, concentration and calculation, memory, fund of knowledge, and abstract thinking. (*Sadock and Sadock, 2002, p. 245*)

64. **(A)** Fatigue is found in amphetamine withdrawal. Arrhythmias, confusion, seizure, and tension are found in amphetamine intoxication. (*Ebert et al, 2000, p. 246*)

65. **(E)** Sleepwalking disorders occur in the first half of the night. Nightmare disorders occur in the last third, sleep terrors in the first third, and REM sleep behavior disorders in the second half of the night. (*Ebert et al, 2000, p. 443*)

66. **(D)** The shift work sleep disorder has symptoms of hypersomnia or insomnia. Complications that can occur are related to high absenteeism, disruption of family and social life, cardiovascular and gastrointestinal disorders, increased alcohol abuse, low morale and low productivity. (*Ebert et al, 2000, p. 445*)

67. **(B)** Aculalia is defined as impaired comprehension and nonsensical speech. Bradylalia is slow speech. Dysprosody is loss of the melody in speech. Dysarthria is difficulty articulating, and cluttering is loss of rhythm in speech—erratic. These are all disorders of speech. (*Sadock and Sadock, 2002, p. 285*)

68. **(A)** All serotonin-dopamine agonists can cause orthostatic hypotension. However, quetiapine is more frequently associated with this symptom. These medications should be used with caution in diabetics, people who have had myocardial infarctions or are taking antihypertensives. Patients with hypotension should also be cautioned. (*Sadock and Sadock, 2002, p. 1108*)

69. **(B)** Rumination is the rechewing or regurgitation of food by an infant or child. The child is usually seen due to failure to thrive. The condition usually starts after normal eating habits have been established which is approximately 3 months of age. The symptoms must be ongoing for at least a month. The problem can be attributed to medical conditions such as hiatal hernia or esophageal reflux. (*Sadock and Sadock, 2002, p. 1242*)

70. **(E)** The mnemonic used for criteria to diagnose depression in the geriatric population is SIGECAPS: S, sleep changes; I, decreased interest; G, excessive guilt; E, decreased energy; C, decreased concentration; A, appetite changes; P, psychomotor agitation or retardation; and S, suicidal ideation. (*Toy and Klamen, 2004, p. 96*)

REFERENCES

American College of Physicians. ACP's PIER: Physicians' Information and Education Resource: Domestic Violence; 2005. Retrieved 30 July 2005, from http://online.statref.com/document.aspx?fxid=50&docid=947

Auth PC, Kerstein MD (eds). *Physician Assistant Review*, 2nd ed. Philadelphia: Lippincott, Williams & Wilkins; 2005.

Ebert MH, Loosen PT, Nurcombe B. *Current Diagnosis and Treatment in Psychiatry*. New York: McGraw-Hill; 2000.

Feibusch KC, Breaden RS, Bader CD, Gomperts SN. *Prescription for the Boards*. Philadelphia: Lippincott, Williams & Wilkins; 2002.

Gabbard GO (ed). *Treatment of Psychiatric Disorders*, 3rd ed. Section 3 Delirium, Dementia, and Amnestic and Other Cognitive Disorders: Vascular Dementia; 2001. Retrieved 1 August 2005, from http://online.statref.com/document.aspx?fxid=7&docid=100.

Kirk HW, Weisbrod JA, Ericson KA. *Psychosocial and Behavioral Aspects of Medicine*. Philadelphia: Lippincott, Williams & Wilkins; 2003.

Labus JB (ed). *The Physician Assistant Medical Handbook*, 2nd ed. Philadelphia: Saunders; 2004.

Moser RL (ed). *Primary Care for Physician Assistants: Clinical Practice Guidelines*, 2nd ed; 2001. Retrieved on 21 July 2005 from http://online.statref.com/document.aspx?fxid=71&docid=738.

Sadock BJ, Sadock, VA. *Synopsis of Psychiatry*, 9th ed. Philadelphia: Lippincott, Williams & Wilkins; 2002.

Tess A, Smetana GW. Medical consultation for electroconvulsive therapy; 2005. Retrieved 20 June 2005 from http://www.uptodate.com.

Tierney LM, McPhee SJ, Papdakis MA (eds). *Current Medical Diagnosis and Treatment*. New York: Lange Medical Books/McGraw-Hill; 2005.

Toy EC, Klamen D (eds). *Case Files: Psychiatry*. New York: McGraw-Hill; 2004.

SECTION VI
Surgery

CHAPTER 13

Emergency Medicine
Questions
Joel W. Bunn, MMS, PA-C

DIRECTIONS (Questions 1 through 35): Each of the numbered items or incomplete statements in this section is followed by answers or by completions of the statement. Select the ONE lettered answer or completion that is BEST in each case.

Questions 1 through 35

1. Which of the following is the most important factor in surviving an out-of-hospital cardiac arrest?

   (A) immediate airway control with intubation
   (B) early defibrillation
   (C) aggressive management of hypotension
   (D) epinephrine usage
   (E) rapid transport to appropriate facility

2. A 27-year-old Rh-negative 14 week gestation patient presents to the emergency department (ED) with vaginal bleeding and passage of "clots," which is consistent with a spontaneous abortion. Which of the following is the most apprpriate dose of RhoGAM?

   (A) 50-ug RhoGAM
   (B) 75-ug RhoGAM
   (C) 100-ug RoGAM
   (D) 300-ug RhoGAM
   (E) 600-ug RhoGAM

3. A 65-year-old ill-appearing female presents to the ED with tachycardia, tachypnea, and an arterial pH of 7.05. In general, what is the most common cause of metabolic acidosis?

   (A) diabetic ketoacidosis (DKA)
   (B) lactic acidosis
   (C) alcoholic ketoacidosis
   (D) nonketotic hyperosmolar acidosis
   (E) aspirin poisoning

4. A 64-year-old female presents to the ED with dyspnea and exertional fatigue. There is a high clinical suspicion for pulmonary embolism. The ventilation quotient (VO) lung scan was read as "low probability" for a pulmonary embolism. Of the following, which would be the most appropriate next step?

   (A) obtain a pulmonary angiogram if the lower extremity ultrasound is negative for deep vein thrombosis (DVT)
   (B) initiate intravenous (IV) heparin without further testing
   (C) send the patient home with instructions to follow-up with her physician tomorrow for further outpatient work-up
   (D) obtain an echocardiogram to assess right atrial pressures
   (E) repeat the VQ lung scan

5. The most reliable clinical assessment tool to confirm endotracheal intubation is

    (A) endotracheal tube condensation
    (B) symmetrical chest expansion
    (C) breath sounds auscultated equally over the chest
    (D) no breath sounds auscultated over the stomach
    (E) use of a carbon dioxide detection device

6. A 76-year-old female (60 kg) with organic brain syndrome presents to the ED with a serum sodium of 180. What is the approximate calculation of water deficit in this hypernatremic patient?

    (A) 4 L
    (B) 6 L
    (C) 8 L
    (D) 11 L
    (E) 14 L

7. A 65-year-old patient with chronic obstructive pulmonary disease (COPD) taking chronic theophylline therapy presents to the ED with palpitations, chest pain, and the feeling that his heart is beating irregularly after starting erythromycin for bronchitis. What is the likely dysrhythmia?

    (A) multifocal atrial tachycardia (MAT)
    (B) atrial fibrillation (AF)
    (C) atrial flutter
    D) sinus bradycardia
    (E) mobitz type II heart block

8. A 58-year-old male with multiple myeloma presents to the ED with altered mental status, hypertension, back pain, and constipation. These findings are suggestive of which of the following medical conditions?

    (A) hyperkalemia
    (B) hypercalcemia
    (C) hypomagnesemia
    (D) hypoglycemia
    (E) hyponatremia

9. The differential diagnoses of a wide anion gap metabolic acidosis include all of the following EXCEPT

    (A) ethanol poisoning
    (B) methanol poisoning
    (C) ketoacidosis
    (D) uremia associated with renal failure
    (E) ethylene glycol poisoning

10. A 16-year-old long-distance runner suffered an external rotation injury to the ankle. Which of the following ligaments is most likely injured?

    (A) anterior talofibular
    (B) posterior talofibular
    (C) deltoid
    (D) calcaneofibular
    (E) tibiofibular

11. A 68-year-old male with a previous medical history of coronary artery disease presents to the ED with a 2-day history of intermittent chest tightness. The pain was not relieved with three nitroglycerin sublingual tablets. What would be the initial assessment if the ECG demonstrated 2 mm ST-segment elevations in leads II, III, and AVF?

    (A) acute anterior wall myocardial infarction
    (B) acute lateral wall myocardial injury
    (C) subendocardial inferior wall myocardial infarction
    (D) subendocardial anterior wall myocardial ischemia
    (E) acute inferior wall myocardial injury

12. All of the following would be considered immediate first-line therapy in a patient with acute coronary ischemia EXCEPT

    (A) oxygen
    (B) aspirin
    (C) glycoprotein IIb/IIIa receptor inhibitors
    (D) nitroglycerin
    (E) morphine

13. A 28-year-old pregnant patient in her third trimester presents with a BP of 164/98. Which of the following medications is the agent of choice in this scenario?

(A) nitroglycerin
(B) magnesium
(C) hydralazine
(D) captopril
(E) hydrochlorothiazide

14. Cardiac enzymes in a patient with a 2-hour history of chest pain secondary to an acute myocardial infarction would commonly demonstrate which of the following findings?

(A) normal creatine kinase (CK-MB) and troponin I
(B) elevated troponin I and normal CK-MB
(C) elevated CK-MB and normal troponin I
(D) normal myoglobin with elevated CK-MB
(E) elevated myoglobin, troponin I, and CK-MB

15. The most specific myocardial injury enzyme marker is

(A) CK-MB
(B) myoglobin
(C) troponin I
(D) troponin T
(E) lactate dehydrogenase (LDH)

16. All of the following are indicators for intravenous thrombolytic therapy in a patient with an acute coronary syndrome EXCEPT

(A) S-T-segment elevation in the inferior wall leads
(B) true posterior wall myocardial infarction
(C) new left bundle branch block
(D) S-T-segment elevation in the anterior/lateral wall
(E) S-T-segment depression

17. A 42-year-old female was brought to the ED from a psychiatric facility for an evaluation following a brief "seizure." The psychiatric staff reports she has been confused and complaining of thirst for the past 5 days. What is the most likely diagnosis?

(A) idiopathic hypoglycemia
(B) psychogenic polydipsia
(C) brain tumor
(D) new-onset epilepsy
(E) psychogenic cerebritis

18. A 44-year-old AIDS patient being treated for pneumocystis carinii pneumonia (PCP) presents to the ED with a relatively acute onset of confusion, pallor, diaphoresis, and tachycardia. What is the most likely cause of the patient's symptoms?

(A) hypoglycemia
(B) meningitis
(C) subarachnoid hemorrhage
(D) hypoxemia
(E) mucous plugging

19. All of the following are ECG findings of hyperkalemia EXCEPT

(A) prolonged Q-T interval
(B) sine wave pattern
(C) flattening P waves
(D) prolonged PR interval
(E) tall peaked T waves

20. A 72-year-old female is brought to the ED after being found on her kitchen floor comatose with a BP of 280/150 and pinpoint reactive pupils. What is the most likely diagnosis?

(A) thalamic hemorrhage
(B) cerebellar hemorrhage
(C) pontine hemorrhage
(D) subarachnoid hemorrhage
(E) intracerebral left occipital hemorrhage

21. A 68-year-old patient presents to the ED with palpitations and dizziness. The ECG demonstrates three or more differently shaped P waves, varying PP, PR, and RR intervals; and atrial rhythm usually between 100 and 180. What is the most likely dysrhymia?

(A) MAT
(B) AF
(C) ventricular tachycardia
(D) sinus dysrhythmia
(E) supraventricular tachycardia

22. A 58-year-old male presents to the ED with palpitations and chest pain. The ECG reveals a narrow complex tachycardia at 180 bpm. Which of the following medications is the agent of choice in this scenario?

(A) amiodarone
(B) lidocaine
(C) adenosine
(D) alprazolam
(E) bretyllium

23. The most immediate management priority in a patient with septic shock is

(A) empiric antimicrobial therapy
(B) inotropic support
(C) oxygenation and ventilation
(D) fluid therapy
(E) acid–base status

24. The antidotal agent for benzodiazepine overdose is

(A) naloxone
(B) Narcan
(C) ketamine
(D) flumazenil
(E) flutamide

25. A patient presented to the ED with a possible foreign body to the hand. Identify the item that would be the least radiopaque.

(A) glass
(B) metal
(C) gravel fragment
(D) plastic
(E) painted wood

26. A 19-year-old female presents to the ED with a 4-day history of a warm, swollen, erythematous hand following a cat bite. Which of the following is the most likely causative pathogen in this scenario?

(A) *Staphylococcus intermedius*
(B) *Haemophilus aprophilus*
(C) *Eikenella corrodens*
(D) *Pasturella multocida*
(E) *Staphylococcus aureus*

27. A 59-year-old cancer patient presents to the ED with fever, pneumonia, hypotension, and tachycardia. Investigative studies include hyperkalemia, hyonatremia, and hypoglycemia. What is the most likely concomitant diagnosis in this scenario?

(A) adrenal insufficiency
(B) syndrome of inappropriate antidiuretic hormone (SIADH)
(C) Cushing's syndrome
(D) hypothyroidism
(E) hyperparathyroidism

28. Which of the following is the most common cause of nontraumatic cardiac tamponade?

(A) metastatic malignancy
(B) uremia
(C) acute idiopathic pericarditis
(D) hemorrhage (anticoagulant use)
(E) bacterial or tubercular pericarditis

29. The peripheral wedge-shaped consolidation on the pleural surface in a patient with a pulmonary embolism is defined as a

(A) Hampton hump
(B) pleural effusion
(C) atelectatic lesion
(D) Westermark sign

30. What are the indications for thrombolytic therapy in a patient with acute pulmonary embolism?

   (A) severe dyspnea
   (B) poor tissue perfusion
   (C) hypertension
   (D) circulatory collapse and refractory hypoxemia
   (E) severe right heart pressures

31. The drug of choice for hypertensive encephalopathy is

   (A) sodium nitroprusside
   (B) labetalol
   (C) esmolol
   (D) intravenous nitroglycerin
   (E) hydralazine

32. Which of the following best describes the presentation of a dissecting thoracic aortic aneurysm?

   (A) syncope, abdominal pain, back pain, and shock
   (B) esophageal, tracheal, bronchial, or neurological disorder
   (C) abrupt and severe pain in the chest or between the scapulae
   (D) lower back pain with radiation into the legs
   (E) dyspnea, orthopnea, and chest tightness

33. A patient with a DVT of his right leg, diagnosed 8 days ago, now presents with a white leg without dorsalis pedis and posterior tibial pulses. Which of the following is the most likely diagnosis?

   (A) phlegmasia alba dolens
   (B) phlebitis areta
   (C) phlegmasia cerulea dolens
   (D) phlebitis fulminans
   (E) phlebitosis dolens

34. An 89-year-old female patient from a nursing home presents to the ED with abdominal pain and distention. The abdominal radiograph demonstrates multiple air-fluid levels and dilated large bowel loops consistent with a large bowel obstruction (LBO). What is the most likely cause of the obstruction?

   (A) diverticulitis
   (B) abdominal wall hernias
   (C) carcinoma
   (D) sigmoid volvulus
   (E) adhesions

35. A 28-year-old male presents to the ED with a back injury following an all terrain vehicle (ATV) crash. The exam reveals a sensory deficit at the nipples. The spinal cord injury level is most likely at which of the following levels?

   (A) T1
   (B) T2
   (C) T3
   (D) T4
   (E) T5

DIRECTIONS (Questions 36 through 40): Each group of items in this section consists of lettered headings followed by a set of numbered words or phrases. For each numbered word or phrase, select the ONE lettered heading that is most closely associated with it. Each lettered heading may be selected once, more than once, or not at all.

Questions 36 through 40

Match the following clinical features of pneumonia to the most likely organism or type of organism.

   (A) consideration in patients with chronic lung disease, patients with laryngeal cancer, immunosuppressed patients, or nursing home patients; insidious onset of disease with low-grade fever, sputum production, and dyspnea
   (B) occurs in compromised patients such as patients at risk for aspiration, alcoholics, the elderly, and other patients with chronic lung disease; acute onset of disease with fevers, rigors, and chest pain

(C) cause of pneumonia in older children, in young adults, and in the elderly; occasionally causes extrapulmonary symptoms, including bullous myringitis, rash, neurologic symptoms, arthritis, and arthralgia

(D) affects all age groups but is particularly prevalent with the extremes of age; patient presents with rigors, bloody sputum, high fever, and chest pain

(E) severe pneumonia with cyanosis, confusion, and other signs of systemic illness; chest radiograph usually shows bilateral lower lobe infiltrates, occasionally associated with empyema

36. *Pseudomonas*

37. Staphyloccocal

38. Pneumococcal

39. *Mycoplasma*

40. *Klebsiella*

DIRECTIONS (Questions 41 through 43): Each of the numbered items or incomplete statements in this section is followed by answers or by completions of the statement. Select the ONE lettered answer or completion that is BEST in each case.

Questions 41 through 43

41. A tall, thin, 26-year-old female presents to the ED with an acute onset of right-sided pleuritic chest pain and dyspnea. What is the most likely diagnosis?

(A) right tension pneumothorax
(B) left pneumothorax
(C) right pleural effusion
(D) right spontaneous pneumothorax
(E) left atelectasis

42. A patient presents with an acute asthmatic attack. Multiple doses of inhaled adrenergic agents are used but the patient continues to have some degree of bronchospasm. Which of the following medications is paramount in the treatment of bronchospasm?

(A) corticosteroids
(B) anticholinergics
(C) theophylline
(D) magnesium
(E) leukotriene modifiers

43. A 46-year-old male presents to the ED with a several hour history of epigastric pain that has localized to the RLQ with associated nausea, vomiting, diarrhea, and anorexia. Which of the following would be the diagnostic study of choice?

(A) abdominal pelvic ultrasound (real time, graded compression, gray scale)
(B) plain abdominal radiograph (flat, upright)
(C) CT abdomen/pelvis (helical, no contrast)
(D) abdominal ultrasound (p.o., IV contrast)
(E) CT abdomen/pelvis (helical, p.o., colonic contrast)

DIRECTIONS (Questions 44 through 48): Each group of items in this section consists of lettered headings followed by a set of numbered words or phrases. For each numbered word or phrase, select the ONE lettered heading that is most closely associated with it. Each lettered heading may be selected once, more than once, or not at all.

Questions 44 through 48

Match the following pathologic conditions to the type of related gastrointestinal (GI) bleeding.

(A) Responsible for 15% of all cases of upper GI bleeding; predisposing factors include alcohol, salicylates, and nonsteroidal anti-inflammatory agents.
(B) Upper GI bleeding secondary to a longitudinal mucosal tear in the cardioesophageal region, usually due to repeated retching.
(C) Usually a painless cause of GI bleeding that is thought to result from erosion into the penetrating artery of the diverticulum.

(D) Arteriovenous malformation, usually in the right colon, which tends to be an obscure cause of lower GI bleeding, particularly in the elderly population.

(E) Most common etiology of upper GI bleeding, encompassing 60% of all cases.

44. Mallory–Weiss syndrome

45. diverticulosis

46. angiodysplasia

47. peptic ulcer disease

48. erosive gastritis and esophagitis

DIRECTIONS (Questions 49 through 58): Each of the numbered items or incomplete statements in this section is followed by answers or by completions of the statement. Select the ONE lettered answer or completion that is BEST in each case.

Questions 49 through 58

49. A 2-year-old was brought to the ED after swallowing a button battery from a watch. Which of the following statements is true regarding button battery ingestion?

(A) A button battery lodged in the esophagus is a true emergency because of the extremely rapid action of the alkaline substance on the mucosa.

(B) Button battery ingestion is essentially a benign ingestion because of the unlikelihood of the battery dissolving.

(C) Button battery ingestion is a minor emergency that can often be treated with a Foley balloon technique extraction.

(D) Most button batteries, even if symptomatic, can be left to pass through the GI tract naturally by peristalsis.

(E) Surgical removal of the button battery is always indicated, even if the patient is asymptomatic.

50. A 62-year-old patient presents to the ED with generalized abdominal pain, nausea, vomiting, and abdominal distention. The radiographs demonstrate multiple loops of dilated small bowel, air-fluid levels, and a string of pearls sign. What is the most likely cause of this clinical senario?

(A) neoplasm

(B) incarceration of abdominal hernias

(C) gallstone ileus

(D) bezoars

(E) adhesions following abdominal surgery

51. A patient presents to the ED with frequent, mucoid, watery stools, nausea, and lower abdominal pain. The patient has been on a cephalosporin-type antibiotic for about 3 months. The most likely diagnosis would be

(A) diverticulitis

(B) fissure in ano

(C) pseudomembranous entercolitis

(D) anorectal tumor

(E) ulcerative colitis

52. A 48-year-old patient presents to the ED with tachycardia, palipitations, and restlessness. The diagnosis of thyroid storm is confirmed and general supportive care is provided. Which of the following is the correct sequence of medications to treat thyroid storm?

(A) propylthiouraci (PTU)—propranolol—iodine

(B) propranolol—PTU—iodine

(C) propranolol—iodine—PTU

(D) iodine—propranolol—PTU

(E) iodine—PTU—propranolol

53. A 6-year-old child (20 kg) presents to the ED after being struck by a car. The child suffered chest, head, and abdominal trauma. The vital signs demonstrate a blood pressure of 80/40, a pulse of 170/min, and a respiratory rate of 40/min. After the airway is managed, which is the most appropriate initial fluid therapy?

(A) D5W at 100 cc/h

(B) NSS 5-cc/kg bolus, then 100 cc/h

(C) LR 20-cc/kg bolus

(D) LR at 20 cc/h

(E) NSS 200-cc bolus

54. A patient presents to the ED with a dislocated shoulder. Nitrous oxide is the drug selected for sedation and analgesia during reduction. Which of the following is true with regard to the administration of nitrous oxide for short-term painful procedures in the ED?

(A) a 50:50 concentration of nitrous and oxygen should be used

(B) never administer oxygen with nitrous oxide

(C) nitrous oxide concentrations should always be <30%

(D) higher altitudes require lower concentrations of nitrous oxide

(E) nitrous oxide is not approved for ED use

55. A 1-month-old infant presents to the ED with lethargy, tachycardia, fever, rash, and leukocytosis. The diagnosis of bacterial meningitis is suspected and a lumbar puncture was performed. What organisms should the antibiotic cover in this case?

(A) *Listeria monocytogenes*, group B strep, *Escherichia coli*

(B) *E. coli*, klebsiella, psuedomonas

(C) group B strep, enterococcus, chlamydia

(D) Listeria, staph, campylobacter species

(E) group A strep, salmonella species

56. A pregnant patient, at 25 weeks' gestation, is involved in a motor vehicle accident. She suffers blunt abdominal trauma. The vital signs are a pulse 100/min, respiratory rate 40/min, and a blood pressure 78/40. Which of the following is a true statement regarding the management of trauma in pregnancy?

(A) intubation should be avoided in the mother due to barotrauma complications

(B) the first resuscitative efforts should be directed toward the mother

(C) the fetus is less susceptible to hypoxia because of uterine reserve

(D) a stat C-section should be considered in every patient

(E) fetal distress is not easily recognized

57. Which of the following disorders may present with a patient experiencing anxiety, tremors, palpitations, fatigue, and hemiplegia?

(A) thyroid storm

(B) hypothyroidism

(C) addisonian crisis

(D) Cushing's syndrome

(E) hypoglycemia

58. A 45-year-old female presents to the ED with photophobia associated with a smaller unilateral pupil on the involved side. Which of the following is the most likely diagnosis?

(A) central retinal artery occlusion

(B) central retinal vein occlusion (CRVO)

(C) iritis/uveitis

(D) retrobulbar hematoma

(E) optic neuritis

DIRECTIONS (Questions 59 through 66): Each group of items in this section consists of lettered headings followed by a set of numbered words or phrases. For each numbered word or phrase, select the ONE lettered heading that is most closely associated with it. Each lettered heading may be selected once, more than once, or not at all.

Questions 59 through 63

Match the following conditions related to traumatic brain injury.

(A) usually results from a skull fracture across the middle meningeal artery

(B) formed deep within the brain tissue and usually caused by shearing or tensile forces that mechanically stretch and tear deep small-caliber arterioles

(C) traumatic blood within the cerebrospinal fluid (CSF) and meningeal intima caused by small tears of subarachnoid vessels

(D) collection of clear, xanthochromic blood-tinged fluid in the dural space

(E) rupture of superficial bridging vessels with rapid movement of the head, as in acceleration–deceleration injuries

59. subdural hematoma

60. epidural hematoma

61. subarachnoid hemorrhage

62. subdural hygroma

63. intracerebral hematoma

Questions 64 through 66

Match the Le Fort fracture classification with its corresponding definition.

  (A) The fracture involves the maxilla, the nasal bones, and the medial aspects of the orbits.

  (B) The fracture involves the maxilla at the level of the nasal fossa.

  (C) The fracture involves the maxilla, zygoma, nasal bones, ethmoids, vomer, and all lesser bones of the cranial base.

64. Le Fort I

65. Le Fort II

66. Le Fort III

DIRECTIONS (Questions 67 through 76): Each of the numbered items or incomplete statements in this section is followed by answers or by completions of the statement. Select the ONE lettered answer or completion that is BEST in each case.

Questions 67 through 76

67. A 42-year-old male presents to the ED with a right-sided facial injury after an assault with a wooden club. The patient complains of diplopia and pain to the right side of the face. The exam reveals enophthalmos, impaired ocular motility, and infraorbital hypoesthesias. What is the most likely diagnosis?

  (A) maxilla fracture involving the superior orbital ridge

  (B) orbital blow-out fracture with herniation of contents into the frontal sinus

  (C) maxillary blow-out fracture with herniation into the soft palate

  (D) orbital blow-out fracture with herniation of contents into the maxillary sinus

  (E) orbital blow-out fracture without herniation

68. A patient is involved in a motor vehicle accident and suffered a fractured neck. The fracture lines extend through the pedicles of C2. Which of the following describes this unstable hyperextension fracture to the cervical spine?

  (A) Jefferson's fracture

  (B) extension teardrop fracture

  (C) clay shoveler's fracture

  (D) Johnson's fracture

  (E) hangman's fracture

69. A 68-year-old female presents to the ED with an exacerbation of chronic low-back pain. Which of the following indicates the patient has developed cauda equina syndrome?

  (A) lower leg weakness, paresthesias to both legs, and incontinence

  (B) loss of deep tendon reflexes bilaterally and urinary retention

  (C) bilateral leg weakness, loss of peripheral pulses, and incontinence

  (D) bilateral leg pain, saddle anesthesia, urinary incontinence, and fecal incontinence

  (E) anesthesia to entire leg, bilateral leg weakness, and loss of deep tendon reflexes

70. A 64-year-old male presents to the ED with decreased visual acuity, red eye, and a "steamy" or hazy cornea. What is the most likely diagnosis?

  (A) acute narrow-angle glaucoma

  (B) iritis/uveitis

  (C) orbital cellulitis

  (D) photopsia

  (E) episcleritis

71. A 6-year-old boy presents to the ED with abdominal pain, blood in the stools, and arthritis. The exam reveals multiple dark erythematous lesions on his legs and buttocks. These findings are characteristic of which disease?

(A) Kawasaki's disease

(B) impetigo

(C) erythema nodosum

(D) Henoch–Schonlein purpura

(E) pneumococcal meningitis

72. A 71-year-old female presents to the ED with malaise, headache, and a rapidly decreasing visual acuity. Which of the following best describes this condition?

(A) glaucoma

(B) multiple sclerosis

(C) temporal arteritis

(D) myasthenia gravis

(E) viral encephalitis

73. A 40-year-old male presents to the ED with acute blunt chest and abdominal trauma following a motor vehicle crash. The patient presented with jugular venous distention, decreased blood pressure, and muffled heart tones. Which of the following is the most likely diagnosis?

(A) pericardial tamponade

(B) tension pneumothorax

(C) myocardial rupture

(D) aortic rupture

(E) myocardial contusion

74. Spontaneous esophageal rupture following forceful vomiting after overindulging in food and alcohol is known as

(A) Budd–Chiari syndrome

(B) Boerhaave's syndrome

(C) Brunarri's syndrome

(D) Brudzinski's syndrome

(E) Brushfield's syndrome

75. A patient presents to the ED after suffering a significant pelvic injury following a fall. The patient has a grade III pelvic fracture and blood at the tip of the meatus. How should one proceed in evaluating urethra and/or bladder injuries?

(A) gently pass a 14- or 16-Fr. Foley catheter

(B) gently pass a 14- or 16-Fr. Coudé catheter

(C) notify the urologist for immediate cystoscopy

(D) gently pass a 10- or 12-Fr. (pediatric) Foley catheter

(E) perform a retrograde urethrogram

76. A 34-year-old male patient presents to the ED following an episode of "rough" sex with his girl friend. He complains of a painful swollen penis. Which of the following best describes a penile rupture?

(A) rupture of the corpus cavernosum when the tunica albuginea is torn

(B) rupture of the dorsal penile artery into the tunica albuginea

(C) rupture of the corpus spongiosum from a tear in the dorsal penile vein

(D) rupture of the tunica albuginea from a tear into the corpus cavernosum

(E) rupture of the corpus cavernosum when the corpus spongiosum is torn

DIRECTIONS (Questions 77 through 81): Each group of items in this section consists of lettered headings followed by a set of numbered words or phrases. For each numbered word or phrase, select the ONE lettered heading that is most closely associated with it. Each lettered heading may be selected once, more than once, or not at all.

Questions 77 through 81

Match the diagrams in Fig. 13–1 with the appropriate Salter–Harris classification of epiphyseal plate injuries.

77. Salter–Harris I

78. Salter–Harris II

79. Salter–Harris III

80. Salter–Harris IV

81. Salter–Harris V

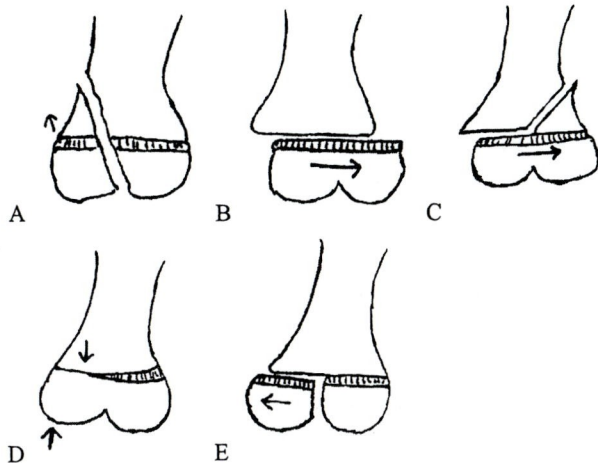

Fig. 13–1. Salter-Harris classification

DIRECTIONS (Questions 82 through 100): Each of the numbered items or incomplete statements in this section is followed by answers or by completions of the statement. Select the ONE lettered answer or completion that is BEST in each case.

Questions 82 through 100

82. A 41-year-old male injures his finger while playing basketball. He is unable to extend the distal interphalnageal (DIP) joint. The radiograph shows an avulsion fracture to the proximal dorsal region of the distal phalanx. What is the diagnosis?

  (A) Bennett fracture
  (B) Rolando's fracture
  (C) mallet finger fracture
  (D) Colles fracture

83. A child falls on an outstretched hand. She complains of pain and swelling to the wrist. The radiograph demonstrates a buckling of the cortex to the distal radius. What is your diagnosis?

  (A) torus fracture
  (B) greenstick fracture
  (C) nightstick fracture
  (D) tuft fracture

84. A 40-year-old male slips on the ice, injuring his left arm. He complains of pain and swelling to the midshaft humeral region. The physical exam reveals a wrist drop on the injured side. Which nerve is most likely injured?

  (A) ulnar
  (B) radial
  (C) median
  (D) axillary
  (E) subclavian

85. After viewing the picture in Fig. 13–2, identify the proper nomenclature of this elbow injury.

  (A) anterior elbow dislocation
  (B) posterior elbow dislocation
  (C) anterior humeral dislocation
  (D) posterior humeral dislocation

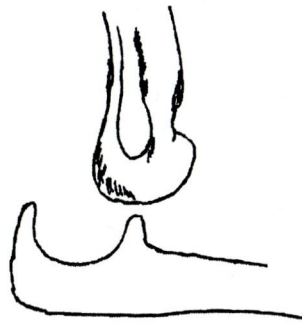

Fig. 13–2. Elbow dislocation

86. A 7-year-old child presents to the ED with fever, neck pain, and a "duck-like" voice. Which of the following is the most likely diagnosis?

  (A) peritonsillar abscess
  (B) Streptococcus pharyngitis
  (C) epiglottitis
  (D) Ludwig's angina
  (E) retropharyngeal abscess

87. What is the mechanism of injury for a posterior shoulder dislocation?

  (A) shoulder internal rotation and adduction
  (B) shoulder internal rotation with abduction
  (C) shoulder external rotation with adduction
  (D) shoulder external rotation with abduction
  (E) fall on an outstretched hand

88. Which of the following medications is responsible for the most drug-related deaths?

(A) benzodiazepines

(B) tricyclic antidepressants (TCAs)

(C) stimulants

(D) monoamine oxidase inhibitors

(E) lithium

89. A 30-year-old male patient presents to the ED with an acute change in mental status. The exam reveals a patient who is sleepy but arousable to loud verbal stimuli. His airway is intact and the vital signs are stable. Investigative studies indicate an alcohol level 150 mg/dL, an anion gap of 30, a metabolic acidosis, an osmolar gap of 20, and calcium oxalate crystalluria. What is the most likely diagnosis?

(A) methanol poisoning

(B) ethanol poisoning

(C) ethylene glycol poisoning

(D) isopropanol poisoning

(E) buspirone poisoning

90. A 20-year-old male presents to the ED following a lethal overdose of acetaminophen. What is the antidote for acetaminophen toxicity?

(A) flumazenil

(B) Narcan

(C) vitamin K

(D) *N*-acetylcysteine

(E) ethanol

91. Which of the following clinical findings differentiates periorbital from orbital cellulitis?

(A) erythema

(B) fever

(C) lid edema

(D) worsening pain with eye movements

(E) development of a rash on the face

92. A 47-year-old male presents to the ED comatose after ingesting an unknown liquid substance. Investigative studies include: pH 7.45, Na 140, Cl 110, HCO_3 19, glucose 180, BUN 30, Cr 1.5, ETOH 0.0, high serum ketones, and a measured osmolality of 380. These findings are most consistent with which of the following toxin ingestions.

(A) methanol

(B) ethylene glycol

(C) daibetic ketoacidosis

(D) isopropanol

(E) alcoholic ketoacidosis

93. A 58-year-old male presents to the ED hypothermic after an environmental exposure to cold weather and snow. The patient's core temperature is 85.5°F. Which of the following is the most accurate statement regarding this scenario?

(A) shivering is common

(B) an Osborne (J) wave is pathognomic for hypothermia

(C) rough handling can produce serious dysrhythmias

(D) a nasogastric tube should be inserted to protect the airway from regurgitation

(E) the patient is in an excitation phase of hypothermia

94. A patient presents to the ED after being bitten by an unknown "insect" while camping. The pain began as a pinprick sensation at the bite site and spread quickly to include the entire bitten extremity. The bite wound became erythematous 45 minutes after the bite. The bite evolved into a target lesion and the patient complains of muscle cramp-like spasms in the large muscle groups. Which of the following is the most likely cause?

(A) black widow spider

(B) hobo spider

(C) brown recluse spider

(D) tarantula

(E) scorpion

95. Which of the following is the most important treatment option in a patient with moderate acute mountain sickness (AMS)?

    (A) oxygen therapy
    (B) dexamethasone
    (C) hyperbaric therapy
    (D) acetazolamide
    (E) immediate descent

96. A patient presents to the ED after being trapped in a house fire. The patient suffered partial thickness burns over the entire anterior chest and abdomen, entire right arm, and the entire right leg. Using the rule of nines, what is the estimated percent of burn?

    (A) 40%
    (B) 44%
    (C) 48%
    (D) 56%
    (E) 62%

97. Which of the following is the most common cause of death by hemorrhage in patients with hemophilia A?

    (A) gastrointestinal hemorrhage
    (B) retroperitoneal hemorrhage
    (C) pulmonary hemorrhage
    (D) renal hemorrhage
    (E) intracranial hemorrhage

98. A 29-year-old logger was struck in the back with a load of logs. The evaluation reveals abscence of patellar reflexes. This finding is consistent with an injury at which of the following dermatone levels?

    (A) L1
    (B) L2
    (C) L3
    (D) L4
    (E) S1

99. A 79-year-old male presents to the ED with a heart rate of 50 bpm, second degree A–V block Mobitz at 50 bpm, BP 90/60, potassium of 5.8, and a digoxin level of 6.9 ng/mL. What is the treatment of choice in this scenario?

    (A) calcium chloride
    (B) potassium infusion
    (C) procainamide
    (D) magnesium
    (E) digoxin immune fab fragments

100. A 39-year-old female presents to the ED with agitation, tremors, visual hallucinations, fever, and tachycardia. The eye exam reveals nystagmus and a sixth cranial nerve palsy. Which of the following conditions best describes this clinical scenario?

    (A) Korsakoff's psychosis
    (B) Wernicke's encephalopathy
    (C) acute dystonia
    (D) acute cocaine toxicity
    (E) trigeminal neuralgia

Answers and Explanations

1. **(B)** Survival of prehospital cardiac arrest is most notably improved by defibrillation. Emergent airway management, the use of epinephrine, prompt treatment of hypotension, and rapid transport to the most appropriate facility only moderately increase survival rates when compared to early defibrillation. *(Tintinalli et al, 2000, p. 6)*

2. **(D)** Rh-negative females who are exposed to Rh-positive blood either through pregnancy, delivery, threatened or spontaneous hemorrhage, surgery for ectopic pregnancy, or amniocentesis may become sensitized and require Anti-D immune globulin (RhoGAM). Patients who are Rh-negative should be administered RhoGAM in threatened or spontaneous abortions. Rh-negative females in the setting of ectopic pregnancies, theatened abortions, and/or complete abortions should be given 50 ug if they are at <12 weeks' gestation and 300 ug if they are at ≥12 weeks' gestation. *(Marx, 2002, pp. 2415, 2425)*

3. **(B)** Metabolic acidosis is characterized by either increased production of acids, decreased excretion of acids, or loss of bicarbonate. The etiology of metabolic acidosis is divided into those with a normal anion gap and those associated with an increased anion gap. Metabolic acidosis with an increased anion gap include lactic acidosis, ketoacidosis, and renal failure. Lactic acidosis is due to decreased oxygen delivery to tissues and associated anaerobic metabolism, which results in an increased production of lactate. This lactate production accompanies severe metabolic acidosis. Low tissue perfusion, characteristic of lactic acidosis, may include shock and sepsis. Metabolic acidosis with a normal anion gap is known as hyperchloremic metabolic acidosis. The primary causes of normal anion gap acidosis include renal loss of bicarbonate through either proximal tubular acidosis, distal tubular acidosis, hyperkalemic renal tubular acidosis, renal insufficiency, or carbonic anhydrase inhibition, and gastrointestinal loss of alkali through either diarrhea, pancreatic fistulas, or ureterosigmoidostomy. *(Marx, 2002, pp. 1714–1723)*

4. **(A)** Pulmonary thromboembolism (PTE) is primarily the result of clot migration from DVT. PTE is a life-threatening and often fatal complication of venous thrombosis ranking as the third leading cause of death in the United States. Even with current technology, the diagnosis of DVT and PTE is rather evasive and difficult. Moreover, approximately 400,000 cases of PTE are missed annually in the United States, resulting in the death of more than 100,000 patients who may have survived with the proper diagnosis and treatment. Identification of risk factors for DVT remains an important diagnostic tool when thinking about the diagnosis of PTE. Many of these risk factors are in some way associated with Virchow's triad of venous stasis, hypercoagulability, and endothelial injury. Risk factors include AIDS (lupus anticoagulant),

acute myocardial infarction, antithrombin III deficiency, Behcet's disease, blood type A, burns, indwelling infusion catheters, chemotherapy, CHF, IV drug abuse, drug-induced lupus anticoagulant, past history of DVT, estrogen replacement therapy, fractures, hemolytic anemias, heparin-associated thrombocytopenia, homocystinuria, hyperlipidemias, immobilization, malignancy, obesity, oral contraceptives, history of PTE, phenothiazines, plasminogen abnormality, polycythemia, postoperative state, postpartum period, protein C and protein S deficiency, systemic lupus erythematosis (SLE), superficial thrombophlebitis, trauma, varicose veins, venography, venous pacemakers, and venous stasis. Ventilation/perfusion scanning (V/Q) is relatively nondiagnostic in most cases of PTE. Only 41% of patients with PTE confirmed through pulmonary angiography will have a high-probability lung scan. In general, a patient has a less than 5% chance of having a PTE if the scan is read as "normal." A "high-probability" scan has a greater than 85% chance that a PTE is present. A scan interpreted as "low-probability" or "nondiagnostic" will have a 15% to 85% chance of having a PTE. Therefore, a nondiagnostic or low-probablity scan is useless in ruling in or ruling out a PTE. Computed tomography offers relatively good way of diagnosing PTE, however, the sensitivity ranges from 40% to 65% and the negative predictive value is around 82% when compared to pulmonary angiography. The pulmonary angiogram is considered the last resort for diagnosing a PTE. A "positive" angiogram provides essentially 100% certainty of the diagnosis of PTE. A "negative" angiogram provides greater than 90% certainty that PTE is excluded. However, technical and patient factors such as dye concerns and movement can significantly alter the diagnostic ability of angiogram. *(Marx, 2002, pp. 1210–1233)*

5. **(E)** Direct visualization of the endotracheal tube passing through the vocal cords is the most reliable indicator for endotracheal tube placement. Auscultation of the chest and epigastric areas may reveal transmitted sounds from the endotracheal tube in the stomach. Condensation in the tube can be an unreliable indicator of proper endotracheal tube placement. *(Tintinalli et al, 2000, p. 87)*

6. **(C)** The definition of hypernatremia is a serum sodium greater than 145 meq/L. Hypernatremia is classified as either isovolemic (diabetes insipidus, skin loss through hyperthermia, and iatrogenic), hypervolemic (administration of hypernatremin solutions, mineralcorticoid excess as in Conn's or Cushing's syndrome, and salt ingestion), and hypovolemic (renal losses through diuretics or glycosuria, GI, respiratory, or skin losses, and adrenal deficiencies). Water deficit in hypernatremic patients is calculated by the following formula:

Water deficit (L) = 0.6 (body weight (kg) $\times$ (measured serum sodium/normal serum sodium) -1

Water deficit = 0.6 (60) = 36 (180/140) -1 = 36 (0.3) = 10.8 L. *(Marx, 2002, pp. 1726–1727)*

7. **(A)** MAT is defined as a chaotic, irregular rhythm with atrial rates of 100 to 150 bpm. Typically, there are more than two foci of impulse formation with at least three distinctly different P waves with varying P″ R, RR, and P′ P′ intervals. MAT is commonly associated with COPD, theophylline toxicity, and beta-adrenergic agonist therapy. Treatment is directed at improving oxygenation and correcting underlying conditions. Rarely, MAT may require a calcium channel blocker, beta-blocker, or amiodarone. AF is a totally chaotic atrial rhythm with multiple microreentry circuits of atrial rates from 300 to 600 impulses/min. Common causes of AF include ischemic heart disease, valvular heart disease, pericarditis, hyperthyroidism, sick sinus syndrome, myocardial contusion, acute ethanol intoxication (i.e., holiday heart syndrome), idiopathic, hypertensive heart disease, cardiomyopathy, cardiac surgery, pulmonary embolism, congestive heart failure, and accessory pathway diseases. Atrial flutter is characterized by regular atrial depolarization rates of 250 to 350 bpm with varying degrees of atrioventicular block. Common causes of atrial flutter include atherosclerotic heart disease, myocardial

infarction, thyrotoxicosis, pulmonary embolism, mitral valve disease, congestive heart failure, and metabolic derangements. Sinus bradycardia is a regular rhythm with atrial and ventricular rates of fewer than 60 bpm with normal P-wave morphology and P–R duration. Sinus bradycardia can be found in healthy adults or it may be associated with pathologic conditions such as hypothermia, excessive parasymparathetic tone, carotid sensitivity, or myocardial infarction. A type II second-degree AV block or Mobitz II block is characterized by a sudden interruption of AV conduction without prior prolongation of the P–R interval. Mobitz II is often associated with a variety of acute and chronic diseases such as anterior wall ischemia. *(Marx, 2002, pp. 1053–1098)*

8. **(B)** Hypercalcemia associated with malignancies is commonly due to increased bone resorption through osteoclastic factors, parathyroid hormone (PTH) factors, prostoglandins, direct erosion by tumor cells, steroids, and peptides. Common neoplasms include multiple myeloma, lymphosarcoma, adult T-cell lymphoma, and Burkitt's lymphoma. Symptoms of hypercalcemia are variable depending on the degree elevation. Typical symptoms include constipation, anorexia, vomiting, confusion, obtundation, psychosis, nephrolithiasis, renal insufficiency, myopathy, back pain, weakness, and hypertension. Hyperkalemia may produce manifestations of weakness, irritability, paresthesias, paralysis, cardiac arrhythmia, and decreased deep tendon reflexes. Hypomagnesemia symptoms include weakness, fasciculations, tremors, convulsions, delirium, coma, hyperreflexia, and cardiac arrhythmias. Hypoglycemia commonly presents with varying degrees of diaphoresis, anxiety, tremors, tachycardia, palpitations, fatigue, syncope, headache, visual disturbances, hemiplegia, and seizures. Hyponatremia may present as confusion, muscle cramps, anorexia, nausea, lethargy, seizures, and coma depending on the degree and rapidity of onset. *(Marx, 2002, pp. 1707–1708, 1724–1726, 1730–1731, 1736–1738, 1748–1750)*

9. **(A)** Ethanol is usually not associated with a clinically significant anion gap metabolic acidosis. Ethanol metabolism may lead to very mild lactic acidosis and is often associatied with alcoholic ketoacidosis. The differential diagnosis for a high anion gap metabolic acidosis includes uremia from renal failure, lactic acidosis, ketoacidosis (DKA, alcoholic ketoacidosis, starvation ketoacidosis), and ingestions (methanol, ethylene glycol, salicylates). *(Tintinalli et al, 2000, p. 135)*

10. **(C)** The medial ankle support comprises the deltoid ligaments, which include tibionavicular, anterior tibiotalar, tibiocalcaneal, and posterior tibiotalar parts. The most common mechanism of injury is an external rotational force. The lateral portion of the ankle is supported by the anterior talofibular, anterior inferior tibiofibular, interosseous, posterior tibiofibular, and the calcaneofibular ligaments. Approximately two thirds of all ankle injuries are isolated anterior talofibular ligament injuries. About 20% involve both anterior talofibular and calcaneofibular ligament injuries. Fewer than 5% of the ankle injuries are isolated deltoid ligament sprains. *(Marx, 2002, pp. 707–714)*

11. **(E)** The ECG criterion used to define an acute myocardial injury pattern is ST-segment elevation of 1 mm or more above the baseline. This should be measured 0.04 seconds past the J point. ST-segment depression and T wave changes are indicative of myocardial ischemia. Abnormal Q waves are consistent with myocardial infarction. Q waves that are 2-mm wide or $25% of the height of the R wave in that lead are indicative of dead heart muscle. The following are the anatomical sites of coronary ischemia related to the ECG leads: anterior septal wall is leads V1 to V4; high lateral wall is leads V5, V6, plus I, and AVL; inferior wall are leads II, III, and AVF; posterior wall leads demonstrate marked depression in leads V1 to V4 (mirror image of anterior wall); and right ventricular infarction will demonstrate ST-segment changes in lead V4R. *(Cummins; AHA pp. 9-23–9-30)*

12. **(C)** In a patient with unstable angina, glycoprotein IIb/IIIa receptor inhibitors are considered adjunctive therapy. Glycoprotein IIb/IIIa

receptor inhibitors should be considered only after routine antianginal therapies have been tried unsuccessfully. Oxygen, aspirin, nitroglycerin, and heparin should continue to be the mainstay treatments. Cardiac catheter patients undergoing a percutaneous coronary intervention may benefit the most from the use of glycoprotein IIb/IIIa receptor inhibitors. *(Braunwald, 2000, pp. 1193–1209)*

13. **(C)** Pregnancy-induced hypertension (PIH) is defined as a blood pressure (BP) reading of 140/90 or higher. The subtypes of PIH include hypertension without proteinuria or edema, preeclampsia (hypertension with proteinuria or edema), and ecclampsia (seizures in the pregnant patient with signs of preeclampsia). PIH occurs in about 5% of pregnancies and eclampsia occurs in less than one in 2,000 deliveries. Risk factors associated with PIH include primigravidas, age less than 20 years, twin or molar pregnancies, hypercholesterolemia in the mother, cigarette smokers, and those with a history of PIH. Hydralazine is the most common antihypertensive used in PIH. The typical dose is 5 mg IV and repeated in a dose of 5 to 10 mg IV every 20 minutes as needed to keep the diastolic bp less than 110 mm Hg. Other agent used with some degree of success include nifedipine, nitroprusside, and labetalol. Magnesium sulfate is used primarily in pregnancy to terminate ongoing seizures and prevent further seizures. This is usually accomplished by keeping the serum magnesium levels at 4 to 7 mg/dL. In general, nitroglycerin and hydrochlorothiazide are not indicated in PIH. *(Marx, 2002, pp. 2421–2424)*

14. **(A)** Two hours after the onset of an acute myocardial infarction, the cardiac enzymes would most commonly demonstrate a normal troponin and CK-MB. Cardiac troponin I and CK-MB elevate in 3 to 12 hours after the onset of myocardial infarction. Serum myoglobin elevates 1 to 4 hours after the onset of myocardial infarction. *(Tintinalli et al, 2000, p. 361)*

15. **(C)** Myocardial necrosis can be identified with a great degree of specificity by troponin I, par-

ticularly in settings of cocaine use, recent surgery, and chronic renal failure. Troponin T and serum myoglobin have a very high sensitivity, but the specificity is poor with regard to myocardial injury. *(Tintinalli et al, 2000, pp. 361–362)*

16. **(E)** Indications for IV thrombolytic therapy include acute myocardial infarction less than 6 to 12 hours old, new or presumed new left bundle branch block, and an ECG that has at least 1 mm of ST-segment elevation in two or more contiguous leads. ST-segment depression is not an indication for thrombolytic therapy. *(Tintinalli et al, 2000, p. 367)*

17. **(B)** In this scenario, the patient's sodium level dropped severely and rapidly secondary to excessive water intake. In this setting, patients may present with confusion, muscle cramps, lethargy, anorexia, nausea, seizures, and coma. Other causes of euvolemic hyponatremia include syndrome of inappropriate secretion of antidiuretic hormone (SIADH), renal failure, glucocorticoid deficiency (hypopituitarism), hypothyroidism, and multiple medications such as thiazide diuretics. *(Marx, 2002, pp. 1720–1726)*

18. **(A)** The symptoms described are due to hypoglycemia caused by pentamidine isethionate. Pentamidine is a common treatment for PCP in the AIDS patient. Pentamidine is an antiprotozoal agent that inhibits synthesis of DNA, RNA, phospholipids, and proteins. Common side effects include hypoglycemia, renal impairment, leukopenia, hepatotoxicity, nausea, anorexia, hypotension, fever, and rash. Monitor metabolic parameters such as BUN, creatinine, glucose, CBC, platelet count, liver function tests, and calcium regularly while on pentamidine therapy. *(Marx, 2002, pp. 1846–1849)*

19. **(A)** The ECG findings of hyperkalemia include the following: 6.5 to 7.5 meq/L—tall peaked T waves, short QT interval, prolonged PR interval; 7.5 to 8.0 meq/L—QRS widening, flattening of the P wave; and 10 to 12 meq/L—prolonged QT interval is also associated with hypocalcemia. *(Tintinalli et al, 2000, pp. 159–162)*

20. **(C)** The typical presentation of pontine hemorrhage is coma, pinpoint reactive pupils, impaired lateral ocular motility, and quadriplegia with decerebrate posturing. Thalamic hemorrhage characteristically leads to impaired consciousness, contralateral motor and sensory loss, and gaze preference to the side of the hemorrhage. Cerebellar hemorrhages typically present with impaired gait, vertigo, lim ataxia, impaired consciousness, and cranial nerve palsies. Subarachnoid hemorrhage presents as a severe acute onset of a headache with associated neurological deficits of varying degrees depending on the extent and location of the hemorrhage. Lobar hemorrhages may present with symptoms of headache, nausea, vomiting, change in mental status, visual disturbance, seizures, and coma depending on the extent and location of the bleed. *(Goldman, 2004, pp. 2301–2304)*

21. **(A)** MAT is associated with the following ECG characteristics: (1) three or more differently shaped P waves; (2) varying PP, PR, and RR intervals; and (3) atrial rhythm usually between 100 and 180. AF is associated with the following ECG characteristics: (1) fibrillatory waves of atrial activity, best seen in leads V1, V2, V3, and aVf; and (2) irregular ventricular response, usually around 170 to 180 in patients with a healthy AV node. Ventricular tachycardia is associated with the following ECG characteristics: (1) wide QRS complexes; (2) rate greater than 100; (3) usually regular rhythm; and (4) a constant QRS axis. A sinus dysrhythmia is associated with the following ECG characteristics: (1) normal sinus P waves and PR intervals; (2) 1:1 AV conduction; and (3) variation of at least 0.12 second between the shortest and longest P-P interval. Supraventricular tachycardia usually occurs at a rate of 100 to 250 with a regular rhythm. *(Tintinalli et al, 2000, pp. 170–180)*

22. **(C)** Adenosine 6 mg, rapid IV push over 1 to 3 seconds, is the first-line drug for PSVT. If conversion to NSR is unsuccessful after 1 to 2 minutes, an additional dose of adenosine 12 mg, rapid IV over 1 to 3 seconds, may be given. The first-line therapy for VT is lidocaine. If the patient is free of carotid bruits, va-gal maneuvers such as carotid sinus massage may be tried. In patients with ischemic heart disease, ice water immersion could be detrimental and should be avoided. *(Cummins; AHA, 1-32–1-35)*

23. **(C)** The first priority in the management of septic shock is assessment of the airway, oxygenation, and ventilation. Oxygen should be administered at 100% via mask or endotracheal tube. Fluid resuscitation is the second priority in the patient with septic shock. Tissue and organ perfusion can be assessed by parameters such as the patient's mental status, blood pressure, respiratory rate, pulse rate, skin color and temperature, central venous pressure, and urine output greater than 30 mL/h (1 mL/kg/h in pediatric patients). Other important areas of assessment and management include acid–base status and antimicrobial therapy. *(Tintinalli et al, 2000, pp. 234–236)*

24. **(D)** Flumazenil competitively blocks the effects of benzodiazepines on GABAergic pathway-mediated inhibitors in the central nervous system (CNS). Naloxone HCl (Narcan) is a narcotic antagonist. Ketamine is a rapid-acting general anesthetic. Flutamide is a nonsteriodal, antiandrogenic agent used for prostate carcinoma. *(Drug Facts and Comparisons, pp. 1802, 3383, 3638)*

25. **(D)** Organic material is generally not visible on plain radiographs. However, certain materials such as wood and plastic that are painted may be visible. Gravel and metal that are reasonable size (.1 mm) also should be visible. *(Tintinalli et al, 2000, p. 285)*

26. **(D)** The most common pathogen found in infected cat bite wounds is *P. multocida*. Pathogens like *Staphylococcus intermedius*, *Eikenella corrodens*, *Haemophilus aphrophilus*, and *Staphylococcus aureus* are commonly seen in infected dog bite wounds. *(Tintinalli et al, 2000, pp. 334–335)*

27. **(A)** Primary adrenocortical insufficiency, also known as Addison's disease, is characterized by inadequate secretion of cortisol, aldos-

terone, or both resulting from destruction of the adrenal glands. Autoimmune destruction of the adrenal glands occurs in about 80% of the cases; however, other causes include tuberculosis, viral infections, iron deposition, carcinomatous destruction of the adrenals, adrenal infarction from arteritis or thrombosis, and adrenal hemorrhage. Other less common causes include postoperative state, fungal infection, AIDS, sarcoidosis, megestrol acetate therapy, and amyloidosis. The typical symptoms include weakness, fatigue, nausea, vomiting, weight loss, increased pigmentation, hypotension, abdominal pain, constipation, diarrhea, salt craving, syncope, confusion, and psychosis. Laboratory results characteristically include hyperkalemia, hyponatremia, hypochloremia, hypoglycemia, elevated BUN/creatinine ratio (prerenal azotemia), anemia, decreased 24-hour urinary cortisol, 17-OHCS, and 17-KS and increased ACTH (primary adrenocorticol insufficiency). SIADH is a syndrome of antidiuretic hormone (ADH) excess, which causes water retention and sodium loss. Common causes of SIADH include malignant tumors, intracranial hemorrhage, hydrocephalus, meningitis, brain abscess, chlorpropamide, thiazide diuretics, vasopressin, and chemotherapeutic agents. Laboratory values of SIADH include hyponatremia, urinary osmolarity greater than serum osmolarity, and urinary sodium usually greater than 30 meq/L. Cushing's syndrome is characterized by glucocorticoid excess secondary to exaggerated adrenal cortisol production or chronic glucocorticoid therapy. Causes of primary glucocorticoid excess include idiopathic, tuberculosis, fungal infections, adrenal hemorrhage, congenital adrenal hyperplasia, sarcoidosis, amyloidosis, HIV/AIDS, and metastatic disease. Secondary causes include exogenous glucocorticoid use, isolated ACTH deficiency, and hypothalamic/pituitary lesions. Clinical manifestations of Cushing's syndrome include hypertension, obesity, menstrual irregularities, hypogonadism, infertility, hirsutism, diabetes mellitus, osteoporosis, bone pain, psychosis, emotional lability, poor wound healing, hair loss, weight gain, and growth retardation. Common laboratory results include hypokalemia,

hypochloremia, metabolic alkalosis, hyperglycemia, and hypercholesterolemia. Primary hypothyroidism (i.e., thyroid gland dysfunction) is the cause of greater than 90% of the cases of hypopthyroidism. Secondary hypothyroidism include pituitary dysfuction, postpartum necrosis, neoplasm, and infiltrative diseases causing a deficiency of TSH. Tertiary causes of hypothyroidism include hypothalamic diseases such as granuloma, neoplasm, or irradiation causing deficiency of thyroid releasing hormone. Common laboratory results of hypothyroidism are increased TSH, hyponatremia, increased cholesterol triglycerides, and liver function tests. Primary hyperparathyroidism is the result of oversecretion of PTH, which in turn causes hypercalcemia. A parathyroid adenoma is the primary etiology of hyperparathyroidism. Clinical manifestations of hyperparathyroidism include urinary calculi, renal failure, osteitis fibrosa cystica, bone demineralization, osteopenia, anorexia, weight loss, constipation, nausea, vomiting, and emotional instability. Laboratory findings include hypercalcemia, hypophosphatemia, hyperchloremia, elevated serum alkaline phosphatase, and hypercalcuria. *(Noble, 2001, pp. 845–849, 869–871, 887–898, 1086–1088; Marx, 2002, pp. 1707–1709)*

28. **(A)** The most common cause of nontraumatic cardiac tamponade is metastatic malignancy. Common symptoms include dyspnea and profound exercise intolerance. Physical exam findings include tachycardia, low systolic arterial blood pressure with a narrow pulse pressure, and pulsus paradoxus. Less common causes of nontraumatic tamponade include acute or chronic idiopathic pericarditis, uremia, bacterial or tubercular pericarditis, hemorrhage (from anticoagulant use), systemic lupus erythematosus, radiation treatments, and myxedema. *(Tintinalli et al, 2000, pp. 393–394)*

29. **(A)** A Hampton hump generally represents a focal area of hemorrhage within the lung or an actual pulmonary infarction. It is a wedge-shaped, dense, consolidated area on the pleural surface of the chest wall. A Westermark sign is a regional area of decreased pulmonary vascularity. Other more common findings of pulmonary embolism on a chest radiograph include atelectasis, elevated hemidiaphragm, patchy consolidation, and pleural effusions. *(Rosen et al, 1992, p. 289)*

30. **(D)** Massive pulmonary embolism associated with hypotension, refractory hypoxemia, circulatory collapse, and right ventricular dysfunction may be treated with thrombolytic therapy. Thrombolytics have proven to be effective in normalizing pulmonary artery pressures, improving right ventricular dysfunction, stabilizing hemodynamics, and correcting hypoxia. Recombinant tissue plasminogen activator (r-TPA) has been shown to be the fastest thrombolytic, but others such as urokinase and streptokinase have been proven to be effective. *(Tintinalli et al, 2000, pp. 400–401)*

31. **(A)** Sodium nitroprusside, a rapidly acting arterial and venous dilator, is the drug of choice for hypertensive emergencies. Labetolol also is an excellent drug for hypertensive emergencies. It is a competitive, selective α_1-blocker and a competitive, nonselective beta-blocker, with the beta-blocking action four to eight times that of alpha blocking. Esmolol is an ultra-short-acting β_1 selective adrenergic blocker with rapid distribution and elimination. Nitroglycerin causes both arterial and venous dilation, with a greater effect on the venous system. The onset of action with nitroglycerine is almost immediate when given intravenously, and the half-life is 4 minutes. Hydralazine is a direct arterial dilator, with the onset of action within 10 minutes when given intravenously and duration of action 4 to 6 hours *(Tintinalli et al, 2000, pp. 405–409)*

32. **(C)** Severe, abrupt chest pain that also may be located between the scapula is common in aortic dissection. Pain in the anterior chest or back may represent involvement of the ascending or descending aorta. *(Tintinalli et al, 2000, pp. 412–416)*

33. **(C)** Phlegmasia alba dolens, "milk leg," is an uncommon presentation of DVT in which there is massive iliofemoral thrombosis. The leg is usually white or pale secondary to associated arterial spasm. When the dorsalis pedis and posterior pulses are diminished or absent, a false diagnosis of arterial occlusion may be made. A patient with phlegmasia cerulea dolens presents with an extensively swollen, cyanotic leg from venous engorgement due to massive iliofemoral thrombosis. This high-grade obstruction can compromise perfusion to the foot from high compartment pressures and lead to venous gangrene. *(Tintinalli et al, 2000, pp. 417–418)*

34. **(C)** Carcinoma of the colon is the most common cause of LBOs in adults. Diverticulitis can also cause LBOs, and patients often give a history of intermittent left lower quadrant pain. Sigmoid volvulus is a less common cause of LBO. It is seen most often in the elderly with poor bowel habits and chronic constipation. *(Diethelm and Stanely, 1991, pp. 736–755)*

35. **(D)** Thoracic T4 dermatone runs across the nipple line. T2 dermatone involves the upper medial bicep region. T3 level runs just above the nipple line and T5 runs just below the nipple line. *(Ferri, 2005, pp. 5–6)*

36. **(E)** *Pseudomonas* pneumonia is commonly associated with hypoxia, confusion, fever, sepsis, and signs of systemic illness and lower lobe infiltrate on chest x-ray. *(Tintinalli et al, 2000, pp. 453–455)*

37. **(A)** *Staphylococcus aureus* pneumonia has an insidious onset with low-grade fever, dyspnea, and sputum production. This etiologic agent should be considered in immunosuppressed patients, those with chronic lung disease, or nursing home patients. *(Tintinalli et al, 2000, pp. 453–455)*

38. **(D)** Pneumococcal pneumonia patients commonly present with sudden onset of rigors, high fever, chest pain, and bloody sputum. The very young and the very old are the most susceptible to pneumococcal pneumonia. *(Tintinalli et al, 2000, pp. 453–455)*

39. **(C)** *Mycoplasma* pneumonia is most prevelant in older children, young adults, and the elderly.

Bullous myringitis, rash, neurologic symptoms, arthritis, and arthralgia are common extrapulmonary symptoms found in patients with *Mycoplasma* pneumonia. *(Tintinalli et al, 2000, pp. 453–455)*

40. **(B)** *Klebsiella* pneumonia usually occurs in patients at risk for aspiration, alcoholics, the elderly, and those with chronic lung disease. Patients usually have an acute onset of severe disease with fever, rigors, and chest pain. *(Tintinalli et al, 2000, pp. 453–455)*

41. **(D)** Spontaneous pneumothorax most commonly affects tall, thin males, between the ages of 20 to 40 years, who are heavy cigarette smokers. The pain is usually pleuritic and localizes to the affected side. Most patients have decreased breath sounds on the affected side, but few have a significant tachypnea or tachycardia. *(Tintinalli et al, 2000, p. 471)*

42. **(A)** Corticosteriods remain the cornerstone of treatment for asthma. Steroids are thought to decrease airway inflammation and restore beta-adrenergic responsiveness. The peak onset of inflammatory effects are delayed at least 4 to 8 hours following oral or intravenous administration. Theophylline is no longer considered a first-line therapy for acute asthma because of its high risk for toxicity, especially when combined with beta-adrenergic drugs. Magnesium does have some bronchodilating effects and can be used in the management of acute asthma. Magnesium should be used only after standard therapy has been tried unsuccessfully. Leukotriene modifiers decrease inflammation, edema, mucous secretion, and bronchoconstriction, thereby diminishing the need for short-acting β_2 agonists. *(Tintinalli et al, 2000, pp. 479–483)*

43. **(E)** A helical, colonic, IV, and p.o. contrast-enhanced CT of the abdomen and pelvis has a sensitivity and specificity of 100% and 98%, respectively. Abdominal pelvic ultrasound (real time, graded compression, gray scale) has a sensitivity and specificity of 82% and 93%, respectively. Plain films have a sensitivity and specificity of 75% and 58%, respectively. A CT abdomen/pelvis with p.o. or colonic contrast decreases the sensitivity and specificity to 88% and 97%, respectively. *(Tintinalli et al, 2000, pp. 500–501)*

44. **(B)** Repeated retching can cause longitudinal tears in the cardioesophageal portion of the stomach. GI bleeding associated with this tear is known as Mallory–Weiss syndrome. *(Tintinalli et al, 2000, p. 520)*

45. **(C)** Diverticular bleeding usually results from an erosion into a penetrating artery of the diverticulum. The GI bleeding associated with diverticular bleeding is usually painless and profuse. *(Tintinalli et al, 2000, p. 520)*

46. **(D)** Arteriovenous malformations or angiodysplasia can be a common source of obscure GI bleeding. It is common in the elderly and usually affects the right colon. *(Tintinalli et al, 2000, p. 520)*

47. **(E)** The most common etiology of upper GI bleeding (60%) is peptic ulcer disease. This includes gastric, duodenal, and stomal ulcers. *(Tintinalli et al, 2000, p. 520)*

48. **(A)** Collectively, 15% of all cases of upper GI bleeding are due to erosive gastritis, esophagitis, and duodenitis. Salicylates, alcohol, and NSAIDs are the most common predisposing factors. *(Tintinalli et al, 2000, p. 520)*

49. **(A)** A button battery ingestion may cause significant complications in as little as 4 to 6 hours due to the rapid action of alkaline in the battery. Severe burns of the esophagus or perforation may occur. A plain radiograph of the abdomen should be obtained first to localize the battery. A battery lodged in the esophagus should be removed emergently with endoscopy. A surgical consult may be indicated for symptomatic ingestions past the esophagus. *(Tintinalli et al, 2000, pp. 530–531)*

50. **(E)** Small bowel obstruction (SBO) is most often due to adhesions following surgery. Incarcerated groin hernias are the second most common causes of SBO. Other hernias that are responsible for SBOs are umbilical, femoral, and obturator foramen. Less common causes

of SBOs are polyps, lymphoma, and adeno-carcinoma. Gallstone ileus is an unusual cause of intraluminal SBO. The most common cause of LBO is neoplasm. *(Tintinalli et al, 2000, pp. 539–540)*

51. **(C)** Pseudomembranous entercolitis is an inflammatory bowel disorder caused by *Clostridium difficile.* The disorder is associated with antibiotic use and is marked by membrane-like plaques of exudates that overlie and replace necrotic intestinal mucosa. The use of broad-spectrum antibiotics, notably clindamycin, cephalosporins, and ampicillin/amoxicillin, is a common cause of *C. difficile* colonization. The treatments of choice include supportive measures and antibiotics such as metronidazole and vancomycin. *(Tintinalli et al, 2000, pp. 553–554)*

52. **(B)** Thyroid storm is characterized by an abrupt, severe, exacerbation of hyperthyroidism. Hyperthyoidism (i.e., thyrotoxicosis, thyrotoxic crisis, and thyroid storm) all refer to varying degrees of thyroid hyperfunction. Common causes of thyroid storm include major stress (e.g., infection, surgery, DKA, myocardial infarction) in a patient with undiagnosed hyperthyroidism, and inadequate therapy in a hyperthyroid patient. Patients typically present with fever, anxiety, agitation, psychosis, hyperhidrosis, heat intolerance, weakness, muscle wasting, palpitations, diarrhea, and vomiting. Laboratory findings show an increased free T4 and/or a decreased TSH. Initial therapy is aimed at reducing the peripheral effects of thyroid hormone with beta-blockers such as propranolol 80 to 120 mg p.o. every 4 to 6 hours. The next objective in thyroid storm is to inhibit hormonal synthesis of thyroid by administering propylthiouracil (PTU) 400 to 600 mg initially, then 400 to 600 mg p.o. every 8 hours. Lastly, iodide is given to inhibit the release of stored thyroid hormone. Iodide is typically given as sodium iodide 250 mg IV every 6 hours or potassium iodide (SSKI), 5 gtt p.o. every 8 hours. Always administer PTU 1 hour before the iodide to prevent the oxidation of iodide and its incorporation in the synthesis of additional thyroid hormone. *(Marx, 2002, pp. 1773–1775)*

53. **(C)** Estimates of weight by age in years for children can follow these general parameters: 10 kg, 1 year old; 20 kg, 6 years old; 30 kg, 10 years old. Use crystalloid to rapidly replace at least 25% of the calculated blood volume (8% or 80 mL/kg and estimated weight) in pediatric patients. A bolus dose of 20 mL/kg (25% if 80 mL/kg) may be administered with an additional 20 mL/kg of crystalloid if signs of shock persist. *(Rosen, 1998, p. 364)*

54. **(A)** Nitrous oxide may be used for both sedation and analgesia in the emergency room, as long as it is mixed with at least 30% oxygen to prevent hypoxia. Therapeutic concentrations of nitrous oxide include those in the 30% to 50% range (maximum 70%). Concentrations below 30% may not be effective in this setting. Younger children (below 8 years old) may not gain therapeutic effect from nitrous oxide. *(Rosen, 1998, p. 306)*

55. **(A)** The most common causes of bacterial meningitis in the infants aged 0 to 4 weeks include group B streptococci, *Escherichia coli,* and *Listeria monocytogenes.* Pathogens comonly infecting infants 4 to 12 weeks include group B streptococci, *E. coli, L. monocytogenes, Haemophilus influenzae,* and *Streptococcus pneumoniae.* Pathogens infecting children and young adults 3 months through 17 years include *S. pneumoniae, Neisseria meningitidis,* and *H. influenzae.* Finally, likely pathogens in adults 18 years and older include *S. pneumoniae* and *N. meinigitidis. (Marx, 2002, pp. 2344–2350)*

56. **(B)** The first priority is resuscitation of the mother. A secure airway is very important because aspiration is common. Oxygen therapy is critical because of the reduced oxygen reserve and increased oxygen consumption in the mother. A trauma patient can quickly become hypoxic, making the fetus very vulnerable to any reduction in oxygen delivery. *(Rosen, 1998, p. 373)*

57. **(E)** Hypoglycemia is defined as a plasma glucose level less than 50 mg/dL; however, the criteria for the diagnosis should inlcude the presence of symptoms, low plasma glucose level in a symptomatic patient, and relief of

symptoms after ingestion of carbohydrates. Contributing factors to symptoms of hypoglycemia include the rate at which the glucose decreases, patient's overall size, underlying health conditions, and previous hypoglycemic reactions. A majority of the symptoms are the result of excessive secretion of epinephrine and CNS dysfunction. Common symptoms include anxiety, diaphoresis, tremors, tachycardia, palpitations, fatigue, syncope, headache, mental status changes, visual disturbances, and hemiplegia. Management of hypoglycemia depends partly on how awake and cooperative the patient is to take nutrition by mouth safely. If the patient is awake and cooperative, administer sugar-containing food or beverage. However, if the patient is unable to take by mouth safely, administer 25 to 75 g of glucose IV as D50W. The dose for children is 0.5 to 1.0 g/kg as D10W. If unable to obtain IV access, administer 1 to 2 mg of glucagon IM or SC. *(Marx, 2002, pp. 1748–1750)*

58. **(A)** Central retinal artery occlusion is characterized by visual loss when thrombus, thromboemboli, cholesterol plaque, calcium, or vasospasm interferes with the major blood supply to the retina. Typically, the patient presents with sudden, painless, monocular loss of vision. Physical exam findings include significant decrease in visual acuity, relative afferent pupillary defect (i.e., Marcus Gunn pupil), and a pale retina with a red spot that is visible on fundoscopic exam. Therapy is directed at reducing the intraocular pressure. Specific treatments include gentle massage of the globe to help force aqueous fluid into the canals of Schlemm, increasing the patient's pCO_2 to decrease vasospasm to the globe (i.e., rebreathing into a bag), carbonic anhydrase inhibitors and/or beta-blockers to decrease intraocular pressure, and anterior chamber paracentesis by an ophthalmologist. CRVO is characterized by painless vision loss of varying severity, slower onset of decreased vision than with arterial occlusion, retinal hemorrhages, cotton wool spots, and macular edema. In addition, CRVO is characterized by dilated retinal venous system consistent with a "squashed tomato" appearance of the

retina. Anterior uveitis includes iritis (inflammation that involves only the iris) and iridocyclitis (inflammation of both the iris and ciliary body). Common etiologies include infection, systemic diseases (i.e., sarcoidosis, lymes disease, ankylosing spondilitis, Reiter's syndrome, systemic lupus erythematosis, Sjogren's syndrome, interstitial nephritis), idiopathic, and trauma. Physical exam findings include ciliary flush (i.e., circumcorneal perilimbal injection of the episcleritis and scleral vessels) conjunctival injection and cells may be present in the anterior chamber. The pupil on the affected side is often small and irregular. Direct and consensual light reflex will cause pain on the affected side to increase. Retrobulbar hemorrhage causes pressure on the globe, which raises intraocular pressure. The high pressures decrease retinal artery perfusion, which results in retinal ischemia. The patient presents with decreased visual acuity, proptosis, and a dilated nonreactive pupil. Treatment includes measures to decrease intraocular pressure and lateral canthotomy. Optic neuritis is inflammation of the optic nerve. Common etiologies include multiple sclerosis, sarcoidosis, leukemia, recent viral illness, collagen vascular dieases, tuberculosis, and heavy metal intoxication. Treatment is directed at the underlying cause. *(Marx, 2002, pp. 910–921, 1195–1197; Yanoff, 2004, pp. 1209–1212)*

59. **(E)** Subdural hematomas are usually the result of venous bleeding, causing blood clots to form between the dura and the brain. The alcoholics and the elderly commonly develop brain atrophy, predisposing them to subdural hematomas. The most common mechanisms are acceleration–deceleration injuries, which usually cause the superficial bridging vessels to rupture. *(Rosen, 1998, p. 439)*

60. **(A)** Epidural hematomas are usually the result of arterial hemorrhage, causing blood clots to form between the inner table of the skull and the dura. Most are due to a direct impact against the skull, causing temporal and parietal bone fractures. Eighty percent are associated with lacerations to the middle meningeal artery or dural sinus. Classically,

the epidural hematoma presents with a head trauma, producing a decreased level of consciousness followed by a "lucid" interval. *(Rosen, 1998, pp. 437–438)*

61. **(C)** Subarachnoid hemorrhage caused by trauma is secondary to small tears of the subarachnoid vessels. Blood will collect within the CSF and meningeal intima. A CT scan will demonstrate increased density within the basilar cisterns, sulci, and interhemispheric fissures. *(Rosen, 1998, p. 441)*

62. **(D)** A subdural hygroma is formed by clear xanthochromic dural space fluid. Although the pathogenesis is unknown, it is thought to be from a tear in the arachnoid space that permits CSF to escape into the dural space. These effusions may collect when injured vessels increase the permeability of the meninges or the underlying parenchyma. *(Rosen, 1998, p. 441)*

63. **(B)** Intracerebral hematomas are the result of mechanical stretching and tearing of deep small-caliber arterioles of the brain. These mechanical forces usually are the result of the brain being propelled against irregular surfaces in the cranial vault. Most of the intracerebral hematomas are in the frontal and temporal lobes. The clinical effects of the intercerebral hemorrhage (ICH) will depend on factors such as size, location, and whether the bleeding is continuing. Most patients will have a loss of consciousness at the time of impact and subsequent ongoing changes in mental status. *(Rosen, 1998, p. 441)*

64. **(B)** Le Fort I fractures involve the maxilla at the level of the nasal bones. *(Rosen, 1998, pp. 457–458)*

65. **(A)** A Le Fort II fracture involves several facial bones, including the maxilla, the nasal bones, and the medial aspects of the orbits. *(Rosen, 1998, pp. 457–458)*

66. **(C)** A Le Fort III fracture involves the maxilla, zygoma, nasal bones, ethmoids, vomer, and lesser bones of the cranial base. It is described as a craniofacial dysfunction. *(Rosen, 1998, pp. 457–458)*

67. **(D)** Direct and compressive forces to the eye may cause a blow-out fracture to the orbital floor with herniation of the contents into the maxillary sinus. Blow-out fractures may produce enophthalmos, diplopia, impaired ocular motility, and infraorbital hypoesthesias. Many orbital floor fractures resolve spontaneously and only require close follow-up with consultants. A decision to operate may be delayed 10 to 14 days, depending on persistent diplopia or enophthalmos. *(Rosen, 1998, pp. 458–459)*

68. **(E)** An unstable, hyperextension fracture through the pedicles of C2 is known as a hangman's fracture. Fortunately, cord damage is usually minimal because the anteroposterior diameter of the neural canal is greatest at the C2 level. Furthermore, less neurological damage occurs because bilateral pedicle fractures tend to decompress themselves, allowing more space for the spinal cord. A Jefferson fracture of C1 is produced by an axial loading injury to the cervical spine, transmitting a force through the occipital condyles to the superior articular surfaces of the lateral masses of the atlas. A clay shoveler's fracture is an avulsion fracture of the spinous process of the lower cervical vertebrae. This oblique fracture of the base of the spinous process, classically C7, derived its name in the 1930s when Australian miners lifted a heavy shovelful of clay causing an abrupt flexion of the head, in opposition to the stabilizing force of the strong supraspinous muscle, resulting in an avulsion fracture of the spinous process. An extension teardrop fracture involves a hyperextension injury in which the anterior longitudinal ligament avulses the inferior portion of the anterior vertebral body at its insertion. The second cervical vertebra is the most common location for an extension teardrop fracture. *(Rosen, 1998, pp. 466–476)*

69. **(D)** The most severe neurological dysfunction, as a result of inadequate or delayed treatment of disk herniation, is cauda equina syndrome. The most common presenting symptoms are saddle anesthesia, bilateral leg pain, urinary incontinence or retention, and fecal incontinence or retention. Most cases of

cauda equina syndrome and cord compression develop over a matter of hours. If the symptoms are delayed, these patients are at high risk for chronic neurological deficits. *(Rosen, 1998, p. 897)*

70. **(A)** Acute narrow angle glaucoma is characterised by a sudden onset of severe pain localized to the affected eye. Common associated visual symptoms include halos around lights, blurriness, and scotomas. Other associated sypmptoms include nausea and vomiting. The primary pathophysiology of narrow angle glaucoma is a congenital narrowing of the anterior chamber. Therefore, certain conditions that narrow this angle may result in a significant rise in intraocular pressure. Situations such as entering a dark room and medications (mydriatics) results in pupillary dilatation and further narrowing the angle of the anterior chamber angle. The typical physical exam findings reveal a red eye with fixed, mid-dilated pupil, corneal clouding, and a shallow anterior chamber. The diagnosis is confirmed by demonstrating markedly elevated intraocular pressure in the range of 60 to 90 mm Hg (normal less than 21 mm Hg). Treatment of narrow angle glaucoma include (1) hyperosmotic agents such as glycerin 50%, isosorbide, mannitol 20%, (2) carbonic anhydrase inhibitors such as acetazolamide, (3) beta-blockers, (4) miotics topical, (5) corticosteriods topically, and (6) antiemetics. Anterior uveitis is inflammation of the anterior segment of the eye. Anterior uveitis includes iritis (inflammation that involves only the iris) and iridocyclitis (inflammation of both the iris and ciliary body). Common etiologies include infection, systemic diseases (i.e., sarcoidosis, lymes disease, ankylosing spondilitis, Reiter's syndrome, systemic lupus erythematosis, Sjogren's syndrome, interstitial nephritis), idiopathic, and trauma. Physical exam findings include ciliary flush (i.e., circumcorneal perilimbal injection of the episcleritis and scleral vessels) conjunctival injection and cells may be present in the anterior chamber. The pupil on the affected side is often small and irregular. Direct and consensual light reflex will cause pain on the affected side to increase. Orbital cellulits is a soft tissue infection that extends deep into the fascia and eye orbit. *Haemophelus influenzae* is found in over 50% of the cases. Approximately, 75% of patients with orbital cellulitis have recently had sinusitis, an upper respiratory infection, or otitis media. Clinical findings include ocular pain, limitation of eye movement, lid edema, proptosis, tenderness of the globe, decreased visual acuity, increased ocular pressure, and pupillary paralysis. Photopsia is the subjective sensation of sparks or flashes of light in retinal, optic, or brain diseases. Episcleritis is inflammation of the connective tissue between the sclera and conjunctiva. Episcleritis is a self-limiting condition where there is much less pain than scleritis. Episcleritis is commonly described as an irritation rather than a true pain. In addition, the orbital vessels blanch with topical neosynephrine. Most cases do not require treatment, however, some physicians elect to use topical steriods. *(Yanoff, 2004, pp. 511–512, 738–739, 1144–1148, 1209–1212, 1492–1496)*

71. **(D)** Henoch–Schonlein purpura is characterized by the triad of abdominal pain, arthritis, and nonthrombocytopenic purpura. This condition is typically immunologically mediated vasculitis by a stimulus that often cannot be identified. Occasionally, a drug or bacterial agent can be identified as the source. Approximately 75% of the cases are white males in the winter months between the ages of 2 to 11 years. Patients characteristically develop a slightly raised symmetrical petechial rash, which is most prominent on the lower extremities. In addition, patients develop colicky abdominal pain, bloody diarrhea, intussception, migratory large joint arthritis. Renal manifestations may present as in the form of hematuria proteinuria, and nephrosis. Therapy is directed at identifying and treating the underlying problem. Kawasaki's disease is an inflammatory vasculitis characterized by 5 days fever plus four out of five of the following criteria: conjuctival injection (bilateral), strawberry tongue and mouth fissures, desquamation and swelling of the fingers and toes, erythematous rash starting on the palms and soles, and enlarged lymph nodes. In addition, Kawasaki's disease is associated with

leukocytosis, increased erythematous seda-tion rate, increased IgE, anemia, and coronary artery aneurysms (20%). Treatment includes aspirin and IV gamma-globulin. Impetigo is a highly contagious skin infection caused by *Streptococcus pyogenes* or *Staphylococcus aureus*. Patients are typically preschool children or young adults with poor hygiene who present erythematous, moist facial vesicles with pain-less honey-crusted lesions. Erythema no-dosum is an inflammatory disease of the skin and subcutaneous tissue characterized by ten-der red nodules. Etiologies include bacterial infections (e.g., Streptococcus, Salmonella, *Neisseria gonorrhoeae*, *Mycobacterium tuberculo-sis*, Chlamydia), deep fungal infections (e.g., Histoplasmosis, coccidioidomycosis), viral diseases (e.g., mononucleosis), drugs (e.g., sulfonamides, oral contraceptives), and idio-pathic. The rash is described as multiple raised, warm, tender nodules with bluish dis-coloration that most commonly involves the pretibial region, however, the forearms or thighs may be involved as well. Therapy con-sists of bedrest, elevation of the extremity, and treatment of the underlying disorder. Pneumo-coccal meningitis does not typically present with a petechial rash or purpura. Meningococ-cemia is a capsulated Gram-negative diplococci that presents with 1 to 2 mm petechiae to full-blown ecchymoses. (*Marx, 2002, pp. 1616–1617, 1638–1639, 1805–1806, 2307, 2344–2350*)

72. **(C)** Temporal arteritis is a vasculitis usually occuring in the elderly involving the temporal and external carotid artery. Left untreated, temporal arteritis may result in bilateral blindness. Patients typically present with uni-lateral, excruciating, burning pain over the af-fected artery. The disease is often associated with polymyalgia rheumatica and may pres-ent with systemic involvement including fever, polymyalgia, malaise, weight loss, and anorexia. Patients complain of decreased vi-sual acuity and the exam reveals a tender, in-flammed temporal artery. Therapy consists of high-dose steroids that are tapered over a pe-riod of months. Acute narrow angle glaucoma is characterised by a sudden onset of severe pain localized to the affected eye. Common associated visual symptoms include halos around lights, blurriness, and scotomas. Other associated symptoms include nausea and vomiting. The primary pathophysiology of narrow angle glaucoma is a congenital nar-rowing of the anterior chamber. Therefore, certain conditions that narrow this angle may result in a significant rise in intraocular pres-sure. Situations such as entering a dark room and medications (mydriatics) results in pupil-lary dilatation and further narrowing the an-gle of the anterior chamber angle. Typical physical exam findings reveal a red eye with fixed, mid-dilated pupil, corneal clouding, and a shallow anterior chamber. The diagno-sis is confirmed by demonstrating markedly elevated intraocular pressure in the range of 60 to 90 mm Hg (normal less than 21 mm Hg). Treatment of narrow angle glaucoma include (1) hyperosmotic agents such as glycerin 50%, isosorbide, mannitol 20%, (2) carbonic anhy-drase inhibitors such as acetazolamide, (3) beta-blockers, (4) miotics topical, (5) corticos-teriods topically, and (6) antiemetics. Multiple sclerosis is a demylinating disease that affects the CNS and is characterized by recurrent at-tacks of focal and multifocal neurologic deficits. Multiple sclerosis may manifest as an optic neuritis, which is an inflammatory con-dition of the optic nerve. Optic neuritis typi-cally manifests as eye pain and visual impairment. Myasthenia gravis is character-ized by episodic muscle weakness caused by loss or dysfuction of acetylcholine receptors. Common symptoms related to ocular muscle involvement include ptosis, diplopia, and muscle fatigability after exercise. Viral en-cephalitis is an acute inflammatory disease of the brain caused by direct viral invasion (e.g., arbovirus, poliovirus, echovirus, coxsack-ievirus). Common symptoms include fever, malaise, headache, vomiting, stiff neck, seizures, and cranial nerve abnormalities. (*Marx, 2002, pp. 919–920, 1462, 1493–1495, 1522–1530*)

73. **(A)** Any patient who has sustained a pene-trating wound or blunt trauma to the thorax or upper abdomen should be suspected of hav-ing a diagnosis of pericardial tamponade. The most common signs of pericardial tamponade are hypotension and tachycardia-associated

elevation in central venous pressure. Beck's triad of pericardial tamponade consists of hypotension, distended neck veins, and distant heart sounds. A tension pneumothorax is an accumulation of air under pressure within the pleural cavity. The air under pressure shifts the mediastinum to the opposite hemithorax and compresses the contralateral lung and great vessels. A myocardial rupture refers to an acute traumatic perforation of the ventricles and atria. Acute myocardial rupture also includes rupture of the interventricular septum, pericardium, chordae, interatrial septum, and papillary muscles and valves. The most common vessel injured in an acute blunt trauma is the thoracic aorta. Deceleration injuries most commonly injure the thoracic aorta because the descending aorta is relatively fixed by the attachments of the intercostal arteries and ligamentous arteriosum. Myocardial contusion will usually demonstrate direct areas of hemorrhage in the anterior wall of the right ventricle and atria. *(Rosen, 1998, pp. 527–542)*

74. (B) Boerhaave's syndrome, postemetic rupture, and spontaneous esophageal rupture are synonymous terms. The most common site of injury is the distal esophagus, which demonstrates a longitudinal tear occurring in the left posterolateral aspect. Most cases occur in middle-aged males after they have indulged in food and alcohol. *(Rosen, 1998, p. 547)*

75. (E) One should proceed to a retrograde urethrogram before invasive interventions if there is any possibility of urethral disruption. Signs of urethral disruption include a high-riding prostate and the presence of blood at the tip of the meatus. Sixty milliliters (or 0.6 mL/kg) of full-strength or half-strength iothalmate meglumine (Conray II) is injected over 30 to 60 seconds. A radiograph is taken during the last 10 mL of contrast material. Retrograde flow through the urethra and into the bladder without extravasation ensures continuity of the urethra and absence of urethral injury. *(Rosen, 1998, pp. 584–585)*

76. (A) A penile rupture is a traumatic rupture of the corpus cavernosum when the tunica albuginea is torn. During vigorous sexual inter-

course, a patient commonly will hear a snapping sound followed by localized pain, detumescence, and slowly progressive penile hematoma. *(Tintinalli et al, 2000, p. 634)*

77. (B) Salter–Harris I fractures involve injuries to the site of the epiphyseal plate. It is most commonly a clinical diagnosis by evidence of tenderness and soft tissue swelling at the growth plate. Most radiographs are normal except for soft tissue swelling and occasionally widening of the epiphyseal space. Complications are rare. *(Rosen et al, 1992, pp. 200–201)*

78. (C) Salter–Harris II fractures are metaphyseal injuries that fracture into the epiphyseal plate. Complications rarely occur. *(Rosen et al, 1992, pp. 200–201)*

79. (E) Salter–Harris III fractures involve the epiphysis that extends into the articular surface. Growth disturbance complications may occur. *(Rosen et al, 1992, pp. 200–201)*

80. (A) Salter–Harris IV fractures are serious growth-disrupting injuries that extend through the epiphysis and metaphysis. Complications of growth disturbances are not uncommon. *(Rosen et al, 1992, pp. 200–201)*

81. (D) Salter–Harris V fractures involve crush injuries to the epiphyseal plate. Growth disturbances and complications commonly occur. *(Rosen et al, 1992, pp. 200–201)*

82. (C) Mallet finger is a disruption of the distal tendon resulting in a flexion deformity at the DIP. It is the most common zone I injury. *(Rosen, 1998, p. 654)*

83. (A) The developing bones of the child are more pliable and flexible than an adult mature bone. In a torus fracture, there is a buckling of the cortex of the bone without complete disruption of the cortical segment. Multiple radiographic views may be necessary to make the diagnosis in small nondisplaced fractures. *(Rosen et al, 1992, p. 175)*

84. (B) The most common nerve injured with a humeral shaft fracture is the radial nerve. The radial nerve runs in close proximity to the posterior midhumeral shaft. A radial nerve injury is evident by a wrist drop. *(Rosen, 1998, pp. 604–605)*

85. **(B)** A dislocation is described by comparing the most distal portion of the joint dislocated to the most proximal. The mechanism for a posterior elbow dislocation is a fall on an outstretched hand or wrist, the elbow being either extended or hyperextended at the time of impact. These patients hold the elbow in flexion at approximately 45° and have marked prominence of the olecranon. *(Rosen, 1998, p. 705)*

86. **(E)** Retropharyngeal abscess is a infected fluid collection in the fascial plane between the posterior pharyngeal muscles and the paraspinous muscles. Primarily, retropharyngeal abscess is a pediatric problem because there are lymph nodes in the retropharyngeal space that can become suppurative. Clinical manifestations include an ill-appearing child with fever, sore throat, neck pain, and voice changes (i.e.,"duck-like voice"). A CT scan with IV contrast of the soft tissues of the neck and upper chest is the best diagnostic test. Therapy is directed at airway stabilization, followed by incision and drainage in the operating room, and IV antibiotics. Peritonsillar abscess is an infected fluid collection in the pharyngeal pillar. The most common etiology is beta-hemolytic Streptococcus, but may also be *S. pneumoniae, H. influenzae,* Staphylococcus, and *Bacteroides fragilis.* Symptoms include fever, sore throat, and odynophagia. The throat pain is usually localized to one side. In addition, the patient drool and find it hard to handle his/her own secretions. Physical exam findings include trismus (i.e., spasm of the muscles of mastication) and pharyngeal pillar swelling that pushes the uvula to the opposite side of the abscess. Streptococcal pharyngitis is an infection of the pharynx and tonsils due to Group A Beta-hemolytic streptococci. Clinical features include sudden onset of fever and sore throat with enlargement of the cervical lymph nodes. Headache, vomiting, abdominal pain, meningismus, and torticollis can occur as well. Epiglottitis is an inflamma-

tory disorder of the supraglottic laryngeal region. Etiologies of epiglottitis include bacterias, viruses, chemical damage (e.g., aspiration of fuel), and mechanical damage (e.g., trauma, burns). The onset of symptoms is sudden with no history of prodromal upper respiratory tract infection. Symptoms include sore throat, fever, a muffled voice, dysphagia, and respiratory distress. Clinical features include drooling, dyspnea, tachypnea, inspiratory stridor, tripod position (i.e., patient leans forward, supporting himself/herself with both hands), and toxic appearance. Ludwig's angina is an abscess formation of the submaxillary, sublingual, and submental spaces accompanied by elevation of the tongue. The cause is due to an infection of the lower second and third molars usually due to beta-hemolytic streptococcus, staphylococcus, and mixed anaerobic and aerobic infections. Patients commonly present with swelling beneath the chin, which is often tense and brawny without fluctuance. The tongue is dislplaced up and posteriorly. In adddition, trismus often makes opening the mouth for exam difficult. Late presentation may cause significant airway compromise. *(Marx, 2002, pp. 972–980, 2249–2250)*

87. **(A)** The most common mechanism of injury for an anterior shoulder dislocation is abduction and external rotation. The lateral edge of the acromion process is prominent and the arm is held in slight abduction and external rotation by the opposite extremity. Anterior shoulder dislocations account for 95% to 97% of all glenohumeral dislocations. *(Rosen, 1998, pp. 726–727)*

88. **(B)** The class of prescription medications responsible for the most drug-related deaths is TCAs. The clinical toxicity is due to the complex pharmacologic activity, low therapeutic index, and general availability. The clinical toxicity is quite variable, ranging from mild antimuscarinic activity to severe cardiotoxicity. *(Tintinalli et al, 2000, pp. 1063–1066)*

89. **(C)** Patients with ethylene glycol ingestion usually present with an acute change in mental status, high anion gap metabolic acidosis,

osmolar gap, and calcium oxalate crystals in the urine. Ethylene glycol is commercially available as preservatives, glycerine substitutes, and antifreeze. Ethylene glycol may be ingested in suicide attempts, accidentally by children, and by alcoholics as an alcohol substitute. The toxic metabolites formed by ethylene glycol metabolism are primarily formaldehyde, formic acid, and oxalic acid. *(Tintinalli et al, 2000, pp. 1103–1107)*

90. **(D)** Treatment priorities of acetaminophen toxicity consist of supportive care, gastrointestinal decontamination, and the use of the antidote *N*-acetylcysteine (NAC). If given early (less than 8 hours after ingestion), NAC can prevent toxicity by inhibiting the binding of the toxic metabolite *N*-acetyl-*p*-benzoquinoneimine to hepatic proteins. In acetaminophen toxicity, more than 24 hours after ingestion, NAC diminishes hepatic necrosis by nonspecific mechanisms. The standard 72-hour oral NAC regimen used in the United States is a loading dose of 140 mg/kg followed by maintenance doses of 70 mg/kg every 4 hours for 17 doses. *(Tintinalli et al, 2000, pp. 1125–1129)*

91. **(D)** Periorbital cellulitis is characterized by warmth, redness, swelling, and tenderness over the affected eye, along with conjunctival injection, eyelid swelling, chemosis, and fever. Orbital cellulitis includes all the symptoms of periorbital (preseptal) cellulitis with the addition of ocular pain and limitation of eye movement. Other physical exam findings may include lid edema, proptosis, marked tenderness to the globe, decreased visual acuity, and pupillary paralysis. *(Marx, 2002, pp. 1945–1949)*

92. **(D)** Isopropyl alcohol (isopropanol), commonly referred to as rubbing alcohol, is a solvent and disinfectant used in many household items such as hair and skin products, antifreeze, and window cleaning solutions. The toxic dose is 1 mL/kg of a 70% solution. Isopropanol is metabolized to acetone. Mild acidosis may occur due to the formation of acetate and formate. Clinical features include CNS depression, acetone

smell on the breath, intoxication, dizziness, headache, confusion, abdominal pain, nausea, vomiting, hypotension, tachycardia, and respiratory depression. This toxicity is associated with a high serum and urine ketone level, however, there is not an increased osmolal gap or anion gap acidosis. Therapy consists of airway management, mechanical ventilation (if necessary), cardiovascular resuscitation, intravenous hydration, and supportive care. Hemodialysis is only indicated for patients with uncorrectable hypotension, deep coma, deteriorating vital signs, and isopropanol levels greater than 400 to 500 mg/dL. Methanol, also referred to as wood alcohol, is commonly used in products such as solvents, antifreeze, windshield washer fluid, Sterno canned heat, paints remover, and varnishes. The lethal ingested dose is approximately 15 to 30 mL in adults. Methanol is oxidized in the liver to formaldehyde and formate, which produces a severe lactic acidosis. These metabolites concentrate in the vitreous humor and optic nerve, causing ocular toxicity and blindness. Clinical manifestations include CNS depression, intoxication, headache, vertigo, confusion, blurred vision, decreased visual acuity ("snowstorm" effect), dilated minimally responsive pupils, retinal edema, and hyperemia of the optic disc. This toxicity is associated with a osmolal gap and an anion gap acidosis, but no ketosis. DKA is a disorder found in insulin dependent patients that is characterized by hyperglycemia, ketonemia, and acidosis. Serum glucose levels are typically greater than 300 mg/dL. Metabolic acidosis is demonstrated by a serum bicarbonate concentration of less than 15 meq/L and a pH of less than 7.2. Ketonemia results from beta-hydroxybutyrate and acetoacetate. This toxicity results in an anion gap acidosis, a ketotic state, but no osmolal gap. Alcoholic ketoacidosis is typically seen in alcoholic patients who are forced to stop drinking shortly after a drinking binge. Beta-hydroxybutyric acid is the predominant ketone formed in alcoholic ketoacidosis. A metabolic acidosis may occur from vomiting, dehydration, and respiratory alkalosis. Therefore, this toxicity is characterized by an anion gap acidosis and a high ketone level, but an osmolal gap will not be seen. (*Marx, 2002, pp. 1750–1751, 2127–2137, 2524*)

93. **(C)** Mild hypothermia is defined as a temperature from 32°C to 35°C (89.6°F to 95°F). In mild hypothermia, the body responds by increasing metabolic activity to produce heat. This is known as the excitation or responsive phase. When the temperature drops below 32°C (89.6°F), bodily functions slow down, giving way to the adynamic phase. As metabolism slows, there is a decrease in both oxygen utilization and carbon dioxide production. As the body temperature falls below 30°C to 32°C (86°F to 89.6°F), shivering will cease. Hypothermia may induce life-threatening dysrhythmias and ECG changes. A characteristic, but not pathognomonic, ECG finding in hypothermia is the Osborne (J) wave. This abnormal wave is a slow, positive deflection at the end of the QRS complex. (*Tintinalli et al, 2000, pp. 1231–1233*)

94. **(A)** The black widow spider (Latrodectus) is found in many areas of the United States. Its bite produces immediate pain and pinprick sensations that soon encompass the entire extremity. Erythema of the bite area develops usually within 1 hour and in about half of the cases quickly evolves into a target pattern. Patients frequently complain of cramp-like spasms in the large muscle groups. The physical exam rarely exhibits muscle rigidity, and serum creatine kinase concentrations usually are not elevated significantly. The brown recluse (*Loxosceles*) spider bites are difficult to identify. The bite lesion is usually mildly erythematous and may become firm and heal with little scarring over several days to weeks. Occasionally, the lesion may become necrotic over 3 to 4 days with subsequent eschar formation. The hobo spider (*Tegenaria*) usually causes a painless local reaction similar to that of the brown recluse spider. Blisters eventually develop that rupture, leaving an encrusted cratered wound. A tarantula bite typically causes pain and local swelling at the site. Treatment consists of local wound care. Scorpions (Scorpionida) present with a multitude of local and systemic manifestations. Some of these manifestations include pain,

paresthesia, cranial nerve and somatic motor dysfunction, uncontrolled jerking, restlessness, pharyngeal incoordination, and respiratory compromise. (*Tintinalli et al, 2000, pp. 1244–1250*)

95. **(E)** The three principles of treatment regarding AMS are (1) to stop the ascent, (2) to descend to lower altitude, and (3) to treat immediately in the presence of change in normal mental status, ataxia, or pulmonary edema. Emergent treatments include oxygen, acetazolamide, nifedipine, dexamethasone, hyperbaric therapy, and continuous positive airway pressure. (*Tintinalli et al, 2000, pp. 1263–1267*)

96. **(B)** The answer is 44% burn. The rule of nines to estimate percentage of burns is as follows: head 9%, anterior trunk 18%, posterior trunk 18%, each leg 18%, each arm 9%, and perineum 1%. (*Tintinalli et al, 2000, p. 1282*)

97. **(E)** Hemophilias A and B are X-linked recessive disorders that are deficiencies in factor VIII and factor IX, respectively. Approximately 85% of patients with hemophilia have hemophilia A. Severity of the disorder depends on the level of factor deficiency. Common clinical findings include hemarthroses, soft tissue bleeding, muscular hematomas, and intracranial bleeding. Intracranial bleeding is the leading cause of death in people with hemophilia. (*Marx, 2002, pp. 1694–1697*)

98. **(D)** An L4 injury causes weakness or paralysis to the quadriceps and thigh adductor muscles, sensory loss to the medial leg, and loss of patellar reflexes. (*Marx, 2002, pp. 1496–1498*)

99. **(E)** Digoxin is the most common digitalis prepararion in the United States. Ingestion of 0.05 mg/kg of digoxin can produce toxic levels. Digoxin toxicity results in enhanced excitability and contractility in myocardial muscle, and decreased conduction velocity in conduction tissue. Therapy is directed at airway management, cardiovascular resiscitation, and continous cardiac monitoring. Ventricular ectopy is treated with lidocaine or phenytoin and symptomatic bradycardia is treated with atropine. Antidote treatment is with digoxin-specific antibiodies, which consist of Fab fragments that bind digoxin, removing it from cardiac receptors and reversing toxicity. Indications include life-threatening dysrhythmias, a serum potassium level greater than 5.0 meq/L, a serum digoxin level greater than 10 to 15 ng/mL, and advanced age. (*Marx, 2002, pp. 2103–2108*)

100. **(B)** Wernicke's encephalopathy is a potentially fatal neurologic disorder, found in alcoholics with poor nutritional status, that is caused by chronic vitamin B_6 deficiency. Alcoholism interferes with gastrointestinal absorption of vitamin B_6 and impairs conversion of vitamin B_6 to its active metabolite. In many patients, concomitant liver disease impairs storage of vitamin B_6. The administration of glucose to an alcoholic patient with an inadequate supply of thiamine may precipitate this disorder. Clinical features inlcude the triad of abnormal mental status, ophthalmoplegia, and gait ataxia. Patients are often disoriented, forgetful, and unable to recognize familiar objects. With prompt therapy, the ophthalmoplegia usually resolves within hours and the coma resolves in hours to days, but the memory deficit may never resolve. Thiamine 100 mg administered intravenously is the treatment of choice. Thiamine 100 mg intravenously is continued daily until the patient has achieved proper oral nutritional status. It is essential that thiamine be given prior to the administration of glucose. (*Marx, 2002, pp. 1469–1476*)

REFERENCES

Tintinalli JE, Kelen GD, Stapczynski JS. *Emergency Medicine: A Comprehensive Study Guide*, 5th ed. New York: McGraw-Hill; 2000.

Cummins R, American Heart Association. *Textbook of Advanced Cardiac Life Support–Emergency Cardiovascular Care Programs*. 1999.

Braunwald E, ACC/AHA Practice Guidelines for the Management of Patients With Unstable Angina and Non-ST-Segment Elevation Myocardial Infarction: Executive Summary and Recommendations. *Circulation*. 102:1193–1209, 2000.

Drug Facts and Comparisons 53rd. *Facts and Comparisons;* 1999.

Marx R.S. *Rosen's Emergency Medicine: Concepts and Clinical Practice*, 5th ed. Mosby; 2002.

Rosen P, Doris P, Barkin S, Barkin R, Markovick V. *Diagnostic Radiology in Emergency Medicine*. St. Louis: Mosby; 1992.

Goldman. *Cecil Textbook of Medicine*, 22nd ed. Saunders; 2004, pp. 2301–2304.

Rosen P. *Emergency Medicine, Concepts and Clinical Practice*. St. Louis: Mosby; 1998.

Diethelm AG, Stanley RJ. The acute abdomen. In Sabiston DS (ed), *Textbook in Surgery*. Philadelphia, PA: Saunders; 1991: 736–755.

Yanoff M. *Opthalmology*, 2nd ed. Mosby; 2004.

Ferri F.F. *Ferri's Clinical Advisor: Instant Diagnosis and Treatment*. St. Louis, MO: Mosby; 2005.

Noble J. *Textbook of Primary Care Medicine*, 3rd ed., St. Louis, MO: Mosby; 2001.

CHAPTER 14

General and Vascular Surgery
Questions

Frank Acevedo, MS, PA-C, and Michel Statler, MLA, PA-C

DIRECTIONS (Questions 1 through 85): Each of the numbered items or incomplete statements in this section is followed by answers or by completions of the statement. Select the ONE lettered answer or completion that is BEST in each case.

Questions 1 through 85

1. Which of the following is associated with worsening hyponatremia due to excess infusion of hypotonic fluid in a postoperative patient?

    (A) oliguria
    (B) paralytic ileus
    (C) cardiac irritability
    (D) hepatic encephalopathy
    (E) central nervous system dysfunction

2. What is the most common cause of fever for a postoperative patient in the first 48 hours following surgery?

    (A) wound infection
    (B) atelectasis
    (C) urinary retention
    (D) bacteremia
    (E) anesthetic reaction

3. Which pulmonary function parameter is the most helpful in predicting potential postoperative complications, including the inability to wean from ventilatory support?

    (A) tidal volume
    (B) functional residual capacity
    (C) expiratory reserve volume
    (D) closing volume
    (E) forced expiration volume/one second

4. A 44-year-old obese white female is noted to have a paralytic ileus and muscle weakness on postoperative day 3. What is the most likely cause of her symptoms?

    (A) hypokalemia
    (B) hypochloremia
    (C) hyponatremia
    (D) hypocalcemia
    (E) hyperkalemia

5. What is the best choice of intravenous fluids for a patient with gastric losses due to prolonged nasogastric aspiration?

    (A) lactated Ringer's with 20 meq KCl/L
    (B) 5% dextrose water with 20 meq KCl/L
    (C) 5% dextrose with 0.5% normal saline with 20 meq KCl/L
    (D) 5% dextrose with 0.9% normal saline with 20 meq KCl/L
    (E) 0.9% normal saline with 20 meq KCl/L

6. What complication is seen with too rapid administration of intrajejunal feedings via a continuous infusion pump?

(A) vomiting
(B) gastric reflux
(C) aspiration of feedings
(D) gastric retention
(E) hyperperistalsis and diarrhea

7. In addition to fingerstick glucose monitoring, what additional testing is important to prevent postoperative complications in the diabetic patient?

(A) serum potassium
(B) urinary ketones
(C) serum osmolality
(D) urinary protein
(E) serum sodium

8. A 35-year-old male is postoperative day 4 status post exploratory laparotomy for a gunshot wound to the abdomen. At the time of exploration, a perforation to the left colon was found and he underwent repair with proximal colostomy. He now is confused, agitated, and has developed oliguria over the past 8 hours. His vital signs are temperature 104°F, respiratory rate 24/min, heart rate 134/min, blood pressure 85/60. What type of shock is most likely in this situation?

(A) hypovolemic
(B) cardiogenic
(C) septic
(D) neurogenic
(E) obstructive

9. A 22-year-old male is brought to the emergency department by emergency medical service after having sustained a single stab wound to the right chest in the fourth intercostal space at the right sternal border. While attempting to resuscitate the patient he becomes hypotensive with marked jugular venous distension. Auscultation of the chest reveals moderately diminished breath sounds on the right side with muffled heart sounds. The most appropriate initial intervention is

(A) right tube thoracostomy
(B) pericardiocentesis
(C) fluid resuscitation
(D) immediate intubation
(E) emergency open thoracotomy

10. A 32-year-old female presents to the surgical clinic with a fluctuant mass of her left breast. The area directly above the lesion is erythematous, warm to touch, and localized point tenderness is present. You make the diagnosis of localized breast abscess. What is the most likely organism?

(A) *Staphylococcus aureus*
(B) *Streptococcus viridens*
(C) blastomycosis
(D) *Pseudomonas aeuriginosa*
(E) *Escherichia coli*

11. Which of the following findings is indicative of increased intracranial pressure from an associated closed head injury?

(A) hypotension, bradycardia, and tachypnea
(B) hypertension, bradycardia, and bradypnea
(C) hypotension, tachycardia, and tachypnea
(D) hypertension, tachycardia, and tachypnea
(E) hypotension, tachycardia, and bradypnea

12. The most common type of gallstone in the United States is

(A) mixed
(B) calcium
(C) brown pigmented
(D) black pigmented
(E) cholesterol

13. Which population has the highest incidence of gallstones in this country?

(A) Caucasian women under the age of 50 years
(B) Caucasian women over the age of 50 years
(C) Hispanic men over the age of 50 years
(D) African-American men under the age of 50 years
(E) Native American women before the age of 60 years

14. Which of the following best describes the underlying pathology of acute cholecystitis?

    (A) intermittent obstruction of the cystic duct without inflammation
    (B) sustained obstruction of the cystic duct with inflammation
    (C) obstruction of the common bile duct without inflammation
    (D) obstruction of the common bile duct with inflammation

15. A 63-year-old white male is seen in the ambulatory outpatient clinic with complaints of midepigastric pain, weight loss, and jaundice. On examination you find his sclerae are icteric. On palpation of the abdomen you find a distended nontender gallbladder. What is the most likely diagnosis?

    (A) gastric carcinoma
    (B) chronic pancreatitis
    (C) acute cholecystitis
    (D) pancreatic carcinoma
    (E) choledocholithiasis

16. What are the expected findings on an abdominal ultrasound that are consistent with choledocholithiaisis?

    (A) pericholecystic fluid
    (B) thickened gallbladder wall
    (C) dilated hepatic ducts
    (D) air in the lumen of the gallbladder

17. A 46-year-old African-American male is seen in the emergency room with upper right quadrant pain that radiates to the right infrascapular area. The pain is colicky and was precipitated by a meal of fried fish and fried potatoes. What is the initial study of choice for this patient?

    (A) plain abdominal x-ray
    (B) ultrasonography
    (C) radionuclide scan (HIDA scan)
    (D) computerized tomography
    (E) oral cholecystogram

18. Which organ is most commonly injured as result of blunt abdominal trauma?

    (A) liver
    (B) spleen
    (C) kidney
    (D) pancreas
    (E) colon

19. A 73-year-old jaundiced female is noted to have a posthepatic obstruction on ultrasound. What is the best test to evaluate the level of obstruction and type of pathology present?

    (A) plain abdominal x-ray
    (B) radionuclide scan (HIDA scan)
    (C) computerized tomography
    (D) oral cholecystogram
    (E) intravenous cholangiography

20. A 58-year-old man presents with the acute onset of abdominal pain associated with fever and shaking chills. The patient is hypotensive and febrile with a temperature of 102.2°F. Although he is confused and disoriented, he complains of right upper quadrant pain during palpation of the abdomen. His sclerae are icteric and the skin is jaundiced. What is the most likely diagnosis?

    (A) biliary colic
    (B) acute cholecystitis
    (C) choledocholithiais
    (D) acute pancreatitis
    (E) ascending cholangitis

21. A 43-year-old Native Indian female presents with a 3-month history of recurrent episodes of right upper quadrant pain that occur a few hours after eating. The episodes are associated with dyspepsia but no fever or chills. Ultrasound is consistent with cholelithiasis. What is the treatment of choice for this patient?

    (A) follow-up ultrasound in 6 months
    (B) ERCP with sphincterotomy
    (C) laparascopic cholecystectomy
    (D) extracorporeal shock wave lithotripsy
    (E) percutaneous transhepatic cholangiogram and stone extraction

22. A 54-year-old male presents to the emergency department with a complaint of severe epigastric pain radiating to the back. The pain has been present for the past 8 hours and is associated with nausea and vomiting which has not relieved the pain. Laboratory data reveal a WBC of 14,000/mm^3, and a serum amylase of 500 U/L (reference range 0 to 286 U/L). The most likely diagnosis is

    (A) bleeding duodenal ulcer
    (B) cholecystitis
    (C) acute pancreatitis
    (D) ischemic colitis
    (E) renal colic

23. Patients with acute pancreatitis may present with varying degrees of severity. In order to triage patients appropriately, what is the most commonly used scale of prognostic indicators?

    (A) Charcot's triad
    (B) Ranson's criteria
    (C) Glasgow scale
    (D) Child–Turcotte classification
    (E) Reynold's pentad

24. A 54-year-old male is diagnosed with chronic pancreatitis. Of the following complications which is most commonly seen in association with this diagnosis?

    (A) respiratory insufficiency
    (B) disseminated intravascular coagulopathy
    (C) necrosis of the gland
    (D) renal insufficiency
    (E) pancreatic pseudocyst

25. Which physical exam finding is associated with Courvoisier's sign?

    (A) periumbilical ecchymosis
    (B) left shoulder pain with left upper quadrant palpation
    (C) palpable, nontender gallbladder
    (D) flank ecchymosis
    (E) inspiratory arrest on palpation of the abdomen

26. What is an appropriate screening test for hepatocellular carcinoma in patients with cirrhosis?

    (A) alkaline phosphatase
    (B) alpha-fetoprotein
    (C) transaminases
    (D) total and fractionated bilirubin
    (E) carcinoembryonic antigen

27. A 48-year-old male alcoholic presents to the emergency department with a complaint of increasing abdominal girth for the past 2 months. Physical examination reveals caput medusa, palmar erythema, gynecomastia, and spider angiomata. Percussion of the abdomen reveals shifting dullness with a positive fluid wave. There is no respiratory distress and the vital signs are otherwise stable. The best initial management of this patient would be

    (A) gastroenterology consult for endoscopy
    (B) surgical consult for portocaval shunt
    (C) abdominal paracentesis
    (D) transjugular intrahepatic portosystemic shunt
    (E) diuretics and sodium restriction

28. What is the most important factor in determining overall survival rates for patients with breast cancer?

    (A) tumor size
    (B) estrogen receptor status
    (C) tumor histology
    (D) axillary lymph node status

29. Chronic intestinal ischemia is most likely to have abdominal pain that is associated with

    (A) guarding and rigidity
    (B) fear of eating
    (C) nausea and vomiting
    (D) bloody diarrhea
    (E) positive obturator and psoas signs

30. What features are commonly associated with lower extremity ulcers that are due to chronic arterial insufficiency?

(A) ulcers are associated with hyperpigmentation changes in the skin

(B) ulcers are most commonly seen around the medial and lateral malleoli

(C) ulcers have a "punched out" appearance with a pale or necrotic base

(D) ulcers are associated with painless lower extremity edema

31. A 22-year-old obese white female is seen with a complaint of a mass in the upper outer quadrant of the left breast. The lesion is smooth, firm, and freely movable, approximately 3 cm in size. The most likely diagnosis is

(A) breast cyst

(B) lipoma of the breast

(C) fibroadenoma

(D) Paget's disease of the breast

(E) fibrocystic disease of the breast

32. Using the TNM (tumor, nodes, metastasis) staging system for breast cancer, how would you classify a lesion that measured greater than 5 cm with suspicious nodes that were fixed to each?

(A) stage I

(B) stage IIA

(C) stage IIB

(D) stage IIIA

(E) stage IIIB

33. What is the most common pathogen associated with postsplenectomy sepsis?

(A) *Staphylococcus aureus*

(B) *Streptococcus pneumoniae*

(C) *Escherichia coli*

(D) *Pseudomonas aeroginosa*

(E) *Proteus mirabilis*

34. What is the most common type of hernia affecting both sexes and all age groups?

(A) direct inguinal hernia

(B) indirect inguinal hernia

(C) femoral hernia

(D) umbilical hernia

(E) incisional hernia

35. Which symptom associated with an acute arterial occlusion to the lower extremities is most associated with the time of occlusion?

(A) pain

(B) pallor

(C) paresthesias

(D) paralysis

(E) pulselessness

36. A 62-year-old male presents to the office concerned about an abdominal aortic aneurysm (AAA). He states that his father died from one at the age of 50 and his brother was diagnosed last week with an AAA. What is the most appropriate screening tool in this situation?

(A) abdominal radiograph

(B) computerized tomography (CT)

(C) palpation

(D) ultrasound

(E) aortography

37. A 56-year-old female presents to the office with complaint of left lower extremity pain, particularly at night. She states that she can ambulate six to eight blocks without difficulty. Examination reveals a 3 × 4 cm ulceration on the medial aspect of her left lower leg, proximal to the medial malleolus. The ulcer base is erythematous with good granulation tissue and it is surrounded by a border of induration. Varicosities are identified along the distribution of the greater saphenous vein. These findings are most likely due to

(A) arteriosclerosis

(B) diabetes mellitus

(C) scleroderma

(D) venous stasis

(E) deep venous thrombosis

38. A 66-year-old male, with a 20-year history of hypertension and 80 pack-year smoking history, presents with progressive claudication affecting both lower extremities. Recently, he has begun to waken at night with leg pain. What would be the expected ankle/brachial index for this patient?

(A) greater than 1.0

(B) 0.8 to 1.0

(C) 0.6 to 0.8

(D) 0.4 to 0.6

(E) less than 0.4

39. What is the most common site of an acute arterial occlusion due to embolic disease?

(A) iliac artery

(B) aortic bifurcation

(C) mesenteric arteries

(D) femoral artery

(E) popliteal artery

40. A 50-year-old male presents with persistent hypertension that has been difficult to control with medications. On exam, there is evidence of hypertensive retinopathy on fundoscopic exam and bilateral flank bruits. What is the most common cause of renovascular hypertension?

(A) atherosclerosis

(B) fibromuscular dysplasia

(C) renal artery dissection

(D) cardiac emboli

(E) renal artery aneurysm

41. A 52-year-old male presented with the acute onset of severe abdominal pain that was aggravated by the ride to the hospital. The patient reported a prior history of a "gnawing type" of epigastric pain that was previously relieved with antacids. On exam, there was generalized abdominal pain with rebound and guarding. What is an expected radiographic finding unique to this clinical presentation?

(A) evidence of gastric distension on an abdominal plain film

(B) filling defect extending beyond the gastric lumen on upper gastrointestinal series

(C) pneumoperitoneum seen on upright chest radiograph

(D) fixed deformity projecting into the gastric lumen on upper gastrointestinal series

42. A 54-year-old male with recurrent duodenal ulcer disease has a 2-week history of repeated vomiting of ingested food and fluids. A UGI confirms the presence of gastric outlet obstruction. What type of metabolic disturbance is most likely associated with this diagnosis?

(A) hypochloremic, hypokalemic metabolic alkalosis

(B) hyperchloremic, hyponatremic metabolic acidosis

(C) hypochloremic, hyponatremic metabolic alkalosis

(D) hyperchloremic, hyperkalemic metabolic alkalosis

(E) hypochloremic, hypocalcemic metabolic acidosis

43. What is the most sensitive and specific diagnostic radiographic test used in the evaluation of acute appendicitis?

(A) plain film of the abdomen

(B) barium enema

(C) ultrasound

(D) spiral CT scan

(E) magnetic resonance imaging (MRI)

44. While there are multiple options for the surgical repair of an inguinal hernia, what is the primary benefit associated with mesh repairs?

(A) decreased postoperative pain

(B) early return to work

(C) reduced risk of recurrence

(D) decreased risk of surgical complications

45. What type of complication is seen with an injury to the ilioinguinal nerve during a hernia repair?

   (A) impotency
   (B) ischemic orchitis
   (C) urinary incontinence
   (D) numbness on the medial aspect of the scrotum

46. A 6-year-old female presents to the emergency department with abdominal distention of 1-day duration. She has not had a bowel movement or passed flatus in 72 hours. Examination reveals markedly diminished bowel sounds with tympany to percussion. She has also passed bloody mucus from her rectum. There is no evidence of hernia and past surgical history is negative. The most likely cause of her clinical picture is

   (A) adhesions
   (B) diverticulitis
   (C) pyloric stenosis
   (D) Meckel's diverticulum
   (E) colon carcinoma

47. Which are the most common symptoms of Crohn's disease?

   (A) abdominal pain, diarrhea, and weight loss
   (B) diarrhea, anorectal lesions, and fever
   (C) weight loss, fever, and vomiting
   (D) abdominal pain, constipation, and fever
   (E) abdominal distention, hemorrhoids, and constipation

48. A 45-year-old male presents with progressive painless dysphagia and regurgitation of undigested food. The patient has tried drinking large amounts of fluids with meals in an attempt to wash down his food. What is the most likely diagnosis?

   (A) achalasia
   (B) esophageal leiomyoma
   (C) reflux esophagitis
   (D) esophageal carcinoma

49. What is the characteristic finding seen on a contrast study of the esophagus for a patient diagnosed with achalasia?

   (A) string sign
   (B) apple core lesion
   (C) bird beak deformity
   (D) lead pipe deformity

50. A patient presents with abdominal distension associated with nausea and vomiting. Which of the following is consistent with a paralytic ileus?

   (A) crampy abdominal pain
   (B) hyperactive bowel sounds
   (C) obstipation and failure to pass flatus
   (D) gas in small intestine only on KUB (kidney, ureter, bladder)

51. What is the first priority in the management of a proven or suspected small bowel obstruction?

   (A) correction of fluid and electrolyte abnormalities
   (B) surgery at the earliest opportunity
   (C) relief of the obstruction
   (D) conducting barium radiograph studies
   (E) further confirmation of diagnosis with supportive laboratory data

52. A 54-year-old male undergoes repair of an abdominal aortic aneurysm. At the time of surgery the inferior mesenteric artery is found to be thrombosed and is not reimplanted. The left hemicolon is observed to be viable at the completion of surgery with good pulsations of the arterial arcade. This finding is possible because of which vascular structure?

   (A) ileocolic artery
   (B) left colic artery
   (C) middle colic artery
   (D) superior rectal artery
   (E) marginal artery of Drummond

53. A 64-year-old male has been experiencing signs and symptoms compatible with diverticular disease for the past 3 weeks. He now presents to the emergency department malnourished with severe left-sided lower abdominal pain. After appropriate workup and hydration, he is taken to the operating room where a perforated sigmoid colon is discovered with gross contamination. What is the most appropriate surgical intervention at this time?

    (A) left colectomy with primary anastomosis
    (B) Hartmann's procedure
    (C) proctocolectomy
    (D) abdominoperineal resection
    (E) low anterior resection

54. What is the most common fistula that develops as a consequence of colonic diverticular disease?

    (A) colovaginal
    (B) colovesicular
    (C) coloenteric
    (D) colocutaneous

55. The most common cause of massive lower gastrointestinal bleeding is

    (A) hemorrhoids
    (B) colon cancer
    (C) diverticular disease
    (D) upper gastrointestinal hemorrhage
    (E) Meckel's diverticulum

56. In order to make the diagnosis of "complicated diverticulitis" which of the following clinical manifestations should be present?

    (A) advanced patient age
    (B) fever
    (C) left lower quadrant pain and tenderness
    (D) bleeding
    (E) abscess formation

57. What is the best advice you can give a patient to decrease the incidence of diverticular disease?

    (A) to lose weight
    (B) to obtain yearly colonoscopy
    (C) to obtain yearly fecal occult blood testing
    (D) to eat a diet high in fiber
    (E) to use stool softeners on a regular basis

58. Which type of colon polyp should be treated by surgical excision because of a high risk of malignant degeneration?

    (A) hamartoma
    (B) hyperplastic
    (C) inflammatory
    (D) tubular
    (E) villous

59. Annual colonoscopic screening in patients with familial adenomatous polyposis (FAP) should begin at what age if the adenomatosis polyposis coli (APC) gene is present?

    (A) 10
    (B) 24
    (C) 34
    (D) 44
    (E) 50

60. What is the most important risk factor in the development of colon cancer?

    (A) dietary content
    (B) inflammatory bowel disease
    (C) age
    (D) cigarette smoking
    (E) hereditary

61. Colorectal carcinoma is most commonly spread through which mechanism?

    (A) veins
    (B) regional lymphatics
    (C) contiguous organ involvement
    (D) distant metastasis

62. An 82-year-old female presents to the office with a complaint of right lower quadrant pain, a 15-pound weight loss over the past month, and fatigue. Examination reveals conjunctival pallor, and a palpable mass in the right lower quadrant. These findings are most compatible with

(A) gastric carcinoma

(B) cecal carcinoma

(C) acute appendicitis

(D) primary hepatoma

(E) pancreatric carcinoma

63. A 56-year-old male is diagnosed with a carcinoma of the sigmoid colon by colonoscopy. As part of the preoperative evaluation for distant metastasis which of the following tests should be performed?

(A) carcinoembryonic antigen level

(B) CT of the chest

(C) endorectal ultrasound

(D) CT scan of the abdomen

(E) bone scan

64. A 63-year-old female undergoes a minimilly invasive surgical approach utilizing laparoscopy to electively resect a sigmoid carcinoma. Of the following which has been shown to occur in association with this approach?

(A) inadequate tumor resection margins

(B) inadequate resection of acceptable number of lymph nodes

(C) increased hospital stay

(D) tumor recurrences at the port sites

(E) increased mortality when compared to other procedures

65. What is the classic radiographic barium enema finding associated with sigmoid colon cancer?

(A) apple core lesion

(B) string sign

(C) haustral sign

(D) skip lesions

(E) lead pipe sign

66. A 56-year-old female has had a left hemicolectomy for resection of an adenocarcinoma of the colon. Pathology reveals that the lesion has penetrated into but not through the muscularis propia of the bowel wall. Positive lymph nodes are also identified. According to the Duke's classification with the Astler–Coller modification what stage is this lesion?

(A) stage A

(B) stage B1

(C) stage B2

(D) stage C1

(E) stage C2

67. The greatest risk for developing colorectal cancer is having been treated for a previous colorectal cancer. As part of the postoperative surveillance in patients treated for colorectal cancer, a blood test is frequently employed every 2 to 3 months for a period of 2 years. This blood test is

(A) PSA (prostate specific antigen)

(B) CBC (complete blood count)

(C) BUN (blood urea nitrogen)

(D) APC gene (adenomatosis polyposis coli gene)

(E) CEA (carcinoembryonic antigen)

68. What is the major clinicopathologic finding that helps to differentiate ulcerative colitis from Crohn's disease?

(A) toxic megacolon

(B) bleeding

(C) fatty infiltration of the liver

(D) jejunal involvement

(E) bimodal age distribution

69. Extracolonic manifestations of inflammatory bowel disease typically do NOT include

(A) ankylosing spondylitis

(B) erythema marginatum

(C) uveitis

(D) pyoderma gangrenosum

(E) arthritis

70. A 32-year-old female was recently diagnosed with mild Crohn's disease. What is the most appropriate first-line therapy in the management of this disease?

(A) surgical resection of the colon

(B) azathioprine

(C) metronidazole

(D) sulfasalazine

(E) infliximab (Remicade)

71. A 55-year-old male has been suffering from ulcerative colitis for the past 22 years and colonoscopy has now revealed a low-grade dysplasia in the left colon. The most appropriate surgical intervention at this time would be

(A) left hemicolectomy

(B) subtotal colectomy

(C) proctocolectomy with ileal pouch-anal anastamosis

(D) local resection of the lesion with 2 cm margins

(E) colonscopic ablation

72. A 45-year-old male presents to the office with the complaint of perianal pain and bleeding. Examination reveals an anal/perianal mass complex. Biopsy is taken and the results are positive for epidermoid carcinoma of the anus. The most appropriate therapy would be

(A) local resection, chemotherapy, and external beam radiation

(B) abdominoperoneal resection

(C) chemotherapy only

(D) local resection only

(E) radiation only

73. A 34-year-old female with ulcerative colitis has been frequently symptomatic from proctitis and proctosigmoiditis. The best management for this particular problem would be

(A) stool bulking agents

(B) nutritional support

(C) corticosteroid enemas

(D) sulfasalazine

(E) systemic immunosuppressive agents

74. A 66-year-old female presents to the emergency department with a complaint of abdominal pain and distension for the past 3 days. Examination reveals a protuberant abdomen with diminished bowel sounds and tympany to percussion. Flat and upright abdominal radiographs reveal distended loops of bowel with prominent haustral markings. The most likely etiology of these findings is

(A) volvulus

(B) adenocarcinoma

(C) diverticular disease

(D) hernia

(E) adhesions

75. Radiographic findings most compatible with large bowel obstruction include

(A) distended proximal colon with air-fluid levels

(B) free air under the diaphragm

(C) large volume of rectal air

(D) pneumobilia

76. A 54-year-old male presents to the emergency department with abdominal distension and pain. A plain radiograph of the abdomen reveals cecal distension to 12 cm. What is the most appropriate initial management for this patient?

(A) intravenous antibiotics

(B) nasogastric suction

(C) observation

(D) surgical exploration

(E) fiberoptic colonoscopy

77. An 80-year-old male nursing home patient is brought to the emergency department with abdominal distension. Plain radiographs of the abdomen reveal a large air-filled kidney-shaped mass in the left upper quadrant. This finding is most compatible with

(A) small bowel obstruction

(B) cecal volvulus

(C) transverse colon volvulus

(D) sigmoid volvulus

(E) toxic megacolon

78. A 34-year-old female presents to the office complaining of bleeding per rectum in association with defecation. Examination reveals a large internal hemorrhoid that required manual manipulation for reduction. What classification is used for this type of hemorrhoid?

(A) first degree
(B) second degree
(C) third degree
(D) fourth degree

79. A 10-year-old male is brought into the office by his mother complaining of anal pain. The child describes a sensation of tearing pain associated with defecation. He has noticed bright red blood on the toilet paper after wiping himself. This presentation is most compatible with

(A) perianal abscess
(B) pilonidal cyst
(C) fistula in ano
(D) hidradenitis suppurativa
(E) anal fissure

80. A 49-year-old male presents to the hospital with right upper quadrant pain, fever, and mild jaundice. An ultrasound is ordered and reveals an intrahepatic cystic mass. Past medical history is positive for ulcerative colitis for the past 20 years. The lesion most likely represents

(A) hepatic adenoma
(B) focal nodular hyperplasia
(C) pyogenic liver abscess
(D) hepatoma

81. The organism most frequently associated with nosocomially acquired diarrhea is

(A) *Bacteroides fragilis*
(B) *Escherichia coli*
(C) *Clostridium tetani*
(D) *Clostridium difficile*
(E) *Bacteroides vulgatus*

82. Hernias are classified as direct or indirect based upon which of the following?

(A) physical examination findings
(B) relationship to the inferior epigastric artery
(C) superior or inferior position to the inguinal ligament
(D) barium enema results
(E) CT scan

83. A patient who has undergone a truncal vagotomy and Billroth II reconstruction for gastric ulcer disease returns postoperatively with complaints of lightheadedness, palpitations, and diaphoresis that develops approximately 30 minutes after eating. What is the most likely explanation of his symptoms?

(A) early dumping syndrome
(B) afferent loop syndrome
(C) blind loop syndrome
(D) alkaline reflux gastritis

84. What is considered to be an important risk factor in the development of gastric carcinoma?

(A) cigarette smoking
(B) high-fat diet
(C) sodium nitrite ingestion
(D) *Heliobacter pylori* infection
(E) high caffeine intake

85. A 56-year-old man presents with severe midepigastric pain that is refractory to antacids and H2 blockers. What is the first-line test to establish the diagnosis of Zollinger–Ellison syndrome?

(A) urease breath test
(B) serum calcium
(C) serum gastrin level
(D) endoscopy for brush biopsies
(E) MRI of the abdomen looking for a gastrinoma

Answers and Explanations

1. **(E)** Hyponatremia with serum levels of 120 to 130 meq/L is commonly associated with central nervous system dysfunction. In particular, irritability, weakness, fatigue, and increased deep-tendon reflexes are seen. If the serum sodium levels drop rapidly, i.e. 10 to 15 meq/L in less than 40 hours, muscle twitching can be seen. Paralytic ileus and hepatic encephalopathy may be seen with hypokalemia; cardiac irritability (peaked T waves, complete heart block, ventricular fibrillation) is associated with hyperkalemia; signs of dehydration and oliguria are associated with hypernatremia. (*Lawrence, 2006, pp. 53–56*)

2. **(B)** The most common cause of fever in the postoperative patient during the first 48 hours after surgery is atelectasis. Because atelectasis occurs so commonly, it is generally not necessary to obtain any diagnostic studies during the first 2 days following surgery. Atelectasis develops secondary to the residual effects of anesthesia, postoperative pain management, and incisional pain. (*Townsend et al, 2004, pp. 306–307*)

3. **(E)** Forced expiration volume/one second (FEV1) is the amount of air exhaled in 1 second during a forced expiration. It is a parameter used to evaluate for problems with ventilation and intrinsic lung disease. FEV1 values less than 1 are indicative of an increased risk of postoperative pulmonary complications and ventilator dependence. (*Lawrence, 2006, p. 26*)

4. **(A)** Potassium is an extremely important cation of the body. It is the main cation of the intracellular compartment. This is one of the predominant electrolytes to determine intracellular volume. Hypokalemia can result in alterations of neuromuscular function and can be responsible for cardiac arrhythmias. There are many reasons for the development of hypokalemia postoperatively. Among these would be gastrointestinal losses from vomiting or diarrhea, fistulous tracts after biliary or pancreatic surgery, and nasogastric suction. In any postoperative patient with prolonged paralytic ileus it is important to evaluate the patient's potassium to see if the etiology of this condition is hypokalemia. (*Lawrence, 2006, pp. 55–56*)

5. **(C)** Five percent dextrose with 0.5% normal saline supplemented with potassium best approximates the electrolyte composition of the gastric losses associated with prolonged nasogastric aspiration. Lactated Ringer's should not be used due to the inadequate amounts of chloride plus the conversion of lactate to bicarbonate does not correct the hypochloremic, hypokalemic metabolic alkalosis. (*Lawrence, 2006, p. 51*)

6. **(E)** Instillation of enteral feeding directly into the small bowel, distal to the ligament of Treitz eliminates the problems of gastric retention, reflux, vomiting, and aspiration that can be seen with feedings that delivered directly into the stomach. Complications associated

with intrajejunal feedings relate to the rate of administration and the caloric content. If feedings are infused too rapidly, the patient may develop abdominal distention, hyperperistalsis, cramping, diarrhea, weakness, and sweating. (*Lawrence, 2006, pp. 79–81*)

7. **(B)** In addition to fingerstick glucose monitoring postoperatively, urinary ketones are important to watch for the development of ketoacidosis which can occur in either type 1 or 2 diabetes. Diabetic ketacidosis is often overlooked in the postoperative patient since it can mimic a postoperative ileus by presenting with nausea, vomiting, and abdominal distension. Measurement of urinary ketones is faster and cheaper than measuring serum ketones. (*Lawrence, 2006, p. 29*)

8. **(C)** The clinical scenario reveals contamination of the abdomen at the time of injury with a potential source of Gram-negative bacteria. Cases of septic shock number over 750,000/year, with an associated mortality of 30% to 50%. Typically patients with septic shock will have an identifiable source of infection, and systemic manifestations of inflammation. Therapy will require emperic antibiotic use guided by a knowledge of the source of infection and most likely pathogens. Usually surgery or interventional radiology will be necessary to effect drainage of abscess formation. Although hypovolemic or hemorrhagic shock is the most commonly encountered clinical cause of shock in the surgical/trauma patient, the delayed presentation speaks against it as a cause. Cardiogenic shock represents pump failure and this patient is too young for this consideration. Neurogenic shock is usually found in association with spinal cord injuries at the cervical or high thoracic region. Obstructive shock is a relatively new term and applies to that shock seen in association with cardiac tamponade, tension pneumothorax, or pulmonary embolism. (*Brunicardi, 2005, pp. 95–102*)

9. **(B)** Cardiac tamponade is classically described by the triad of venous hypertension (JVD), arterial hypotension, and muffled heart sounds. In the emergency department, suspicion of this clinically entity is usually confirmed by ultrasonography and is acutely treated by pericardiocentesis. Removal of as little as 100 mL may relieve symptoms and buy time for definitive surgical exploration, repair of injury, and cardiac window. A right tube thoracostomy may be indicated in this patient but would not relieve symptoms or raise blood pressure. Fluid resuscitation though applied to all trauma patients would also not be of initial benefit in this case. Immediate intubation, even if indicated, would require a prophylactic tube thoracostomy to prevent the development of tension pneumothorax in the event of an unrecognized lung injury. Emergency thoracotomy should be reserved for those patients who do not respond to resuscitation or have unresponsive blood pressure with pressures below 70 mm Hg. (*Brunicardi, 2005, pp. 101, 133, 683*)

10. **(A)** Bacterial infection of the breast is most commonly caused by *Staphylococcus aureus* and *Streptococcus*. Localized abscesses as described in this patient are more commonly seen with *S. aureus* infections. Streptococcal infections usually present with superficial involvement of the skin and cellulitic streaking. Mycotic infections are extremely rare but when they do occur usually blastomycosis or sporotrichosis are the offending infections. *Escherichia coli* and *Pseudomonas* species are infrequent causes of breast abscess formation and are more likely to be seen in immunocompromised or hospitalized patients. Breast abscesses are treated with local wound care and intravenous antibiotics. Penicillins or cephalosporins are most commonly utilized. In hospitalized patients methicillin-resistant *S. aureus* may be encountered and antibiotics should be adjusted accordingly. (*Brunicardi, 2005, p. 462*)

11. **(B)** As intracranial pressure increases, the body attempts to maintain cerebral perfusion pressure (CPP equals the difference between mean arterial pressure and intracranial pressure) by raising the systolic blood pressure; this response is known as Cushing's reflex. In addition to hypertension, the Cushing's reflex is associated with bradycardia and a decreased respiratory rate. Rapid, deep breath-

ing can be seen along with hypertension and bradycardia in association with an impending herniation. (*Lawrence, 2006, p. 200*)

12. **(A)** Approximately 75% of the gallstones found in Western civilization are of the mixed variety. The mixed variety contains cholesterol and calcium. Most of the mixed stones do not contain enough calcium to be appreciated on plain films. Black-pigmented stones account for 20% of the stones and are often associated with hemolysis and cirrhosis. Brown-pigmented stones are most commonly associated with infected bile. (*Lawrence, 2006, pp. 337–338*)

13. **(E)** Native Americans have the highest incidence of gallstones. By the age of 60 the Native American male runs a rate of 50%, while the female of the same age and population will develop gallstones 80% of the time. The prevalance in white females younger than 50 years is 5% to 15%, and those older than 50, the prevalence is 25%. For white males younger than 50, the prevalence is 4% to 10%, and for those older than 50, it is 10% to 15%. (*Lawrence, 2006, p. 338*)

14. **(B)** Sustained obstruction of the cystic duct from cholelithiasis leads to dilation and inflammation in acute cholecystitis. Biliary colic is characterized by intermittent obstruction without inflammation. Choledocholithiasis is characterized by jaundice secondary to obstruction of the common bile duct; in ascending cholangitis the common bile duct obstruction is complicated by infection. (*Lawrence, 2006, pp. 343–345*)

15. **(D)** Pancreatic carcinoma presents with weight loss, jaundice, and midepigastric pain. A palpable, nontender gallbladder (Courvoisier's sign) is more often associated with a pancreatic malignancy than cholelithiasis, especially if the tumor is in the head of the pancreas. In acute cholecystitis, the obstruction in the cystic duct is associated with inflammation, resulting in a tender gallbladder on palpation of the right upper quadrant (Murphy's sign); obstruction of the common bile duct in choledocholithiasis will result in jaundice, but not

weight loss. Gastric carcinoma will present with midepigastric pain and weight loss, but not jaundice or a palpable gallbladder. Midepigastric pain is the most common symptom seen in chronic pancreatitis and weight loss may be seen in association with malabsorption secondary to exocrine insufficiency. (*Lawrence, 2006, pp. 264, 343–345, 361–362*)

16. **(C)** The abdominal ultrasound will show dilated intrahepatic and extrahepatic ducts secondary to obstruction of the common bile duct in choledocholithiasis. Ultrasound findings of a thickened gallbladder wall and pericholecystic fluid are seen with acute cholecystitis. Air in the lumen of the gallbladder is seen in acute emphysematous cholecystitis. (*Lawrence, 2006, pp. 343–345*)

17. **(B)** Ultrasonography has been proven to be the most sensitive of the imaging studies in biliary tract disease. Some studies have stated that ultrasound is approximately 95% accurate in detecting disease in the biliary tree. It can detect stones, dilation of biliary ducts, thickening of the gallbladder, and pericolic collections of fluid and can also provide information pertaining to associated liver or pancreatic pathology. (*Lawrence, 2006, p. 339*)

18. **(B)** Although blunt abdominal trauma may injure any intraabdominal organ, the spleen is most commonly affected. Unless patients are hemodynamically unstable most splenic injuries are treated nonoperatively, with the goal being splenic salvage. Overwhelming postsplenectomy infection with encapsulated bacteria (*Streptococcus pneumoniae, Haemophilus influenzae,* and *Neisseria meningitidis*) is a major complication occurring most commonly in children and immunocompromised hosts. (*Brunicardi, 2005, p. 166*)

19. **(C)** Computerized tomography is an excellent noninvasive procedure to determine not only the level of obstruction but also the pathologic process. In the event a carcinomatous condition is identified; this procedure will also aid in the staging of the disease as well as guide the surgeon in evaluating the resectability of the condition. (*Lawrence, 2006, pp. 349–342*)

20. (E) The presenting symptoms associated with ascending cholangitis include fever, chills, right upper quadrant pain, and jaundice (Charcot's triad); the symptoms are secondary to an infected obstruction of the common bile duct. With spread of the infection, the patient may also develop hypotension and mental status changes; these additional symptoms in conjunction with Charcot's triad are known as Reynold's pentad. Additional symptoms of common bile duct obstuction include light-colored stools and dark, tea-colored urine. (*Lawrence, 2006, pp. 344–345*)

21. (C) Once cholelithiaisis is confirmed in patients with biliary colic, the treatment of choice is an elective cholecystectomy, which is performed laparoscopically in the majority of cases. (*Lawrence, 2006, p. 343*)

22. (C) Patients who present with acute pancreatitis are usually diagnosed by exclusion. Other conditions that must be excluded include mesenteric infarction, perforated duodenal ulcer disease, and acute cholecystitis. Typically patients present with epigastric pain that radiates to the back and is described as "stabbing" or "boring" in quality. Although there is no one test pathognomonic for acute pancreatitis, elevations in serum lipase levels have been found to have the highest specificity in making the diagnosis. (*Brunicardi, 2005, pp. 1233–1235*)

23. (B) Ranson's criteria were developed to grade the severity of pancreatitis by utilizing laboratory and clinical findings. These are measured when the patient is admitted. Within the next 48 hours, in addition to the original five criteria, an additional six variables are employed. Upon admission the patient's age, WBC, glucose, LDH, and AST are evaluated. Within the next 48 hours the HCT, BUN, calcium, PO_2 on room air, base excess, and estimated fluid sequestration are measured. When less than two Ranson's signs are present, mortality is virtually zero; however, it increases to >50% when seven or more are present. The Acute Physiology and Chronic Health Evaluation II (APACHE II) is another classification of severity of disease. This system evaluates variables in temperature, mean arterial pressure, heart rate, respiratory rate, oxygenation, arterial pH, serum sodium, serum potassium, serum creatinine, hematocrit, WBC, and Glasgow Coma Scale (neurologic evaluation). (*Brunicardi, 2005, p. 1236*)

24. (E) Patients with acute pancreatitis are subject to many complications. Metabolic complications include hyperglycemia, hypocalcemia, and renal insufficiency. Cytokines elaborated during acute pancreatitis can lead to adult respiratory distress syndrome and significant glandular necrosis. Other acute complications include disseminated intravascular coagulopathy and associated hemorrhagic diathisis. Although pancreatic pseudocyst may also be found in association with acute pancreatitis (10%), it is recognized as the most frequent complication associated with chronic pancreatitis (20% to 38%). Patients with chronic pancreatitis are also at a significantly increased risk for the development of pancreatic carcinoma. This risk is 10-fold greater than that seen in comparable patient populations. (*Brunicardi, 2005, pp. 1240–1256*)

25. (C) A palpable, nontender gallbladder in a patient with jaundice is known as Courvoisier's sign This finding is seen in patients with pancreatic carcinoma, especially with lesions involving the head of the pancreas. Flank ecchymosis (Grey—Turner sign) and periumbilical ecchymosis (Cullen's sign) are seen in association with acute hemorrhagic pancreatitis. Pain in the RUQ associated with inspiratory arrest is known as Murphy's sign; pain in the left shoulder on palpation of the left upper quadrant is seen with splenic injury. (*Lawrence, 2006, pp. 356, 362, 432*)

26. (B) Hepatocellular carcinoma (HCC) should be suspected with any patient with a known history of cirrhosis who presents with an acute deterioration in their condition. Alpha-fetoprotein is a marker that is elevated in 60% to 80% of patients with HCC. While the alpha-fetoprotein may be elevated up to 400 mg/dL in patients with cirrhosis alone, elevations more than 500 to 1000 mg/dL are almost always associated with HCC. (*Lawrence, 2006, p. 370*)

27. (E) The development of ascites in patients with portal hypertension is multifactorial and involves increases in hydrostatic pressure, neuroendocrine responses of the renin–angiotensin–aldosterone system, and decreased oncotic pressure due to hepatic insufficiency. The use of endoscopy, portocaval shunting with or without transjugular intrahepatic portosystemic shunt is indicated primarily for hemorrhage. Due to the pathophysiology of ascites development, abdominal paracentesis is indicated for tense ascites that is symptomatic. This is primarily due to the recurrent nature of ascites in patients with portal hypertension. Medical management utilizing sodium restriction, loop diuretics, or potassium sparing diuretics is effective in over 90% of patients. Renal function should be closely monitored as well as serum electrolytes so as to identify and correct any abnormalities that may develop. (*Brunicardi, 2005, p. 1157*)

28. (D) Axillary lymph node status is the most important prognostic factor in breast cancer. Patients with evidence of spread of disease have a significant decrease in 5-year survival; patients with stage I disease have a 96% 5-year survival rate compared to patients with stage III disease and evidence of lymph node involvement who have a 53% 5-year survival rate. The next most important factors are estrogen receptor status and tumor size. (*Lawrence, 2006, p. 397*)

29. (B) The clinical symptoms associated with chronic intestinal ischemia include severe epigastric pain following meals, which results in weight loss and fear of eating. (*Lawrence, 2006, p. 457*)

30. (C) Ulcers secondary to chronic arterial insufficiency are painful and have a punched-out appearance with a pale or necrotic base. Arterial ulcerations may occur on the toes, heel, or dorsum of the foot as the result of minor trauma. By contrast, venous ulcers that occur at the level of the malleoli are associated with significant lower extremity edema and pigmentation changes due to chronic venous insufficiency. Additionally, venous ulcerations have granulation tissue at the base. Diabetic

ulcerations are painless, secondary to diabetic neuropathy. (*Lawrence, 2006, p. 451*)

31. (C) Fibroadenomas are among the most common benign lesions found in young female patients. They occur usually from the late teens into the early thirties, although they have been found to a lesser degree in all age groups. This lesion is firm, ovoid, freely movable, and usually 1 to 3 cm in size. In most instances when the lesion is greater than 3 cm, observation is recommended since in the younger patient many of these lesions will have spontaneous resolution. Surgery is recommended, after fine-needle aspiration, on those lesions that increase in size on observation. Fibrocystic disease usually occurs between the ages of 30 and 50. Breast cysts and lipomas are soft. (*Lawrence, 2006, p. 392*)

32. (D) The American Joint Committee on Cancer established the TNM system for the clinical staging of cancer. Utilizing this system, a tumor that is greater than 5 cm with suspicious nodes that were fixed to each other would be classified as a stage IIIA lesion. Depending on the node involvement and other metastasis, this lesion could become a stage IIIB. Any distant metastasis of the tumor, no matter what size, would automatically change the stage to a stage IV. Treatment is designed according to the staging of a lesion along with its cell type. (*Lawrence, 2006, p. 395*)

33. (B) *Streptococcus pneumoniae* accounts for 75% of the cases of postsplectomy sepsis, followed in decreasing frequency by *Haemophilus influenzae*, *Neisseria meningitidis*, beta-hemolytic streptococcus, *Staphylococcus aureus*, *Escherichia coli*, and *Pseudomonas*. Occasionally viral and parasitic infections can lead to sepsis as well. (*Lawrence, 2006, p. 438*)

34. (B) Indirect hernias are the most common type of hernia affecting 50% of males and 70% females. Indirect inguinal hernias represent almost all inguinal hernias in children; direct inguinal hernias and femoral hernias are rare in children. (*Lawrence, 2006, pp. 230–231*)

35. (A) The acute onset of pain seen with ischemia in an acute arterial occlusion is associated with the time of occlusion in 80% patients. Pain is often followed by paresthesias, pallor, and paralysis. When these symptoms are present for longer than 12 hours, it is unlikely that the limb will be salvageable. (*Doherty et al, 2005, p. 74*)

36. **(D)** Anterior–posterior and lateral abdominal radiographs may reveal calcification of an AAA as an incidental finding. CT scans have replaced aortography in the preoperative imaging of aneurysms. Abdominal palpation on physical examination may be reliable in thin patients but cannot accurately provide information about the presence or absence of aneurysms in all patients. Ultrasonography is cost-effective and is the most commonly utilized screening modality for AAAs. It can be utilized for initial detection of an AAA or for yearly follow-up of progression. (*Brunicardi, 2005, pp. 733–734*)

37. **(D)** Chronic venous insufficiency (CVI) can result in many characteristic skin changes to the affected limb. Typically patients will develop edema, induration, pigmentation, and ulceration. Whereas arterial disease typically results in ulcerations located on the distal toes or lateral aspect of the affected extremity, CVI will most commonly produce ulcers proximal to the medial malleolus. (*Brunicardi, 2005, p. 810*)

38. **(E)** An ankle/brachial index of 1.0 is considered to be normal; values less than 1.0 are consistent with chronic occlusive disease. Values less than 0.8 are consistent with claudication. Rest pain is associated with values less than 0.4. Rest pain is an indicator of advanced arterial insufficiency and may also be associated with tissue necrosis. (*Doherty et al, 2005, p. 722; Lawrence, 2006, p. 452*)

39. **(D)** The most common site for an acute embolic occlusion is the femoral artery. Other common sites include the axillary, popliteal, and iliac arteries as well as the aortic bifurcation and mesenteric vessels. The majority (80%) of arterial embolic originate in the heart in patients with atrial fibrillation or from mural thrombi in the left ventricle from an aki-

netic or dyskinetic portion of the myocardium following a myocardial infarction. (*Lawrence, 2006, p. 459*)

40. **(A)** Atherosclerosis account for 67% of the cases of renovascular hypertension, which is seen more commonly in males older than 45 years; it can be bilateral in 95% of cases. Fibromuscular dysplasia accounts for 33% of cases and can also be bilateral (50%); however it is seen predominately in women and the hypertension develops before the age of 45. Rare causes of renovascular hypertension include renal artery aneurysms, dissections, emboli, and hypoplastic renal arteries. (*Doherty et al, 2005, p. 590*)

41. **(C)** Duodenal ulcers typically present with midepigastric pain may be described as gnawing in quality and radiating to the back. The pain is worse 1 to 3 hours after eating and is worse when the patient is fasting. The epigastric pain is usually relieved with eating or antacids. If a duodenal ulcer is complicated by perforation, the epigastric pain will acutely worsen; the patient will be tachycardic and have a rigid abdomen with rebound and guarding. Upright chest x-ray will show evidence of free air in conjunction with a perforated ulcer. Gastric distension is seen with gastric outlet obstruction; a fixed deformity projecting into the lumen of the stomach is seen more commonly with gastric carcinoma. Filling defects may be seen beyond the lumen of the stomach in patients with gastric ulcers; however, the clinical presentation in this vignette is consistent with duodenal ulcer disease. (*Lawrence, 2006, pp. 260–269*)

42. **(A)** Hypokalemia is associated with gastrointestinal losses, such as diarrhea, vomiting, fistulae, and malabsorption. In particular, in cases with prolonged vomiting or losses to nasogastric suctioning, there are additional losses of chloride and hydrogen ions that produce a hypochloremia, hypokalemic metabolic alkalosis. (*Lawrence, 2006, p. 55*)

43. **(D)** Spiral CT scan is the most sensitive and specific diagnostic radiographic test which shows an enlarged appendix with peri-

appendiceal fat in 90% to 95% of cases of acute appendicitis. Spiral CT is especially helpful with patients presenting with atypical findings on either physical exam or laboratory testing. Abdominal ultrasound may show a dilated tubular structure in the right lower quadrant, but this technique is user dependent and less sensitive in adults than children. Plain films may show localized air–fluid levels or localized ileus, but generally are not helpful. (*Doherty et al, 2005, p. 70; Lawrence, 2006, p. 301*)

44. **(C)** Following a review of 20 randomized clinical trials comparing the merits of mesh repairs over nonmesh repairs, it was concluded that there was 50% to 75% decrease in the risk of a recurrent hernia following a mesh repair. (*Lawrence, 2006, p. 232*)

45. **(D)** After the ilioinguinal nerve passes through the internal oblique muscle (superior and lateral to the internal ring), it runs along the spermatic cord. Injury to this nerve results in numbness to the groin, scrotum, and anterior thigh. (*Lawrence, 2006, p. 226*)

46. **(D)** Meckel's diverticulum is prevalent in 2% of the population, has a 2:1 female predominance and is usually located 2 ft from the ileocecal valve. 50% of the patients are less than 2 years of age, and two tissue types (gastric and pancreatic) may be found within its confines. The most common clinical presentations are bleeding, intestinal obstruction, and diverticulitis. Bleeding is the most frequent complication in children. Obstruction in children without a history of prior surgery may be due to intussusception where a Meckel's diverticulm acts as the lead point. When intussusception develops past 24 months of age, a pathologic starting point caused by polyps, duplication cysts, or a Meckel's diverticulum should be considered. (*Brunicardi, 2005, pp. 1493–1494*)

47. **(A)** Although certain clinical features are more commonly associated with specific locations of the disease along the gastrointestinal tract, most Crohn's disease patients have the triad of abdominal pain, diarrhea, and weight loss. Abdominal pain is the most common presenting symptom. It may be intermittent or constant. (*Lawrence, 2006, p. 289*)

48. **(A)** Achalasia is characterized by progressive dysphagia, which is painless in contrast to esophageal cancer, which is characterized by odynophagia. While patients with achalasia have regurgitation of food, there is minimal loss of weight. Esophageal cancer is associated with anorexia and weight loss. Patients with achalasia typically drink large amounts of liquids to force their food down and have problems with aspiration pneumonia. Patients with reflux esophagitis will complain of epigastric or substernal pain that is worse when supine or leaning forward. Leiomyomas are generally asymptomatic. (*Lawrence, 2006, pp. 244–249*)

49. **(C)** Patients with achalasia have constriction at the level of the distal esophagus leading to progressive dilation of the proximal esophagus. On contrast study this has a bird's beak appearance. The bird's beak appearance can also be seen in patients with a sigmoid volvulus. Apple core lesions are commonly seen with colorectal carcinoma; and lead pipe deformity is seen with loss of normal haustral marking in ulcerative colitis. String sign is seen in association with small bowel obstruction in Crohn's disease. (*Lawrence, 2006, pp. 247, 318, 323, 324, 327*)

50. **(C)** Obstipation and failure to pass flatus are symptoms of both paralytic ileus and a small bowel obstruction (SBO). In paralytic ileus, the patient usually has minimal abdominal pain, and hypoactive or absent bowel sounds due to hypomotility. Patients with an SBO will have crampy abdominal pain and increased bowel sounds with high-pitched sounds and rushes due to increased peristalsis. Plain films in paralytic ileus will show gas throughout the small and large bowel on plain films as opposed to air confined to the small intestine only in SBO. (*Lawrence, 2006, pp. 297–299*)

51. **(A)** The first priority in proven or suspected small bowel obstruction is the correction of

fluid and electrolyte abnormalities. Often, large volumes of fluid must be infused. The patient must be given sufficient fluid not only for maintenance requirements, but also to correct losses from vomiting and nasogastric output and third-space loss. Urine output should be closely monitored for the adequacy of hydration. If the patient has a partial small bowel obstruction, no detectable hernia on exam, and a history of operation, resolution may occur with fluid replacement and nasogastric tube placement, making an operation unnecessary. If the patient has no apparent etiology for obstruction, a cause should be determined by upper gastrointestinal and small bowel x-ray series. Laboratory data cannot confirm the diagnosis of bowel obstruction, but are useful to rule out other diagnoses. A patient with a complete small bowel obstruction should undergo operation at the earliest opportunity, once the fluid and electrolyte repair is sufficient to establish adequate urine output. (*Lawrence, 2006, pp. 299–300*)

52. **(E)** The superior mesenteric artery supplies the right side of the colon while the inferior mesenteric artery, and its branches, supplies the left. Where the inferior mesenteric artery is occluded or sacrificed during surgery, collateral blood flow from the superior mesenteric artery reaches through anastamoses of terminal branches of arteries that connect via the marginal artery of Drummond. This arterial arcade is fully developed in only 15% to 20% of patients. (*Brunicardi, 2005, p. 1057*)

53. **(B)** This is classified as an emergent resection in an unprepared patient. It should be noted that some surgeons may attempt a primary resection and anastomosis along with aggressive abdominal lavage. However, the most appropriate therapy involves resection of the affected segment of colon, end colostomy with the creation of a distal mucus fistula if the segment is long enough to reach the anterior abdominal wall. Conversely where the distal segment is too short a Hartmann's procedure should be performed (resection, end colostomy, distal rectal stump oversewn, and left in the pelvis for later reanastomosis). Abdominoperioneal resection is used in the treatment of malignant disease of the lower rectum. In this procedure a permanent colostomy is created and the entire rectum, anal canal, and anus are removed. In the management of benign disease of the lower rectum a proctocolectomy is appropriate to preserve anal function. (*Brunicardi, 2005, pp. 1066–1071*)

54. **(B)** In patients with complicated diverticular disease of the colon approximately 5% will develop some kind of fistula. The most common fistula developed is the colovesicular fistula. Colocutaneous fistulas have been known to occur as a complication of diverticular disease but are extremely rare. When encountering a fistula as a complication of diverticular disease you must define the anatomical relationships of the fistula and exclude other causes. Other causes of fistula formation in association with colon disease include malignancy, radiation therapy, or inflammatory bowel disease. (*Brunicardi, 2005, p. 1084*)

55. **(C)** Although hemorrhoids are the most common cause of lower gastrointestinal hemorrhage, they do not cause massive hemorrhage. Massive lower gastrointestinal hemorrhage is most commonly due to diverticular disease. Upper gastrointestinal hemorrhage may present as massive lower hemorrhage. This is due to the cathartic effect of blood. Colon cancer usually presents with occult bleeding. Meckel's diverticulum may also present as massive lower gastrointestinal hemorrhage but is not as common a disease entity as diverticular disease of the colon. (*Brunicardi, 2005, pp. 1081–1082*)

56. **(E)** Although advanced age and bleeding can complicate the management of diverticular disease, "complicated diverticulitis" is a term reserved for patients who in addition to diverticular disease present with abscess formation, obstruction, perforation, or fistulas between adjacent structures. Staging using the Hinchey system will further delineate the extent of disease. (*Brunicardi, 2005, p. 1083*)

57. **(D)** The only factor that appears to decrease the incidence of diverticular disease is the

eating of a diet high in fiber. A commonly accepted theory in the formation of diverticula is that high intraluminal pressure causes herniation of the mucosa and muscularis mucosa at the point where vessels penetrate the colon. Lack of dietary fiber results in diminished stool volume, which in turn requires higher intraluminal pressures and wall tension for distal propulsion. Fecal occult blood testing and colonoscopy have been shown to accurately screen and detect for colon cancer. (*Brunicardi, 2005, pp. 1081–1082*)

58. **(E)** Villous adenomas may contain cancer in up to 40% of cases and when greater than 2 cm in size this risk goes up to 35% to 50%. Tubular adenomas infrequently are associated with malignancy. When the pathology is mixed, tubulovillous adenomas, there is an intermediate risk of 22% for carcinoma. Hyperplastic polyps and hamartomatous polyps are not premalignant but are very difficult to distinguish from adenomatous polyps and are often removed at colonoscopy. (*Brunicardi, 2005, pp. 1086–1087*)

59. **(A)** This is an autosomal dominant condition that only accounts for 1% of colon cancer cases. Starting at 10 to 15 years of age, flexible sigmoidoscopy had been the recommended screening tool for FAP patients. Today, genetic screening of patients for the APC gene is the standard of care. If the APC gene is identified then flexible sigmoidoscopy is employed as before starting at ages 10 to 15. This approach is also utilized when testing is refused. If APC genetic testing is negative then screening can begin at age 50, utilizing average-risk guidelines. (*Brunicardi, 2005, p. 1087*)

60. **(C)** Colon cancer is the most common malignancy of the gastrointestinal tract. Although individuals of any age can develop colon cancer, increasing age is the most dominant risk factor associated with its development. Only 20% of colon cancers are found in patients with a known family history of colorectal carcinoma. Ulcerative colitis and Crohn's disease also increase the risk of acquiring colon cancer, with the greatest risk being found in patients with ulcerative colitis for greater than

30 years. Cigarette smoking has been identified as conveying an increased risk for the development of colonic adenomas as do diets high in animal fat and low in fiber. (*Brunicardi, 2005, pp. 1084–1085*)

61. **(B)** Involvement of the regional lymph nodes is the most common initial form of disease dissemination in colorectal carcinoma. Nodal involvement is correlated with the size of tumor, cellular histology, and depth of invasion. This form of spread precedes distal metastasis where hepatic lesions are most commonly encountered in colorectal carcinoma. (*Brunicardi, 2005, pp. 1089–1090*)

62. **(B)** Right-sided colon lesions can grow to large sizes due to the liquid characteristic of stool in this region. These large exophytic lesions can result in occult blood loss with the subseqent development of iron deficiency anemia. The triad of weight loss, anemia, and a palpable mass in the right lower quadrant should raise suspicion for right colon carcinoma. (*Lawrence, 2006, p. 277*)

63. **(D)** Abdominal/pelvic CT scans and chest radiographs should be obtained as part of the preoperative staging of colon carcinoma for the evaluation of distant metastasis. CT scan of the chest is indicated only if the chest radiograph is abnormal. Endorectal ultrasound is useful in further staging rectal carcinoma. Bone scan is not indicated as a routine diagnostic study in the preoperative staging of colon cancer. Although carcinoembryonic antigen levels are performed preoperatively, they are not useful in staging and are useful only in the postoperative follow-up of patients. (*Brunicardi, 2005, p. 1091*)

64. **(D)** Data are still being accumulated comparing minimally invasive and conventional surgical technique survival rates. Studies have shown that an adequate number of lymph nodes, comparable to that obtained with an open procedure, can be obtained. Furthermore, resection margins are not compromised with laparascopic resection. Hospital stay, morbidity, and mortality are also diminished using a minimally invasive surgical approach.

Of concern are reports of trochar site cancer implantation. (*Brunicardi, 2005, pp. 393–394*)

65. **(A)** Barium enema finding of carcinoma of the sigmoid colon causing high-grade obstruction shows the classic "apple core" lesion. The string sign, also known as the string sign of Kantor, is an area of stricture or stenosis that shows up as a narrow line of contrast, giving the appearance of a string associated with the stricture. This sign is seen commonly in association with Crohn's disease of the terminal ileum. The lead pipe sign seen on barium enema is due to loss of haustral markings of the colon in association with ulcerative colitis. (*Brunicardi, 2005, pp. 1062, 1079*)

66. **(D)** The Dukes' classification and its Astler–Coller modification are still used in general surgery but have been mostly replaced by the American Joint Committee on Cancer TNM staging system. Nevertheless, Dukes' classification/Astler—Coller modification is as follows: stage A confined to mucosal penetration, and B1 and B2 both have negative lymph nodes, with B1 penetrating into but not through the muscularis propia and B2 penetrating through the muscularis propia. C1 and C2 both have positive lymph nodes and C1 penetrates into but not through the muscularis propia and C2 penetrating through the muscularis propia. Stage D denotes distant metastasis. (*Brunicardi, 2005, pp. 1090–1091*)

67. **(E)** The use of carcinoembryonic antigen (CEA) is well established for monitoring recurrent colon cancer, with recurrence suggested not by the absolute level of this antigen, but rather by a progressive rise from the postoperative baseline. It is important to understand that despite surveillance an increased survival benefit has never been proven. Prostate specific antigen (PSA) can be utilized in screening for de novo prostate cancer as well as recurrences. Complete blood count (CBC) can be influenced by chemotherapy and/or radiation treatments. The APC gene is utilized in screening of first-degree relatives of patients who have familial polyposis coli. (*Brunicardi, 2005, p. 1094*)

68. **(D)** Toxic megacolon is more common in ulcerative colitis but can also occur in association with Crohn's disease. Bleeding is common in both ulcerative colitis and Crohn's disease as is the bimodal distribution of the disease and fatty infiltration of the liver. Typically ulcerative colitis does not involve the small bowel except in cases where a backwash ileitis is present. Involvement of the jejunum does not occur in ulcerative colitis. Another helpful distinguishing characteristic includes the continuous involvement of the colon and rectum compared to "skip lesion" involvement seen in Crohn's disease. (*Brunicardi, 2005, pp. 1076–1077*)

69. **(B)** Extracolonic manifestations of inflammatory bowel disease include fatty liver infiltration, primary sclerosing cholangitis, cirrhosis, bile duct carcinoma, arthritis, sacroilitis, ankylosing spondylitis, erythema nodosum, pyoderma gangrenosum, uveitis, iritis, episcleritis, and conjunctivitis. Erythema marginatum is seen in association with rheumatic fever. (*Brunicardi, 2005, p. 1077*)

70. **(D)** Traditionally sulfasalazine and related medications are the first-line agents utilized in treating mild to moderate inflammatory bowel disease. Some evidence exists to support the use of antibiotics like metronidazole for the purpose of decreasing intraluminal bacteria. Immunosuppressive agents are used for patients who have failed salicylate therapy and/or are refractory or dependent upon corticosteroids. As Crohn's disease can involve any part of the gastrointestinal tract from the mouth to the anus, surgical intervention is reserved for the management of complications of the disease. (*Brunicardi, 2005, p. 1078*)

71. **(C)** Total proctocolectomy with an end ileostomy has been the "gold standard" for the management of low-grade dysplasia in patients with ulcerative colitis. Invasive carcinoma may be present in up to 20% of these lesions. Restorative proctocolectomy with ileal pouch-anal anastamosis is the procedure of choice in order to preserve anal sphincter function and avoid a permanent ileostomy. The other procedures given as choices are insufficient in dealing with the confluent

involvement of the colon so often found in ulcerative colitis. (*Brunicardi, 2005, p. 1079*)

72. **(A)** Epidermoid carcinoma of the anal canal is a slow-growing tumor that often presents as an anal or perianal mass. Wide escision, followed by 5-fluorouracil, mitomycin, and external beam radiation (Nigro Protocol), typically results in a greater than 80% cure rate. The presence of inguinal lymph node metastasis is a poor prognostic indicator. Management of recurrences is typically achieved by performing an abdominoperineal resection. (*Brunicardi, 2005, p. 1096*)

73. **(C)** Systemic corticosteroids have many associated serious side effects and as such their use should be restricted to the shortest possible course. Corticosteroid enemas provide effective local therapy for proctocolitis and proctosigmoiditis with much fewer side effects than systemic steroid administration. Other preparations may help with this particular issue but local therapy affords the best opportunity at symptomatic relief with the fewest side effects. (*Brunicardi, 2005, p. 1078*)

74. **(B)** Large bowel obstruction is most commonly caused by an adenocarcinoma. This is followed in decreasing incidence by diverticular scarring and volvulus. Adhesions are the most common cause of small-bowel obstruction and are rare as a cause of large bowel obstruction. The presence of haustral markings on radiographic evaluation helps to differentiate between small and large bowel involvement. (*Lawrence, 2006, pp. 284–285*)

75. **(A)** Large bowel obstruction appears radiographically as proximal colonic distention with air–fluid levels. Typically there is a paucity of total absence of air in the rectum. Free air under the diaphragm may be seen with any perforation of a hollow viscus. Pneumobilia is typically seen in association with gallstone ileus where an anastamosis between the bowel and the biliary tree exists. (*Lawrence, 2006, pp. 256, 284–285*)

76. **(D)** Massive distention of the cecum, as detected on plain radiograph, is typically seen in "closed loop" obstructions where the ileocecal valve is competent. When distention approaches 12 cm, there is an increased risk of perforation and/or gangrene. Expedient surgical intervention is indicated. Although intravenous fluids and antibiotics as well as nasogastric decompression are important adjuncts to management, surgical exploration is the only way to rapidly address this emergent situation. Fiberoptic colonoscopy is reserved for the occasional case of volvulus where it can be both diagnostic and therapeutic. (*Lawrence, 2006, p. 284*)

77. **(B)** Cecal volvulus is a result of nonfixation of the right colon. Radiographically it appears as a large air-filled kidney-shaped mass appearing on the opposite side of the obstruction. Sigmoid and transverse colon volvulus both share the same radiographic appearance, bent inner tube. Toxic megacolon will appear as a diffuse colonic distention and is due to chronic functional or mechanical obstruction. (*Brunicardi, 2005, p. 1099*)

78. **(C)** Hemorrhoids are classified as external (distal to the dentate line and covered with anoderm) and internal (proximal to the dentate line and covered with insensate anorectal mucosa). Internal hemorrhoids are further classified based upon their extent of prolapse. First-degree hemorrhoids bulge into the anal canal and may prolapse in association with straining. Second-degree hemorrhoids prolapse through the anus but reduce spontaneously. Third-degree hemorrhoids prolapse through the anal canal and require manual manipulation for reduction. Fourth-degree hemorrhoids prolapse and cannot be reduced, as such they are at increased risk for strangulation. (*Brunicardi, 2005, p. 1101*)

79. **(E)** Anal fissure is a common disease entity that presents with the characteristic symptoms of "tearing pain" during defecation and hematochezia. The tear is in the anoderm and can be visualized when the buttocks are spread apart. Digital rectal examination and other invasive studies should be avoided during the acute phase due to the patient's inability to tolerate these procedures. The majority

of these will heal with conservative medical management. Hidradenitis suppurativa may mimic an anal fissure. Perirectal abscesses present with pain and occasionally fever and urinary retention. In immunocompromised hosts and diabetic patients perianal abscess can pose a life-threatening infection. (*Brunicardi, 2005, pp. 1103–1105*)

80. **(C)** The lesion is described as cystic and associated with fever, right upper quadrant pain, and mild jaundice. In light of the history of inflammatory bowel disease the most likely diagnosis is pyogenic liver abscess. Pyogenic liver abscess can also be seen in association with biliary tract manipulation, diverticular disease, and systemic infections such as endocarditis. The other lesions listed are classified as solid lesions of the liver. (*Brunicardi, 2005, pp. 1159–1162*)

81. **(D)** *Clostridium difficile* colitis is the most common cause of nosocomially acquired diarrhea. The depletion of normal colonic bacteria through antibiotic administration allows for an overgrowth of *C. difficile*. Almost any antibiotic can cause pseudomembranous colitis and the risk rises with prolonged antibiotic use. Treatment includes immediate withdrawal of the offending antibiotic. First-line pharmacotherapy is oral metronidazole for 10 days. In patients allergic to metronidazole, oral vancomycin may be used as a second-line therapeutic option. (*Brunicardi, 2005, p. 1100*)

82. **(B)** Direct and indirect hernias can only be classified based upon the relationship of the origin of the hernia and the location of the inferior epigastric artery. If the hernia is medial to the inferior epigastric artery then it is a direct hernia. When the hernia originates lateral to the inferior epigastric artery, it is an indirect inguinal hernia. Most indirect inguinal hernias are due to a patent processus vaginalis, whereas direct inguinal hernias are largely due to a weakness of the posterior inguinal wall. (*Brunicardi, 2005, p. 1357*)

83. **(A)** Early dumping syndrome is seen following ingestion of high osmolarity foods, i.e. milk products. Shortly after eating, the patient develops tachycardia, palpitations, diaphoresis, anxiety, and weakness. Patients may also experience abdominal cramping and diarrhea. Afferent loop syndrome is the result of the spontaneous decompression of the obstructed afferent limb following a Billroth II reconstruction and is associated with severe abdominal pain with nausea and vomiting of dark brown material that looks like motor oil. Blind loop syndrome also occurs following a Billroth II procedure; proliferation of bacteria in the afferent loop leads to diarrhea, weight loss, and anemia from a vitamin B_{12} deficiency. Alkaline reflux gastritis is characterized by weight loss, weakness, abdominal pain, and persistent nausea. (*Lawrence, 2006, pp. 273–274*)

84. **(D)** Risk factors for the development of adenocarcinoma of the stomach include *Heliobacter pylori* infection, pernicious anemia, achlorhydria, and chronic gastritis. *H. pylori* infection has a 3.6–18-fold increased risk of gastric cancer. (*Lawrence, 2006, p. 262; Doherty et al, 2005, p. 262*)

85. **(C)** High gastrin levels, greater than 1000 pg/mL, are considered to be diagnostic for Zollinger–Ellison syndrome. When serum gastrin levels are greater than 5000 pg/mL, it is suggestive of metastatic disease. A secretin test can also prove to be provocative if serum gastrin levels are borderline high (200 to 500 pg/mL); an increase in gastrin levels more than 150 pg/mL within 15 minutes is considered to be diagnostic. Serum calcium levels are helpful in the work-up of MEN-1 (multiple endocrine neoplasia type 1), which is associated with Zollinger–Ellison syndrome. While endoscopy and MRI are helpful in the diagnostic evaluation, gastrinomas are generally very small and hard to localize. (*Lawrence, 2006, pp. 271–272; Doherty et al, 2005, pp. 272–273*)

REFERENCES

Brunicardi FC, Anderson DK, Billiar TR, Dunn DL, Hunter JG, Pollock RE. *Principles of General Surgery*, 8th ed. New York: McGraw-Hill; 2005.
Doherty GM, Ailawadi G, Binkley CE, DuBay DA, Lin TR, McGillicuddy JW, Saunders BD, Welling

TH. *Current Consult Surgery.* New York: Lange Medical Books; 2005.

Lawrence PF. *Essentials of General Surgery,* 4th ed. Philadelphia: Lippincott Williams & Wilkins; 2006.

Townsend CM, Beauchamp RD, Evers BM, Mattox K. *Sabiston Textbook of Surgery: The Biological Basis of Modern Surgical Practice,* 17th ed. Philadelphia: Elsevier Saunders; 2004.

CHAPTER 15

Orthopedics
Questions

Cathy A. Gillespie, DHSc, PA-C

DIRECTIONS (Questions 1 through 30): Each of the numbered items in this section is followed by possible answers. Select the ONE lettered answer that is BEST in each case.

Questions 1 through 30

1. Nonsteroidal anti-inflammatory agents are frequently utilized in treating the patient with osteoarthritis. In addition to the potential for bleeding and gastrointestinal effects, the primary concern, especially in the elderly patient, is irreversible damage to which of the following?

   (A) eyes
   (B) heart
   (C) kidneys
   (D) peripheral vascular system
   (E) central nervous syndrome

2. Which of the following is more likely to occur as a transient side effect following a corticosteroid joint injection?

   (A) paresthesia at joint injection site
   (B) joint infection
   (C) anaphylactic shock
   (D) mild allergic reactions
   (E) postinjection flare

3. The prophylactic antibiotic of choice for use in perioperative total joint replacement is best accomplished with which of the following?

   (A) penicillin and fluoroquinolone
   (B) macrolide
   (C) vancomycin
   (D) aminoglycoside
   (E) first or second generation cephalosporins

4. Which of the following is the most common etiology of osteomyelitis associated with prosthetic joint replacement or trauma?

   (A) *Pseudomonas aeruginosa*
   (B) *Staphylococcus aureus*
   (C) *Streptococcus*
   (D) candidiasis
   (E) *Enterococcus*

5. A 42-year-old male presents with complaints of progressive pain and limitation of motion involving his right shoulder for the past 2 months. He states that his shoulder was mainly painful at night with referral of pain to the deltoid region until his last tennis match yesterday when he noticed a marked increase in his pain and limitation of motion. On physical examination, there is tenderness to palpation of the anterior right shoulder, with maximum tenderness over the supraspinatus insertion. Active range of motion is decreased and there is weakness in abduction and forward flexion. Passive range of motion is full with complaints of increased pain with abduction. Which of the following is the most likely diagnosis?

(A) adhesive capsulitis

(B) rotator cuff rupture

(C) degenerative joint disease

(D) acromioclavicular dislocation

(E) proximal tear of the biceps tendon

6. A 7-year-old male is brought to the emergency department after sustaining a fall onto his outstretched hand. He complains of pain involving the entire arm and refuses to move his arm, which is held in anatomical position with the elbow flexed at 90°. On physical examination there is notable tenderness over the elbow with associated swelling and pain on attempted rotation. There is no apparent tenderness to palpation involving the wrist or shoulder. The child refuses to participate with range of motion evaluation. Radiographic evaluation of the elbow shows the presence of a positive posterior fat pad sign. What is the most likely diagnosis with this patient's presentation?

(A) nursemaid's elbow

(B) lateral epicondylitis

(C) medial epicondylitis

(D) radial head dislocation

(E) occult fracture of the radial head

7. A 53-year-old female presents with pain in her right wrist. The pain is aggravated by movement of the thumb and when she makes a fist. She also notes that when she moves her thumb there is an occasional locking sensation in the radial aspect of her wrist. Physical examination of the wrist reveals swelling and tenderness over the distal radius, and full flexion of the thumb into the palm, with ulnar deviation of the wrist produces pain. Radiographic evaluation of the wrist shows no bone abnormalities. Which of the following would be the treatment of choice in this patient presentation?

(A) immobilization of the wrist with a thumb spica splint

(B) corticosteroid injections over the course of three return visits

(C) operative treatment to restore functionality

(D) prompt neurological evaluation

(E) proceed to bone scan to evaluate the area of pain

8. A 35-year-old male presents with complaints of swelling and pain in left knee. The patient states he sustained a twisting injury in a basketball game 3 days ago. The injury did not take him out of the game; he was able to participate with minimal difficulty. Over the last 2 days the pain has progressed. He notes a catching sensation and pain that is more medially located. On physical examination the patient is found to have tenderness over the medial joint line and limited range of motion. Forced flexion and circumduction of the joint causes a painful click. What is the most likely diagnosis in this patient presentation?

(A) anterior cruciate ligament tear

(B) medial meniscus tear

(C) pes anserine bursitis

(D) tibial plateau fracture

(E) medial collateral ligament tear

9. Which of the following motor, sensory, and reflex finding are most likely to be found in a patient with lumbar radiculopathy of the L4–L5 disc?

(A) weakness of the anterior tibialis, numbness of the shin, and an asymmetric knee reflex

(B) weakness of the great toe flexor and gastrocsoleus, inability to sustain tiptoe walking and an asymmetrical ankle reflex

(C) weakness of the great toe extensor, numbness on the top of the foot and first web space, no reflex findings

(D) perianal numbness, urinary and bowel incontinence

(E) ankle clonus

10. Which of the following characteristics help to distinguish the "pseudoclaudication" of a patient with spinal stenosis from true claudication?

    (A) insidious onset of symptoms
    (B) worsening of pain by lumbar flexion
    (C) radiation of pain to the upper back
    (D) preservation of pedal pulses
    (E) localizing maximum area of discomfort to the lower back

11. Evaluating for glenohumeral joint instability consists of evaluating the joint for anterior, posterior, and inferior instability. Which of the following is the most common test to perform in the evaluation of joint laxity and inferior stability?

    (A) apprehension test
    (B) relocation test
    (C) sulcus sign
    (D) Jahnke test
    (E) drop arm test

12. A 15-year-old male was playing football and was hit during a play, causing an abduction injury of his left lower leg. He locates the pain along the medial aspect of the knee and there is a minimal level of joint effusion. Which of the following test would assess for stability of the medial collateral ligament?

    (A) valgus stress test
    (B) varus stress test
    (C) apprehension sign
    (D) Lachman test
    (E) anterior drawer sign

13. Evaluation of the spine in patient presumed to have scoliosis should include the forward bend test. In addition to this which of the following should be included in the evaluation of scoliosis?

    (A) evaluation for joint meniscal injury
    (B) evaluation for neuromuscular abnormalities
    (C) evaluation for congenital cardiac disorder
    (D) evaluation for cranial nerve abnormalities
    (E) evaluation for growth hormone deficiency

14. A 12-year-old obese male presents with pain in the right thigh and medial knee. The pain has been over a 6-week time period. The pain is described as aching in nature. Over the last month the patient has had a limp present. On physical examination the right knee is found to be unremarkable, but there is a slight limp noted with gait. Radiographs of the right knee are normal. Which of the following is the most appropriate step in the evaluation of this patient?

    (A) examine and x-ray the right hip
    (B) x-ray the left knee for comparison
    (C) obtain a CT scan of the right knee
    (D) obtain a magnetic resonance image of the right knee
    (E) reassure the parents and observe the patient for progression

15. Treatment of scoliosis is usually employed for patients with curvature beyond which of the following curve magnitudes:

    (A) 20°
    (B) 30°
    (C) 40°
    (D) 50°
    (E) 60°

16. An 18-year-old male sustains a traumatic dislocation of his patella in a rugby match, which spontaneously reduced with extension of the knee. The patient states that this has never happened before. He has some swelling of the knee and no findings of joint instability or crepitus. There are no radiographic findings associated with the knee. Which of the following is proper management in this presentation?

(A) operative repair for treatment

(B) brace immobilization for 6 to 8 weeks

(C) application of heat for the next 2 weeks

(D) maintain reduction in a brace for 2 to 3 weeks

(E) full leg casting for 6 to 8 weeks

17. A 24-year-old male presents with low back pain of 2 days duration. The patient is a manual laborer and reports lifting a heavy box while at work yesterday. Initially the patient had no complaints, but the following day stiffness and pain began. The patient denies radiation of the pain, numbness, or difficulty with urination. He denies previous complaints of back pain or injury. On physical examination there is noted paravertebral muscle spasm and slight decrease in range of motion of the spine. Deep tendon reflexes are equal bilaterally and there are no sensory deficits noted. Which of the following is the most appropriate intervention?

(A) MRI of the lumbar spine

(B) plain radiographs of the lumbar spine

(C) return the patient to work with no limitations

(D) refer the patient for trigger point injections

(E) initiate a short period of rest, analgesia, and progressive functional program

18. A new military recruit is in his third week of boot camp and is seen in the infirmary with complains of anterior tibial pain of 3 weeks duration. On physical examination there is noted tenderness on palpation over the lower portion of the anterior tibia. Radiographs of the lower leg are negative for fracture. The patient is treated conservatively, and returns in 4 days time with persisting pain. What would be the next step in the management of this patient?

(A) repeat plain radiographs

(B) order a CT scan of the lower leg

(C) order an MRI of the lower leg

(D) order an ultrasound of the lower leg

(E) order a venous Doppler evaluation of the lower leg

19. A 44-year-old female presents with complaints of numbness and tingling of her right second and third fingers for the past 2 months. She recently began with nighttime wakening with pain in her right hand and wrist. She is a secretary, and notes that typing aggravates the symptoms along with grasping the steering wheel and holding her coffee mug. The patient notes a past history of a neck injury 3 years ago, that has been associated with continual complaints of intermittent neck pain. She has had a previous MRI of the cervical spine that revealed the presence of a bulging disc at C6–C7. Which of the following diagnostic evaluations is most appropriate to determine the etiology of the patient's paresthesias?

(A) psychological testing

(B) plain radiograph of the right wrist

(C) plain radiograph of the cervical spine

(D) electromyography/nerve conduction velocity

(E) selective nerve root blocks

20. Which of the following is most diagnostic of a septic joint?

(A) synovial fluid analysis

(B) plain radiograph

(C) ultrasound of the joint

(D) CT scan of the joint

(E) MRI of the joint

21. An 8-year-old male presents with complaint of a painful right wrist of 2 days duration. Mother of the child reports that the child jumped off of a swing landing on his outstretched arms. He immediately complained of pain in the right wrist and now has some mild swelling on the radial aspect of the wrist. Radiographic evaluation of the wrist presents an area of impaction on the distal radius, with a slight bend in the opposing cortex. Which of the following best describes this type of pediatric fracture?

   (A) greenstick fracture
   (B) torus fracture
   (C) plastic deformation
   (D) radial neck fracture
   (E) Monteggia fracture

22. Which of the following is the most common injured structure in a varus ankle sprain?

   (A) deltoid ligament
   (B) calcaneofibular ligament
   (C) anterior talofibular ligament
   (D) posterior talofibular ligament
   (E) syndesmosis ligament

23. A 39-year-old female presents with complaint of pain in her left foot of 4 weeks duration. The patient works as a cashier in a department store, which requires her to be on her feet for long periods of time. She notes that the pain is most severe on the bottom of her foot and is worse upon arising in the morning, and then it subsides with ambulation. The patient has a benign past medical history and no other complaints. Which of the following is the most likely diagnosis of this patient?

   (A) heel spur
   (B) achillis tendonitis
   (C) tarsal tunnel syndrome
   (D) plantar fascitis
   (E) posterior tibial nerve entrapment

24. Which of the following characteristics may be seen in a patient who has osteoarthritis?

   (A) bony enlargement of the interphalangeal joints
   (B) morning stiffness that persists for over 30 minutes
   (C) prodromal systemic symptoms of malaise and fever
   (D) symmetrical joint swelling with warmth and tenderness
   (E) subcutaneous nodules over the extensor surfaces

25. A 17-year-old male presents with complaints of pain located in his 5th digit. He was involved in an altercation and states his hand was injured from punching someone. On physical examination of the patient's hand, there is tenderness, swelling, and pain with extension. The patient is diagnosed with a "boxer's fracture." What radiographic finding would be present to diagnose this patient?

   (A) spiral fracture of the 3rd metacarpal
   (B) fracture of the 4th metacarpal
   (C) fracture of the 5th metacarpal
   (D) comminuted fracture of the distal phalanx of the 5th digit
   (E) comminuted fracture of the distal phalanx of the 4th digit

26. Which of the following best defines the deformity that causes a "mallet finger."

   (A) rupture or avulsion of the insertion of the extensor tendon at the base of the distal phalanx
   (B) rupture or avulsion of the insertion of the flexor tendon at the base of the distal phalanx
   (C) fracture of the distal phalanx
   (D) dislocation of the distal interphalangeal joint
   (E) fracture of the proximal phalanx

27. A 6-year-old male presents with complaints of a limp affecting the left lower leg of 3 weeks duration. There is no association of pain. The mother of the child notes the limp is more noticeable with increased activity. There is no associated fever or swelling of the lower extremity. The child has progressed on the growth chart with no delays. On physical examination there is mild restriction of hip motion. Which of the following findings on radiographs of the hip and pelvis would confirm the diagnosis of Legg–Calve–Perthes disease?

    (A) normal plain film
    (B) normal MRI findings
    (C) MRI finding of osteonecrosis of the femoral head
    (D) MIR finding of bilateral spondyloepiphyseal dysplasia
    (E) MRI finding of multiple epiphyseal dysplasias

28. A 10-year-old male presents to the emergency room status post a fall from his bicycle. The patient complains of pain located in his right knee with an associated 2 cm × 2 cm abrasion just inferior to the patella. There is no swelling noted of the knee. The child is not cooperative with examination of the extremity. Radiographs are taken of the right knee and there is no finding of fracture or joint changes. Incidentally a lesion is noted at the distal femur, described as a pedunculated bone mass capped in cartilage. With this finding, what is the most likely diagnosis?

    (A) osteoid osteoma
    (B) chondroblastoma
    (C) osteosarcoma
    (D) osteochondroma
    (E) Ewing sarcoma

29. A 39-year-old female presents with complaints of left anterior knee pain of 4 weeks duration. She has noted difficulty with going up and down stairs. The patient also notes increased pain in the knee upon arising after being seated for a period of time. The pain may then improve with walking. The patient denies joint crepitus or locking sensation. On physical examination there is no swelling or obvious joint distortion. The pain is reproduced with placing the knee in slight flexion and gentle pressure placed on the patella as the patient contracts the quadriceps. The knee appears stable, with no signs of crepitus, joint laxity, or internal derangement. Radiographs of the left knee are essentially benign. What course of treatment is best for this patient?

    (A) crutches for 6 weeks, keeping the joint nonweight bearing
    (B) cortisone injection
    (C) physical therapy to strengthen the quadriceps
    (D) physical therapy to strengthen the lower back
    (E) progress to orthopedic evaluation for consideration of internal derangement of the knee

30. A 4-year-old male presents with complaints of right hip pain of 4 days duration and an associated limp. The patient is recovering from an upper respiratory infection that appears to be resolving. The child is currently afebrile. On physical examination there is notable limitation of movement with internal rotation. Radiographs reveal minor soft tissue swelling around the joint, with no bony findings. CBC and erythrocyte sedimentation rate are not elevated. What would be the most appropriate long-term complication to consider for this patient?

    (A) osteoarthritis of the hip
    (B) septic arthritis
    (C) pyogenic arthritis
    (D) osteomyelitis
    (E) avascular necrosis of the hip

Answers and Explanations

1. **(C)** Nonsteroidal anti-inflammatory agents (NSAIDS) are metabolized in the liver and excreted via the kidneys. Elderly patients are more at risk of developing irreversible damage to the renal system. Renal function physiologically decreases with advancing age. With decreased clearance of the medication, renal damage ensues and leads to accumulation of the drug and further renal damage. Renal function should be monitored in the elderly patient receiving high doses of any NSAID. Hepatic failure is also a concern with use of NSAID, especially where there is potential for overdose. There is no documented evidence of damage to the eyes, heart, peripheral vascular system, or central nervous system. (*Katzung, 2001, p. 762; Tierney et al, 2005, p. 63*)

2. **(E)** Postinjection flare or inflammation may occur in 10% of patients for 24 to 48 hours after the injection. This reaction is characterized by increased pain and responds to ice, rest, and analgesics. Allergic and anaphylactic reactions may occur, but are extremely rare. Facial flushing may be seen with steroid joint injections, but is only an occasional side effect. Joint infection is a potential complication from incorrect technique and not a direct side effect secondary to the use of the corticosteroid. (*Greene, 2001, pp. 22–23*)

3. **(E)** The prophylactic antibiotic of choice for use in perioperative total joint replacement is best accomplished with the use of first generation cephalosporins. The use of antibiotics prior to total joint replacement has been shown to decrease the incidence of postoperative infection. First and second generation cephalosporins are effective against staphylococci and many Gram-negative organisms. Aminoglycosides are also potentially effective, but come with the greater risk of hearing loss and renal damage. Vancomycin does have good coverage against staphylococcal organisms, but is not effective against Gram-negative organisms. Macrolides have some coverage against staphylococcal organisms, but they have no effect on the more likely Gram-negative organisms involved with postoperative joint infections. Penicillins have no clinical effectiveness with staphylococcal or Gram-negative organisms. (*Katzung, 2001, p. 762*)

4. **(B)** *Staphylococcus aureus* is the most common etiology with the history of a prosthetic joint replacement. *Staphylococcus* epidermis is also more likely to be seen as a result of prosthetic joint replacement, decubitus ulcer association, or trauma. *Pseudomonas aeruginosa* may be seen in the tissues of a wound from a puncture. *Streptococcus* is not a common etiology associated with osteomyelitis. Candidal osteomyelitis more commonly develops in the immunocompromised patient. Enterococcal would more likely be associated with colonic flora and less likely from a puncture wound as described. (*Tierney et al, 2005, pp. 830–831*)

5. **(B)** The clinical presentation of progressive pain associated with decreased motion and

weakness involving abduction and forward flexion in a 42-year-old is most suggestive of a rotator cuff tear. Contributing to the diagnosis is the history of repetitive use and night pain, most likely from lying on the affected area. Adhesive capsulitis presents with pain and limitation of movement, both active and passive range of motion are equally limited. Degenerative joint disease involving the glenohumeral joint is relatively uncommon and seen more likely with patient's with rheumatoid arthritis, avascular necrosis, or long-standing chronic rotator cuff disease. Acromioclavicular dislocation is more likely seen in association with a result of trauma directly onto the joint and is characterized by tenderness and swelling over the acromio-clavicular joint. Proximal tear of the biceps tendon is more commonly diagnosed by the distinctive finding of a bulge of the biceps muscle in the lower arm. Rotator cuff tear often coexists with biceps tendon rupture. (*Skinner, 2003, pp. 193–196; Tierney et al, 2005, pp. 797–798; Greene, 2001, pp. 144–146*)

6. **(E)** The most likely diagnosis in this patient presentation is an occult fracture of the radial head. This is supported by the mechanism of injury, physical examination, and radiographic findings. On physical examination, tenderness over the radial head with local swelling and pain with rotation and flexion of the forearm is usually present. Fractures of the radial head may be subtle on initial radiographs. The finding of an anterior fat pad may be a normal finding, but the finding of a posterior fat is pathological and usually indicates an occult fracture of the radial head. Nursemaid's elbow is more commonly seen in children 1 to 3 years of age and associated with injury that is pulling in nature on the hand with the elbow in full extension. Lateral and medial epicondylitis are typically overuse injuries that occur in patient's 35 to 50 years of age. Radial head dislocation may be associated with fracture of the radial head; the supporting evidence in this case does not support dislocation. Radial head dislocation is typically posteriorly and evident on radiographs. (*Hay et al, 2005, pp. 818–819; Greene, 2001, pp. 654–657*)

7. **(A)** This patient presentation is most consistent with De Quervain tendonitis. Inflammation or tenosynovitis of the abductor pollicis longus and extensor pollicis brevis thickening of the tendon sheath results in pain, swelling, and a triggering phenomenon of locking or sticking. This disorder is more common in middle-aged women and repetitive motion injuries. On physical examination the finding of a positive Finkelstein test, which is pain with full flexion of the thumb into the palm, with ulnar deviation of the wrist is diagnostic of De Quervain tendonitis. Initial treatment is aimed at immobilization of the wrist to allow for pain and inflammatory relief. A course of nonsteroidal anti-inflammatory drugs (NSAIDs) is helpful for pain relief as well. Corticosteroid injection is reserved for patients who fail with immobilization and NSAID use. Operative treatment should only be considered if injections are not helpful. Radiographic evaluation is not helpful in the evaluation or treatment of this condition. (*Greene, 2001, pp. 230–234; Skinner, 2003, p. 546*)

8. **(B)** This patient presentation is most consistent with a medial meniscus tear. Medial meniscus tears are more likely to present with a twisting injury of the knee. Patients usually are ambulatory after the injury, with pain and swelling progressing 2 to 3 days after the injury. The pain is usually located in the medial or lateral side of the knee and associated with a catching or locking sensation caused by swelling or mechanical blockage from torn meniscus. On physical examination there is tenderness over the medial or lateral joint line. The McMurray test is positive when forced flexion and circumduction of the joint causes a painful click. Anterior cruciate ligament can result from a twisting injury as well, but would be more likely associated with hemarthrosis and a positive Lachman test or anterior drawer sign. Pes anserine bursitis more commonly presents with tenderness distal to the medial joint line and more likely associated with overuse. Tibial plateau fracture would present with bony tenderness and a result of high energy fracture. Medial collateral ligament tear would present with pain and instability with valgus stress on the joint.

(*Greene, 2001, pp. 379–381; Skinner, 2003, pp. 161–163*)

9. **(C)** The radiculopathy found with L4–L5 disc herniation presents with weakness of the great toe extensor, numbness on the top of the foot and first web space, and no reflex findings. Radiculopathy of the L3–L4 disc presents with weakness of the anterior tibialis, numbness of the shin, and an asymmetric knee reflex. Radiculopathy of the L5–S1 disc presents with weakness of the great toe flexor and gastrocsoleus, inability to sustain tiptoe walking, and an asymmetrical ankle reflex. Cauda equina syndrome is associated with perianal numbness and urinary and bowel incontinence. Ankle clonus is more likely to be associated with demyelinating conditions. (*Greene, 2001, pp. 559–562*)

10. **(D)** The pain of spinal stenosis presents in the lower back, radiating to the buttocks and thighs and is aggravated with walking and alleviated with rest or lumbar flexion. Distinguishing "pseudoclaudication" of a patient with spinal stenosis from true vascular insufficiency is best supported by the preservation of pedal pulses and the location of pain in the thighs. (*Skinner, 2003, pp. 234–237; Tierney, 2005, pp. 793–794*)

11. **(C)** Evaluating for inferior instability and overall joint laxity is best evaluated by the sulcus test. This test is performed with the athlete in a seated position with the arm at their side or in abduction at 30°. Distractive force is then placed longitudinally along the humerus. A positive finding is discomfort or apprehension of instability. The apprehension test evaluates for anterior instability, and the relocation test evaluates for relief of anterior instability. Jahnke test evaluates for reduction of posterior instability. The drop arm test is used in evaluation of a rotator cuff tear. (*Skinner, 2003, pp. 182–185*)

12. **(A)** Evaluating the medial collateral ligament is best completed with applying valgus stress to the knee extended and then flexed at 25° and evaluating the stability. If the knee shows exaggerated laxity, there is more likelihood the medial collateral ligament is torn. Varus stress evaluates the integrity of the lateral collateral ligament. The apprehension sign evaluates for patellar instability. The Lachman test and anterior drawer sign are to evaluate for anterior cruciate ligament tears. (*Skinner, 2003, p. 351; Tierney et al, 2005, pp. 134–135*)

13. **(B)** Evaluating a patient with presumed scoliosis would include evaluation for other conditions associated with scoliosis. Assessing the patient for limb length discrepancy, abnormal joint laxity, and most importantly neuromuscular abnormalities is of prime importance. Patients with scoliosis should be evaluated for cerebral palsy, muscular dystrophy, myelomeningocele, and spinal muscular atrophy. Joint meniscal injury, congenital cardiac disorders, cranial nerve abnormalities, and growth hormone deficiency are not necessarily etiologically associated with scoliosis. (*Greene, 2001, pp. 696–699*)

14. **(A)** This patient presentation is most suggestive of slipped capital femoral epiphysis of the right hip. This condition is commonly seen in adolescent's age (11 to 13 years), and obesity is also a contributing factor. The patient more commonly presents with referred pain to the medial knee and thigh with an associated limp. The combination of a thicken growth plate from the influence of growth hormone causing a weaker bone, lack of sexual maturity to stabilize the physis, obesity adding mechanical stress, and the mechanics of the joint adds to the increased likelihood of slippage of the epiphysis. Examination of the hip along with radiographic studies is imperative to further evaluate this patient. Hip examination would reveal loss of abduction and internal rotation of the hip. Radiographically a frog-legged lateral view is best for detecting slippage. Establishing the degree of slippage is imperative to determining the treatment. In this patient presentation, an x-ray of the left knee is not necessary. Further radiographic evaluation of the knee with CT scan or MRI is not necessary. Reassuring the parents and observing this patient is not advisable, as prompt evaluation and treatment is imperative due to the progressiveness of this disease.

(Skinner, 2003, pp. 603–603; Hay et al, 2005, pp. 815–816)

15. **(A)** The treatment of scoliosis depends on the magnitude of the curvature of the spine and the risk of progression. Curvatures less than 20° usually do not require intervention. Curvature at 20° to 40° in a skeletally immature patient may respond to bracing. Curvatures greater than 60° may require surgical intervention. *(Hay et al, 2005, p. 815)*

16. **(D)** Acute traumatic dislocation of the knee commonly follows an injury of direct force or activity of the quadriceps. In most cases reduction occurs spontaneously when the knee is extended. Appropriate treatment is to maintain reduction for 2 to 3 weeks, and isometric exercises of the quadriceps and strengthening of the vastus medialis. Immobilizing the joint either with a brace or casting is not necessary, and the application of heat would be not as therapeutic as the anti-inflammatory effect of ice. Operative repair would only be considered in patients with recurrent episodes of dislocations. *(Skinner, 2003, p. 141)*

17. **(E)** The initial treatment of a patient with low back pain without neurological deficit consists of conservative management despite the causation. Muscle strain, ligament sprain, or early disc disease are all treated with rest, analgesia, and progressive functional activities. Diagnostic evaluation to include radiographs, and MRI of the lumbar spine is reserved for the patient who does not respond to conservative management. Returning the patient to work, especially manual labor, would be counterproductive for the pain. Trigger point injections are not proven to show benefit in the treatment of acute low back pain. *(Skinner, 2003, pp. 239–230)*

18. **(C)** This patient presents with "shin splints," a descriptive term for pain in the shin. Shin pain is usually associated with activity, such as vigorous training. Pain and tenderness is typical in the anterior shin and usually disappears in 1 to 2 weeks time as conditioning improves. Continued pain as the patient is experiencing should be evaluated for stress fractures. Plain radiographs are often normal at first; MRI or technetium bone scans are indicated for diagnosis of stress fractures. CT scan, ultrasound, and venous Doppler evaluations are not indicated in this patient presentation. *(Skinner, 2003, p. 174)*

19. **(D)** The presentation of numbness and tingling in the second and third fingers, nocturnal pain, and the precipitating factors of typing, grasping the steering wheel, and holding a coffee mug is suggestive of carpal tunnel syndrome. However, with the patient's past history of neck injury and bulging disc of C6–C7, further evaluation is necessary to pinpoint the etiology. Electromyography and nerve conduction velocity studies will assist in differentiating the causation of the numbness and tingling. Radiographs of the wrist are not indicated for the evaluation of numbness and there is no trauma noted to the area. Radiographs of the cervical spine will not show progression of disc bulging, or locate nerve involvement. Nerve root blocks are not indicated for diagnostic purposes. Psychological testing is not warranted with the patient presentation. *(Skinner, 2003, pp. 550–552)*

20. **(A)** The evaluation of septic arthritis is best accomplished with synovial fluid analysis and culture. Radiological imaging can be normal. Ultrasound evaluation can demonstrate fluid in the joint, but is not specific to the diagnosis. CT scan and MRI of the joint are not specific to the diagnosis. *(Skinner, 2003, p. 439)*

21. **(B)** This patient scenario is consistent with a torus fracture of the radius. Torus fractures commonly present as a "buckle" of the cortex and are due to force or compression of the bone. This type of fracture is more common to occur in a pediatric patient due to the "softer" nature of the bone. Torus fractures usually do not create alignment issues and heal within 3 weeks with simple immobilization. A greenstick fracture involves disruption of one side of the cortex with angulation of the bone; this type of fracture does not separate the ends of the bone. Plastic deformation is the change in the natural shape of the bone with a detectable suture line; there is no "buckle" with this type of fracture. Radial neck fracture would present with angulation of the radial head, and is proximally located. Monteggia fracture refers to an ulnar fracture with associated radial head dislocation from the capitulum. (*Skinner, 2003, pp. 628–631; Hay et al, 2005, p. 820*)

22. **(C)** An inversion injury to the ankle causes disruption of the lateral ligament complex that consists of the anterior talofibular ligament, calcaneofibular ligament, and the posterior talofibular ligament. The majority of inversion or varus ankle sprains first involve the anterior talofibular ligament. The calcaneofibular ligament is only involved in more serious injuries, and the posterior talofibular ligament is rarely injured. The deltoid ligament is more likely to be injured with an eversion and rotational injury of the medial ankle. The syndesmosis ligament joins the tibia and fibula together and is more likely injured by an external rotational force to the foot, what commonly is known as a "high sprain." (*Skinner, 2003, pp. 511–512*)

23. **(D)** This patient presentation is typical of the pain associated with plantar fascitis, where the pain is located on the bottom of the foot and more commonly is severe on initially getting up in the morning and lessens with ambulation. Most cases of plantar fascitis there is maximal pain along the plantar medial aspect of the heel, corresponding to the origin of the plantar fascia at the medial calcaneal tuberosity. Heel spurs are more likely to be associated with continued pain. Achillis tendonitis is more likely to occur over the bony prominence of the calcaneus. Tarsal tunnel syndrome is associated with compression of the posterior tibial nerve and with diffuse pain, paresthesias, and burning of the medial ankle, and is worse after walking and occurs at night. (*Tierney et al, 2005, p. 826*)

24. **(A)** Bony enlargements of the interphalangeal joints (Heberden's and Bouchard's nodes) are associated with osteoarthritis. Morning stiffness may be seen initially in patients with osteoarthritis, but it seldom lasts longer than 15 minutes. Morning stiffness that persists for over 30 minutes, prodromal systemic symptoms of malaise and fever, symmetrical joint swelling with warmth and tenderness, and subcutaneous nodules over the extensor surfaces are more characteristic of a patient with rheumatoid arthritis. (*Tierney et al, 2005, pp. 801–807*)

25. **(C)** Boxer's fracture refers to a fracture of the 5th metacarpal. This is the most common fracture of the hand and is seen with injuries associated with a closed fist striking an object. With all of the potential fractures the patient will typically have a history of trauma, local tenderness, swelling, deformity, and/or decreased range of motion. (*Skinner, 2003, p. 563*)

26. **(A)** Mallet finger is caused by rupture or avulsion of the insertion of the extensor tendon. It is also known as baseball finger due to the cause of injury commonly associated with a ball striking the finger, causing sudden passive flexion of the actively extended distal interphalangeal joint. The presentation is a DIP joint that is unable to extend at the joint. Treatment of this extensor tendon injury is best accomplished with continuous splinting of the DIP joint in extension for 6 to 8 weeks. (*Greene, 2001, p. 271*)

27. **(C)** The diagnosis of Legg–Calve–Perthes disease (LCPD) is associated with MRI findings of osteonecrosis of the femoral head. LCPD most commonly presents with the classic "painless limp" and typically in 4- to 8-year-olds, with a fourfold increased likelihood in males. Prompt diagnosis is essential to avoid growth deficit and to preserve limb function. Initial plain films maybe normal; this does not confirm the diagnosis of LCPD. MRI findings are more specific to evaluate for osteonecrosis. The finding of bilateral spondyloepiphyseal and epiphyseal dysplasia is more likely to be associated with bilateral presentation and short stature. (*Greene, 2001, pp. 675–677*)

28. **(D)** This patient presentation is more consistent with osteochondroma, which is the most common bone tumor in children and is typically associated with a pain-free mass. The tumor appears as a pedunculated or sessile lesion that resembles a cartilaginous cap on a boney stalk. This tumor has a very rare malignant tendency and is excised only if it interferes with function. (*Hay et al, 2005, pp. 826–827*)

29. **(C)** This patient presentation is most likely patellofemoral syndrome. The typical presentation includes anterior knee pain of vague location; the pain is increased by flexion load such as stair climbing and the patient has a positive "theater sign." Theater sign consist of pain after being seated for prolonged period of time. Treatment of patellofemoral syndrome is initially conservative and aimed at strengthening the quadriceps. Referral to physical therapy is helpful with regaining strength and implementing therapeutics. Injection of the joint with corticosteroid would be less likely associated with the initial approach and weight-bearing exercises should be avoided in the acute phase. Immobilizing the joint is counterproductive. (*Tierney et al, 2005, pp. 798–799*)

30. **(E)** This patient presentation is most consistent with transient synovitis of the hip. This is the most common cause of limping with pain in children 3 to 10 years of age. Transient synovitis presents more commonly in males and usually follows a self-limiting upper respiratory infection. Radiographic findings are nonspecific and there is no elevation of white blood cell count (WBC) or erythrocyte sedimentation rate (ESR). Treatment is aimed at keeping the hip in slight flexion to avoid avascular necrosis of the femoral head. Acute precipitation to osteoarthritis is not the focus of this presentation. Septic arthritis would more likely be associated with infection and have elevated WBC and ESR. Pyogenic arthritis may present with infection or adjacent osteomyelitis, purulent joint effusion, and an elevated WBC and ESR. (*Hay et al, 2005, pp. 823–824*)

REFERENCES

Greene W (ed). *Essentials of Musculoskeletal Care*, 2nd ed. Rosemont, IL: American Academy of Orthopaedic Surgeons; 2001.

Hay WW, Levin MJ, Sondheimer JM, Deterding RR (eds). *Current Pediatric Diagnosis & Treatment*, 17th ed. New York: McGraw-Hill; 2005.

Katzung BG (ed.). *Basic & Clinical Pharmacology*, 8th ed. New York: McGraw-Hill; 2001.

Skinner HB. *Current Diagnosis and Treatment in Orthopedics*, 3rd ed. New York: McGraw-Hill; 2003.

Tierney LM, McPhee, SJ, Papadakis, MA (eds). *2005 Current Medical Diagnosis & Treatment*, 44th ed. New York: McGraw-Hill; 2005.

Otolaryngology and Eye
Questions

Gary R. Uremovich, MS, MPAS, PA-C

DIRECTIONS (Questions 1 through 45): Each of the numbered items or incomplete statements in this section is followed by answers or by completions of the statement. Select the ONE lettered answer or completion that is BEST in each case.

Questions 1 through 45

1. Melissa is 7-year-old female who is brought to her pediatrician by her mother for evaluation of a 2-day history of fever to 101°F, sore throat, and redness and tearing in both eyes. She denies any cough, nasal congestion, or any pain or photophobia in her eyes. Melissa has been taking swimming lessons 2 days a week for the past month. Findings on physical exam include copious watery discharge and scanty exudate in both eyes, prominent follicles present on both her conjunctiva and pharyngeal mucosa, and nontender preauricular lymphadenopathy. The most appropriate treatment for Melissa at this time is which of the following?

    (A) penicillin to be taken four times a day by mouth
    (B) topical or systemic antiviral such as acyclovir
    (C) no specific treatment required at this time
    (D) instillation of a mast cell stabilizer to each eye
    (E) culture of ocular exudate

2. A 35-year-old male presents to your office complaining of a painless, localized swelling of his left, lower eyelid that has developed over a period of weeks. He comes in today because it is now producing a foreign body sensation in his left eye. On physical exam, his visual acuity is normal and there is no evidence of injection or discharge. There is a nontender, localized nodule on the lower eyelid. What is the likely diagnosis?

    (A) hordeolum
    (B) chalazion
    (C) pterygium
    (D) dacrocystitis
    (E) blepharitis

3. A 50-year-old male presents with an acute and painless onset of a bright red blood patch along the lateral part of his sclera. His visual acuity is normal and blood pressure is within normal limits. He has had a cough which is getting better. What is the most appropriate treatment?

    (A) no treatment is needed
    (B) CT scan to rule out intracranial hemorrhage
    (C) complete blood count (CBC) and bleeding studies
    (D) emergent consultation with an ophthalmologist
    (E) a complete intraocular examination with dilation

4. A 43-year-old male presents with complaint of a 3-day history of localized pain, redness, and swelling of his upper eyelid. He denies fever, visual changes, or photophobia. On physical exam, the patient's eyelid is diffusely red, with a tender, localized area of swelling that points outward. He appears to have an infection of the glands of the upper eyelid. The most common pathogen associated with this infection is which of the following?

(A) *Staphylococcus aureus*

(B) *Streptococcus pneumoniae*

(C) *Haemophilus influenzae*

(D) *Candida albicans*

(E) *Aspergillus species*

5. A 38-year-old man presents to the emergency room complaining of persistent double vision after being hit in the left eye during a fist fight the night before. On physical exam, his left perioribital area is markedly edematous and ecchymotic. Based on his history, what other abnormal finding might you expect to find as you complete your ophthalmic exam, and what diagnostic study would you order to best confirm your diagnosis?

(A) hyphema; Schiotz tonometer

(B) hyphema; plain x-ray

(C) restricted ocular movement; CT scan

(D) restricted ocular movement; plain x-ray

(E) ruptured globe, retinal angiography

6. A 45-year-old female presents with sudden onset of excruciating pain in the right eye, blurred vision, nausea, and vomiting. Physical exam reveals decreased visual acuity, intraocular pressure of 70 mm Hg, shallow anterior chamber, steamy cornea, and a moderately dilated right pupil. Which of the following is the most likely diagnosis?

(A) retinal detachment

(B) retinal artery occlusion

(C) uveitis

(D) primary open angle glaucoma

(E) primary acute angle closure glaucoma

7. A patient is experiencing visual loss in the temporal half of each eye. Where do you suspect the lesion is?

(A) right optic radiation

(B) left optic radiation

(C) optic chiasm

(D) right optic tract

(E) left optic tract

8. A 75-year-old male presents with painless, sudden loss of vision in one eye. A careful history reveals previous episodes of vision loss that resolved spontaneously. A workup for these previous episodes included a carotid ultrasound, which confirmed a diagnosis of bilateral carotid stenosis. Given this patient's current symptoms and past medical history, which of the following findings would be expected on funduscopic examination?

(A) retinal lines that have the appearance of a "ripple on a pond" or a "billowing sail"

(B) a pale or milky retina with a cherry red fovea

(C) enlarged physiologic cup, occupying more than half of the disc's diameter

(D) swollen disc with blurred margins; physiologic cup is not visible

(E) yellowish-orange to creamy-pink disc with sharp margins and a centrally located physiologic cup

9. A 35-year-old woman presents with a history of a self-limited upper respiratory illness 3 weeks prior to this clinic visit. She now complains of persistent weakness and malaise, which worsens near the end of the day. She complains that she has a difficult time keeping her right eye open during the later part of the day. Taking a nap often helps. You notice that her right eyelid covers the top portion of her pupil. Pupillary reactions are normal. A complete neurological evaluation is otherwise negative. Which evaluation is most likely to confirm your preliminary diagnosis?

(A) CT scan of the brain

(B) lumbar puncture

(C) fundoscopic examination

(D) tensilon test

(E) psychiatric evaluation

10. A 26-year-old male presents with bilateral conjunctivitis, dysuria, and pain in his lower back, and right Achilles tendonitis. What is the probable diagnosis?

(A) ankylosing spondylitis

(B) Reiter's syndrome

(C) Behçet's disease

(D) polyarteritis nodosa

(E) gonococcal disease

11. A 2-year-old presents with mild but obvious crossed-eyes since birth. Unless this is treated by an ophthalmologist what is the likely outcome?

(A) amblyopia

(B) esotropia

(C) exotropia

(D) hypophoria

(E) strabismus

12. A 62-year-old woman presents with a 3-week history of progressively more painful and worsening external otitis. She is a type 2 diabetic patient and has been poorly controlled on oral hypoglycemics. Examination demonstrates a foul-smelling purulent drainage and the presence of granulation tissue within the auditory canal. The tympanic membrane appears to be normal and mobile to pneumatic testing. What is the most appropriate management decision at this time?

(A) debride the canal and start on oral antipseudomonal antibiotics (i.e., ofloxacin)

(B) perform a Gram stain and culture of the discharge

(C) request an emergent CT of the head

(D) prescribe oral antibiotics, topical otic antibacterial drops, and effective pain management

(E) improve management of the diabetes to improve efficacy of conservative therapy

13. A 16-year-old male presents with a history of injury to his left pinna while competing at a wrestling match. The superior outer portion of the pinna is edematous and fluctuant to palpation (Fig. 16–1). There is minimal tenderness to palpation. Which of the following management decisions is most appropriate?

(A) refer the patient for I&D and pressure dressing

(B) have the patient return only if he develops a fever to 101°F

(C) apply a soft, bulky, and loose-fitting dressing to protect the pinna

(D) prescribe a 10-day course of amoxicillin and schedule for a clinic follow-up

(E) perform an I&D only if the pinna becomes red and tender

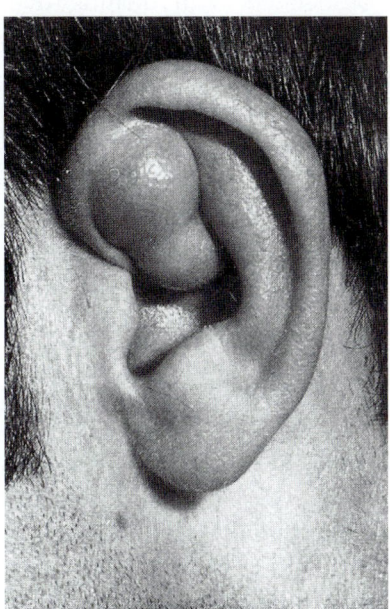

Fig. 16–1. From Becker W, Naumann HH, Pfaltz CR, Buckingham RA, *Atlas of Ear Nose and Throat Diseases*, 2nd ed, Thieme Medical Publisher, New York, 1994, with permission.

14. A 65-year-old male with a history of diabetes mellitus presents with an acute episode of left facial paralysis. He is still able to wrinkle and elevate both sides of his forehead. He denies recent viral illness or ear pain. His diabetes has been well-controlled. Examination of the tympanic membranes and the external pinnae are normal. The Weber and Rinné tuning fork assessments are normal. Visual acuity, extraocular movement, and pupillary responses are all normal and equal bilaterally. Which of the following is the most likely diagnosis?

(A) Bell's palsy
(B) Ramsey–Hunt syndrome
(C) cerebrovascular accident
(D) peripheral facial nerve palsy
(E) diabetic neuropathy

15. A patient presents with a 3-day history of vertigo associated with turning over in bed, which lasts for several minutes. There are no other symptoms of the ear. Positional testing shows rotary nystagmus, which diminishes with repeated testing. Which of the following is the most likely diagnosis?

(A) central nervous system lesion
(B) positional vertigo
(C) labyrinthitis
(D) Meniere's disease
(E) vestibular neuronitis

16. A 33-year-old female presents with episodes of vertigo lasting about 20 minutes and associated with fluctuating hearing loss and a low-frequency nonpulsatile tinnitus in the affected ear. After these episodes of vertigo the patient states that her hearing improves and the tinnitus resolves. Which of the following illnesses is suggested by these symptoms?

(A) Meniere's disease
(B) eustachian tube dysfunction
(C) vestibular neuronitis
(D) paroxysmal positional vertigo
(E) none of the above

17. A 55-year-old female patient presents with a lengthy history of chronic ear infections and episodic purulent drainage from the right ear canal. The patient is without symptoms at this time. Examination of the tympanic membrane shows it to be retracted with a pocket of white material within the pars flaccida (Fig. 16–2). What is this finding called?

(A) tympanosclerosis
(B) otosclerosis
(C) cholesteatoma
(D) keratosis obliterans
(E) chronic otitis media

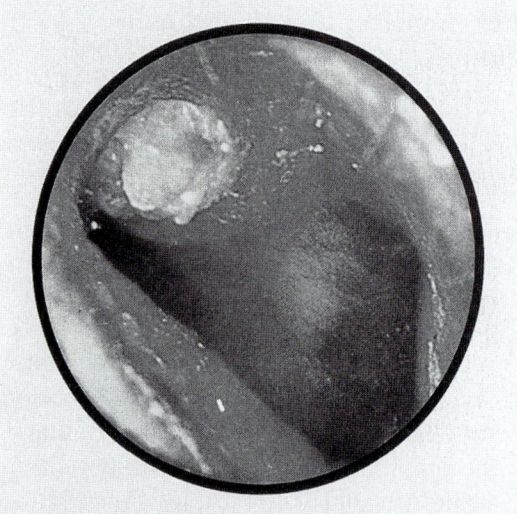

Fig. 16–2. From Becker W, Naumann HH, Pfaltz CR, Buckingham RA, *Atlas of Ear Nose and Throat Diseases*, 2nd ed, Thieme Medical Publisher, New York, 1994, with permission.

18. A 35-year-old male presents with a 1-week history of a marked decrease of hearing in his right ear. He denies trauma, otorrhea, or vertigo. The physical examination appears to be normal except for his tuning fork tests. The Weber test lateralizes to the better ear and the Rinne test shows air conduction to be better than bone conduction in both ears. After confirmation of your findings with an audiometric evaluation which would be the most appropriate treatment?

(A) broad-spectrum antibiotic
(B) antiviral medication
(C) decongestant
(D) oral steroids
(E) all of the above

19. A 60-year-old female presents with an acute onset of left facial nerve paralysis. She has severe pain. You notice that she has vesicles on the pinna. What is the name of this syndrome?

(A) Bell's palsy
(B) Ramsey–Hunt
(C) Mobius
(D) Millard–Gubler
(E) Melkersson–Rosenthal

20. A 4-year-old presents with a history of right otitis media, which was treated with amoxicillin for the past 4 days. Today the parent has noted that the child is complaining of worsening pain and a 103°F fever. The outer ear appears to be displaced forward and the outer posterior portion of the ear is tender to palpation. Your examination demonstrates a bulging right tympanic membrane with purulent effusion. What is your diagnosis?

(A) suppurative otitis media
(B) otitis media with effusion
(C) external otitis
(D) mastoiditis
(E) cellulitis of the pinna

21. A 50-year-old female presents with a progressive sense of decreased hearing in her right ear over several years. Her father had hearing problems at a young age but never was evaluated. She denies trauma, noise exposure, or ear disease as a child. Your examination demonstrates a completely normal appearing tympanic membrane which is mobile to pneumatic testing. Tuning fork tests show a Weber test which lateralizes to the affected (right) ear. Air conduction is greater than bone conduction of the left; on the right bone conduction is greater than air conduction. What is your diagnosis?

(A) serous otitis media
(B) otosclerosis
(C) presbycusis
(D) tympanosclerosis
(E) idiopathic hearing loss

22. A 14-year-old male presents with a history of "swimmer's ear," which was treated with cortisporin otic suspension 3 days prior. He now presents with increased erythema and crusting around the outer ear canal and a weeping somewhat vesicular area that extends below the tragus. His pain has increased. What is the likely diagnosis?

(A) *Psuedomonas* otitis externa
(B) mastoiditis
(C) Ramsey–Hunt syndrome
(D) neomycin allergy
(E) necrotizing otitis externa

23. A 59-year-old female presents with severe right ear pain for the last week. She also complains that the ear hurts most when chewing. Her hearing has not been affected. Examination shows tenderness to palpation of the external canal meatus anteriorly. The tympanic membrane is clear. What is your diagnosis?

(A) otitis externa
(B) otitis media
(C) temporomandibular joint dysfunction
(D) furuncle of the canal
(E) chondritis

24. Which of the following conditions is the most common for predisposing someone to developing acute sinusitis?

(A) viral infection of the upper respiratory tract
(B) dental infections
(C) intranasal foreign body
(D) barotrauma from deep-sea diving or airplane travel
(E) nasal steroid use

25. A 45-year-old male presents with decreased nasal flow from either nostril. He first noticed this when smoking and saw a decrease in the volume of air coming from one nostril and then reversing. Otherwise, he does not feel as if he is having problems breathing. He denies purulent drainage or facial pain. What treatment is most appropriate?

    (A) nasal steroid sprays
    (B) topical nasal decongestants
    (C) oral decongestant
    (D) saline irrigation
    (E) no treatment necessary

26. A 3-year-old male presents with a 2-week history of purulent rhinorrhea from his right nostril. Mother complains that the child's nose has a bad odor. What is the most likely diagnosis?

    (A) maxillary sinusitis
    (B) ethmoid sinusitis
    (C) foreign body
    (D) nasal polyp
    (E) acute viral rhinitis

27. A young woman in her second trimester of pregnancy complains of chronic nasal congestion. She denies rhinorrhea, facial pain, or fever. She has not had previous problems with nasal symptoms until the last several weeks. It seems to be getting worse. Your examination of the nose and throat is normal. What is your diagnosis?

    (A) allergic rhinitis
    (B) perennial rhinitis
    (C) vasomotor rhinitis
    (D) rhinitis of pregnancy
    (E) chronic rhinitis

28. Which nasal condition, if found in young children, is suggestive of cystic fibrosis?

    (A) chronic rhinorrhea
    (B) nasal polyps
    (C) choanal atresia
    (D) perennial allergic rhinitis
    (E) acute sinusitis

29. Parents bring their 14-year-old son in for several severe nose bleeds from his left nostril over the past 2 weeks. There is a large reddish-brown mass within the left posterior nasal cavity. What is this mass?

    (A) blood clot
    (B) inverting papilloma
    (C) hemorrhagic polyp
    (D) septal hematoma
    (E) juvenile angiofibroma

30. Which is the most common site of epistaxis in adults?

    (A) anterior septum
    (B) posterior septum
    (C) inferior turbinate
    (D) superior nasal vault
    (E) floor of nose

31. An elderly patient with a history of hypertension, diabetes mellitus, and supraventricular tachycardia presents with a brisk episode of epistaxis from the left nostril and a mild amount of bleeding from the right nostril. The bleeding first occurred last night and lasted for about 10 minutes and then stopped. It has now been continuously bleeding for about 20 minutes. You are in the emergency department and are unable to visualize the bleeding site because of the extent of bleeding from the left nostril. What is the most appropriate next step in your evaluation?

    (A) Get a detailed history of medications, prior surgery, prior episodes of epistaxis, and possible nasal disease. Review prior medical records if available
    (B) Perform diagnostic laboratory work including complete blood counts, hemoglobin, hematocrit, and clotting factors. Prepare the patient for vitamin K administration
    (C) Assess the hemodynamic state of the individual by obtaining blood pressures including a "tilt" test to rule out hypovolemia, pulse, and electrocardiogram, and cardiac monitoring

(D) Start a large bore intravenous line and provide at least 1 L of lactated Ringer's solution. Start oxygen by mask with a flow of at least 2 L/min

(E) Focus your attention on the bleeding. Carefully insert a cotton pledget soaked in a topical vasoconstricter (i.e., oxymetazoline) and pinching the nose. If this fails to slow down the bleeding, insert a nasal tampon or one of the many commercially prepared emergency nasal packs

32. Which of the following is one of the signs or symptoms most useful in predicting acute bacterial sinusitis and the decision to treat with antibiotics?

(A) acute symptoms for at least 7 days

(B) bilateral facial pain made worse by bending forward

(C) copious green nasal discharge

(D) unilateral facial or maxillary dental pain

(E) gradual worsening of symptoms

33. A 26-year-old healthy appearing male presents with rhinorrhea since having a nondisplaced nasal fracture 3 weeks prior. According to the patient, his nose has completely healed and feels fine now. He complains of a short gushes of a clear salty tasting liquid out his right nostril several times a day. He states that he can sometimes precipitate the drainage by leaning his head forward. Which test would you run on this liquid?

(A) "bull's-eye" test

(B) specific gravity

(C) Gram stain

(D) culture and sensitivity

(E) glucose dipstick

34. A 20-year-old male sustains a blow to his nose during a disagreement with some friends 5 or 6 days prior to his visit today. He complains that his breathing progressively worsened despite the outward swelling decreasing. Your examination shows soft fluctuant swelling of the septum bilaterally. This area is not tender to palpation. What is your treatment plan?

(A) nasal steroids for a couple of weeks to reduce intranasal swelling

(B) broad-spectrum antibiotic to prevent abscess formation

(C) emergent referral to an ENT provider

(D) CT scan to rule out a complex nasal fracture

(E) needle aspiration of the fluctuant area with cultures

35. The most common cause of chronic cough in adults is which of the following?

(A) common cold

(B) sinusitis

(C) asthma

(D) postnasal drip syndrome

(E) gastroesophageal reflux disease

36. An elderly patient presents with slurred speech. You have her protrude her tongue and it deviates to the right. Which cranial nerve (CN) is involved?

(A) left CN XII

(B) right CN XII

(C) left CN X

(D) right CN X

(E) left CN IX

37. A 45-year-old white male presents with a history of persistent fatigue throughout the day despite a full night of sleep. He complains of a sore throat and headache each morning. He has used short-acting sleeping pills, which only seem to worsen his symptoms. He is being treated for poorly controlled hypertension. The patient is morbidly obese. Which of the following conditions is most likely for this patient?

(A) endogenous depression

(B) diabetes mellitus

(C) hypothyroidism

(D) obstructive sleep apnea

(E) Cushing's syndrome

38. A 14-year-old male presents with a history of unilateral tonsillitis from a previous visit. His mother has noticed that his right tonsil has continued to enlarge over a period of 6 weeks despite a 10-day course of treatment with amoxicillin. The pharynx is normal except for a unilaterally enlarged tonsil on the right. There is no exudate or inflammation noted. Careful oral palpation and comparison of the tonsils demonstrates a firm nontender right tonsil that is 50% larger than the tonsil on the left. He has nontender right anterior cervical adenopathy. A complete blood count and differential is within normal limits. Which of the following is most appropriate in managing this patient?

(A) obtain an urgent surgical consult for tonsillectomy

(B) prescribe an alternative antibiotic and schedule for routine follow-up

(C) perform a monospot test

(D) reassure the patient and his mother that this is normal after tonsillitis and that the tonsil will eventually decrease in size as the patient ages

(E) request a soft tissue lateral radiograph to rule out a retropharyngeal abscess

39. A 30-year-old male presents for a routine physical examination and has an incidental finding of a flat, white, painless lesion on the buccal and gingival mucosa of the lower lip that does not rub off with a tongue blade. He states that this is the area where he usually "parks" his chewing tobacco. The patient denies any local or systemic symptoms. What is this lesion called?

(A) candidiasis

(B) mucous patch

(C) Fordyce's spot

(D) basal cell carcinoma

(E) leukoplakia

40. A patient presents with episodic painful swelling of the right submandibular salivary gland associated with eating. The swelling eventually dissipates over the course of a couple of hours. Examination of the floor of the mouth demonstrates clear secretions from Wharton's duct. Which of the following conditions is the most likely the cause of this patient's complaint?

(A) viral

(B) bacterial

(C) calculi

(D) fungal

(E) cancer

41. A 12-year-old male presents with pain and swelling along the floor of his mouth. Examination shows elevation of the patient's tongue, edema, and exquisite bilateral tenderness of the submandibular triangle of the neck. The patient complains of dysphagia and is drooling because of inability to swallow secretions. What is the diagnosis?

(A) ranula

(B) retropharyngeal abscess

(C) sialadenitis

(D) dental abscess

(E) Ludwig's angina

42. A 35-year-old acutely ill–appearing male presents with a rapidly worsening sore throat and odynophagia over the course of 3 days. Examination of the pharynx shows minimal erythema. You suspect epiglottitis based on the severity of clinical presentation out of proportion to the minimal findings of the oropharyngeal examination. Which of the following statements is correct concerning the care of this patient?

(A) epiglottitis in adults is extremely rare and should not be considered in this patient

(B) visualization of the epiglottis by indirect laryngoscopy (using a laryngeal mirror and head lamp) is safe in adults

(C) intubation is mandatory in all patients with epiglottitis

(D) adults with epiglottitis can be treated as outpatients

(E) oral antibiotics are very effective in treating adult cases of epiglottitis

43. In laryngopharyngeal reflux, which symptom is the least likely to be cited by the patient?

(A) heartburn

(B) hoarseness

(C) cough

(D) globus sensation

44. An 18-year-old male presents with sore throat which has worsened over the past several days. He complains of pain that is now localizing to the left side of his throat. He is talking with a muffled "hot potato" voice and appears to be acutely ill. He complains of pain radiating into his left ear. He has a tender 2 cm jugulodigrastric node. What other complaint would you most likely find in this patient?

(A) rash

(B) trismus

(C) dentalgia

(D) purulent rhinorrhea

(E) halitosis

45. A 15-year-old female presents with exudative tonsillitis, fever, and adenopathy for the last 5 days. Her primary care provider placed her on amoxicillin when the rapid strep test was positive. Within 24 hours she develops a non-pruritic maculopapular rash. What is the most likely cause of the rash?

(A) allergic reaction

(B) scarlatiniform lesions

(C) mononucleosis rash

(D) photosensitivity

(E) drug eruption

Answers and Explanations

1. **(C)** Melissa's symptoms (fever, pharyngitis, and conjunctivitis) and findings on exam, particularly nontender preauricular lymphadenopathy, are characteristic of a viral conjunctivitis. This condition is found more commonly in children, and contaminated swimming pools are sometimes the source of infection. There is no specific treatment, but the conjunctivitis is self-limited, usually lasting about 10 days. Application of topical antibiotics may prevent secondary infection. Penicillin, indicated for streptococcal pharyngitis, would not be appropriate because there are no physical exam findings such as pharyngeal erythema, tonsillar exudate, or tender cervical adenopathy to support the diagnosis. Acyclovir may be helpful in the treatment of herpes simplex virus conjunctivitis, which is a disease characterized by unilateral injection, irritation, mucoid discharge, pain, and mild photophobia. A mast cell stabilizer would be helpful in allergic conjunctivitis to alleviate symptoms of itching, a symptom that Melissa did not complain of. *(Vaughan et al, 1999, pp. 100–101; Tierney et al, 2001, pp. 192–194, 1348)*

2. **(B)** A chalazion is a sterile granulomatous inflammation of a meibomian gland usually characterized by a hard, painless, localized swelling on the upper or lower eyelid that develops over weeks. It can be differentiated from hordeolum by the absence of acute, inflammatory signs. Most chalazia point toward the conjunctival surface and if large enough can produce a foreign body sensation and/or distort vision. A pterygium is a disorder of the conjunctiva, not the eyelid itself. Dacrocystitis also involves inflammation and is characterized as a warm, tender, localized infection of the lacrimal sac. Blepharitis is usually bilateral and involves inflammation of the entire lid margins. *(Vaughan et al, 1999, pp. 74–76, 85, 113)*

3. **(A)** No treatment is needed for a subconjunctival hemorrhage. The sudden onset and bright red appearance can be quite alarming for the patient. The hemorrhage is caused by rupture of a small conjunctival vessel and may be associated with sneezing or coughing. The best treatment is reassurance. The blood is reabsorbed within 2 weeks. *(Vaughan et al, 1999, p. 104)*

4. **(A)** The symptoms and findings described above are associated with a hordeolum, which is most often caused by a staphylococcal infection, usually *Staphylococcus aureus*. *(Vaughan et al, 1999, pp. 74–75)*

5. **(C)** A history of facial/orbital trauma that results in diplopia is suggestive of an orbital blowout fracture causing entrapment. As a result, one would expect to find restriction of extraocular movements. Although plain x-rays may be helpful in the initial identification of bony injury, CT scanning with axial and coronal views provides the best assessment of orbital trauma. A hyphema is a possible abnormal finding in this patient as well, but

would not require radiographs or tonometry. *(Vaughan et al, 1999, pp. 352–353; Noble et al, 2001, p. 1681)*

6. **(E)** The patient's symptoms, abnormal findings noted on the eye exam, and her significantly elevated intraocular pressure of 70 mm Hg (normal range of intraocular pressure is 10 to 24 mm Hg) are all consistent with a diagnosis of acute angle closure glaucoma. This type of glaucoma is an ophthalmic emergency requiring immediate reduction in the intraocular pressure. Primary open angle glaucoma is the most common form of glaucoma; it is a chronic condition that is often asymptomatic until the disease is far advanced. Both retinal detachment and retinal artery occlusion are painless disorders with abnormal findings on exam that are different than those stated. *(Vaughan et al, 1999, pp. 204, 210; Noble et al, 2001, p. 1667)*

7. **(C)** A lesion of the optic chiasm will produce bitemporal hemianopsia. Lesions of the optic tract or optic radiation will produce visual loss on the same side of both eyes. *(Bickley and Hoekelman, 1999, p. 212)*

8. **(B)** A central retinal artery occlusion occurs as a result of a small emboli breaking loose from sclerotic plaque and lodging in retinal arterioles. Ophthalmoscopy reveals a pale retina with a cherry-red spot at the fovea. The funduscopic exam findings described in answer (A) are consistent with retinal detachment; in answer (C), the findings are consistent with glaucoma; in answer (D), the findings are consistent with papilledema; and in answer (E), the findings are normal. *(Bickley and Hoekelman, 1999, p. 220; Vaughan et al, 1999, p. 281)*

9. **(D)** Tensilon (edrophonium) testing will confirm that this patient has a classic presentation of myasthenia gravis. The usual adult test dose of 0.2 cm^3 edrophonium chloride is given intravenously. The eyelids are assessed for improvement in function. Additional dosing provided in 0.2 cm^3 increments to total of 1.0 cm^3. Unilateral ptosis is often a presenting sign and worsens with fatigue and can improve with a nap. Often, the ptosis will be-

come bilateral. The weakness increases and often shows diurnal variation. This disease most often affects young adults aged 20 to 40 years and often occurs after an illness, stress, injury, or pregnancy. It involves cholinesterase destroying acetylcholine at the myoneural junction. It may be an autoimmune disease with the production of antiacetylcholine antibodies causing reduction in the replacement of acetylcholine. Cholinesterase-inhibiting drugs can reverse the ptosis and fatigue associated with myasthenia gravis. The differential diagnosis in this case could include multiple sclerosis and brainstem lesions. Respectively, absence of sensory deficits or pupil abnormalities rule against these. *(Vaughan et al, 1999, pp. 275–276)*

10. **(B)** Reiter's syndrome is a disorder that consists of the triad of arthritis, conjunctivitis, and urinary tract symptoms. Reiter's syndrome is sometimes referred to as a reactive arthritis, which is responding to an infection elsewhere in the body. Reiter's syndrome develops in 1% to 3% of men after a nonspecific urethritis, up to 4% of persons after enteric infections caused by *Shigella, Salmonella,* and *Campylobacter,* and in a higher proportion of patients with Yersinia enteric infections. The major criteria include polyarthritis, conjunctivitis or anterior uveitis, urethritis or cervicitis, and balanitis circinata or keratoderma blennorrhagicum. The minor criteria include plantar fasciitis, Achilles tendonitis, lower back pain, sacroiliitis, and spondylitis; keratitis; cystitis and prostatitis; psoriasiform eruptions, oral ulcers, and nail changes; and diarrhea, leukocytosis, increased serum globulins, and evidence of inflammation in the synovial fluid. The diagnosis of Reiter's syndrome is based on history and medical examination. *(Szilard Kiss et al, 2003, pp. 1764–1765)*

11. **(A)** Amblyopia is the permanent loss of visual acuity in a child from abnormal visual experience during the maturation phase of sight development. During this maturation phase it is critical for the retina and central nervous system to become integrated. Strabismus ("crossed-eyes") or any disorder that causes a blurred retinal image in one or both eyes can

lead to this permanent visual disorder. The eye causing the blurred image is ignored by the central nervous system, thereby preventing neurological integration of that eye. Treatments center on forcing the ignored eye to be actively involved in perception. Interventions range from patching the good eye to force use of the amblyopic eye, use of special glasses, or surgical correction of the ocular muscles. The other answers are descriptions of muscles weakness. *(Vaughan et al, 1999, pp. 216–219)*

12. **(C)** The most pressing need at this time is to confirm the diagnosis of malignant external otitis (osteomyelitis of the skull base) by documenting osseous erosion with a CT scan. Persistent external otitis in a diabetic or any immunocompromised patient can evolve into osteomyelitis and extend into the skull base. Patients complain of a deep excruciating pain and foul drainage. Finding granulation tissue within the ear canal and the presence of cranial nerve palsies are suggestive of this condition. Occasionally, surgical debridement of infected bone is needed if aggressive medical treatment does not control the infection. *(Tierney et al, 2001, p. 217)*

13. **(A)** The skin of the pinna is tightly bound to the perichondrium of the cartilage. The cartilage depends on the perichondrium for vascular nourishment. Blunt trauma to the pinna can result in a hematoma or seroma and can cause the perichondrium to become detached from the cartilage. The devascularized cartilage dies and can eventually cause a permanent "cauliflower" deformity of the pinna. Strict aseptic technique during the I&D and a tightly formed compressive dressing is necessary to allow effective blood supply to the cartilage of the pinna without the advent of a postoperative infection. Antibiotics are often prescribed after the procedure to prevent an infection since perichondritis worsens the cosmetic damage. *(O'Donoghue et al, 2000, p. 27)*

14. **(C)** This patient has a central lesion causing facial paralysis instead of the typical peripheral lesion seen in Bell's palsy. Sparing of forehead movement in patients with facial paralysis is evidence of a lesion superior to the nucleus of the seventh cranial nerve (i.e., a brain tumor or stroke). A central lesion causes paralysis of the lower face on the contralateral side with sparing of the forehead since ipsilateral fibers provide enervation of the forehead. When the facial paralysis is caused by a peripheral lesion (i.e., middle ear infection) there is ipsilateral paralysis involving all subsections of the seventh cranial nerve including the forehead. *(Schuller and Schleuning, 1994, p. 523)*

15. **(B)** This patient has positional vertigo, which is assumed to be caused by movement of a small canalith within the inner ear. This is a benign process that is often self-limited. Positional exercises are helpful in quickening its resolution. Canalith repositioning procedures are effective at resolving the vertigo in about 80% of cases with just one outpatient treatment. All of the other clinical causes of vertigo would have additional ear symptoms such as tinnitus or hearing loss. *(Schuller and Schleuning, 1994, pp. 237–239)*

16. **(A)** These symptoms are classically associated with Meniere's disease (endolymphatic hydrops). Therefore, any patient presenting with episodic vertigo, tinnitus, and fluctuating hearing loss should have a complete otoneurologic evaluation. The physical examination and laboratory tests are usually normal in Meniere's disease except for vestibular and auditory tests. Treatment initially is dietary with a low sodium diet. *(Gates, 1998, pp. 79–80; Schuller and Schleuning, 1994, pp. 502–506)*

17. **(C)** A cholesteatoma is a squamous epithelium–lined sac that gradually increases in size and by pressure necrosis can eventually erode through bone (i.e., ossicular chain) or nerves (i.e., facial nerve). It often becomes infected and causes an intermittently draining ear. Eustachian tube dysfunction causes the tympanic membrane to become retracted and invaginate upon itself within the pars flaccida. Squamous epithelium becomes entrapped and gradually leads to the formation of a cholesteatoma. Cholesteatomas can also result from perforation of the tympanic membranes involving the margin or pars flaccida.

Treatment includes marsupialization of the cyst and reconstructive surgery. *(Tierney et al, 2001, p. 220)*

18. **(D)** This patient has sudden neurosensory hearing loss. The neurosensory nature of this disorder is suggested by the tuning fork tests. Weber testing lateralizing to the affected ear would be suggestive of a conductive hearing loss (otitis media or canal obstructed with cerumen). The etiology of sudden neurosensory hearing loss is unknown but may be viral or vascular. The only treatment that has shown effectiveness is the use of corticosteroids as soon as possible after the onset of symptoms. Providing therapeutic doses of prednisone within 2 weeks of the hearing loss is important. *(Ballenger and Snow, 1996, pp. 1109–1112)*

19. **(B)** Ramsey–Hunt syndrome is associated with intense ear pain, vesicles on the pinna, and facial paralysis. It is caused by the herpes-varicella virus producing a shingles type of cutaneous lesion. Treatment should include steroids, antiviral medications, and pain medication. *(Jafek and Murrow, 2001, p. 177)*

20. **(D)** Mastoiditis is not as common as it was in the preantibiotic era. However, it is still a complication that can be seen with delay in treatment of a suppurative otitis media. Pathognomonic signs of mastoiditis include tenderness or periosteal elevation of the postauricular area over the mastoid cortex, displacement of the ear anteriorly, and edema of the posterior portion of the auditory canal. Treatment requires tympanocentesis for cultures, intravenous antibiotics, and possible surgical debridement of the middle ear and mastoid cavity. *(Wilson et al, 2004 pp. 70–71)*

21. **(B)** Otosclerosis is a genetic condition in which the bones of the inner ear soften and then harden. This causes the three bones of hearing to harden at the joints, preventing them from conducting vibrations into the cochlea. The diagnosis is made by observing a completely normal appearing tympanic membrane with conductive hearing loss as noted by tuning forks. Treatment is dependent on the amount of conductive loss and can be managed with hearing aids or by a surgical procedure called a stapedectomy. *(Woodson, 2000, pp. 46–47)*

22. **(D)** Cortisporin contains neomycin for which 10% to 15% of the population have a topical sensitivity. The patient should have his ear drops changed to non–neomycin-containing drops such as Floxin or Ciprofloxin. If the canal is too edematous for drops to enter, an otowick may need to be inserted. Occasionally, oral steroids are needed if the swelling and allergic reaction are severe. *(Calhoun et al, 2001, p. 38)*

23. **(C)** Temporomandibular joint dysfunction (TMJ) is a common cause of referred ear pain. The cause may be inflammation induced by a recent dental procedure or grinding teeth at bedtime (bruxism). The diagnostic clues are that the patient has pain that is worsened with chewing and she has tenderness over the TMJ within the ear canal with an otherwise normal ear examination. Treatment involves a soft diet, warm compresses, and nonsteroidal anti-inflammatory medication. Dental evaluation is often needed in patients with chronic TMJ disorders. *(Woodson, 2000, pp. 50–51)*

24. **(A)** Upper respiratory infections are the most common disorder leading to acute sinusitis. The infection develops primarily because of ostial obstruction from mucosal edema. Initially, the patients feel as if they are getting over their viral infection when they then develop a worsening of their symptoms with an increase in purulent drainage, facial pain, and fever. *(Fauci et al, 1998, p. 180)*

25. **(E)** No treatment is necessary. This is a normal physiological process called "nasal cycle." Many people become aware of this cycle when sleeping. It allows the nasal mucosa to more effectively produce mucous that can trap particles. *(Wilson et al, 2004, p. 170)*

26. **(C)** Foreign bodies within the nose quickly create a particulary foul smelling, unilateral purulent drainage. The nose should be carefully decongested and anesthetized with topical solution. Care should be taken not to push

the foreign body into the nasopharynx where it can be aspirated. *(Wilson et al, 2004 p. 187)*

27. **(D)** Rhinitis of pregnancy is fairly common. Nasal congestion can peak in the third trimester. No treatment is required since this disorder resolves after delivery. *(Woodson, 2000, p. 106)*

28. **(B)** Nasal polyps in a child should make the clinician suspicious for possible cystic fibrosis. Usually this illness manifests itself in early childhood with predominantly lung involvement. Recurrent sinusitis and otitis media are also frequently seen. The onset of nasal polyps in these patients typically appears between the ages of 5 and 14. Diagnosis of cystic fibrosis is made by a sweat chloride test. *(Woodson, 2000, pp. 106–107)*

29. **(E)** Juvenile angiofibromas are bening vascular tumors that tend to occur in postpubescent adolescent males (13 to 21 years of age). Typically the patient presents with very brisk unilateral epistaxis. Biopsies are not performed in the clinic setting because of the risk of hemorrhage. *(Calhoun et al, 2001, p. 211; Wilson et al, 2004, p. 220)*

30. **(A)** Anterior septal bleeding from Kiesselbach's plexus is by far the most common site of epistaxis in children and adults. Often there is a history of trauma (picking the nose) or hayfever. In adults it is important to rule out clotting disorders, aspirin use, and a family history of epistaxis. Pinching the nose firmly, sitting upright, and leaning slightly forward is often helpful in stopping epistaxis. The site of bleeding should then be sought with a nasal speculum, topical nasal decongestant, and effective light source. *(Wilson et al, 2004, pp. 211–212)*

31. **(E)** Stop the bleeding! Epistaxis can be life-threatening. Fortunately, most nose bleeds are mild and simple to treat; however, patients can still die from a severe nose bleed. While all of the other answers can be appropriate in the right setting, it is critical to stop a vigorous nasal bleed as soon as possible. This patient is at risk of a posterior arterial bleed because of

being elderly, a hypertensive, and taking blood thinners. If a nasal tampon or nasal packing is used, it should stay in place (as long as the bleeding is controlled) for at least 3 days. It should be removed by an ENT specialist. Be sure to place the patient on a broad-spectrum antibiotic to prevent sinusitis (because of the blocked sinus ostia) or toxic shock syndrome from Staphylococcus aureus. *(Calhoun et al, 2001, pp. 212–216)*

32. **(D)** Unilateral facial or dental pain near to the maxillary sinuses is a reliable symptom to differentiate a higher percentage of patients with acute bacterial sinusitis (ABS). Health care providers tend to prescribe antibiotics too often. In fact, most rhinosinusitis is viral and does not require antibiotics. However, even in patients with documented bacterial sinusitis, two-thirds will improve without antibiotic treatment. Therefore, antibiotic therapy should be reserved for patients who have had symptoms for more than 7 days and meet clinical criteria. Four signs and symptoms that are the most helpful in predicting ABS include purulent nasal discharge, maxillary tooth or facial pain (especially unilateral), unilateral maxillary sinus tenderness, and a sudden worsening of symptoms after initial improvement. *(Scheid and Hamm, 2004, pp. 1685–1692)*

33. **(E)** Glucose is present in cerebrospinal fluid (CSF) and can be detected with a urine glucose dipstick (50 to 80 mg/dL). Injuries in the region of the nasal bones and nasal process of the frontal bone may lead to a fracture through the cribiform or ethmoid bones. CSF drainage is most commonly unilateral and may be intermittent, coming in short, rapid gushes, or may present as a steady flow. A clue to a CSF leak can be gained from the characteristic "bull's-eye" test when the fluid is mixed with blood and allowed to dry on a white sheet. That is not helpful after the bleeding has stopped. Often these leaks can seal off spontaneously by having the patient on bed rest, with the head elevated. Leaks that do no stop require more elaborate evaluation and surgical intervention. *(Wilson et al, 2004, pp. 222–223)*

34. **(C)** Emergency referral for definitive treatment of this septal hematoma is critical. The hematoma requires surgical drainage, evaluation of the septal cartilage, and use of a drain to prevent reaccumulation of the hematoma. Failure to treat a septal hematoma may lead to a septal abscess and a saddle deformity by destruction of the septal cartilage. (*Wilson et al, 2004, pp. 224–225*)

35. **(D)** Postnasal drip syndrome (PNDS) is the most common cause of cough in adults. In 30% to 60% of patients, sinusitis is the cause of the PNDS; another major cause is rhinitis of any etiology. Asthma is the second most common cause of chronic cough in adults, and gastroesophageal reflux disease is the third most common. (*Noble et al, 2001, p. 171*)

36. **(B)** The hypoglossal nerve (CN XII) controls movement of the tongue. The tongue deviates toward the side of the lesion. The increase in muscle tone of the innervated portion of tongue pushes it toward the weaker (contralateral) side. Further evidence of hypoglossal nerve damage can be documented by noting fasciculations and atrophy of the denervated portion of the tongue. Subtle defects can be detected by having the patient push his or her tongue against the inside of the cheek while the examiner feels the pressure exerted by the tongue against the outer cheek. The tongue muscles of the unaffected side will push more firmly against the contralateral cheek on the affected side. (*Bickley and Hoekelman, 1999, pp. 201, 574*)

37. **(D)** Obstructive sleep apnea syndrome (OSA) is often the result of a structurally small upper airway combined with a loss of muscle tone, allowing the pharynx to collapse during inspiration. Most patients with OSA are middle-aged men. Often they have poorly controlled systemic hypertension. They frequently complain of daytime drowsiness, persistent fatigue, recent weight gain, and cognitive impairment. Use of alcohol or sedatives can worsen symptoms as seen in this patient. (*Tierney et al, 2001, pp. 332–333*)

38. **(A)** Unilateral tonsillar enlargement can be the presentation of lymphoma. Occasionally one tonsil may appear larger than the other because one is more deeply placed within the tonsillar fossa. However, careful clinical examination can usually differentiate this from a truly enlarged tonsil. A peritonsillar abscess is ruled out by the absence of trismus, peritonsillar swelling, and tenderness to palpation. A diagnostic tonsillectomy is indicated if one tonsil is larger than the other and especially if there is progressive worsening of cervical adenopathy. (*Gates, 1998, pp. 415–416*)

39. **(E)** Leukoplakia can occur anywhere on mucous membranes and is associated with chronic local irritation, such as from tobacco usage. These lesions are simple hyperkeratotic areas caused by chronic irritation. However, they can be precancerous with 2% to 6% of lesions having cellular dysplasia or early squamous cell carcinoma. A similar precancerous lesion is erythroplakia. It is occasionally associated with leukoplakia but has a localized area of erythema. This distinction is important since as many as 90% of erythroplakic lesions are precancerous. (*Bickley and Hoekelman, 1999, p. 238; Tierney et al, 2001, p. 237*)

40. **(C)** Salivary calculi (sialolithiasis) most commonly occur within the submandibular gland because of the length and upward-sloping orientation of Wharton's duct. Calculi obstructing the duct should be considered when swelling and pain are associated with stimulation of salivation, such as occurs with eating. A partially obstructing stone will lead to a gradual reduction in the swelling of the gland. Submandibular stones can usually be palpated within the gland and occasionally can be seen at the orifice of Wharton's duct. Sialogogues (to increase salivary flow) can help force the stone out of the duct. Occasionally, the orifice is enlarged surgically to allow the stone to pass more easily. Persistent pain, swelling, and purulent drainage from the duct orifice is seen when the gland becomes secondarily infected (sialadenitis). Repeated infections caused by chronically obstructed secretions can cause stricture of the duct, which eventually may require surgical removal of the gland. (*Schuller and Schleuning, 1994, pp. 237–239*)

41. **(E)** Ludwig's angina is a cellulitis of the floor of the mouth. This infection causes swelling of the soft tissues of the floor of the mouth. This can lead to rapid obstruction of the airway by pushing the tongue back into the throat. Treatment often includes surgical drainage and intravenous antibiotics. Dental disease is the usual etiology 50% of the time. However, it can also be associated with infected lacerations or injuries to the floor of the mouth. (*O'Donoghue et al, 2000, p. 241; Hay et al, 2001, p. 413*)

42. **(B)** Unlike epiglottitis in children, instrumentation of the pharynx is usually safe for adults and is useful in confirming epiglottitis. This condition is not rare and should be considered in adults with symptoms of throat pain out of proportion to the examination findings. Adult patients with epiglottitis should be admitted for monitoring of the airway while initiating treatment with intravenous antibiotics and steroids. Adults rarely require intubation to secure the airway. However, if symptoms are rapidly progressing, the airway may not respond quickly enough to the treatment regimen and intubation may be required. (*Tierney et al, 2001, p. 245*)

43. **(A)** Symptoms of heartburn are present only in about 43% of patients found to have clinical evidence of laryngopharyngeal reflux. Patients often are unaware of acid coming into the laryngeal area. Endoscopic examination of the larynx often shows erythema and edema of the arytenoid tissue in the posterior laryngeal area where the reflux occurs. (*Jafek and Murrow, 2001, p. 180*)

44. **(B)** The classic signs and symptoms of a peritonsillar abscess include trismus——difficulty opening the mouth. This is caused by spasm of the pterygoid muscles in response to the abscess. Peritonsillar abscess is a complication of tonsillitis. It is most common in adolescents and young adults. Symptoms include low-grade fever, dysphagia, and a characteristic "hot potato" voice. Examination of the oropharynx would demonstrate displacement of the affected tonsil toward the midline and superior and lateral to the tonsil. Diagnosis is confirmed by needle aspiration, which is also therapeutic. Antibiotics without effective drainage are not effective. (*Woodson, 2000, pp. 117–121*)

45. **(C)** Infectious mononucleosis is a generalized disease caused by the Epstein–Barr virus, which has a high incidence of rash associated with amoxicillin use. The appearance of the exudative tonsils can be indistinguishable from that caused by beta-hemolytic strep. Superimposed bacterial infections, as in this case, do occur and require antibiotics. Scarlitiniform rashes associated with strep infections would normally appear early in the disease. This patient is not an allergic to amoxicillin, but has a rash secondary to the reaction of the patient to taking this antibiotic with the virus. The monospot or heterophil antibody test used to diagnose mononucleosis may be negative during the first 2 weeks of the illness. (*Wilson et al, 2004, p. 281*)

References

Ballenger JJ, Snow JB (eds). *Otorhinolaryngology: Head and Neck Surgery*, 15th ed. Baltimore: Williams & Wilkins, 1996.

Bickley LS, Hoekelman RA (eds). *Bates' Guide to Physical Examination and History Taking*, 7th ed. Philadelphia: Lippincott; 1999.

Calhoun KH, Eibling DE, Wax MK (eds). *Expert Guide to Otolaryngology*. Philadelphia: American College of Physicians; 2001.

Fauci AS, Braumwald E, Isselbacher KJ (eds). *Harrison's Principles of Internal Medicine*, 14th ed. New York: McGraw-Hill; 1998.

Gates GA (ed). *Current Therapy in Otolaryngology Head and Neck Surgery*, 6th ed. St. Louis: Mosby; 1998.

Jafek BW, Murrow BW (eds). *ENT Secrets*, 2nd ed. Philadelphia: Hanley & Belfus, Inc; 2001.

Hay WW et al (eds). *Current Diagnosis and Treatment*, 15th ed. New York: McGraw-Hill; 2001.

Noble J, Greene HL, Levinson W (eds). *Textbook of Primary Care Medicine*, 3rd ed. St. Louis: Mosby; 2001.

O'Donoghue GM, Narula MA, Bates GJ. *Clinical ENT*, 2nd ed. San Diego: Singular Publishing Group; 2000.

Scheid DC, Hamm RM. Acute bacterial rhinosinusitis in adults. Part I: Evaluation *Am Fam Physician.* 2004;70:1685–1692.

Schuller DE, Schleuning AJ (eds). *DeWeese and Saunders' Otolaryngology—Head and Neck Surgery,* 8th ed. St. Louis: Mosby; 1994.

Szilard Kiss S, Letko E, Qamruddin S, Baltatzis S, Foster CS. Long-term progression, prognosis, and treatment of patients with recurrent ocular manifestations of Reiter's syndrome. *Ophthalmology* 2003;110:1764–1769.

Tierney LM, McPhee SJ, Papadakis MA (eds). *Current Medical Diagnosis and Treatment,* 40th ed. New York: McGraw-Hill; 2001.

Vaughan D, Asbury T, Riordan-Eva P. *General Ophthalmology,* 15th ed. Stamford, CT: Appleton & Lange; 1999.

Wilson WR, Nadol JB Jr, Randolph GW. *The Clinical Handbook of Ear, Nose and Throat Disorders.* New York: Parthenon Publishing Group; 2004.

Woodson, GE. *Ear, Nose and Throat Disorders in Primary Care.* Philadelphia: WB Saunders Co; 2000.

CHAPTER 17

Urology
Questions

Raymond Eifel, MS, PA-C

DIRECTIONS (Questions 1 through 30): Each of the numbered items or incomplete statements in this chapter is followed by answers or completions of the statement. Select the ONE lettered answer or completion that is BEST in each case.

Questions 1 through 30

1. What is the most common composition of renal calculi?

   (A) cystine
   (B) calcium
   (C) struvite
   (D) uric acid

2. Which diagnostic finding is most indicative of acute pyelonephritis?

   (A) hematuria
   (B) pyuria
   (C) white blood cell casts
   (D) epithelial cells

3. Which procedure is the most helpful screening test for prostate cancer?

   (A) digital rectal exam
   (B) serum prostate specific antigen
   (C) transrectal ultrasound
   (D) prostate biopsy

4. What is the most likely pathogen associated with acute cystitis?

   (A) *Eschericha coli*
   (B) *Pseudomonas* species
   (C) *Staphylococcus epidermidis*
   (D) *Chlamydia trachomatis*

5. What is the chief symptom associated with bladder cancer?

   (A) pyuria
   (B) hematuria
   (C) dysuria
   (D) urinary frequency

6. Which condition is suggested by urethritis, arthritis, and conjunctivitis?

   (A) chlamydial infection
   (B) gonococcal infection
   (C) Reiter's syndrome
   (D) tertiary syphilis

7. Which of the following is a painless lesion of the penis?

   (A) chancre
   (B) chancroid
   (C) granuloma inguinale
   (D) *Lymphogranuloma venereum*

8. Inability to retract the foreskin from the glans penis due to inflammation or infection is often an indication for circumcision. Which condition does this describe?

   (A) phimosis
   (B) paraphimosis
   (C) balanitis
   (D) urethral meatus stricture

9. Which of the following would be of most concern if found while examining a 26-year-old healthy male patient?

   (A) tender epidydimis
   (B) enlarged, fluid-filled scrotum
   (C) nontender mass on the testes
   (D) mass that feels like a "bag of worms"

10. Which scrotal mass will transilluminate?

    (A) varicocele
    (B) spermatocele
    (C) testicular mass
    (D) torsed testicle

11. Which treatment is most effective in a 70-year-old male diagnosed with stage T4 prostate cancer who presents with hip and back pain?

    (A) watchful waiting
    (B) radical prostatectomy
    (C) external beam radiation
    (D) hormonal therapy

12. The anatomical portion of the prostate that becomes hyperplastic with benign prostatic hyperplasia is the

    (A) anterior fibromuscular area
    (B) central zone
    (C) transition zone
    (D) peripheral zone

13. A 38-year-old male presents with an abrupt onset of myalgia and low back/perineal pain. The patient also reports urinary symptoms of frequency, urgency, and dysuria. A urinalysis reveals pyuria; urine culture reveals the presence of Gram-negative bacteria. What is the most reasonable initial therapeutic approach for this patient?

    (A) hospitalization with administration of intravenous antibiotics
    (B) trimethoprim-sulfamethoxazole or a flouroquinolone for 4 weeks
    (C) a flouroquinolone and alpha blocker for 8 to 12 weeks
    (D) nonsteroidal anti-inflammatory agents and hot sitz baths

14. A 20-year-old college football player presents with a chief complaint of a dull ache in his scrotum after prolonged standing on the sideline. It seems to get worse with vigorous activity and is relieved by lying down. Dilated veins are observed on inspection in the left scrotum, and both testicles are palpable and without masses. What is the most likely diagnosis?

    (A) varicocele
    (B) spermatocele
    (C) hydrocele
    (D) testicular mass

15. A 72-year-old man presents to the office with a chief complaint of a 3-month history of nocturia. He states that his urine stream is weak, has been increasingly slow to start during this time, and sometimes he finds himself straining to void. What is the most reasonable initial treatment for this patient?

    (A) watchful waiting
    (B) trial of tamulosin
    (C) trial of finasteride
    (D) TURP

16. A 6-month-old male is brought to the office by his mother for a follow-up check for a right undescended testicle that has been absent since birth. This exam is consistent with previous exams, revealing an empty right hemiscrotum. Even with treatment, which of the following is most likely to occur to this patient in future years?

(A) testicular torsion

(B) epididymitis

(C) orchitis

(D acute appendicitis

17. A 65-year-old female presents with a complaint of blood in her urine, intermittently for the last month. The patient denies any fever, chills, flank pain, or dysuria. Social history is positive for tobacco use: 45 pack years, but patient reports stopping her tobacco use last year. What is the most likely cause of her hematuria?

(A) urinary tract infection

(B) bladder cancer

(C) renal calculi

(D) pyelonephritis

18. A 32-year-old male presents severely worried with a complaint of increased urinary frequency and bladder pain. He states that he has been feeling poorly for the past 4 days with intermittent fever, chills, and persistent malaise. He states never feeling this way before. Physical examination is significant for a temperature of 101°F. Genital examination is normal except a gentle rectal examination reveals an enlarged and tender prostate. What is the most likely diagnosis?

(A) acute bacterial prostatitis

(B) chronic bacterial prostatitis

(C) prostatic abscess

(D) benign prostatic hypertrophy

19. A 66-year-old male with a 15-year history of hypertension and status post inferior myocardial infarction 4 months ago presents for a follow-up office appointment. He has been feeling well, without chest pain or shortness of breath, and has returned to his work as a salesman at a local insurance company. He reports being compliant with his prescription of isosorbide and denies any side effects. He says that he is nervous about resuming sexual activity with his wife since the heart attack because he wonders if sexual relations can hurt his heart. He has tried a couple of times to have sexual relations with his wife but has been unable to achieve a full erection. What is the most reasonable initial therapeutic approach for this patient's erectile dysfunction?

(A) tadalafil

(B) vardenafil

(C) sildenafil

(D) alprostadil

20. A 16-year-old female presents to the emergency department with a 1-day history of severe right flank pain with associated vomiting. She denies any fever, urgency, or dysuria. Her past medical history is unremarkable. Physical exam reveals she has guarding and rebound is present on the right, along with severe right CVA tenderness. Which of the following radiographic studies is indicated for this patient?

(A) KUB (kidneys, ureter, and bladder)

(B) intravenous pyelogram

(C) noncontrast spiral computed tomography

(D) flat plate

21. A 75-year-old female, mother of four, presents to your office to establish care. Appearing healthy, she reports a past medical history positive for hypertension and denies any additional problems. However, when specifically asked she admits to having urinary incontinence for "a couple of years" and now describes symptoms that have recently worsened, with the patient experiencing the urge to void almost hourly. These urges are so severe that she is now using four to five adult incontinence pads per day to manage the urine she leaks. What is the most likely diagnosis?

(A) urge incontinence

(B) stress incontinence

(C) overflow incontinence

(D) functional incontinence

22. A 53-year-old male patient, who has failed several medication treatments for hypertension and has been recently started on captopril, returns to your office reporting a sudden onset of fatigue, nausea, and vomiting. The patient is confused and tachycardic. BUN and creatinine levels are elevated. Which of the following radiographic studies will be most helpful in making the diagnosis?

(A) abdominal x-ray
(B) chest x-ray
(C) renal ultrasound
(D) computed tomography (CT)

23. A 65-year-old male presents with his third episode of kidney stones in the last year. Stone analysis from the previous episodes was positive for calcium stones. Physical exam on this visit is positive for costovertebral tenderness. Laboratory studies for parathyroid hormone are elevated. What is the most likely underlying etiology for the patient's recurrent episodes of nephrolithiasis?

(A) primary hyperparathyroidism
(B) multiple endocrine neoplasia
(C) vitamin D intoxication
(D) hyperthyroidism

24. A patient with a history of multiple episodes of renal calculi secondary to hypercalcemia also has repeatedly corresponding suppressed levels of parathyroid hormone (PTH). What is the most likely cause for the low level of PTH?

(A) malignancy
(B) primary hyperparathyroidism
(C) vitamin D intoxication
(D) hyperthyroidism

25. A 54-year-old female presents with gross hematuria and flank pain. Physical exam is positive for a RUQ palpable mass and negative for costovertebral tenderness. Gross blood is observed in the urine specimen. What is your most likely diagnosis?

(A) renal cell carcinoma
(B) renal cyst
(C) angiomyolipoma
(D) renal abscess

26. A 32-year-old male presents to the urgent care center with a concern of scrotal tenderness that began 3 days ago and has now worsened. Physical exam:
temperature: 100.7°F and positive tenderness in the posterolateral aspect of the right teste and swelling, negative spermatic cord tenderness with palpation, or transillumination. What is this patient's most likely diagnosis?

(A) epididymitis
(B) orchitis
(C) epididymo-orchitis
(D) testicular torsion

27. A 21-year-old sexually active female student presents to the university clinic with recurrent pain with urination. Initially treated with trimethoprim-sulfamethoxazole, her follow-up urine culture was negative. What is the most likely organism causing her discomfort?

(A) *Escherichia coli*
(B) *Chlamydia trachomatis*
(C) *Candida* species
(D) *Proteus* species

28. A 43-year-old female patient presents with back pain and hematuria. The patient reports having this problem earlier this year prior to moving, and recalls the clinician at that time telling her, "they're just cysts." Denying any history of urinary tract infections, the patient reports her mother was on dialysis before passing away. The patient is afebrile and physical exam is positive for diffuse back tenderness and bilateral flank masses with palpation. Urine dip is positive for 3+ blood and is negative for leukocytes and nitrites. What is this patient's most likely diagnosis?

(A) adult polycystic kidney disease
(B) renal cyst
(C) horseshoe kidney
(D) renal cell carcinoma

29. A 37-year-old female returns to your office a week after being treated for a urinary tract infection. She reports her symptoms have not gotten better and have even gotten worse with a fever and flank pain. A urine specimen is obtained and viewed under a microscope. Which type of casts would you expect to observe in this patient's urine sediment?

(A) white blood cell
(B) epithelial cell
(C) red blood cell
(D) hyaline

30. When treating a patient for benign prostatic hypertrophy (BPH), which of the following medical therapies affects the patient's prostatic-specific antigen (PSA) level?

(A) phytotherapy
(B) α-adrenergic antagonists
(C) 5α-reductase inhibitors
(D) saw palmetto

Answers and Explanations

1. **(B)** Eighty to eighty-five percent of all kidney stones are composed of calcium. Another 5% of kidney stones consist of uric acid. Calcium and uric acid stones are more common in males. One to two percent of kidney stones consist mainly of cystine. Less than 2% are made of struvite, a combination of magnesium, ammonium, and phosphate. Struvite stones frequently present as staghorn calculi, are associated with urinary tract infections, and are more common in women. Stones containing calcium are radiopaque; others are radiolucent. (*Tanagho and McAninch, 2004, pp. 259–264*)

2. **(C)** White blood cell casts in the presence of the acute symptoms (fever, chills, flank pain, and dysuria) usually provide strong evidence of acute pyelonephritis. Although observed in many patients, the finding of pyuria is nonspecific and a patient with pyuria may or may not have infection. Hematuria is rarely seen in acute pyelonephritis. The presence of hematuria usually suggests the presence of calculi or tumor. Epithelial cells are not associated with pyelonephritis. (*Rakel and Bope, 2005, p. 806*)

3. **(B)** Only one-quarter to one-third of prostate cancers occur in areas of the gland accessible to palpation by a digital rectal exam (DRE); a negative exam provides little information. True sensitivities and specificities are not known for serum prostate-specific antigen (PSA) because the "gold standard" (i.e., biopsy) for diagnosis of prostate cancer cannot ethically be performed on asymptomatic men with negative PSA testing, but PSA may be helpful in picking up small latent cancers. The utility of transrectal ultrasound (TRUS) in screening is severely limited by the low sensitivity, high cost, and discomfort of the test. (*Rakel, 2002, pp. 173–174*)

4. **(A)** Women experience urinary tract infections at a much higher rate than do their male counterparts. Cystitis most commonly is due to ascending colonization of the lower urinary tract. In females the urethra is shorter and easily contaminated with fecal flora. Other factors that increase the risk of cystitis include extremes of age, sexual intercourse, diaphragm use, and pregnancy. *Escherichia coli* is the most common pathogen in uncomplicated cystitis. *Pseudomonas* is more likely in patients with recurrent urinary tract infections and in hospitalized patients. *Staphylococcus epidermidis* may indicate a contaminated specimen. *Chlamydia trachomatis* is more likely in sexually transmitted urethritis. (*Tanagho and McAninch, 2004, pp. 203–205*)

5. **(B)** The most common presenting symptom of bladder cancer is painless hematuria, which occurs in 85% of patients. Additional symptoms of bladder irritability and urinary frequency, urgency, and dysuria are the second most common presentation and are usually associated with invasive bladder cancer. (*Walsh, 2002, pp. 253–254*)

6. **(C)** Chlamydia and gonorrhea infection can both result in urethritis. Gonococci can disseminate to the joints and cause septic arthritis. Chlamydia is typically asymptomatic but can cause chronic conjunctivitis in adolescents and young adults. Reiter's syndrome is a result of an untreated chlamydia infection and although typically characterized in texts by the triad of urethritis, arthritis, and conjunctivitis, all of the symptoms may not be present or not identified at the time of presentation. Tertiary syphilis is characterized by neurologic and cardiovascular disease, gumma, auditory and ophthalmic involvement, and cutaneous lesions. (*Noble, 2001, pp. 1282–1285*)

7. **(A)** Chancre is the painless lesion caused by *Treponema pallidum* (syphilis). The chancre occurs about 3 weeks after exposure. It often goes unnoticed and resolves without treatment in 3 to 6 weeks. Chancroid is the painful lesion of *Haemophilus ducreyi*. It is a large sloughing ulcer with secondary infection and inflammation of the inguinal lymph nodes. The lesion of granuloma inguinale produces a shallow painful ulcer with a bright red base from which Donovan bodies from *Calymmatobacterium granulomatis* can be found in tissue scrapings and secretions. Lymphogranuloma venereum may be associated with multiple shallow painless lesions caused by *Chlamydia trachomatis*, which heal quickly. A painful unilateral adenopathy may follow the healing of the ulcerations. (*Keck, 2005, pp. 13–30*)

8. **(A)** Phimosis is the condition in which the foreskin (prepuce) cannot be retracted because of adherence or fibrosis with acute or chronic inflammation. Recurrent balanitis, inflammation of the glans penis, is common. Paraphimosis is the inability to return the retracted foreskin over the glans. This is often iatrogenic following instrumentation or Foley catheter insertion. Urethral meatal stricture occurs following inflammation of the urethra. (*Tanagho and McAninch, 2004, p. 620*)

9. **(C)** Although all of these findings might elicit some concern, the most concerning would be the nontender testicular mass since that should be considered testicular cancer until proven otherwise. Testicular cancer affects predominantly young males in the 20- to 35-year-old range. These tumors can metastasize early in their development and almost all will require chemotherapy to treat. A tender epididymis might indicate epididymitis. A fluid-filled scrotum is likely due to a hydrocele and can be surgically repaired. The "bag of worms" mass is classic for a varicocele, a condition that usually does not require treatment unless considered a causative factor for infertility. (*Rakel, 2002, pp. 1277–1278*)

10. **(A)** Spermatoceles are cysts of the epididymis filled with clear watery fluid or sometimes a more creamy fluid filled with spermatozoa. They are translucent. Varicoceles are dilations of one or both of the venous drainage systems of the testicle. They nearly always occur on the left. A testicular mass always should be considered carcinoma. It does not transilluminate. Testicular torsion presents with pain and swelling; it will not transilluminate. (*Noble, 2001, p. 1455*)

11. **(D)** Prostate cancer treatment recommendations vary greatly among experts. The treatment choice will depend on the stage and grade of tumor. Watchful waiting has been suggested for patients with localized disease and a shorter life expectancy. Surgery and radiotherapy have been suggested for patients with localized disease with the intent of curing their cancer. Both have incontinence and impotence as their main side effects. Stage T4 tumors have metastasized beyond the prostatic capsule and therefore would not benefit from surgery or radiation. Since the patient is experiencing symptoms of bony metastasis, palliative care would be recommended. Hormonal therapy with orchiectomy, LH–RH agonists, or antiandrogens would help slow progression of the disease and improve symptoms. (*Noble, 2001, pp. 1427–1428*)

12. **(C)** Benign prostatic hyperplasia develops in the transition zone and involves, to varying degrees, both stromal and epithelial tissue. The hyperplastic process results in increased cell numbers. As enlargement progresses, mechanical obstruction results from intrusion of

the transition zone into the urethral lumen. The peripheral zone is the primary site for prostate carcinoma—approximately 60% to 70% occurs there. The remainder typically are found in the central zone. (*Tanagho and McAninch, 2004, pp. 367–369*)

13. **(B)** Trimethoprim-sulfamethoxazole and flouroquinolones have high drug penetration into prostatic tissue and are recommended for 4 to 6 weeks for patients with acute bacterial prostatitis. Patients presenting as acutely ill, are febrile, and exhibit symptoms of acute urinary retention would benefit from hospitalization with parenteral antibiotics. Patients with chronic bacterial prostatitis may benefit from a longer course of antibiotics combined with an alpha blocker to reduce urinary symptoms. NSAIDs and sitz baths may also relieve symptoms associated with chronic prostatitis. (*Tanagho and McAninch, 2004, pp. 218–220*)

14. **(A)** A varicocele can be recognized by the presence of scrotal enlargement caused by dilation of the pampiniform venous plexus. Varicoceles present as a "bag of worms" in the spermatic cord and are more prominent when the patient stands. Varicoceles occur on the left side more than 80% of the time. Hydroceles and spermatoceles are caused by fluid collection and are usually asymptomatic. Testicular masses must always be included in the differential diagnosis of scrotal masses as they generally present as painless. (*Noble, 2001, p. 1455*)

15. **(B)** Watchful waiting, although an option, is unlikely to resolve the patient's moderate symptoms. A trial of tamulosin, a selective alpha blocker, is most reasonable as it will provide the patient with the quickest improvement in symptoms without the systemic side effects (i.e., orthostatic hypotension) of a nonselective alpha blocker. Finesteride, a 5α-reductase inhibitor requires 6 months of therapy before seeing symptomatic improvement. Transuretheral resection of the prostate (TURP) has higher rates of morbidity and mortality and includes risks of retrograde ejaculation, impotence, and incontinence. (*Tanagho and McAninch, 2004, pp. 369–373*)

16. **(A)** An undescended testis can be brought down into the scrotum with an orchiopexy surgery between 9 and 15 months. Even with treatment there are several consequences associated with cryptochidism including infertility, malignancy, associated hernia, and torsion of the undescended testis. The risk of *malignancy* is approximately 1 in 80 with a unilateral undescended testis. The most common tumor developing in an undescended testis is a seminoma. Orchiopexy does not change the risk of developing cancer of the testis. Cryptorchidism does not increase the likelihood of epididymitis, orchitis, or appendicitis. (*Behrman et al, 2005, pp. 1817–1818*)

17. **(B)** Hematuria in women older than 60 years is consistent with a bladder malignancy. Bladder cancer causes episodic, gross hematuria that is usually painless. Cigarette smoking is a risk factor that also increases the incidence of bladder cancer. Painful hematuria associated with suprapubic discomfort or dysuria (or both) is more indicative of cystitis or calculi. Pyelonephritis is associated with chills, fever, and flank pain. (*Rakel, 2002, pp. 1280–1282*)

18. **(A)** Acute bacterial prostatitis is the most common diagnosis in men younger than 50 years old. Patient presentation includes the sudden onset of constitutional and urinary symptoms. Chronic bacterial prostatitis presents without fever and the digital rectal exam is often normal. Prostatic abscesses are a result of inappropriate treatment for a prior episode of acute bacterial prostatitis. The incidence of benign prostatic hypertrophy is age related with symptoms presenting in the fifth decade. (*Tanagho and McAninch, 2004, pp. 218–220*)

19. **(D)** All phosphodiesterase type 5 (PDE5) inhibitors (tadalafil, vardenifil, sildenifil) are contraindicated in men taking organic nitrates (i.e., isosorbide dinitrate or nitroglycerin). Several second-line therapies exist, including alprostadil, vacuum-constriction devices, and penile implants. Referral to a urologist is recommended when considering these therapeutic options. (*Rakel and Bope, 2005, pp. 820–821*)

20. **(C)** The preferred study for a adolescent with suspected renal colic is the spiral CT. This study is performed quickly, delineates the number and location of calculi, and demonstrates whether there is hydronephrosis in the involved kidney. It can also identify stones too small to be picked up on other diagnostic studies. In the past, an intravenous pyelogram was generally performed. A KUB (kidneys, ureter, and bladder) film may not pick up radiolucent stones. A "flat plate" is an older out-of-date term for a KUB. (*Behrman et al, 2005, p. 1823*)

21. **(A)** Urinary incontinence is defined as involuntary urine loss. Urge incontinence is the result of uninhibited urge sensations that are so strong that the patient experiences an involuntary urine loss. Women particularly experience this problem with the changes associated with aging (weakened pelvic muscles secondary to childbirth). The problem may be worsened by the use of diuretics to treat hypertension. Stress incontinence is associated with increases in intra abdominal pressure (laughing, sneezing, coughing, etc.). Overflow incontinence is associated with leaking small amounts of urine from mechanical factors that affect an already distended bladder. Functional incontinence is associated patients who exhibit cognitive impairment (severe dementia). (*Goldman and Ausiello, 2004, pp. 111–114*)

22. **(C)** Symptoms of nausea, vomiting, fatigue, and confusion are associated with a diagnosis of renal failure. The recent addition of captopril, an angiotensin-converting enzyme inhibitor, may have precipitated these symptoms. A renal ultrasound is the study of choice and is used to rule out urinary obstruction and determine kidney size. A chest x-ray would only be indicated if an associated heart concern is suspected. A CT may not be available in all locations and often requires contrast, which can increase the injury to the kidneys. An abdominal study is not indicated. (*Cheng and Zass, 2003, p. 766*)

23. **(A)** Hypercalcemia secondary to primary hyperparathyroidism can be assessed with a parathyroid hormone (PTH) level. PTH raises calcium levels by increasing bone resorption and increasing renal tubular resorption of calcium. Multiple endocrine neoplasia, vitamin D intoxication, and hyperthyroidism are associated with suppressed PTH levels. (*Carroll and Schade, 2003, pp. 1959–1966*)

24. **(A)** Malignancy and primary hyperparathyroidism account for over two-thirds of the cases of hypercalcemia. Primary hyperparathyroidism is associated with an elevated PTH. Malignancy, like vitamin D intoxication and hyperthyroidism, are associated with suppressed levels of PTH. However, malignancy is the most common of the three. (*Rakel, 2002, pp. 1261–1263*)

25. **(A)** The triad of gross hematuria, flank pain, and palpable mass are the common findings, although rarely seen together, associated with renal cell carcinoma. Of the three, a palpable mass is the least likely to be found, but when present is significant for advanced disease. A majority of renal masses are simple cysts, which require no additional workup. Angiomyolipoma contains large amounts of fat as shown on CT. A renal abscess is associated with a patient presentation that includes fever and flank pain. (*Tanagho and McAninch, 2004, pp. 351–354*)

26. **(A)** Pain and swelling are prominent features of epididymitis; fever and abdominal pain may also be present. Epididymitis is caused by an ascending infection that without treatment will continue to the testicles, causing a significant swelling that will make it difficult for the clinician to distinguish between the epididymis and the testicles (epididymo-orchitis). Orchitis alone is most commonly viral (mumps) and observed in prepubertal males. In males younger than 30 years, epididymitis can be confused with torsion. (*Rakel and Bope, 2005, pp. 797–798*)

27. **(B)** *Chlamydia* should be considered in recurrent episodes of dysuria when urine cultures are found to be negative and the patient has failed to respond to therapy. All of the other organisms are treatable with trimethoprim-sulfamethoxazole. (*Rakel and Bope, 2005, p. 781*)

28. **(A)** Adult polycystic kidney disease is a hereditary condition that almost always has a bilateral presentation (95% of the cases). It does not appear until after the age of 40 and dialysis or kidney transplantation is necessary for survival. Renal cysts and renal cell carcinoma generally present unilaterally. A horseshoe kidney (fusion of the renal tissue) may be palpated bilaterally, otherwise the patient is asymptomatic. (*Tanagho and McAninch, 2004, pp. 511–519*)

29. **(A)** Pyelonephritis results from an ascending urinary tract infection from the bladder via the ureter to kidney. Although not pathognomonic, white blood cell casts are suggestive of pyelonephritis. Red blood cell casts are highly suggestive of glomerulonephritis. Epithelial cell casts are typical in acute tubular necrosis. Hyaline casts in small numbers are insignificant and are commonly seen in patients who regularly exercise. (*Tanagho and McAninch, 2004, p. 54*)

30. **(C)** 5α-Reductase inhibitors (finasteride) can lower a patient's PSA level by 50% and a baseline PSA should be taken prior to beginning therapy. α-Adrenergic antagonists (doxazosin, terazosin) relax prostate and bladder neck smooth muscles and may cause dizziness and orthosatic hypotension, but do not affect PSA levels. Phytotherapy refers to the use of plants or plant extracts for medicinal purposes; saw palmetto is a popular treatment for BPH. (*Rakel and Bope, 2005, p. 816*)

REFERENCES

Behrman RE, Kliegman RM, Jenson HB (eds). *Nelson Textbook of Pediatrics*, 17th ed. Philadelphia, PA: WB Saunders; 2005.

Carroll MF, Schade DS. A practical approach to hypercalcemia. *Am Fam Physician.* 1 May 2003; 1959–1966.

Cheng A, Zass A. *The Osler Medical Handbook.* Philadelphia, PA: Mosby; 2003.

Goldman L, Ausiello D (eds). *Cecil Textbook of Medicine*, 22nd ed. Philadelphia, PA: WB Suanders; 2004.

Keck JW. Ulcerative lesions. In *Clinics in Family Practice*. Philadelphia, PA: WB Saunders; 2005.

Noble J (ed). *Textbook of Primary Care Medicine*, 3rd ed. St. Louis, MO: Mosby; 2001.

Rakel RE (ed). *Textbook of Family Practice*, 6th ed. Philadelphia, PA: WB Saunders; 2002.

Rakel RE, Bope ET (eds). *Conn's Current Therapy*, 57th ed. Philadelphia, PA: Elsevier; 2005.

Tanagho EA, McAninch JW (eds). *Smith's General Urology*, 16th ed. New York: McGraw-Hill; 2004.

Walsh PC (ed). *Campbell's Urology*, 8th ed. Philadelphia, PA: WB Saunders; 2002.

Health Promotion & Disease Prevention

CHAPTER 18

Preventive Medicine
Questions

James F. Cawley, MPH, PA-C

DIRECTIONS (Questions 1 through 28): Each of the numbered items or incomplete statements in this section is followed by answers or by completions of the statement. Select the ONE lettered answer or completion that is BEST in each case.

Questions 1 through 28

1. The rates of prostate cancer are highest among

    (A) Whites
    (B) African Americans
    (C) Latinos
    (D) Native Americans

2. Which of the following is the best example of primary prevention?

    (A) flouridation of drinking water to prevent dental caries
    (B) mammography to detect breast cancer
    (C) testing to detect C- Reactive protein (CRP) for the identification of coronary heart disease
    (D) performing carotid endarterectomy for the prevention of stroke

3. The recommended protocol for screening and prevention of hepatitis B infection

    (A) screening using HBsAg is recommended for all pregnant women at their first prenatal visit
    (B) routine screening using HBsAg is recommended for all adults
    (C) routine screening using HBsAg is recommended only for pregnant women and newborns
    (D) screening using HBsAg is recommended only to detect carriers

4. The most prevalent arboviral disease in the United States

    (A) *Hantavirus*
    (B) Lyme disease
    (C) Eastern equine encephalitis
    (D) West Nile Virus encephalitis

5. The leading cause of death among children aged 0 to 4 years

    (A) sudden infant death syndrome
    (B) birth defects
    (C) unintentional injuries
    (D) infections

6. The rate that is defined as the number of new cases of a disease occurring in a population per unit time

(A) virulence
(B) epidemic
(C) incidence
(D) prevalence

7. The recommended approach to the prevention of colorectal cancer in asymptomatic non-high-risk adults

(A) yearly fecal occult blood tests beginning at age 55
(B) double-contrast barium enema every other year after age 55
(C) annual flexible sigmoidoscopy beginning at age 50
(D) colonoscopy every 10 years and flexible sigmoidoscopy every 5 years beginning at age 50

8. Which of the following standard childhood immunizations requires a booster?

(A) Hib B
(B) MMR
(C) DPT
(D) Varicella

9. Controlled clinical trials that fail to randomize study subjects are prone to

(A) observer bias
(B) recall bias
(C) selection bias
(D) lead-time bias

10. The only major sexually transmitted illness for which a safe and effective vaccine exists

(A) syphilis
(B) chlamydia
(C) hepatitis B
(D) herpes simplex II

11. Which of the following statements related to the identification of family violence is TRUE?

(A) only 10% of battered women are identified by physicians
(B) most cases of domestic violence are sporadic and isolated
(C) in some population groups in the United States, up to 50% of pregnant women experience domestic violence
(D) caregivers are the most common abusers of battered elders

12. If death rates per 1,000 licensed drivers are plotted by age, the distribution of the curve is

(A) bell shaped
(B) J shaped
(C) U shaped
(D) unimodal

13. The leading cause of mortality among African Americans is

(A) cancer
(B) heart disease
(C) unintentional injuries
(D) diabetes mellitus

14. Gastrointestinal infection most likely to be associated with the sequellae of Gillian Barre syndrome (GBS)

(A) salmonellosis
(B) enterohemorrhagic *E. coli*
(C) *Campylobacter jejuni*
(D) listeriosis

15. The most common, bacterial, sexually transmitted disease pathogenin the United States

(A) chancroid
(B) gonorrhea
(C) syphilis
(D) Chlamydia

16. The rate defined as the number of deaths in children under 1 year of age in a given time frame and population divided by the number of live births in the same time frame and population

    (A) neonatal mortality rate
    (B) infant mortality rate
    (C) postneonatal mortality rate
    (D) perinatal mortality rate

17. A graph commonly used in epidemiology where the number of cases of a disease are plotted on the *x*-axis and time units are plotted on the *y*-axis

    (A) infection scatterplot
    (B) epidemic curve
    (C) outbreak diagram
    (D) histogram

18. In the course of investigating a 24-year-old HIV infected male, it was observed that the HbsAg was positive. The patient is asymptomatic, the physical examination normal, and the CD4 count 800. Which test is the most helpful in determining if he is in the acute phase of viral hepatitis?

    (A) HBeAg
    (B) HBsAg
    (C) IgG anti-HBcAg
    (D) IgM anti-HBcAg

19. One of your patients is a 30-year-old male who tells you he is planning to travel to the Dominican Republic for a 3-week hiking trip. The most appropriate medication to use for malarial prophylaxis is

    (A) Atovaquone
    (B) Chloroquine
    (C) Mefloquine
    (D) Doxycycline

20. Based on data from the Framingham Heart Study, indicate that the single most important independent risk factor for the development and progression of atherosclerosis is

    (A) tobacco use
    (B) elevated blood pressure
    (C) elevated cholesterol
    (D) homocystine

21. In the United States, the largest proportion of TB cases occur among

    (A) HIV-infected persons
    (B) foreign-born persons
    (C) IV drug abusers
    (D) the incarcerated

22. Which is the pathogenic pathway in the development of colorectal cancer accounting for 15% of sporadic cases and nearly all cases of hereditary nonpolyposis colorectal cancer?

    (A) chromosomal instability
    (B) FAP mutation
    (C) microsatellite instability
    (D) telomere cutoff

23. In the chemoprevention of breast cancer with Tamoxifen, the major concern is

    (A) lymphedema
    (B) renal failure
    (C) gastrointestinal side effects
    (D) risk of thromboembolism

24. In the health care environment, the most common cause of infectious diarrhea in the United States

    (A) *Giardia lamblia*
    (B) *Clostridium difficile*
    (C) *Cyclospora*
    (D) *Salmonella*

25. Which of the following infections is transmitted chiefly from person to person?

    (A) California encephalitis
    (B) West Nile virus encephalitis
    (C) Eastern Equine encephalitis
    (D) Meningococcal meningitis

26. Which of the following statements most accurately describes depressive disorders?

   (A) they are associated with more frequent visits for physical symptoms
   (B) they can result in suicide in over 50%
   (C) they mostly affect young married men
   (D) they are not an economic burden

27. Which of the following acts as a cofactor in duodenal ulcer?

   (A) use of cigarettes
   (B) blood group O
   (C) nonsteroidal anti-inflammatory drugs (NSAIDs)
   (D) *Helicobacter pylori*

28. A 10-month-old child is brought to your office by her mother because of vomiting and profuse diarrhea for 24 hours. She has a temperature of 100°F and signs of dehydration. No other person in the household is ill. The most likely etiologic agents is

   (A) adenovirus
   (B) rotavirus
   (C) echovirus
   (D) parvovirus

Use the following information to answer questions 29 and 30.

Questions 29 through 30

On a Friday afternoon, a 30-year-old registered nurse is brought to your office in employee health for evaluation following a needlestick injury that occurred in the HIV clinic. The source patient involved is known to be infected with HIV and has advanced AIDS.

29. Which of the following factors carries the greatest risk for the transmission of HIV to the nurse?

   (A) depth of injury
   (B) presence of visible blood on the needle
   (C) entrance of the needle into a vein or artery of the source patient
   (D) stage of illness of the source patient

30. What is the most appropriate course of action for this health worker?

   (A) reassure her of the low risk of infection
   (B) offer 2-drug antiretroviral therapy
   (C) draw HIV antibody test and refer to an infectious disease specialist on Monday
   (D) offer triple-drug antiretroviral therapy

Questions 31 through 40

31. The most important risk factor for heat-related illness is

   (A) age over 65
   (B) age under 1
   (C) history of previous heat stroke
   (D) obesity

32. An intervention study demonstrates that attending a sexual history taking skills building workshop resulted in higher levels of comfort of providers questioning patients about their number of sexual partners (RR = 1.4; 95% confidence intervals 1.2–33.8).

   The major weakness of this study is

   (A) power
   (B) internal validity
   (C) precision
   (D) failure to demonstrate statistical significance

33. For which patient is pneumococcal vaccine (PPV 23) not beneficial?

   (A) a 15-month-old HIV infected child
   (B) a 20-year old about to undergo a splenectomy for thrombotic thrombocytopenic purpura (TTP)
   (C) a 5-year old with sickle cell disease
   (D) a 10-year-old child with nephrotic syndrome

34. Which of the following vaccines are contraindicated during pregnancy?

   (A) rabies vaccine
   (B) influenza vaccine
   (C) varicella vaccine
   (D) hepatitis B vaccine

35. The medical evaluation of a 32-year-old HIV-infected patient reveals a tuberculin skin test reaction at 5 mm and indurated. His chest x-ray is normal. He is currently taking antiretroviral therapy that includes protease inhibitors. He has not previously received antituberculous therapy nor had any known contact with people with TB. Which is the most appropriate intervention at this time?

    (A) isoniazid (INH) for 9 months
    (B) no preventive therapy for TB needed
    (C) rifampin for 9 months
    (D) Streptomycin for 6 months

36. The incidence rate of lung cancer is 120/100,000 person-years for smokers and 10/100,000 per person-year for nonsmokers. What is the risk of developing lung cancer for persons who smoke?

    (A) 5
    (B) 12
    (C) 50
    (D) 100

37. Breast cancer is the most frequently diagnosed neoplasia among women. It is estimated that one woman out of every eight will develop the disease over the course of a lifetime. What is the lifetime risk of developing cancer in a woman in which the *BRCA 1* gene has been detected?

    (A) 20%
    (B) 40%
    (C) 50%
    (D) 70% or more

38. The use of matching as a technique to control for confounding is most appropriate for which type of study?

    (A) a large-scale cohort study
    (B) a case-control study with small numbers
    (C) a clinical trial with factorial design
    (D) cross-sectional study with multiple variables

39. Asthma is a common disease in children and the prevalence of asthma in the United States has risen over the past 20 years. While the prevalence rate of asthma was 3% in 1982, the rate rose to 5% in 1992 with sharp increases noted in early childhood to adolescence. Which of the following factors is most strongly predictive of asthma mortality in children?

    (A) age
    (B) gender
    (C) environmental pollutants
    (D) severity of illness

40. A 10-year-old boy with sickle cell disease presents with headache, anorexia, and fever. He complains of pain in the right tibia and local inflammation is noted. Osteomyelitis is diagnosed; the most likely etiologic agent is

    (A) *Salmonella*
    (B) *Shigellosis*
    (C) *Listeria*
    (D) *Campylobacter*

Answers and Explanations

1. **(B)** Risk factors for prostate cancer include age, race, living in an industrialized country, and family history. The mortality rate for prostate cancer for African American men is 3 times higher than that for White men; the incidence rate for African American men is 1.6 times higher than that for White men. *(Lang and Hensrud, 2004, p. 385)*

2. **(A)** Primary prevention is the concept of preventing disease before it occurs. Floridation of water supplies has been shown to decrease rates of dental caries. Mammography and testing for CRP are forms of secondary prevention as disease already exists in the patient; surgery for carotid artery stenosis is essentially a therapeutic procedure consistent with tertiary prevention. *(Jekel et al, 1997)*

3. **(A)** Children born to hepatitis B infected mothers have a high risk of contracting the infection. Immunization decreases the risk to the newborn by 75% to 95%. *(US Preventive Services Task Force, 1997, p. 269)*

4. **(D)** West Nile virus has become the most common mosquito borne infectious disease in the United States since the 2002 epidemic, far more prevalent than eastern equine encephalitis. Between 2001 and 2004, it spread progressively annually across the United States and is now endemic in most parts of the United States. Hantavirus is transmitted by aerosolized rodent droppings and causes hantavirus pulmonary syndome (HPS). Lyme disease is caused by tick bites and is endemic particularly in states on the Eastern seaboard. (Source: http://www.postgradmed.com/issues/2003/07_03/gelfand.htm)

5. **(C)** Unintentional injuries such as falls, motor vehicle accidents, drownings, burns, and others are the leading causes of death among children aged 1 through 4. (CDC, National Center for Health Statistics, 2005).

6. **(C)** Incidence rates reflect the occurrence of new cases of a disease in the population and are often used to assess the risk of a disease to the public's health. Virulence refers to the pathological properties of infecting microorganisms. Epidemic refers to outbreaks of disease above normal levels. Prevalence is the number of existing cases of a disease in a population per unit time. *(Aschengrau and Seage, 2003, p. 44)*

7. **(D)** Screening to detect colorectal cancer should employ multiple modalities. Fecal occult blood testing has advantages of simplicity, low cost, and cost effectiveness, but has low sensitivity and poor compliance. Evidence suggests that barium enema is often inaccurate for the detection of polyps and early cancers and is suboptimal for CRC as a population screening test. No data exist from randomized trials as to the efficacy of sigmoidoscopy. Colonoscopy has been shown to be effective in detecting premalignant colon polyps and is recommended by The American

Cancer Society and the US Preventive Services Task Force. *(Lang and Hensrud, 2004, pp. 547–548)*

8. **(B)** The length of immune protection for most commonly used childhood vaccines is considered to extend throughout the childhood years. For measles, level of immune protection following initial immunization have been shown to decrease on a yearly basis. School-aged children in the U.K. receive a booster dose between ages 3 and 5. The American Academy of Pediatrics recommends that the appropriate age for routine administration of the second dose of measles-mumps-rubella (MMR) vaccine is between ages 4 to 6 years. The implementation of the two-dose measles vaccine schedule has improved the control of measles, but some outbreaks continue to occur in school children, although 95% of children in school have received one dose of vaccine. Because most measles vaccine failures are attributable to failure to respond to the first dose, all children receive two doses of measles-containing vaccine at school entry (4 to 6 years of age). American Academy of Pediatrics Policy Statement on the Second Administration of MMR. Available at: www.aappolicy.aappublications.org. CDC. MMWR. Recommendations for Immunization of the Advisory Committee on Immunization Practices, February 8, 2002

9. **(C)** Persons who are assigned by the investigator or volunteer to study groups may differ systematically in characteristics other than the intervention itself, thereby limiting the studies' internal validity and the generalizability of the results. *(US Preventive Services Task Force, 1997, Chapter ii, p. xlviii)*

10. **(C)** Hepatitis B is commonly sexually transmitted, accounting for roughly 55% of all cases. Hepatitis B is more efficiently transmitted through sexual contact than HIV. The likelihood of sexual transmission of hepatitis B is reduced with condom use. The hepatitis B immunization is a safe and effective vaccination and has been shown to decrease rates of transmission. No vaccines are available for syphilis or chlamydial infections. An effective vaccine

for herpes simplex II, a viral infection, is still under development. *(Lang and Hensrud, 2004, Chapter 51, p. 597)*

11. **(A)** Several studies have demonstrated very low rates of identification of battered women by physicians, even in hospitals with established protocols for this problem. There are discrete patterns of occurrence of domestic violence, but cases involve persons (mostly women) from all social strata. Domestic violence is prevalent among women (15% of women seen in emergency departments, and 12% to 23% of women in family practice settings). In surveys of pregnant women primarily from urban public clinics, 7% to 18% of women experienced some form of physical abuse (including forced sexual activity) during their pregnancy. The most common abusers of the elderly are family members. *(US Preventive Services Task Force, 1997, Chapter 51 pp. 556–558)*

12. **(C)** Fatalities per 1,000 licensed drivers in the United States are highest among the youngest and oldest drivers, the graph plotting fatalities by age showing a U-shaped distribution. *(Lang and Hensrud, 2004, Chapter 23, p. 267)*

13. **(A)** While hypertension, diabetes, HIV infection, and trauma are more prevalent in African Americans than in other races, heart disease still (as is the case in the general population) is by far the most common cause of deaths. Heart disease among African Americans claims 27% of all deaths in this racial group. *(Lang and Hensrud, 2004, Chapter 35, p. 406)*

14. **(C)** The incidence of Guillian Barre syndrome is about 1 to 2 cases in every 100,000 people per year. In about half of all the cases, the onset of the syndrome follows a viral or bacterial infection, such as the common cold, viral gastrointestinal infections, infectious mononucleosis, viral hepatitis, and campylobacteriosis (usually from eating undercooked poultry). A small number of cases have been known to occur after a medical procedure, such as minor surgery. GBS is believed to be an autoimmune disorder in which the body produces antibod-

ies that damage the myelin sheath. It has also been associated with influenza immunization. *(Lang and Hensrud, 2004, Chapter 53, p. 623)*

15. **(D)** There are an estimated 3 million new cases of Chlamydial infection each year in the United States. This is higher than current rates of either syphilis or gonorrhea. A component of the increase in the number of reported cases observed during the 1990s was the increase in the number of states that made chlamydia a reportable infection. The highest rates of gonococcal infections were observed during the 1980s and the occurrence of syphilis peaked during the 1990s. Chancroid is a rare sexually transmitted disease. *(Lang and Hensrud, 2004, Chapter 51, p. 596)*

16. **(B)** The infant mortality rate, commonly used as an index of the health status of a region or country, is calculated as the number of infant deaths under age 1 in a given time frame and population over the number of live births in the same time frame and population. The neonatal mortality rate is the number of infant deaths under age 28 days or less over the number of live births; the postneonatal mortality rate is the number of deaths of infants aged between 28 days and 365 days over the number of live births minus the neonatal death rate; the perinatal mortality rate is the number of stillbirths plus the number of infant deaths ages 7 days or less over the number of stillbirths in the same time frame plus the number of live births in the same time period. *(Jekel et al, 1997, Chapter 2, p. 34)*

17. **(B)** The epidemic curve is used frequently to graphically depict the case–time relationship of an outbreak of a disease, particularly an infectious disease. The curve is the plot of cases on the *x*-axis and time (in units of hours, days, months, or years depending on the nature of the disease) on the *y*-axis. *(Jekel et al, 1997, Chapter 3, p. 45)*

18. **(D)** Antibodies to the hepatitis B core antigen appear early in the infection with the IgM fraction being the most prominent. The presence of the surface antigen and/or the e antigen do not provide sufficient information

regarding the timing of the acquisition of the infection. *(Kasper et al, 2005)*

19. **(B)** Chloroquine is a standard prophylaxis for the prevention of malaria. The Dominican Republic is a country with a high risk for malaria; it is also a chloroquine-susceptible region as are most parts of Central America and Mexico. It is safe, efficatious, and has few major side effects. Chloroquine is ideal for short visits to endemic regions. Mefloquine and doxycycline are medications used in chloroquine-resistant regions. CDC Travel Website. www.cdc.gov. *(Lang and Hensrud, 2004, Chapter 24, p. 273)*

20. **(B)** Tobacco use is clearly the risk factor with the greatest influence on the pathology of atherosclerosis. Blood pressure elevation and elevations of level of homocystine and cholesterol are also important factors in atherosclerosis progression. *(Lang and Hensrud, 2004, Chapter 53, p. 623)*

21. **(B)** Foreign-born individuals comprise more than a third (36%) of new cases of reported TB in the United States. Individuals in the other categories have a high risk for the development of TB. *(Wallace et al, 1998)*

22. **(C)** There are at least three distinct pathways involving genetic alterations in the development of colon cancer. Chromosomal instability arises from an accumulation of allelic losses or mutation; this accounts for some cases of sporadically occurring colon cancer. The second pathway, microsatellite instability involves inactivating mutations in the genes responsible for DNA repair resulting in widespread mutations at repetitive DNA sequences (microsatellites). The third pathway is hypermethylation of promoter regions of genes. *(Lang and Hensrud, 2004, Chapter 47, p. 544)*

23. **(D)** The report of the National Surgical Adjuvant Breast and Bowel Project P-1 Study (NSABP) showed that Tamoxifen achieved a 49% reduction in the incidence of invasive breast cancer in women at an increased risk of the development of breast cancer. A side effect

noted in the study was an increased risk of thromboembolic disease. *(Lang and Hensrud, 2004, Chapter 30, p. 357)*

24. **(B)** Infectious diarrhea is a common problem causing one to two episodes person annually in the United States. Children under 3 years old are at the highest risk. In the hospital setting, *C. difficile* represents the most frequently occurring form of infectious diarrhea typically through the inappropriate administration of antibiotics. Salmonella is typically a food-borne illness transmitted in the community. Giardia and cyclospora infections are typically water-borne infections also primarily acquired in nonhospital settings. *(Lang and Hensrud, 2004, Chapter 53, p. 623)*

25. **(D)** California encephalitis, West Nile virus encephalitis, and eastern encephalitis are arboviral diseases transmitted primarily by mosquitoes. Meningococcal meningitis is a bacterial infection transmitted by person to person spread. *(Kasper et al, 2005)*

26. **(A)** Depression is most common in persons who are young, female, divorced, single, separated, severely ill, or have a prior history or family history of depression. Persons who are depressed frequently seek medical attention for various physical symptoms. Suicide attempts are most commonly reported among women and men aged 20 to 24 years. The highest rate of completed suicide is among men over the age of 65 years. The most important risk factor for suicide is psychiatric illness. The majority of suicide victims have affective, substance abuse, personality or other mental disorders. *(US Preventive Services Task Force, 1997, Chapter 50, pp. 547–549)*

27. **(D)** Eradication of *Helicobacter pylori* infection heals ulcers except for those caused by NSAID use. *H. pylori* infection is not a cofactor when NSAID use is present. The known risk factors for duodenal ulcers include cigarette use (RR = 2), family history (RR = 3), blood group O (RR = 1.3), and gastric hyperacidity (RR = 7). *(Wallace et al, 1998)*

28. **(B)** Rotavirus is the most common cause of gastrointestinal disease as well as dehydration among small children. It can be a severe infection and is most common in the cooler months of the year. Adenovirus and echovirus infections are much less common causes of diarrheal disease; parvovirus infection is associated with nongastrointestinal symptoms in children. *(Chin, 2000)*

29. **and 30. (29-A)** and **(30-D)**. The overall risk of acquiring HIV following a needlestick injury is 0.03%. A large case control study among recipients of needlestick injuries in three countries (US, U.K., and France) showed that the factor with highest odds ratio for seroconversion was the depth of the injury (RR = 16.1). Guidelines issued by the CDC recommend that triple antiretroviral therapy be instituted immediately. CDC. Mortality and Morbidity Weekly Report, 1998;47 [RR-7], 1–28.

31. **(A)** Older adults are the most susceptible to heat-related illness because of decreased response of the cardiovascular system during hot weather. *(LaDou, 1997, pp. 144–145)*

32. **(C)** Power refers to the ability of the study to detect statistically significant results. This study reached statistical significance as the confidence intervals do not cross 1. Internal validity relates to the lack of systematic bias in a study. Even though this study reached statistical significance, it lacks precision as indicated by the wide range in the confidence intervals suggesting that the sample size was small.

33. **(A)** Pneumococcal vaccine is not recommended for children under age 2 years or less. Protection with pneumococcal vaccination is important in persons with various conditions conferring higher risk of pneumococcal infection such as those who are asplenic, have sickle cell disease, or who have chronic diseases such as renal failure. The spleen is important in the immune defense of infections with polysaccharide antigens. *(Lang and Hensrud, 2004, Chapter 50, pp. 578–579)*

34. **(C)** Varicella (VZV) vaccine is contraindicated as it is a live-virus preparation. In general,

live-virus vaccines should not be used in pregnant women as there is an increased risk of infection of the developing fetus. The vaccines for hepatitis B and influenza are inactivated virus vaccines. There is no evidence that inactivated vaccines or toxoids are harmful in pregnant women. For pregnant women exposed to varicella or zoster, an appropriate prophylactic measure may be the use of varicella immune globulin (VZIG). CDC. MMWR. General Recommendations of Immunzation. Guidelines for Vaccinating PregnantWomen. February 8, 2002, Page 18.

35. **(A)** A positive tuberculin skin test of 5-mm induration or more is considered positive in a person who has HIV infection, has had contact with a person with TB, or who has a positive chest x-ray. HIV-infected persons are at an increased risk of TB and should be screened on a regular basis. Prophylaxis is warranted in this patient and it is recommended that INH be used for 9 months. Rifampin is not recommended for use in patients taking protease inhibitors and this reduces effective levels of the antiretroviral drug. *(Chin, 2000, pp. 526–527)*

36. **(B)** The formula for the calculation of relative risk is I_e/I_{non-e}, where I represents the incidence of disease and e represents exposure. In this case, $120/100,000 /10/100,000 = 12$. This indicates that the risk of developing lung cancer among those exposed is 12 times that of the rate of those not exposed. *(Jekel et al, 1997)*

37. **(D)** The strongest risk factors (RR over 4) for the development of breast cancer include age over 65, prior invasive or in situ breast cancer, family history of two or more relatives with premenopausal or bilateral breast cancer, or atypical hyperplasia on biopsy. Lesser risk factors (RR less than 2) include nulliparity, obesity, family history of a first-degree relative with breast cancer, age at full-term pregnancy greater than 30 years of age, or history of ovarian or endometrial cancer. Known risk factors account for only 20% of breast cancer in younger patients and 30% in older patients. Patients with either the *BRCA 1* or *BRCA 2* gene mutation have a very high risk; charac-

teristics of persons with such gene mutations include breast cancer at an early age, bilateral breast cancer, and both breast and ovarian cancers. *(Lang and Hensrud, 2004, Chapter 30, pp. 353–360; US Preventive Services Task Force, 1997, Chapter 7 pp. 73–81)*

38. **(B)** Matching is a technique used in the conduct of case-control studies to control for confounding. Subjects enrolled in a study are matched for age, gender, smoking, or any other variables not being analyzed in the study. This technique is not used in cohort studies as it is too time consuming and expensive; in such studies, randomization of subjects is used to control for confounding. Matching cannot be used in cross-sectional studies as these are purely descriptive studies and do include a control group. *(Jekel et al, 1997, pp. 150–151)*

39. **(D)** Risk factors for developing asthma include male gender, positive family history, respiratory tract infections, ambient air pollution, environmental tobacco smoke, and bronchial hyperreactivity. In terms of predictors of mortality, large epidemiologic studies reveal that the severity of illness is the most important factor. While increasingly prevalent, overall age-adjusted death rates from asthma are fairly low. *(Wallace et al, 1998)*

40. **(A)** Due to functional asplenia, persons with sickle cell disease are susceptible to a variety of infections with polysaccaride-containing bacterial antigens of which salmonella is a very common agent. *(Kasper et al, 2005)*

REFERENCES

Aschengrau A, Seage GR. *Essentials of Epidemiology for Public Health*. Sudbury, MA: Jones and Bartlett; 2003.

Chin J. *Control of Communicable Diseases Manual*, 17th ed. Washington, D.C.: American Public Health Association; 2000.

Jekel JF, Elmore JG, Katz DL. *Epidemiology, Biostatistics, and Preventive Medicine*. Philadelphia, PA: W.B. Saunders; 1997.

Kasper D., Braunwald E., Fauci AS, et al. *Harrison's Principles of Internal Medicine*, 16th ed. New York: McGraw-Hill; 2005.

LaDou J. *Occupational and Environmental Medicine*, 2nd ed. Stamford, CT: Appleton and Lange; 1997.

Lang RS, Hensrud DD. *Clinical Preventive Medicine*, 2nd ed. Chicago: AMA Press; 2004.

US Preventive Services Task Force. *Guide to Clinical Preventive Services*, 2nd ed. Baltimore, MD: Williams and Wilkins; 1997.

Wallace RB, Doebbling BN, Last JM, et.al. *Maxcy-Rosenau-Last Public Health and Preventive Medicine*, 14th ed., Stamford, CT: Appleton and Lange; 1998.

SECTION VIII

Practice Test

Questions

Questions 1 through 225

1. Which of the following factors places an individual at risk for squamous cell cancer of the esophagus?

   (A) tobacco smoking
   (B) lye ingestion
   (C) achalasia
   (D) excessive alcohol ingestion
   (E) GERD

2. An endoscopy should be performed if a patient does not respond or does not adequately respond to proton pump inhibitors (PPIs) after how many month(s)?

   (A) 24
   (B) 12
   (C) 6
   (D) 3
   (E) 1

3. A 62-year-old male presents to the emergency room complaining of colicky abdominal pain, nausea, and vomiting. The abdomen is distended. There is tympany, and decreased bowel sounds are noted on exam. A large, tender irreducible hernia is found in the right groin. The correct diagnosis is

   (A) indirect inguinal hernia
   (B) direct inguinal hernia
   (C) incarcerated hernia
   (D) strangulated hernia
   (E) ventral hernia

4. Which of the following is more likely to be associated with ulcerative colitis versus Crohn's disease?

   (A) more common in smokers
   (B) small bowel involvement
   (C) associated with perianal disease
   (D) bloody diarrhea

5. The 2005 Dietary Guidelines for Americans recommends sensible and moderate alcohol intake for those who choose to drink, which translates to

   (A) one drink per month for women and two drinks per month for men
   (B) one drink a week for women and two drinks per week for men
   (C) one drink per day for women and two drinks per day for men
   (D) five drinks per day for both men and women
   (E) current guidelines suggest abstaining from alcohol completely

6. Risk factors that remain important clues in the diagnosis of *Clostridium difficile* include

(A) patients of advanced age and comorbid conditions such as diabetes

(B) diabetes with a history of antibiotic use within the past year

(C) travel to third world nations

(D) antibiotic use or a hospital stay within the past 3 months

(E) attending a daycare or preschool center

7. Cullen's sign is associated with

(A) diastasis recti

(B) umbilical calculi

(C) umbilical fistula

(D) umbilical hernia

(E) retroperitoneal bleeding

8. An elderly patient is brought in to the ER complaining of incontinence of liquid "like tea water" stool. He is complaining of rectal pressure and lower abdominal pain. The pain is cramping in quality and the patient's abdomen is "bloated." Digital rectal exam reveals hard stool in the rectum. Which of the following should be selected as the initial treatment for this patient?

(A) passing a nasogastric tube

(B) soapsuds enema

(C) milk of magnesia

(D) administration of opiate analgesics for pain

(E) manual disimpaction

9. Mrs. Jones was found to have colorectal cancer. Her colonoscopy was negative preoperatively. Her surgery was felt to be curative. She should have subsequent surveillance exams every

(A) 1 year

(B) 2 years

(C) 3 years

(D) 5 years

(E) 10 years

10. What is the most common drug to cause acute liver failure?

(A) alcohol

(B) ketoconazole

(C) lisinopril

(D) acetaminophen

(E) methotrexate

11. Which of the following is associated with worsening hyponatremia due to excess infusion of hypotonic fluid in a postoperative patient?

(A) oliguria

(B) paralytic ileus

(C) cardiac irritability

(D) hepatic encephalopathy

(E) central nervous system (CNS) dysfunction

12. What is the most common cause of fever for a postoperative patient in the first 48 hours following surgery?

(A) wound infection

(B) atelectasis

(C) urinary retention

(D) bacteremia

(E) anesthetic reaction

13. What is the best choice of intravenous fluids for a patient with gastric losses due to prolonged nasogastric aspiration?

(A) lactated ringers with 20 meq KCL/L

(B) 5% dextrose water with 20 meq KCL/L

(C) 5% dextrose with 0.5 N saline with 20 meq KCL/L

(D) 5% dextrose with 0.9% N saline with 20 meq KCL/L

(E) 0.9% N saline with 20 meq KCL/L

14. In addition to fingerstick glucose monitoring, what additional testing is important to prevent postoperative complications in the diabetic patient?

(A) serum potassium
(B) urinary ketones
(C) serum osmolality
(D) urinary protein
(E) serum sodium

15. A 22-year-old male is brought to the emergency department (ED) by EMS after having sustained a single stab wound to the right chest in the fourth intercostal space at the right sternal border. While attempting to resuscitate the patient he becomes hypotensive with marked jugular venous distension. Auscultation of the chest reveals moderately diminished breath sounds on the right side with muffled heart sounds. The most appropriate initial intervention is?

(A) right tube thoracostomy
(B) pericardiocentesis
(C) fluid resuscitation
(D) immediate intubation
(E) emergency open thoracotomy

16. Which of the following findings is indicative of increased intracranial pressure from an associated closed head injury?

(A) hypotension, bradycardia, and tachypnea
(B) hypertension, bradycardia, and bradypnea
(C) hypotension, tachycardia, and tachypnea
(D) hypertension, tachycardia, and tachypnea
(E) hypotension, tachycardia, and bradypnea

17. Which population has the highest incidence of gallstones in this country?

(A) Caucasian women under the age of 50 years
(B) Caucasian women over the age of 50 years
(C) Hispanic men over the age of 50 years
(D) African American men under the age of 50 years
(E) Native American women before the age of 60 years

18. A 46-year-old African American male is seen in the emergency room with upper right quadrant pain that radiates to the right infrascapular area. The pain is colicky and was precipitated by a meal of fried fish and fried potatoes. What is the initial study of choice for this patient?

(A) plain abdominal x-ray
(B) ultrasonography
(C) radionuclide scan (HIDA scan)
(D) computerized tomography (CT)
(E) oral cholecystogram

19. A 54-year-old male presents to the ED with a complaint of severe epigastric pain radiating to the back. The pain has been present for the past 8 hours and is associated with nausea and vomiting, which has not relieved the pain. Laboratory data reveal a WBC of $14,000/mm^3$, and a serum amylase of 500 U/L (reference range 0 to 286 U/L). The most likely diagnosis is?

(A) bleeding duodenal ulcer
(B) cholecystitis
(C) acute pancreatitis
(D) ischemic colitis
(E) renal colic

20. What is an appropriate screening test for hepatocellular carcinoma in patients with cirrhosis?

(A) alkaline phosphatase

(B) alpha-fetoprotein

(C) transaminases

(D) total and fractionated bilirubin

(E) carcinoembryonic antigen

21. What features are commonly associated with lower extremity ulcers that are due to chronic arterial insufficiency?

(A) ulcers are associated with hyperpigmentation changes in the skin

(B) ulcers are most commonly seen around the medial and lateral malleoli

(C) ulcers have a "punched out" appearance with a pale or necrotic base

(D) ulcers are associated with painless lower extremity edema

22. What is the most common type of hernia affecting both sexes and all age groups?

(A) direct inguinal hernia

(B) indirect inguinal hernia

(C) femoral hernia

(D) umbilical hernia

(E) incisional hernia

23. A 62-year-old male presents to the office concerned about an abdominal aortic aneurysm (AAA). He states that his father died from one at the age of 50 and his brother was diagnosed last week with an AAA. What is the most appropriate screening tool in this situation?

(A) abdominal radiograph

(B) CT

(C) palpation

(D) ultrasound

(E) aortography

24. What is the most common site of an acute arterial occlusion due to embolic disease?

(A) iliac artery

(B) aortic bifurcation

(C) mesenteric arteries

(D) femoral artery

(E) popliteal artery

25. Which type of colon polyp should be treated by surgical excision because of a high risk of malignant degeneration?

(A) hamartoma

(B) hyperplastic

(C) inflammatory

(D) tubular

(E) villous

26. Which of the following drugs treats HIV disease by blocking viral entry into the cells?

(A) delavirdine

(B) efavirenz

(C) enfuvirtide

(D) fosaprenavir

(E) nevirapine

27. Which drug used to treat tuberculosis is contraindicated in a patient who is taking indinavir?

(A) ethambutol

(B) isoniazid

(C) pyrazinamide

(D) rifampin

(E) zidovudine

28. A 48-year-old female presents with a chief complaint of gradually progressing difficulty in climbing stairs over the past 3 months. On physical exam there is notable proximal muscle weakness of the upper and lower extremities. The remainder of the exam is unremarkable. On laboratory evaluation, a serum creatine phosphokinase (CPK) is elevated and a muscle biopsy reveals lymphoid inflammatory infiltrates. What is the appropriate initial treatment of choice in this patient?

(A) prednisone
(B) methotrexate
(C) azathioprine
(D) hydrochloroquine
(E) cyclophosphamide

29. A 65-year-old male presents with complaints of acute onset of pain and swelling of the right great toe. He denies recent alcohol ingestion or trauma to the area. On physical exam, the patient is afebrile and the first metatarsophalangeal joint is erythematous, swollen, and warm to the touch. Laboratory evaluation reveals a WBC count of 12,000 and a normal differential. Serum uric acid level is 5 mg/dL. Synovial fluid analysis reveals the presence of rhomboid shaped crystals. What is the most likely diagnosis for this patient?

(A) acute gout
(B) pseudogout
(C) psoriatic arthritis
(D) infectious arthritis
(E) rheumatoid arthritis

30. A 50-year-old female with known recent diagnosis of rheumatoid arthritis has begun treatment with celecoxib. She has been on this medication for 1 year and notes that her pain continues. Early signs of joint involvement are present in the patient's hands. What medication is the best choice in addition to the celecoxib?

(A) methotrexate
(B) tumor necrosis factor (TNF) inhibitor
(C) antimalarial
(D) minocycline
(E) aspirin

31. A 65-year-old ill-appearing female presents to the ED with tachycardia, tachypnea, and an arterial pH of 7.05. In general, what is the most common cause of metabolic acidosis?

(A) diabetic ketoacidosis
(B) lactic acidosis
(C) alcoholic ketoacidosis
(D) nonketotic hyperosmolar acidosis
(E) aspirin poisoning

32. The most reliable clinical assessment tool to confirm endotracheal intubation is

(A) endotracheal tube condensation
(B) symmetrical chest expansion
(C) breath sounds auscultated equally over the chest
(D) no breath sounds auscultated over the stomach
(E) use of a carbon dioxide detection device

33. A 58-year-old male with multiple myeloma presents to the ED with altered mental status, hypertension, back pain, and constipation. These findings are suggestive of which of the following medical conditions?

(A) hyperkalemia
(B) hypercalcemia
(C) hypomagnesemia
(D) hypoglycemia
(E) hyponatremia

34. A 16-year-old long-distance runner suffered an external rotation injury to the ankle. Which of the following ligaments is most likely injured?

(A) anterior talofibular
(B) posterior talofibular
(C) deltoid
(D) calcaneofibular
(E) tibiofibular

35. A 68-year-old male with a PMH of coronary artery disease presents to the emergency department with a 2-day history of intermittent chest tightness. The pain was not relieved with three nitroglycerin sublingual tablets. What would be the initial assessment if the ECG demonstrated 2 mm ST segment elevations in leads II, III, and AVF?

   (A) acute anterior wall myocardial infarction

   (B) acute lateral wall myocardial injury

   (C) subendocardial inferior wall myocardial infarction

   (D) subendocardial anterior wall myocardial ischemia

   (E) acute inferior wall myocardial injury

36. The rates of prostate cancer are highest among

   (A) Whites

   (B) African Americans

   (C) Latinos

   (D) Native Americans

37. The recommended protocol for screening and prevention of hepatitis B infection

   (A) screening using HBsAg is recommended for all pregnant women at their first prenatal visit

   (B) routine screening using HBsAg is recommended for all adults

   (C) routine screening using HBsAg is recommended only for pregnant women and newborns

   (D) screening using HBsAg is recommended only to detect carriers

38. The leading cause of death among persons aged 0 to 4 years of age

   (A) sudden infant death syndrome (SIDS)

   (B) birth defects

   (C) unintentional injuries

   (D) infections

39. The recommended approach to the prevention of colorectal cancer in asymptomatic non-high-risk adults.

   (A) yearly fecal occult blood tests beginning at age 55

   (B) double-contrast barium enema every other year after age 55

   (C) annual flexible sigmoidoscopy beginning at age 50

   (D) colonoscopy every 10 years and flexible sigmoidoscopy every 5 years beginning at age 50

40. Which of the following statements related to the identification of family violence is TRUE?

   (A) only 10% of battered women are identified by physicians

   (B) most cases of domestic violence are sporadic and isolated

   (C) in some population groups in the United States, up to 50% of pregnant women experience domestic violence

   (D) caregivers are the most common abusers of battered elders

41. All of the following would be considered immediate first-line therapy in a patient with acute coronary ischemia EXCEPT

   (A) oxygen

   (B) aspirin

   (C) glycoprotein IIb/IIIa receptor inhibitors

   (D) nitroglycerin

   (E) morphine

42. A 42-year-old female was brought to the ED from a psychiatric facility for an evaluation following a brief "seizure." The psychiatric staff reports she has been confused and complaining of thirst for the past 5 days. What is the most likely diagnosis?

   (A) idiopathic hypoglycemia

   (B) psychogenic polydipsia

   (C) brain tumor

   (D) new-onset epilepsy

   (E) psychogenic cerebritis

43. A 44-year-old AIDS patient being treated for PCP pneumonia presents to the ED with a relatively acute onset of confusion, pallor, daiphoresis, and tachycardia. What is the most likely cause of the patient's symptoms?

    (A) hypoglycemia
    (B) meningitis
    (C) subarachnoid hemorrhage
    (D) hypoxemia
    (E) mucous plugging

44. A 72-year-old female is brought to the ED after being found on her kitchen floor comatose with a BP of 280/150 and pinpoint reactive pupils. What is the most likely diagnosis?

    (A) thalamic hemorrhage
    (B) cerebellar hemorrhage
    (C) pontine hemorrhage
    (D) subarachnoid hemorrhage
    (E) intracerebral left occipital hemorrhage

45. The most immediate management priority in a patient with septic shock is

    (A) empiric antimicrobial therapy
    (B) inotropic support
    (C) oxygenation and ventilation
    (D) fluid therapy
    (E) acid–base status

46. A patient presented to the emergency department with a possible foreign body to the hand. Identify the item that would be the least radiopaque.

    (A) glass
    (B) metal
    (C) gravel fragment
    (D) plastic
    (E) painted wood

47. A 59-year-old cancer patient presents to the ED with fever, pneumonia, hypotension, and tachycardia. Investigative studies include hyperkalemia, hyonatremia, and hypoglycemia. What is the most likely concomitant diagnosis in this scenario?

    (A) adrenal insufficiency
    (B) syndrome of inappropriate antidiuretic hormone (SIADH)
    (C) Cushing's syndrome
    (D) hypothyroidism
    (E) hyerparathyroidism

48. The drug of choice for hypertensive encephalopathy is

    (A) sodium nitroprusside
    (B) labetalol
    (C) esmolol
    (D) intravenous nitroglycerin
    (E) hydralazine

49. An 89-year-old female patient from a nursing home presents to the ED with abdominal pain and distention. The abdominal radiograph demonstrates multiple air-fluid levels and dilated large bowel loops consistent with a large bowel obstruction. What is the most likely cause of the obstruction?

    (A) diverticulitis
    (B) abdominal wall hernias
    (C) carcinoma
    (D) sigmoid volvulus
    (E) adhesions

50. A 28-year-old male presents to the ED with a back injury following an ATV crash. The exam reveals a sensory deficit at the nipples. The spinal cord injury level is most likely at which of the following levels?

    (A) T1
    (B) T2
    (C) T3
    (D) T4
    (E) T5

51. The earliest sign of chronic kidney disease (CKD) is

    (A) microscopic hematuria
    (B) hypertension
    (C) proteinuria
    (D) abnormal creatinine
    (E) hyperkalemia

52. How often should patients with diabetes mellitus be screened for microalbuminuria?

(A) once a month
(B) every 3 months
(C) every 6 months
(D) once a year
(E) there is no specific timetable

53. Which of the following urinary findings is suggestive of acute glomerulonephritis?

(A) red cells and red cell casts
(B) white cells and white cell casts
(C) renal tubular epithelial cells
(D) oval fat bodies
(E) hyaline casts

54. Which of the following is an absolute indication to initiate dialysis?

(A) proteinuria >3 g/24 h
(B) glomerular filtration rate <10 mL/min
(C) hyperkalemia >5.0 meq/L
(D) seizures
(E) hyperphosphatemia >6.5 mg/dL

55. A renal ultrasound would be most beneficial for diagnosing which of the following?

(A) nephrotic syndrome
(B) polycystic kidney disease
(C) glomerulonephritis
(D) acute tubular necrosis
(E) lupus nephritis

56. Which of the following types of renal calculi is associated with an infectious cause?

(A) struvite
(B) uric acid
(C) calcium oxalate
(D) cystine
(E) calcium phosphate

57. Prolonged, heavy use of NSAIDs causes which type of kidney damage?

(A) glomerular
(B) tubulointerstitial
(C) autoimmune
(D) macrovascular
(E) NSAIDs do not cause kidney damage

58. Which class of medications is useful to treat renal calculi due to hypercalciuria?

(A) calcium channel blockers
(B) colchicine
(C) allopurinol
(D) citrate
(E) thiazide diuretics

59. Glucose will spill into the urine when the serum glucose reaches what level?

(A) >126 mg/dL
(B) 150 to 175 mg/dL
(C) 180 to 200 mg/dL
(D) >250 mg/dL
(E) >400 mg/dL

60. Which of the following is MOST indicative of urinary tract infection?

(A) positive nitrite on dipstick
(B) positive leukocyte esterase on dipstick
(C) 2 to 3 WBCs/HPF on urine dipstick
(D) urine culture revealing 10,000 to 20,000 colonies of *Lactobacillus*
(E) positive nitrite and leukocyte esterase on dipstick

61. A 62-year-old patient presents to the ED with generalized abdominal pain, nausea, vomiting, and abdominal distention. The radiographs demonstrate multiple loops of dilated small bowel, air-fluid levels, and a string of pearls sign. What is the most likely cause of this clinical scenario?

(A) neoplasm
(B) incarceration of abdominal hernias
(C) gallstone ileus
(D) bezoars
(E) adhesions following abdominal surgery

62. A patient presents to the emergency department with frequent, mucoid, watery stools, nausea, and lower abdominal pain. The patient has been on a cephalosporin-type antibiotic for about 3 months. The most likely diagnosis would be

(A) diverticulitis

(B) fissure in ano

(C) pseudomembranous entercolitis

(D) anorectal tumor

(E) ulcerative colitis

63. A patient presents to the emergency department with a dislocated shoulder. Nitrous oxide is the drug selected for sedation and analgesia during reduction. Which of the following is true with regard to the administration of nitrous oxide for short-term painful procedures in the emergency department?

(A) a 50:50 concentration of nitrous and oxygen should be used

(B) never administer oxygen with nitrous oxide

(C) nitrous oxide concentrations should always be 30%

(D) higher altitudes require lower concentrations of nitrous oxide

(E) nitrous oxide is not approved for emergency department use

64. A pregnant patient, at 25 weeks' gestation, is involved in a motor vehicle accident. She suffers blunt abdominal trauma. The vital signs are a pulse 100/min, respiratory rate 40/min, and a blood pressure 78/40. Which of the following is a true statement regarding the management of trauma in pregnancy?

(A) intubation should be avoided in the mother due to barotrauma complications

(B) the first resuscitative efforts should be directed toward the mother

(C) the fetus is less susceptible to hypoxia because of uterine reserve

(D) a stat C-section should be considered in every patient

(E) fetal distress is not easily recognized

65. Which of the following disorders may present with a patient experiencing anxiety, tremors, palpitations, fatigue, and hemiplegia?

(A) thyroid storm

(B) hypothyroidism

(C) Addisonian crisis

(D) Cushing's syndrome

(E) hypoglycemia

66. A 35-year-old male presents to your office complaining of a painless, localized swelling of his left, lower eyelid that has developed over a period of weeks. He comes in today because it is now producing a foreign body sensation in his left eye. On physical exam, his visual acuity is normal and there is no evidence of injection or discharge. There is a nontender, localized nodule on the lower eyelid. What is the likely diagnosis?

(A) hordeolum

(B) chalazion

(C) pterygium

(D) dacrocystitis

(E) blepharitis

67. A 32-year-old mother complains of pain and photophobia in her right eye after being accidentally poked in the eye by her 2-year-old daughter. On physical exam, the patient appears uncomfortable, is tearing excessively, and keeping the eye closed. Visual acuity in the left eye is 20/20 and in the right eye is 20/100. Application of a topical anesthetic relieves the patient's pain. The right conjunctiva is injected. On fluorescein staining, there is evidence of uptake at the central location of the epithelium of the cornea. Appropriate treatment and follow-up for this patient includes which of the following?

(A) warm compresses and referral to an ophthalmologist

(B) topical antibiotic ointment, oral analgesics for pain, and referral to an ophthalmologist

(C) topical antibiotic ointment, topical anesthetic for repeated use by the patient to control pain, and referral to an ophthalmologist

(D) topical antibiotic ointment, pressure bandage (eye patch) to immobilize the eyelid for 24 hours, oral analgesics for pain control, and advice to return only if she is not getting better over the next 3 to 4 days

(E) instillation of a corticosteriod to relieve ciliary spasm, pressure bandage (eye patch) to immobilize the eyelid, and referral to an ophthalmologist

68. A 55-year-old active female presents for evaluation and possible excision of painless lesions on the upper eyelids of both eyes, which have been present for several years. On physical exam, the lesions are nontender and appear as slightly raised, yellowish, well-circumscribed plaques in the skin along the nasal portion of both eyelids. On the basis of your exam, which of the following blood tests would you most likely expect to be abnormal?

(A) albumin
(B) lipid levels
(C) liver enzymes
(D) alkaline phosphatase
(E) amylase

69. A 14-year-old male presents within several hours of an episode of a friend slapping his left ear that initially caused pain and dizziness. He denies pain, otorrhea, or dizziness at this time but states that his hearing is still a little muffled. Tuning fork testing is normal with a nonlateralizing Weber and air conduction is greater than bone conduction bilaterally. Exam of the tympanic membrane (TM) shows a small clean central perforation. Which of the following is the most appropriate treatment?

(A) antibacterial drops
(B) keeping the ear dry
(C) oral antibiotics
(D) surgical consult
(E) all of the above

70. A patient presents with a 3-day history of vertigo associated with turning over in bed, which lasts for several minutes. There are no other symptoms of the ear. Positional testing shows rotary nystagmus which diminishes with repeated testing. Which of the following is the most likely diagnosis?

(A) CNS lesion
(B) positional vertigo
(C) labyrinthitis
(D) Meniere's disease
(E) vestibular neuronitis

71. In patients with established coronary heart disease, the goal for LDL cholesterol control is

(A) 100 mg/dL
(B) 130 mg/dL
(C) 160 mg/dL
(D) 190 mg/dL

72. First-line therapy for Raynaud's phenomenon should include

(A) diltiazem
(B) reassurance and warm clothing
(C) reserpine
(D) methyldopa

73. Your patient's wife calls asking for advice. Her husband was admitted this morning with acute coronary syndrome and the doctors are recommending he have coronary artery bypass grafting (CABG). What are the indications for bypass versus percutaneous coronary intervention?

(A) patients should have bypass if they have two lesions both with 80% occlusion
(B) patients should have bypass if they have one lesion with 95% occlusion and diabetes
(C) patients should have bypass if they have triple vessel disease
(D) patients have bypass if they have two lesions both with >95% occlusion

74. A 62-year-old female comes into the office complaining of substernal chest pain and diaphoresis. Her ECG indicates ST elevation in leads II, III, and AVF. What is the next step of care for this patient?

    (A) obtain a stat chest radiograph
    (B) start a verapamil drip
    (C) have the patient chew an aspirin
    (D) repeat the ECG

75. Anticoagulation therapy for a mechanical valve should target what international normalized ratio (INR) range?

    (A) 1.0 to 2.0
    (B) 2.1 to 3.0
    (C) 2.5 to 3.5
    (D) 3.5 to 4.5

76. Indications for aortic aneurysm repair include

    (A) an asymptomatic aneurysm greater than 5.5 cm
    (B) 5-cm aneurysm in a patient with coronary artery disease
    (C) an asymptomatic aneurysm of 3.4 cm in diameter
    (D) 4-cm aneurysm in a patient with a recent CVA

77. Conservative management of arterial peripheral vascular disease includes

    (A) papaverine
    (B) pentoxifylline
    (C) calcium channel blockers
    (D) alpha adrenergic blockers

78. A 62-year-old female with pulmonary hypertension called 911 complaining of diaphoresis and severe dyspnea. Upon arrival to her home, the paramedics found her to have pallor, diaphoresis, tachypnea, hypotension, and tachycardia. Her pulse oxymetry was 89% so they gave her a non-rebreather oxygen mask and transported her to the ED. She was not complaining of angina. The ED physician assistant noted her to be in acute distress with elevated jugular venous pressure, a medial heave, a tender palpable liver, a systolic murmur of tricuspid regurgitation, and an S4 gallop. ECG demonstrated right axis deviation and RV hypertrophy with no STT changes. Her ABG demonstrated a low PaO_2 and a low $PaCO_2$. What is her likely diagnosis?

    (A) acute coronary syndrome
    (B) cor pulmonale
    (C) heart failure
    (D) pulmonary embolus

79. A 33-year-old healthy female during a routine physical exam was found to be hypertensive with a blood pressure of 150/98 mm Hg 3 months ago. She has no family history of hypertension but her provider was concerned so she was started on angiotensin converting enzyme inhibitors (ACEIs). Her blood pressure improved slightly, but on a routine blood draw her creatinine is noted to be 2.3. She is asymptomatic but is noted to have an abdominal bruit. On the basis of her history and laboratory evaluation, which of the following is her most likely diagnosis?

    (A) essential hypertension
    (B) isolated systolic hypertension
    (C) secondary hypertension
    (D) pheochromocytoma

80. A 55-year-old college professor complains of recent occipital headaches that are noted in the morning and subside later in the day. She has noted that over the past 6 months she tires easily. She has a family history of hypertension but denies all other risk factors. Her blood pressure in the clinic is noted to be 172/108 mm Hg. How would you classify her hypertension?

    (A) essential hypertension
    (B) secondary hypertension related to primary aldosteronism
    (C) secondary hypertension related to Cushing's syndrome
    (D) accelerated hypertension

81. A 35-year-old male presents with a 1-week history of a marked decrease of hearing in his right ear. He denies trauma, otorrhea, or vertigo. The physical exam appears to be normal except for his tuning fork tests. The Weber test lateralizes to the better ear and the Rinne test shows air conduction to be better than bone conduction in both ears. After confirmation of your findings with an audiometric evaluation which would be the most appropriate treatment?

(A) broad-spectrum antibiotic
(B) antiviral medication
(C) decongestant
(D) oral steroids
(E) all of the above

82. A 4-year-old presents with a history of right otitis media, which was treated with amoxicillin for the past 4 days. Today the parent has noted that the child is complaining of worsening pain and a 103 degree fever. The outer ear appears to be displaced forward and the outer posterior portion of the ear is tender to palpation. Your exam demonstrates a bulging right TM with purulent effusion. What is your diagnosis?

(A) suppurative otitis media
(B) otitis media with effusion
(C) external otitis
(D) mastoiditis
(E) cellulitis of the pinna

83. Which of the following is the most common complication associated with bacterial sinusitis?

(A) Pott's puffy tumor
(B) meningitis
(C) orbital cellulitis
(D) cavernous sinus thrombosis
(E) cerebral abscess

84. Which medication is usually associated with rhinitis medicamentosa?

(A) oxymetazoline
(B) Psuedoephredrine
(C) chlorpheniramine
(D) Fluticasone
(E) guafenesin

85. Which of the following is the most common cause of unilateral left vocal cord paralysis?

(A) laryngeal cancer
(B) stroke
(C) idiopathic
(D) Pancoast's tumor
(E) trauma

86. A 73-year old with a history of rheumatic fever and coronary atherosclerosis presents to the emergency department with dyspnea on exertion and orthopnea. He called 911 because he could not catch his breath. On exam, he has JVD, hepatic congestion, and peripheral edema. A blowing holosystolic murmur along the left sternal border that is intensified during a Valsalva maneuver is noted. Atrial fibrillation is noted on his ECG. What is his most likely diagnosis?

(A) aortic stenosis
(B) mitral regurgitation
(C) mitral stenosis
(D) tricuspid regurgitation

87. A retired operating room nurse comes to the clinic complaining of a dull ache in her legs after prolonged standing. She notes her legs feel heavy and she has mild ankle edema when she spends the day shopping. The aching pain and the edema resolve spontaneously if the patient elevates her legs. She denies calf tenderness or dyspnea. Physical exam reveals +1 ankle edema bilaterally. What is her most likely diagnosis?

(A) deep venous thrombosis
(B) lymphedema
(C) varicose veins
(D) intermittent claudication

88. You suspect your patient has mitral regurgitation. Which of the following tests would be the most helpful to confirm your diagnosis?

    (A) SPECT scan
    (B) exercise stress test
    (C) echocardiogram
    (D) magnetic resonance imaging (MRI) scan

89. Which patient population is most likely to experience giant cell or temporal arteritis?

    (A) African American women
    (B) Caucasian males
    (C) Scandinavian women
    (D) Hispanic men

90. One of the most common and annoying side effects of ACE inhibitor use is

    (A) hypotension
    (B) dry cough
    (C) urinary frequency
    (D) tinnitus

91. An increase in which factor is most likely to increase the preload?

    (A) arterial vascular tone
    (B) stroke volume
    (C) heart rate
    (D) intravascular volume

92. Cardiogenic shock is characterized by profound hypotension. Which of the following Swan–Ganz catheter findings is consistent with this form of shock?

    (A) decreased preload, decreased afterload, and decreased cardiac output
    (B) decreased preload, increased afterload, and increased cardiac output
    (C) normal preload, normal SVR, and decreased cardiac output
    (D) increased preload, increased SVR, and decreased cardiac output

93. Arterial baroreceptors are found in all of the following locations except

    (A) right and left atria
    (B) aortic arch
    (C) pulmonary veins
    (D) external jugular vein

94. Diastolic dysfunction is characterized by

    (A) increased systemic vascular resistance
    (B) decreased ventricular compliance
    (C) increased stroke volume
    (D) decreased afterload

95. A patient arrives in the ED with ST elevation in leads II, III, and AVF. The patient is hemodynamically stable. What measure should you use to limit the size of infarction in this patient?

    (A) nonsteroidal anti-inflammatory medication
    (B) glucocorticoids
    (C) calcium channel blockers
    (D) fibrinolytic agents

96. A 12-month-old child who was involved in a motor vehicle accident was brought into the emergency department. His skin is cool, clammy, and mottled. The neck veins are flat. There is evidence of trauma to the right upper quadrant of the abdomen. Which of the following types of shock is the patient MOST likely to have?

    (A) cardiogenic
    (B) dissociative
    (C) hypovolemic
    (D) vasogenic

97. In regard to the epidemiology of acute otitis media (AOM), all of the following epidemiological statements are correct EXCEPT

    (A) children in daycare settings are at greater risk for AOM.
    (B) the highest peak incidence for AOM is from 6 to 13 months of age.
    (C) the highest rate of AOM occurs in the winter months.
    (D) the prevalence for AOM is greater in Caucasians than in Native Americans

98. A 4-week-old infant presents with generalized lymphadenopathy and hepatosplenomegaly. Upon further questioning, his mother expresses concern that he may be infected with the human immunodeficiency virus (HIV), too, as she was HIV-seropositive prior to the birth of her son. Which of the following is the preferred (most sensitive and specific) test to confirm the diagnosis that her son is positive for HIV?

    (A) HIV Western blot
    (B) HIV DNA polymerase chain reaction test
    (C) HIV RNA polymerase chain reaction test
    (D) HIV p24 antigen test

99. Which of the following has been demonstrated as a significant risk factor for SIDS in developed countries?

    (A) female infants
    (B) large for gestational age infants
    (C) prenatal maternal smoking
    (D) supine sleep position

100. The condition characterized by displacement of the proximal femoral epiphysis due to disruption of the growth plate and in which the head of the femur is usually displaced medially and posteriorly relative to the head is called

    (A) slipped capital femoral epiphysis
    (B) Legg–Calvé–Perthes disease
    (C) congenital hip dysplasia
    (D) femoral anteversion

101. When evaluating a 6-year-old male for sudden onset of right hip pain with an associated limp and no history of trauma, which of the following is the most likely diagnosis?

    (A) developmental dysplasia of the hip
    (B) Legg–Calve–Perthes disease
    (C) slipped capital femoral epiphysis
    (D) transient monoarticular synovitis

102. Up to 50% of patients with Lyme disease will develop arthritis within several weeks to months after exposure. Of the following, which is NOT commonly associated with the arthritis of Lyme disease?

    (A) attacks are recurrent and migratory
    (B) attacks typically last days to weeks
    (C) chronic attacks usually follow multiple attacks
    (D) fevers may be high

103. A 5-year-old child presents to the office with complaints of a sore throat and fever for 2 days. She is diagnosed with acute pharyngitis. Which of the following is the MOST common organism for her infection etiology?

    (A) adenovirus
    (B) group A beta-hemolytic *Streptococcus*
    (C) group C *Streptococcus*
    (D) *Streptococcus pneumoniae*

104. All of the following are cardinal signs of pediatric congestive heart failure EXCEPT

    (A) bradycardia
    (B) cardiomegaly
    (C) hepatomegaly
    (D) tachypnea

105. A 4-month-old infant presents with lethargy, fever, marked irritability, a bulging fontanelle, and positive Kernig's and Brudzinski's signs. A lumbar puncture reveals elevated lymphocytes, normal protein concentration, and normal glucose concentration. Which of the following is the MOST likely diagnosis?

    (A) bacterial meningitis
    (B) infectious mononucleosis
    (C) tuberculous meningitis
    (D) viral meningitis

106. In the revised Jones criteria for the diagnosis of acute rheumatic fever (ARF), which of the following is NOT included among the major manifestations?

(A) subcutaneous nodules

(B) carditis

(C) chorea

(D) fever

(E) polyarthritis

107. An adult male, not previously vaccinated for rabies, presents to the emergency room after being bitten by an aggressive stray dog. The dog was captured, and declared "probably rabid" by a local veterinarian. Which of the following treatment options should you select for this patient?

(A) administer human rabies immune globulin only

(B) administer equine rabies antiserum only

(C) administer human rabies immune globulin and equine rabies antiserum

(D) administer human rabies immune globulin and equine rabies antiserum AND human diploid cell rabies vaccine

(E) administer human rabies immune globulin and human diploid cell rabies vaccine

108. A 35-year-old forest ranger presents with a rash on his back. It started 4 days ago as a red maculopapular lesion about 2 cm in diameter. Now it is 14 cm in diameter with an area of central clearing. In addition to the rash, he has had a headache, fever, chills, and muscle aches. The most likely diagnosis is

(A) cellulitis

(B) wasp sting

(C) rocky mountain spotted fever

(D) poison ivy

(E) Lyme disease

109. An otherwise healthy, immunocompetent healthcare worker converts to a positive PPD. Which of the following drugs is recommended for this person?

(A) rifampin

(B) pyrazinamide

(C) ethambutol

(D) Streptomycin

(E) isoniazid

110. In the treatment of peptic ulcer disease of infectious etiology, which of the following drug combinations will provide the most efficacious therapy?

(A) metronidazole and omeprazole

(B) Bismuth subsalicylate and omeprazole and sucralfate

(C) amoxicillin and bismuth subsalicylate and antacid

(D) omeprazole and amoxicillin and clarithromycin

(E) clarithromycin and metronidazole and sucralfate

111. A patient is seen at the clinic for her health maintenance checkup. She claims to have started her first menstrual period last week. On physical exam, her breast development shows the areola and papilla forming a secondary mound. Her genital exam reveals an abundance of coarse, curly pubic hair covering the labia and mons pubis. According to Tanner's stages of sexual maturation, at what stage would you assess her sexual maturity?

(A) Tanner stage II

(B) Tanner stage III

(C) Tanner stage IV

(D) Tanner stage V

112. During the first year of life, what would be the expected average growth for an infant who weighs 7 lb at birth?

    (A) 6 lb at 2 weeks, 12 lb at 5 months, 18 lb at 12 months
    (B) 6 lb at 3 weeks, 21 lb at 4 months, 30 lb at 12 months
    (C) 7 lb at 2 weeks, 14 lb at 4 months, 21 lb at 12 months
    (D) 7 lb at 2 weeks, 21 lb at 6 months, 30 lb at 12 months

113. A 3-year-old child presents to the emergency department with bruises on his body. His mother claims that her son sustained these bruises when he tumbled down the stairs 8 days ago. Which of the following colors would you expect the bruises to be if this occurred as stated?

    (A) brown
    (B) purple
    (C) red
    (D) yellow

114. With normal growth and development, the angular alignment of children's legs progresses through a series of developmental stages. Which of the following children have angular development in the lower extremities considered to be PATHOLOGIC?

    (A) 12-month-old male with genu varum
    (B) 36-month-old female with genu valgum
    (C) 36-month-old female with genu varum
    (D) 60-month-old male with genu valgum

115. A 9-year-old child, who was diagnosed with a viral upper respiratory infection 2 weeks ago, returns to the clinic with a complaint of a 2-day history of drooping of one side of her mouth. She is afebrile with a blood pressure of 110/60 mm Hg. Her physical exam reveals an inability to completely close her left eye, inability to wrinkle her forehead, and drooping of her mouth on the left side. Her smile is asymmetric. The remainder of her exam is otherwise normal. Which of the following is the MOST likely diagnosis?

    (A) Bell's palsy
    (B) botulism
    (C) brain stem glioma
    (D) Guillain–Barré syndrome

116. A 5-year-old child presents to the office for a school physical exam. His past medical history is unremarkable, including normal growth and development. His physical exam is normal except for a grade II/VI high-pitched, vibratory, systolic ejection murmur heard best at the left lower sternal border with radiation to the apex. When the child is in a supine position, the murmur is louder. Which of the following murmurs is the MOST likely diagnosis?

    (A) physiologic peripheral pulmonic stenosis (PPPS) murmur
    (B) pulmonary ejection murmur
    (C) Still's murmur
    (D) venous hum

117. Which of the following sleeping positions for a healthy infant should be recommended to parents during anticipatory guidance in order to reduce the risk for SIDS?

    (A) prone position
    (B) seated position
    (C) side position
    (D) supine position

118. At 12 hours of age, a physical exam is performed on a neonate with intrauterine growth retardation. He is noted to have microcephaly, jaundice, and hepatosplenomegaly. Which of the following is the MOST likely congenital viral infection in this neonate?

    (A) cytomegalovirus
    (B) herpes simplex virus
    (C) rubella
    (D) syphilis

119. A 2-year-old child presents to the emergency department via ambulance due to a seizure lasting approximately 2 minutes with jerking and somnolence. En route in the ambulance her vital signs are

temperature 39°C rectal
pulse 120/min
respiration 32/min
blood pressure 110/64 mm Hg

Upon further questioning, her mother claimed she had a runny nose yesterday. On physical exam she is sleepy, but arousable with negative Kernig's and Brudzinski's signs. Which of the following seizures is the MOST likely diagnosis?

(A) absence seizure
(B) complex partial seizure
(C) febrile seizure
(D) simple partial seizure

120. A 6-month-old infant presents to the emergency department with a 2-day history of vomiting and diarrhea. Upon physical exam she appears to be intermittently irritable and restless with minimal tearing when crying. Her capillary refill is 3 to 4 seconds. She has decreased skin turgor, sunken eyes, and a depressed anterior fontanel. On the basis of these clinical manifestations, what is the magnitude of her dehydration?

(A) less than 3%
(B) approaching 3% to 5% (mild)
(C) approaching 6% to 10% (moderate)
(D) approaching 11% to 15% (severe)

121. A 36-year-old patient reporting sudden hair loss is found to have a round, well-circumscribed 3-cm area of alopecia on the parietal scalp area with exclamation point hairs. The most likely diagnosis is

(A) anagen effluvium
(B) androgenetic alopecia
(C) alopecia areata
(D) tinea capitis

122. An acute eruption of violaceous, pruritic, polygonal, shiny, flat-topped papules involving the flexor surfaces is suggestive of which of the following?

(A) lichen planus
(B) pityriasis rosea
(C) psoriasis
(D) seborrheic dermatitis

123. Arthropod bites that typically reveal a central blue color of impending necrosis with a surrounding white area of vasospasm and a peripheral red halo of inflammation are associated with

(A) scabies
(B) black widow spiders
(C) brown recluse spiders
(D) deer ticks

124. A patient known to have allergic rhinitis and asthma presents with chronic pruritic inflammatory lesions of the flexor surfaces, wrists, and dorsal areas of the feet. The lesions are excoriated, lichenified, and crusted patches and plaques. The most likely diagnosis is

(A) nummular eczema
(B) psoriasis
(C) seborrheic dermatitis
(D) atopic dermatitis

125. A 65-year-old patient presents with a 4-week history of dark red pruritic urticarial plaques on the flexor surfaces. The plaques begin developing tense bullae on the surface. This clinical presentation is most suggestive of

(A) bullous pemphigoid
(B) bullous impetigo
(C) pemphigus vulgaris
(D) dermatitis herpetiformis

126. A 25-year-old nullipara consults you because she suddenly stopped menstruating. On questioning her further you find she recently has lost 19 pounds after starting long distance running. The most appropriate step in her evaluation is measurement of

(A) serum TSH concentration

(B) serum prolactin concentration

(C) hCG concentration

(D) serum estradiol-17b concentration

(E) serum testosterone concentration

127. Which of the following two causes of non-traumatic vaginal bleeding are seen most frequently in the adolescent and reproductive-aged female?

(A) pregnancy and coagulopathy

(B) thyroid dysfunction and anovulation

(C) exogenous hormone use and polyps

(D) anovulation and pregnancy

128. A 39-year-old woman, G3P3, complains of severe, progressive secondary dysmenorrhea and menorrhagia. Pelvic exam demonstrates a tender, diffusely enlarged uterus with no adnexal tenderness. Endometrial biopsy findings are normal. What is the next diagnostic exam needed?

(A) MRI

(B) transvaginal and abdominal ultrasound

(C) hysterosalpingography

(D) laparoscopy

(E) CT scan of the pelvis

129. A 36-year-old G2P2 comes to your office complaining of heavy menstrual bleeding for the past year. The patient is bleeding through a super tampon and a heavy pad every hour of the first 3 days of her cycle. Her cycle lasts 5 days and cycle length has decreased to having a period every 20 days. She complains of fatigue. Her physical exam and lab workup are normal (negative beta-HCG, LH, FSH, prolactin, clotting times, liver function test (LFT), and renal function test), except for the CBC and further labs indicating she has iron deficiency anemia. The patient's weight is 298

pounds. In addition to iron supplementation, which of the following is the best INITIAL therapy for this patient?

(A) hysterectomy

(B) oral contraceptives

(C) D & C

(D) long-term conjugated estrogen therapy

(E) daily dosing of aspirin

130. The combination of dysmenorrhea, deep dyspareunia, low back pain, and chronic pelvic pain are symptoms that best fit with which of the following conditions?

(A) adenomyosis

(B) ovarian cancer

(C) endometriosis

(D) interstitial cystitis

131. A 47-year-old G3P1 woman comes into the office complaining of heavy, painful, and irregular menstrual bleeding that has been going on for the past 6 months to a year. She has not been sexually active for the past year. On physical exam, her uterus is estimated to be the size of uterus at 12 weeks' gestation. Pelvic ultrasound confirms the presence of a leiomyoma. Her hematocrit is 29%, MCV is 68 fL, and serum ferritin is 10 g/L. What should be the first-line therapy?

(A) myomectomy of leiomyoma

(B) hysterectomy

(C) ablation therapy

(D) oral contraceptive therapy in standard doses

(E) depot methodroxyprogesterone acetate 150 mg IM every 28 days

132. A 49-year-old G2P2 patient has a known history of uterine myomata that are approximately 16-week size. Within the past year, her periods have become progressively heavier and longer. A dilation and curettage performed 6 months earlier showed no pathology and failed to decrease the bleeding. Her hematocrit is 34%. The patient is not orthostatic and does not complain of dizziness. Which of the following would be the best next step?

(A) abdominal myomectomy

(B) laparoscopic-assisted myomectomy

(C) leuprolide acetate (Lupron Depot)

(D) transfusion with two units of packed cells

(E) total abdominal hysterectomy

133. A 20-year-old nulliparous woman presents to the emergency department complaining of pelvic pain and fever and chills. Her symptoms have been going on for 3 days. She has had no new sexual partners, but does not routinely use condoms with her current partner because they "have been dating for 1 year." Clinically, her cervix is erythematous, friable, and there is a mucopurulent discharge. The cervical motion tenderness is significant. Her pregnancy test is negative and there are no adnexal masses. What is the most likely pathogen causing her symptoms?

(A) *Neisseria gonorrhoeae*

(B) *Chlamydia trachomatis*

(C) *Haemophilus influenzae*

(D) *Escherichia coli*

(E) *Gardnerella vaginalis*

134. A very firm ovarian mass, estimated at 8 cm, is found in a 33-year-old female, at her annual exam. Which of the following interventions should be considered first?

(A) combination chemotherapy

(B) radiation therapy

(C) surgical consult

(D) exploratory laparoscopy

135. A 40-year-old patient has not had a Pap smear since the birth of her last baby (15 years ago). Today's Pap smear result for this patient indicates squamous cell carcinoma. The reason she sought medical care was for postcoital bleeding. At the time of the Pap smear there was a friable lesion present. At this point, the most appropriate step in this patient's management is

(A) repeat Pap smear in 4 to 6 months

(B) biopsy visualized lesion and refer patient for gynecologic consult

(C) colposcopy with endocervical curettage and directed biopsy

(D) LEEP or cervical conization

(E) radical hysterectomy and radiation therapy

136. A 62-year-old woman presents with incontinence and urinary frequency. Her only medication is hormone replacement therapy. She is otherwise healthy. Most of her incontinence occurs during physical activity. Exam and urinalysis suggest no urological, rectal, or gynecological abnormalities. Cystometrics demonstrate a bladder capacity of 400 mL and postvoid residual of 10 mL. A full bladder stress test is positive. The most likely diagnosis is

(A) urge incontinence

(B) stress incontinence

(C) overflow incontinence

(D) functional incontinence

137. A mother brings her 3½-year-old daughter to your clinic after feeling a "lump in her belly" while bathing her the previous evening. The child appears playful and absent of discomfort. The patient's mother denies any nausea, vomiting, or hematuria with the child. Physical exam reveals a smooth and firm abdominal mass on the left side. What is the most likely diagnosis?

(A) renal cell carcinoma

(B) neuroblastoma

(C) polycystic kidney disease

(D) Wilm's tumor

138. A 52-year-old male comes to see you for follow-up of a recent right knee injury. During the visit, you ask whether anything else is "going on." He denies any other medical problems, but he mentions that he would like some advice on another issue. He reports that he has been unable to maintain erections in the past year. He has heard the commercials for "erection medications" on television and wonders if one might work for him. What are the most common etiologies for this patient's concern?

(A) neurogenic and arterial disorders

(B) psychologic and neurogenic disorders

(C) vascular and hormonal disorders

(D) hormonal and venous disorders

139. A 48-year-old female presents to your clinic complaining of an increasing frequency of urination. She states, "it feels like I have to urinate every couple of hours." She also reports occasional urine leakage that has caused her some alarm to the point where she now wears a mini pad, "just in case." A catheterized urine specimen is negative. What physical exam finding would support your diagnosis?

(A) uretheral hypermobility

(B) bulging of the anterior vaginal wall

(C) atrophic vaginal changes

(D) normal genito-urinary exam

140. When treating a patient for benign prostatic hypertrophy (BPH), which of the following medical therapies affects the patients prostatic specific antigen (PSA) level?

(A) phytotherapy

(B) α-adrenergic antagonists

(C) 5α-reductase inhibitors

(D) saw palmetto

141. Cervical cysts are noted while performing a Papanicolaou test. The MOST likely diagnosis is

(A) Bartholin's cysts

(B) nabothian cysts

(C) cervicitis

(D) human papillomavirus (HPV)

(E) cervical carcinoma

142. A 25-year-old G1P1 presents to your clinic for her annual exam. She has no history of abnormal Pap smears, but the results from today's test show squamous intraepithelial lesions (SIL), low grade. Which of the following is the best option for what should be done next?

(A) recheck Pap in 1 year

(B) repeat Pap smear in 4 to 6 months, using traditional method

(C) repeat Pap smear in 4 to 6 months, using liquid-based cytology

(D) HPV testing

(E) colposcopy

143. At 8 weeks' gestation, a 24-year-old primipara was seen a week prior complaining of vaginal bleeding and lower abdominal cramping. Her beta-hCG level was 1,000 mlU/mL at that time. Today, she has no abdominal pain or evidence of tissue passed per vagina. Transvaginal ultrasound show no adnexal masses as well as no clear pregnancy. Her repeat beta-hCG level is 1100 mlU/mL. What can be concluded from this information?

(A) the patient has a pregnancy that is non-viable, but its location is unknown

(B) she has had a spontaneous abortion and needs a D & C

(C) the hCG level needs to be repeated in 48 hours for more information on viability

(D) an ectopic pregnancy is probable

(E) this is a molar pregnancy

144. A 26-year-old mother who is nursing presents to clinic complaining of right breast tenderness and fever. Upon physical exam, she has a 2-cm fluctuant mass at the site of erythema and tenderness. The patient had been seen 4 days ago and was placed on oxacillin, which she has been taking. At this point the BEST treatment is

(A) changing antibiotic to vancomycin and discontinuing nursing

(B) surgical drainage and continuation of nursing

(C) discontinuation of nursing and hot soaks

(D) incision and drainage, hot soaks, antibiotics, and breast emptying

(E) hot packs and manual emptying of breasts

145. A 48-year-old woman comes in for her annual physical exam and biannual screening mammogram. Her family history is negative for breast cancer. Her breast physical exam reveals no palpable masses; however, a screening and then diagnostic mammogram demonstrates several coarse calcifications that are suspicious for breast cancer. Which of the following statements is most accurate?

(A) fine needle aspiration would be the best diagnostic method for this finding

(B) since there is no palpable mass on physical exam, the patient may be observed with additional mammography in 3 months

(C) an image-guided, local excisional biopsy provides the most definitive diagnosis

(D) a reasonable option for this patient is a core tissue biopsy done with sterotaxis

(E) ultrasound imaging is the diagnostic method of choice for ductal carcinoma in situ (DCIS)

146. A 19-year-old female presents to the clinic with complaints of vaginal discharge that started 3 weeks ago. Intercourse is uncomfortable and she is experiencing postcoital bleeding. Her periods have been normal with her last period ending yesterday. She and her new partner use spermicidal foam, but no condoms. Pelvic exam shows mucopurulent discharge from the cervix, left adnexal fullness, and mild cervical motion tenderness. Her pregnancy test is negative. Given the above information, the MOST likely diagnosis is

(A) urinary tract infection

(B) *Trichomonas* vaginitis

(C) intrauterine pregnancy

(D) pelvic inflammatory disease

(E) cervical dysplasia

147. Following a gunshot wound to the lower abdomen, a 29-year-old male is hospitalized and treated with clindamycin for a potential anaerobic infection. After 3 days of clindamycin therapy while recuperating in the hospital, he develops severe diarrhea, dehydration, and lower abdominal cramping. A stool culture is ordered and later discovered to contain *C. difficile*. After discontinuing the clindamycin, which of the following would be the most appropriate treatment?

(A) cefaclor (Ceclor)

(B) doxycycline (Monodox)

(C) amoxicillin (Amoxil)

(D) metronidazole (Flagyl)

(E) cephalexin (Keflex)

148. Which of the following medications is most appropriate for the treatment of an initial case of acute uncomplicated cystitis in a 23-year-old female?

(A) amoxicillin (Amoxil)

(B) ciprofloxacin (Cipro)

(C) doxycycline (Monodox)

(D) azithromycin (Zithromax)

(E) gentamicin (Garamycin)

149. All of the following are generally effective at quickly managing an acute asthma attack in the adult patient EXCEPT

(A) albuterol

(B) levalbuterol (Xopenex)

(C) metaproterenol (Alupent)

(D) salmeterol (Serevent)

(E) pirbuterol (Maxair)

150. Which of the following type 2 diabetes medications is INCORRECTLY paired with its mechanism of action?

(A) glyburide (Diaβeta), increases pancreatic secretion of insulin

(B) metformin (Glucophage), decreases hepatic glucose production

(C) acarbose (Precose), increases cellular uptake of glucose

(D) rosiglitazone (Avandia), increases insulin sensitivity of tissues

(E) repaglinide (Prandin), increases pancreatic secretion of insulin

151. The preferred methods for monitoring warfarin therapy and unfractionated heparin (UFH) therapy is to measure the _____ and _____, respectively

- (A) aPTT (activated partial thromboplastin time); INR
- (B) ACT (activated clotting time); INR
- (C) INR; aPTT
- (D) INR; ACT
- (E) ACT; aPTT

152. A 61-year-old male arrives at the emergency department suffering an acute myocardial infarction as a result of coronary artery thrombosis. One of the agents administered to the patient is a thrombolytic agent. From the choices below, which drug is a thrombolytic agent?

- (A) abciximab (ReoPro)
- (B) alteplase (tPA)
- (C) warfarin
- (D) heparin
- (E) clopidogrel (Plavix)

153. A patient on a 16 mg daily dose of hydromorphone is being switched to morphine sulfate for pain control. If 7.5 mg of hydromorphone is equianalgesic with 30 mg of morphine sulfate, what dose of morphine sulfate should be prescribed if you account for 25% cross-tolerance?

- (A) 30 mg
- (B) 36 mg
- (C) 48 mg
- (D) 64 mg
- (E) 80 mg

154. It is recommended that baseline LFTs be ordered before starting therapy with all of the following medications EXCEPT

- (A) pioglitazone (Actos)
- (B) simvistatin (Zocor)
- (C) extended-release niacin (Niaspan)
- (D) gemfibrozil (Lopid)
- (E) clopidogrel (Plavix)

155. One of the most common adverse effects with spasmolytics like carisoprodol (Soma) and cyclobenzaprine (Flexeril) is their tendency to cause

- (A) rash
- (B) drowsiness
- (C) hypertension
- (D) myalgia
- (E) hyperglycemia

156. A 44-year-old male has periodic attacks of gout that are secondary to hyperuricemia. Plasma uric acid levels can be decreased with

- (A) allopurinol (Zyloprim) or prednisone
- (B) allopurinol (Zyloprim) or probenecid (Benemid)
- (C) colchicine or probenecid (Benemid)
- (D) indomethacin (Indocin) or colchicine
- (E) aspirin or prednisone

157. Which of the following are consistent with lead poisoning?

- (A) profound anemia
- (B) severe complaints of mild and persistent muscle weakness
- (C) acute difficulty concentrating after exposure
- (D) basophilic stippling
- (E) treatment with chelating agent is always required

158. A 48-year-old previously healthy, African American man presents to his local emergency center with acute onset of dyspnea on exertion while mowing the grass. He has no past medical history. Laboratory studies reveal a WBC 6.1, Hgb 5.8, Hct 20.1, MCV 68, and Plt count 254,000. What diagnosis is most likely the cause of his symptoms?

- (A) sickle cell anemia
- (B) thalassemia
- (C) iron deficiency
- (D) hemolytic anemia
- (E) TTP

159. Which of the following is true of macrocytic anemias?

   (A) causes include poor absorption of vitamin B_{12} in the stomach due to prior gastrectomy

   (B) Schilling's test is used to diagnose folate deficiency

   (C) folate supplementation should be started empirically to prevent worsening anemia, while further studies are being performed

   (D) when associated with the loss of taste and atrophy of the tongue mucosa, it suggests vitamin B_{12} deficiency.

   (E) strict vegetarians are at risk of folate deficiency and may need chronic supplementation.

160. One day, while covering the internal medicine floor, you evaluate a patient who was admitted for pneumonia. Upon reviewing the routine laboratory studies ordered for that day, you note that the patient has developed an anemia. The chemistry profile reveals a total bilirubin of 2.6 with an elevated LDH. Potential causes of the anemia and hyperbilirubinemia may include all of the following EXCEPT

   (A) malaria

   (B) drug use

   (C) folate deficiency

   (D) recent blood transfusion

   (E) disseminated intravascular coagulopathy

161. A 76-year-old woman presents to the ER after experiencing severe pain in the left hip, worse upon standing or walking. She denies any falls or trauma precipitating the pain. Physical exam reveals enlarged suboccipital and cervical lymph nodes. Electrophoresis studies were positive for serum M. Subsequent urinalysis was positive for Bence-Jones proteins. Which of the following would NOT be expected in this patient, given the probable diagnosis?

   (A) hypercalcemia

   (B) anemia

   (C) renal failure

   (D) splenomegaly

   (E) fever

162. Which of the following is the primary emergency treatment for anaphylaxis?

   (A) epinephrine

   (B) antihistamines

   (C) atropine

   (D) aminophylline

   (E) dopamine

163. A 12-year-old boy reaches under his friend's porch to retrieve a baseball and suffers a small puncture wound to his left hand as a result of a bite by the friend's cat. Within a few hours, he becomes febrile and complains of chills. Which drug would be the most appropriate to give this patient?

   (A) amoxicillin + clavulanate (Augmentin)

   (B) erythromycin

   (C) doxycycline (Monodox)

   (D) levofloxacin (Levaquin)

   (E) gentamicin (Garamycin)

164. Which of the following regimens has superior efficacy in treating acute nausea and vomiting associated with high doses of cyclophosphamide?

   (A) metoclopramide (Reglan)

   (B) metoclopramide (Reglan) + dexamethasone (Decadron)

   (C) ondansetron (Zofran) + dexamethasone (Decadron)

   (D) lorazepam (Ativan)

   (E) prochlorperazine (Compazine)

165. A 52-year-old male is brought to the emergency department by his daughter because she recently notices that he gets extremely tired, has periodic tremors in his hands, and suffers from increasing memory lapses. Initial lab work shows a serum creatinine of 2.2 mg/dL. His past medical history is significant for bipolar disorder, for which he has been taking the same drug for the past 32 months. Which of the following is most likely responsible for the patient's symptoms?

(A) valproic acid (Depakote)

(B) lithium carbonate (Lithobid)

(C) carbamazepine (Tegretol)

(D) olanzapine (Zyprexa)

(E) risperidone (Risperdal)

166. Angiotensin receptor blockers (ARBs) are not as likely to produce cough and angioedema compared to ACEIs because they do not

(A) cause hyperkalemia

(B) cause hyponatremia

(C) increase bradykinin levels

(D) undergo a first pass effect

(E) cross the blood–brain barrier

167. Which of the following drugs used for the management of obesity increases the fat content of the stool and can potentially cause fecal urgency and incontinence?

(A) dexfenfluramine (Redux)

(B) orlistat (Xenical)

(C) sibutramine (Meridia)

(D) phentermine (Adipex-P)

(E) benzphetamine (Didrex)

168. What is the most common cause of chronic obstructive pulmonary disease (COPD)?

(A) air pollution

(B) recurrent infection

(C) cigarette smoking

(D) asthma

(E) pneumoconiosis

169. What is the most common histological form of lung cancer?

(A) adenocarcinoma

(B) large cell carcinoma

(C) small cell carcinoma

(D) squamous cell carcinoma

170. What is the most common cause of acute bronchiolitis in a child under 2 years of age?

(A) adenovirus

(B) respiratory syncytial virus (RSV)

(C) coronavirus

(D) parainfluenza virus

171. Which occupation carries the highest risk for developing silicosis?

(A) alloy manufacturers

(B) insulators

(C) coal miners

(D) quarry workers

172. A young child presents to the emergency department with the sudden onset of fever, dysphagia, drooling, and soft respiratory stridor. A lateral neck x-ray demonstrates a "thumbprint" sign. What is the most likely diagnosis?

(A) bronchiolitis

(B) bronchitis

(C) croup

(D) epiglottitis

(E) laryngeal trauma

173. What is considered first-line drug therapy for patients with COPD?

(A) corticosteroids

(B) ipratropium bromide

(C) terbutaline

(D) theophylline

174. A 3-year-old child presents to the emergency room with a "seal-like" or barking cough along with rhinorrhea for several days. Exam reveals an afebrile child who exhibits stridor with expiratory wheezing while at rest. What is the recommended treatment?

(A) IM dexamethasone
(B) IM diphenhydramine
(C) nebulized albuterol
(D) nebulized epinephrine

175. In which gender and age group is a spontaneous pneumothorax most likely to occur?

(A) male between 2 and 10 years of age
(B) female between 2 and 10 years of age
(C) male between 20 and 40 years of age
(D) female between 20 and 40 years of age

176. A 25-year-old male presents for preadmission testing (PAT) to correct a ventral hernia. The PAT includes a chest x-ray, which reveals a single, smooth, calcified, well-defined node of approximately 2 cm in diameter. What is the most appropriate next step in the management of this patient?

(A) obtain a CT scan
(B) obtain old films for comparison
(C) proceed directly to biopsy
(D) watchful waiting

177. A 55-year-old smoker with lung cancer presents with ptosis and miosis. What is the third clinical finding that comprises this syndrome found in patients with lung cancer?

(A) anhidrosis
(B) pericarditis
(C) pneumonitis
(D) systemic acidosis

178. A 7-year-old previously healthy patient presents with acute onset of respiratory distress following ingestion of a piece of candy. Which of the following signs or symptoms is most ominous?

(A) aphonia
(B) cough
(C) drooling
(D) stridor

179. Imaging of the chest is an essential part of the work-up of a patient with suspected occupational interstitial lung disease. What is the most likely diagnosis in a patient with a CXR that reveals a reticular linear pattern with basilar predominance?

(A) asbestosis
(B) coal works pneumoconiosis
(C) silicosis
(D) talcosis

180. A child presents to the office with respiratory symptoms consistent with influenza. What would be most helpful in supporting the diagnosis?

(A) chest x-ray with air bronchograms
(B) elevated WBC
(C) epidemiologic and overall clinical data
(D) history of no influenza immunization
(E) presence of pneumonia

181. The most common etiology for a subarachnoid hemorrhage is which of the following?

(A) trauma
(B) ruptured aneurysm
(C) bleeding arteriovenous malformation
(D) embolic stroke
(E) primary intracerebral hemorrhage

182. A 34-year-old male presents to your office with the complaint of pain and fatigue in his right wrist. He states that the pain can sometimes wake him up at night and feels as if his thumb is "falling asleep." He reports the problem started since he has been writing a chapter for a review book. On physical exam, you note a positive Tinel sign but no response to a Phalen maneuver. While sending him for a nerve conduction study, you tell him the most likely diagnosis is

(A) ulnar nerve compression

(B) radial nerve compression

(C) thoracic outlet syndrome

(D) median nerve compression

(E) peroneal nerve compression

183. The physical exam test of placing a vibrating tuning fork in the middle of a patient's forehead to test for sensorineural hearing loss is called

(A) rinne

(B) tinel

(C) dix-Hallpike

(D) babinski

(E) weber

184. A 48-year-old female presents with new onset headache which she describes as nonspecific, worse on awakening, intermittent throughout the day but can worsen with bending over or coughing. Her husband reports that she has not been herself since before the headaches started about 4 to 6 weeks ago. Which of the following tests would be best for determining the etiology of her presenting symptoms?

(A) noncontrast head CT scan

(B) lumbar puncture

(C) contrast enhanced brain MRI

(D) noncontrast brain MRI

(E) cerebral angiography

185. An 18-year-old female is transferred to your emergency department from a local college infirmary. She presented yesterday with a complaint of headache but became confused and is now febrile. You notice a petechial rash on physical exam and her cerebrospinal fluid (CSF) comes back with increased WBCs, increased protein, and decreased glucose. What is the most likely organism responsible for her meningitis?

(A) *H. influenzae*

(B) *L. monocytogenes*

(C) *N. meningitidis*

(D) *Mycobacterium tuberculosis*

(E) Coxsackievirus B

186. Huntington's disease is a movement disorder characterized by involuntary writhing of muscle groups. It is characterized by a clincial triad which includes the following

(A) progressive dementia, chorea, and a pattern of inheritance

(B) progressive dementia, tremor, and no pattern of inheritance

(C) depression, tremor, and no pattern of inheritance

(D) depression, chorea, and no pattern of inheritance

(E) depression, chorea, and tremor

187. A 40-year-old male presents to your office with the complaint of tinnitus and vertigo, which is intermittent and does not seem to be effected by position. The episodes can vary in length from minutes to hours and have been occuring over the past week. This has never happened to him before. His neurological exam is unremarkable except for decreased sensorineural hearing loss in his left ear. This is most consistent with which of the following?

(A) benign positional vertigo

(B) Ménière disease

(C) otosclerosis

(D) acute peripheral vestibulopathy

(E) salicylate toxicity

188. Wernicke's encephalopathy can be a complication of chronic alcoholism. It is caused by which of the following?

    (A) vitamin B_{12} deficiency
    (B) vitamin B_1 deficiency
    (C) cirrhosis
    (D) uremia
    (E) hypoventilation

189. A 62-year-old male presents to the ED with aphasia and right lower extremity weakness, which started about 4 hours ago. You now notice progressing right upper extremity weakness, worsening right lower extremity weakness, and decreased sensation throughout his right side. This cerebral ischemia is best characterized as

    (A) transient ischemic attack
    (B) stroke in evolution
    (C) completed stroke
    (D) subarachnoid hemorrhage
    (E) global cerebral ischemia

190. A 58-year-old male presents to your office with a complaint of tremor in his right hand. Upon questioning, you discover that the tremor is getting worse and he is having trouble eating with a fork and buttoning his shirt. On your physical exam you notice bradykinesia, rigidity, and a shuffling gait. What is your initial assesment?

    (A) essential tremor
    (B) Wilson disease
    (C) Huntington disease
    (D) Parkinson disease
    (E) progressive supranuclear palsy

191. A 55-year-old right-handed male presents with a 4-hour history of weakness and tingling of his right hand and numbness of the right side of his mouth. Mild difficulty was noted with word finding. His symptoms have improved since onset but have not fully resolved. There is no significant past medical history. Physical exam revealed flat right nasolabial fold, subjective numbness of the right hand, right pronator drift, clumsiness of finger tapping on the right hand, increased deep tendon reflexes on the right as well as a present Babinski. What is the most likely etiology for this patient's problem?

    (A) migraine headache
    (B) peripheral neuropathy
    (C) syncope
    (D) transient ischemic attack
    (E) seizure

192. A 73-year-old male is brought into your office by his adult children with a concern of memory loss. They report their father's memory has been declining since the death of their mother a few months ago but are now concerned because he is loosing weight, sleeping during the daytime, and is not keeping up with the current events like he usually does. This type of behavior is most associated with which of the following?

    (A) Pick disease
    (B) Creutzfeld–Jakob disease
    (C) depression
    (D) Alzheimer disease
    (E) vitamin B_{12} deficiency

193. Which of the following is more likely to occur as a transient side effect following a corticosteroid joint injection?

    (A) paresthesia at joint injection site
    (B) joint infection
    (C) anaphylactic shock
    (D) mild allergic reactions
    (E) post-injection flare

194. A 15-year-old male was playing football and was hit during a play, causing an abduction injury of his left lower leg. He locates the pain along the medial aspect of the knee and there is a minimal level of joint effusion. Which of the following test would assess for stability of the medial collateral ligament?

(A) valgus stress test
(B) varus stress test
(C) apprehension sign
(D) Lachman test
(E) anterior drawer sign

195. Evaluation of the spine in patient presumed to have scoliosis should include the forward bend test, in addition to this which of the following should be included in the evaluation of scoliosis?

(A) evaluation for joint meniscal injury
(B) evaluation for neuromuscular abnormalities
(C) evaluation for congenital cardiac disorder
(D) evaluation for cranial nerve abnormalities
(E) evaluation for growth hormone deficiency

196. A 12-year-old obese male presents with pain in the right thigh and medial knee. The pain has been for over a 6-week time period. The pain is described as aching in nature. Over the last month, the patient has had a limp present. On physical exam, the right knee is found to be unremarkable, but there is a slight limp noted with gait. Radiographs of the right knee are normal. Which of the following is the most appropriate step in the evaluation of this patient?

(A) examine and x-ray the right hip
(B) x-ray the left knee for comparison
(C) obtain a CT scan of the right knee
(D) obtain a magnetic resonance image of the right knee
(E) reassure the parents and observe the patient for progression

197. A new military recruit is in his third week of boot camp and is seen in the infirmary with complaints of anterior tibial pain of 3-week duration. On physical exam, there is noted tenderness on palpation over the lower portion of the anterior tibia. Radiographs of the lower leg are negative for fracture. The patient is treated conservatively, and returns in 4 days time with persisting pain. What would be the next step in the management of this patient?

(A) repeat plain radiographs
(B) order a CT scan of the lower leg
(C) order an MRI of the lower leg
(D) order an ultrasound of the lower leg
(E) order a venous Doppler evaluation of the lower leg

198. A 44-year-old female presents with complaints of numbness and tingling of her right second and third fingers for the past 2 months. She recently began with night time wakening with pain in her right hand and wrist. She is a secretary, and notes that typing aggravates the symptoms along with grasping the steering wheel and holding her coffee mug. The patient notes a past history of a neck injury 3 years ago, that has been associated with continual complaints of intermittent neck pain. She has had a previous MRI of the cervical spine that revealed the presence of a bulging disc at C6-C7. Which of the following diagnostic evaluations is most appropriate to determine the etiology of the patient's paresthesias?

(A) psychological testing
(B) plain radiograph of the right wrist
(C) plain radiograph of the cervical spine
(D) electromyography/nerve conduction velocity
(E) selective nerve root blocks

199. Which of the following is most diagnostic of a septic joint?

(A) synovial fluid analysis
(B) plain radiograph
(C) ultrasound of the joint
(D) CT scan of the joint
(E) MRI of the joint

200. Which of the following characteristics may be seen in a patient who has osteoarthritis?

(A) bony enlargement of the interphalangeal joints
(B) morning stiffness that persists for over 30 minutes
(C) prodromal systemic symptoms of malaise and fever
(D) symmetrical joint swelling with warmth and tenderness
(E) subcutaneous nodules over the extensor surfaces

201. A 17-year-old male presents with complaints of pain located in his fifth digit, he was involved in an altercation and states his hand was injured from punching someone. On physical exam of the patient's hand, there is tenderness, swelling, and pain with extension. The patient is diagnosed with a "boxer's fracture." What radiographic finding would be present to diagnose this patient?

(A) spiral fracture of the third metacarpal
(B) fracture of the fourth metacarpal
(C) fracture of the fifth metacarpal
(D) comminuted fracture of the distal phalanx of the fifth digit
(E) comminuted fracture of the distal phalanx of the fourth digit

202. Which of the following best defines the deformity that causes a "mallet finger?"

(A) rupture or avulsion of the insertion of the extensor tendon at the base of the distal phalanx
(B) rupture or avulsion of the insertion of the flexor tendon at the base of the distal phalanx
(C) fracture of the distal phalanx
(D) dislocation of the distal interphalangeal joint
(E) fracture of the proximal phalanx

203. A 39-year-old female presents with complaints of left anterior knee pain of 4-week duration. She has noted difficulty with going up and down stairs. The patient also notes increased pain in the knee upon arising after being seated for a period of time. The pain may then improve with walking. The patient denies joint crepitus or locking sensation. On physical exam there is no swelling or obvious joint distortion. The pain is reproduced with placing the knee in slight flexion and gentle pressure placed on the patella as the patient contracts the quadriceps. The knee appears stable, with no signs of crepitus, joint laxity, or internal derangement. Radiographs of the left knee are essentially benign. What course of treatment is best for this patient?

(A) crutches for 6 weeks, keeping the joint non-weight-bearing
(B) cortisone injection
(C) physical therapy to strengthen the quadriceps
(D) physical therapy to strengthen the lower back
(E) progress to orthopedic evaluation for consideration of internal derangement of the knee

204. A 4-year-old child presents with complaints of right hip pain of 4 days duration and an associated limp. The patient is recovering from an upper respiratory infection that appears to be resolving. The child is currently afebrile. On physical exam, there is notable limitation of movement with internal rotation. Radiographs reveal minor soft tissue swelling around the joint, with no boney findings. CBC and erythrocyte sedimentation rate are not elevated. What would be the most appropriate long-term complication to consider for this patient?

(A) osteoarthritis of the hip

(B) septic arthritis

(C) pyogenic arthritis

(D) osteomyelitis

(E) avascular necrosis of the hip

205. Which of the following medications interact to decrease lithium levels?

(A) indomethacin

(B) potassium sparing diuretics

(C) theophylline

(D) valproic acid

(E) COX-2 inhibitors

206. What disorder may have an abnormal dexamethasone suppression test?

(A) personality disorder

(B) anxiety disorder

(C) dissociative disorder

(D) adjustment disorder

(E) mood disorder

207. What personality type may have "slow" activity seen on EEG?

(A) avoidant personality

(B) paranoid personality

(C) histrionic personality

(D) schizoid personality

(E) borderline personality

208. A patient presented to your office with multiple somatic complaints. During the mental status exam you notice that the patient loses the thread of conversation and discusses irrelevant topics based on an external stimuli. The patient never gets back to the main point they were trying to express. What is this thought process called?

(A) tangentiality

(B) circumstantiality

(C) looseness of association

(D) word salad

(E) neologisms

209. Which of the following personality disorders is listed in Cluster C?

(A) avoidant

(B) antisocial

(C) borderline

(D) schizoid

(E) paranoid

210. Which of the following is the most common thyroid carcinoma?

(A) anaplastic carcinoma

(B) follicular carcinoma

(C) medullary thyroid carcinoma

(D) papillary carcinoma

(E) primary thyroid carcinoma

211. A 39-year-old woman presents to the office for evaluation of a palpable nodule in the neck of 2 years duration. She has no other symptoms. She takes levothyroxine for Hashimoto's disease diagnosed 5 years ago. She has a history of low-dose chest irradiation for an enlarged thymus gland during infancy. On exam, a firm, nontender, 2.5-cm nodule is palpable in the left lobe of the thyroid. What is the next diagnostic step?

(A) ultrasound of the neck

(B) thyroid scintiscan

(C) MRI of the neck

(D) CT scan of the neck and chest

(E) fine-needle aspiration of the nodule

212. What lipid-lowering agent reduces the production of VDRL particles and secondary reduction of LDL particles in the blood but may cause a prostaglandin-induced flushing reaction?

   (A) Colestipol
   (B) Ezetimibe
   (C) Lovastatin
   (D) Niacin

213. A 35-year-old obese man presents with type 2 diabetes. This patient has a BMI of 32. After discussing diet and exercise as part of the treatment plan, it is decided that the patient should be started on an oral medication. Which of the following medications could have a beneficial effect on this patient's weight?

   (A) metformin
   (B) glyburide
   (C) rosiglitazone
   (D) repaglinide

214. A 58-year-old type 2 diabetic patient was started on a new medication 2 weeks ago to improve blood sugar levels. This patient presents with increased flatulence, abdominal discomfort, and, at times, severe diarrhea. Which of the following medications is characteristic for causing these side effects?

   (A) rosiglitazone
   (B) Glucovance
   (C) glyburide
   (D) acarbose

215. Which of the following statements is incorrect related to the treatment of bipolar disorder?

   (A) start lithium and have levels checked frequently
   (B) start psychotherapy
   (C) add an antipsychotic medication
   (D) continue drug therapy for 2 to 4 months
   (E) hospitalize if the patient is in full manic state

216. What type of schizophrenia is characterized by self injury, harm to others, mutism, or rigidity?

   (A) paranoid
   (B) undifferentiated
   (C) disorganized
   (D) catatonic
   (E) schizophreniform

217. Which disorder is characterized by episodes of hypomania and depression for greater than 2 years?

   (A) dysthmia
   (B) major depressive disorder
   (C) cyclothymia
   (D) bipolar
   (E) mood disorder

218. Which of the following disorders is not treated with an SSRI?

   (A) post traumatic stress disorder
   (B) anorexia
   (C) panic attacks
   (D) general anxiety disorder
   (E) obsessive compulsive disorder

219. A 9-year-old child presents to the urgent care center with her mother. The child is complaining of dark colored urine. The mother mentions that the child was complaining of cough and cold symptoms a few weeks ago. The urine shows gross hematuria without nitrites or leukocytes. Which of the following is the best test to help the clinician confirm the diagnosis?

   (A) monospot
   (B) antistreptolysin O titer
   (C) immunoglobulin electrophoresis
   (D) renal biopsy

220. Upon performing a newborn exam, the clinician notes a widened pulse pressure, paradoxical splitting of S_2, and a "machine" like murmur heard best at the second intercostal space, left sternal border, and inferior to the clavicle. Which of the following is the most likely diagnosis?

(A) tetralogy of fallot

(B) ventricular septal defect

(C) atrial septal defect

(D) patent ductus arteriosus

221. Extracolonic manifestations of inflammatory bowel disease typically do not include

(A) ankylosing spondylitis

(B) erythema marginatum

(C) uveitis

(D) pyoderma gangrenosum

(E) arthritis

222. A 34-year-old female with ulcerative colitis has been frequently symptomatic from proctitis and proctosigmoiditis. The best management for this particular problem would be

(A) stool bulking agents

(B) nutritional support

(C) corticosteroid enemas

(D) sulfasalazine

(E) systemic immunosuppressive agents

223. The organism most frequently associated with nosocomially acquired diarrhea is?

(A) *Bacteroides fragilis*

(B) *Escherichia coli*

(C) *Clostridium tetani*

(D) *Clostridium difficile*

(E) *Bacteroides vulgatus*

224. A 56-year-old man presents with severe mid-epigastric pain that is refractory to antacids and H2 blockers. What is the first line test to establish the diagnosis of Zollinger–Ellison syndrome?

(A) urease breath test

(B) serum calcium

(C) serum gastrin level

(D) endoscopy for brush biopsies

(E) MRI of the abdomen looking for a gastrinoma

225. A 77-year-old male walks to work every day. One month ago he developed buttock and thigh pain after walking two blocks The patient is now limited to one block and then he must sit down to alleviate symptoms. He denies pain with weight bearing but notes the pain only after he walks. He denies any recent injury or fall. What is the most likely diagnosis for this patient?

(A) spinal stenosis

(B) aortoiliac occlusive disease

(C) myalgias

(D) popliteal occlusive disease

Answers and key item phrases

<table>
<tr><td>1.</td><td>(D) Risk factors for cancer of the esophagus</td><td>19.</td><td>(C) Diagnosis of pancreatitis</td></tr>
<tr><td>2.</td><td>(E) Use of protein pump inhibitors</td><td>20.</td><td>(B) Screening for hepatocelluar cancer</td></tr>
<tr><td>3.</td><td>(D) Diagnosis of acute abdominal pain</td><td>21.</td><td>(C) Findings in arterial insufficiency</td></tr>
<tr><td>4.</td><td>(D) Features of inflammatory bowel disease</td><td>22.</td><td>(B) Incidence of hernia</td></tr>
<tr><td>5.</td><td>(C) Dietary guidelines alcohol consumption</td><td>23.</td><td>(D) Diagnosis of aneurysm</td></tr>
<tr><td>6.</td><td>(D) Risk factors of C. difficile infection</td><td>24.</td><td>(D) Arterial occlusion</td></tr>
<tr><td>7.</td><td>(E) Physical exam of the abdomen</td><td>25.</td><td>(E) Polyps in colon cancer</td></tr>
<tr><td>8.</td><td>(E) Treatment of fecal impaction</td><td>26.</td><td>(C) Pharmacologic treatment of HIV</td></tr>
<tr><td>9.</td><td>(B) Follow-up for colon cancer</td><td>27.</td><td>(D) Pharmacologic treatment of HIV</td></tr>
<tr><td>10.</td><td>(D) Hepatotoxicity caused by medication</td><td>28.</td><td>(A) Diagnosis of polymyositis</td></tr>
<tr><td>11.</td><td>(E) Findings in hyponatremia</td><td>29.</td><td>(B) Diagnosis of pseudogout</td></tr>
<tr><td>12.</td><td>(B) Causes of postoperative fever</td><td>30.</td><td>(A) Treatment of rheumatoid arthritis</td></tr>
<tr><td>13.</td><td>(C) Choice of intravenous fluids</td><td>31.</td><td>(B) Causes of acidosis</td></tr>
<tr><td>14.</td><td>(B) Surgical complications of diabetes</td><td>32.</td><td>(E) Placement of endotracheal tube</td></tr>
<tr><td>15.</td><td>(B) Findings in cardiac tamponade</td><td>33.</td><td>(B) Findings in hypocalcemia</td></tr>
<tr><td>16.</td><td>(B) Signs of increased intracranial pressure</td><td>34.</td><td>(C) Common ankle sprains</td></tr>
<tr><td>17.</td><td>(E) Characteristics of gallbladder disease</td><td>35.</td><td>(E) Diagnosis of myocardial infarction</td></tr>
<tr><td>18.</td><td>(B) Diagnosis of gallbladder disease</td><td>36.</td><td>(B) Rates of prostate cancer</td></tr>
</table>

37. **(A)** Hepatitis screening

38. **(C)** Causes of death in children

39. **(D)** Colon cancer screening

40. **(A)** Rates of family violence

41. **(C)** Therapy of ischemic heart disease

42. **(B)** Diagnosis of seizure disorder

43. **(A)** Pneumonia in HIV disease

44. **(C)** Presentation of pontine hemorrhage

45. **(C)** Management of septic shock

46. **(D)** Recognition of foreign body

47. **(D)** Syndrome of inappropriate ADH secretion

48. **(A)** Treatment of hypertensive emergency

49. **(C)** Causes of abdominal distention

50. **(D)** Acute trauma

51. **(C)** Causes of CKD

52. **(D)** Screening for nephropathy

53. **(A)** Markers of glomerular injury

54. **(D)** Contraindications for dialysis

55. **(B)** Use of ultrasound

56. **(A)** Types of calculi

57. **(B)** Side effects of NSAID use

58. **(E)** Treatment of hypokalemia

59. **(C)** Glucosuria

60. **(E)** Diagnosis of urinary tract infection

61. **(E)** Causes of small bowel obstruction

62. **(C)** Pseudomembranous colitis

63. **(A)** Use of nitrous oxide

64. **(B)** Trauma in pregnancy

65. **(C)** Presentation of hypoglycemia

66. **(B)** Diagnosis of ocular lesions

67. **(B)** Treatment of corneal abrasion

68. **(B)** Diagnosis of ocular lesions

69. **(B)** Ear trauma

70. **(B)** Diagnosis of vertigo

71. **(A)** Recommendations for LDL cholesterol

72. **(B)** Raynaud's therapy

73. **(C)** Indications for coronary bypass

74. **(C)** Treatment of myocardial infarction

75. **(C)** Therapeutic range INR

76. **(A)** Indications for aneurysm treatment

77. **(B)** Treatment of peripheral vascular disease

78. **(B)** Diagnosis of cor pulmonale

79. **(C)** Diagnosis of hypertension

80. **(A)** Diagnosis of hypertension

81. **(D)** Treatment of sudden hearing loss

82. **(D)** Diagnosis of mastoiditis

83. **(C)** Complications of bacterial sinusitis

84. **(A)** Causes of rhinitis medicamentosa

85. **(C)** Vocal cord paralysis

86. **(D)** Diagnosis of mitral regurgitation

87. **(C)** Symptoms of venous insufficiency

88. **(C)** Diagnosis of mitral regurgitation

89. **(C)** Risk for temporal arteritis

90. **(B)** Side effects of ACEIs

91. **(D)** Pathophysiology of cardiac function

92. **(D)** Findings in cardiogenic shock

93. **(D)** Pathophysiology of cardiac function

94. **(B)** Diastolic dysfunction

95. **(D)** Treatment of myocardial infarction

96. **(C)** Hypovolemic shock in children

97. **(D)** Characteristics of otitis media

98. **(B)** Diagnosis of HIV

99. **(C)** Risk factors for sudden infant death

100. **(A)** Findings in slipped capital femoral epiphysis

101. **(D)** Diagnosis of hip pain

102. **(C)** Characteristics of Lyme disease

103. **(A)** Causes of pharyngitis

104. **(A)** Congestive heart failure in children

105. **(D)** Finding in meningitis

106. **(D)** Diagnosis of ARF

107. **(E)** Rabies prophylaxis

108. **(E)** Presentation of Lyme disease

109. **(E)** Prophylaxis for tuberculosis

110. **(D)** Treatment of peptic ulcer disease

111. **(C)** Tanner stages

112. **(C)** Normal growth and development

113. **(D)** Recognition of child abuse

114. **(C)** Normal growth and development

115. **(A)** Diagnosis of Bell's palsy

116. **(C)** Characteristics of innocent murmurs

117. **(D)** Prevention of SIDS

118. **(A)** Congenital viral infections in neonate

119. **(C)** Diagnosis of seizures

120. **(C)** Assessment of dehydration

121. **(C)** Diagnosis of alopecia areata

122. **(A)** Diagnosis of lichen planus

123. **(C)** Characteristics of arthropod bites

124. **(D)** Characteristics of atopic dermatitis

125. **(A)** Diagnosis of pemphigoid

126. **(C)** Presentation of amenorrhea

127. **(D)** Causes of vaginal bleeding

128. **(B)** Workup of dysmenorrheal

129. **(B)** Abnormal uterine bleeding

130. **(C)** Characteristics of endometriosis

131. **(E)** Irregular menstrual bleeding

132. **(C)** Treatment of myomata

133. **(B)** Etiology of pelvic inflammatory disease

134. **(C)** Treatment of ovarian mass

135. **(B)** Abnormal pap smear

136. **(B)** Stress incontinence

137. **(D)** Presentation of Wilm's tumor

138. **(B)** Erectile dysfunction

139. **(D)** Diagnosis of incontinence

140. **(C)** PSA levels

141. **(B)** Diagnosis of cervical cysts

142. **(E)** Abnormal pap smear

143. **(A)** Vaginal bleeding during pregnancy

144. **(D)** Treatment of mastitis

145. **(C)** Workup of breast mass

146. **(D)** Vaginal discharge

147. **(D)** Treatment of *Clostridium difficile*

148. **(B)** Treatment of urinary tract infection

149. **(D)** Treatment of acute asthma

150. **(C)** Euglycemic agents

151. **(C)** Monitoring anticoagulation

152. **(B)** Thrombolytic agents

153. **(C)** Equianalgesic dosing

154. **(E)** Initiation of lipid agents

155. **(B)** Medication side effects

156. **(B)** Treatment of gout

157. **(D)** Findings in lead poisoning

158. **(C)** Etiology of anemia

159. **(D)** Vitamin B_{12} deficiency

160. **(C)** Diagnosis of anemia

161. **(D)** Characteristics of multiple myeloma

162. **(A)** Treatment of anaphylaxis

163. **(A)** Treatment of cat bite

164. **(C)** Treatment of nausea

165. **(B)** Medication side effects

166. **(C)** Medication side effects

167. **(B)** Medication side effects

168. **(C)** Etiology of COPD

169. **(A)** Pathology of lung cancer

170. **(B)** Features of bronchiolitis

171. **(D)** Risk of occupational lung disease

172. **(D)** Presentation of epiglottitis

173. **(B)** Treatment of COPD

174. **(D)** Management of croup

175. **(C)** Characteristics of pneumothorax

176. **(B)** Solitary pulmonary nodule

177. **(A)** Findings in Horner's syndrome

178. **(A)** Recognition of airway obstruction

179. **(A)** Diagnosis of asbestosis

180. **(C)** Diagnosis of influenza

181. **(B)** Cause of subarachnoid hemorrhage

182. **(D)** Symptoms of median nerve compression

183. **(E)** Physical exam of the neruologic system

184. **(C)** Presentation of intracranial mass

185. **(C)** Etiology of meningitis

186. **(A)** Diagnosis of Huntington's disease

187. **(B)** Presentation of Meinere's disease

188. **(B)** Diagnosis of Wernicke's encephalopathy

189. **(B)** Stroke in evolution

190. **(D)** Presentation of Parkinson's disease

191. **(D)** Features of transient ischemic attack

192. **(C)** Diagnosis of depression

193. **(E)** Post-injection flare

194. **(A)** Physical exam of the knee

195. **(B)** Detection of scoliosis

196. **(A)** Diagnosis of hip pain

197. **(C)** Diagnosis of lower extremity pain

198. **(D)** Work up of wrist pain

199. **(A)** Evaluation of septic arthritis

200. **(A)** Characteristics of osteoarthritis

201. **(C)** Boxer's fracture

202. **(A)** Definition of mallet finger

203. **(C)** Presentation of patellofemoral syndrome

204. **(E)** Diagnosis of hip pain

205. **(D)** Effects on lithium levels

206. **(A)** Dexamethasone suppression test in psychiatric disorders

207. **(E)** Characteristics of personality types

208. **(A)** Mental status exam

209. **(A)** Characteristics of personality disorders

210. **(D)** Pathology of thyroid cancer

211. **(E)** Presentation of thyroid nodule

212. **(D)** Effects of lipid lowering agents

213. **(A)** Euglycemic agents in diabetes

214. **(D)** Side effects of euglycemic agents

215. **(D)** Treatment of bipolar disorder

216. **(D)** Characteristics of schizophrenia

217. **(C)** Symptoms of depression

218. **(B)** Use of SSRIs

219. **(B)** Presentation of glomerulonephritis

220. **(D)** Presentation of patent ductus arteriosis

221. **(B)** Manifestations of inflammatory bowel disease

222. **(C)** Management of ulcerative colitis

223. **(D)** Etiology of diarrhea

224. **(C)** Diagnosis of Zollinger–Ellison syndrome

225. **(B)** Diagnosis of peripheral vascular disease

Index